Books Are for Talking, Too!

Books Are for Talking, Too!

THIRD EDITION

✤ Jane L. Gebers ✤

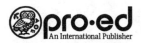
pro·ed
An International Publisher

8700 Shoal Creek Boulevard
Austin, Texas 78757-6897
800/897-3202 Fax 800/397-7633
www.proedinc.com

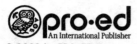
An International Publisher

© 2003 by PRO-ED, Inc.
8700 Shoal Creek Boulevard
Austin, Texas 78757-6897
800/897-3202   Fax 800/397-7633
www.proedinc.com

Library of Congress Cataloging-in-Publication Data

Gebers, Jane L.
    Books are for talking, too! / Jane L. Gebers—3rd ed.
       p. cm.
    Includes bibliographical references and indexes.
    ISBN 0-89079-902-4
    1. Children—Books and reading.   2. Children's literature—Bibliography.   3. Picture books
  for children—Bibliography.   4. Language arts.   I. Title.

Z1037.A1 G394   2003
011'.62—dc21   2002068053

This book is designed in Stone Sans and Lucida Sans Narrow

Printed in the United States of America

1 2 3 4 5 6 7 8 9 10   07 06 05 04 03

Dedicated to the memory of
Jason Haerter Smedley
(May 5, 1978–March 22, 2000)
who loved the arts of listening, reading, writing, and speaking

❧

and to his father,
Bill

Contents

Section 4

Section 5

Preface

Fifteen years ago I began *Books Are for Talking, Too!* from a collection of picture books I had used with speech- and language-delayed children and the resources of several good libraries in Monterey, California. The sourcebook of children's literature promoted interaction and language learning within a literate context. Simultaneous with its publication, the philosophy of whole-language instruction emerged and the field of children's literature burgeoned with picture books. Educators began to view literature in terms of its expanded potential and ask questions such as, How can I use books in planning lessons around the seasons of the year? and Which books will tie in to a unit on American history? Five years later, *Books Are for Talking, Too!* was expanded and revised with more books and extended activities for classroom use to reflect these changes in education and learning.

Today, consensus findings from two decades of scientific research have further shaped literacy instruction, and the ways parents and educators can use children's picture books may be broadened still. Although we can retain important aspects of the whole-language theory—such as children's active participation in the learning process—current trends highlight the fundamental sound elements of language to better ensure that all children achieve the ultimate goal of literacy. When I have browsed through great bookstores such as Rizzoli and Borders in San Francisco or Barnes & Noble in my hometown of Walnut Creek, California, or small, independent bookstores across the country, I have always been delighted to see new children's books. Now I am doubly delighted, convinced that the writers, artists, and publishing houses appreciate these findings. So many children's books reflect an understanding of the importance of a child's awareness of language (from the sounds of language—its melody, rhythm, and rhyme—to the uses of language, whether it is in the metalinguistic sense of metaphors and similes or in the pragmatic sense as they focus on the social uses of language).

These author/illustrator teams provide enormously rich experiences to children. Children can learn about the beginnings of the women's rights movement in the United States in *You Forgot Your Skirt, Amelia Bloomer.* The delightful illustrations show how fancy, floor-length, "proper" dresses swept the garbage off the streets and into their hemlines, causing one woman to question such "properness" and inspire a change in women's thinking about the style of the day. Children, adolescents, and adults can enjoy the much-beloved folk song by Woody Guthrie, *This Land Is Your Land,* illustrated by the well-known Americana artist Kathy Jacobsen. Her paintings of the industrialization of America, the Great Depression, and the varied expanse of land across the United States add meaning to the words of the song. Children can also learn about a little-publicized event in the lives of Amelia Earhart and Eleanor Roosevelt, who dined together at the White House and ended their evening with a thrilling flight over Washington, D.C. The artist's detailed black-and-white illustrations in *Amelia and Eleanor Go for a Ride* are authentically replicated, right down to the White House china.

There is value in the whimsy of many children's stories. For example, Martha, the dog that learns to read and speak from a bowl of alphabet soup in *Martha Speaks,* shows children there are good uses for literacy (especially for dogs) and good reasons for turn-taking in conversation. Lilly, the kindergartner who adores her teacher, learns important lessons in classroom behavior when she decides to show-and-tell her special new purchases at the wrong time in *Lilly's Purple Plastic Purse.* And everyone can learn a lesson in the art of compromise from Farmer Brown, who refuses to budge when his cows type a demand letter for electric blankets because it's cold in the barn in *Click, Clack Moo: Cows That Type.*

As you pause to reflect on the many titles found in the catalogs, I hope you are as inspired as I am by this literature. It is a medium so rich with possibilities, so broad in its scope of language experience, so amazing in its talent for creating new approaches to teaching children about life and the human beings who have shaped our world that it needs every opportunity to be presented.

I am grateful to those who have provided support for this third edition. Special thanks go to my dear friend and colleague Lisa Winslow, speech-language pathologist, for her generous sharing of information, ideas, and children's books. I also thank those who have given me feedback over the years about the usefulness of the book and for giving me suggestions for the kinds of books and themes they would like to see in new editions.

Literature can please us, delight us, touch us, inform us, and, most of all, connect us to life through the experiences of others. We can easily read these books to children, preadolescents, and adolescents. All we need to do is seek them out. With a little preparation, we can just as easily expand books' traditional use by bringing about discourse for language learning, speech production, and literacy as we underscore their messages about life.

Jane L. Gebers, MA
Speech-Language Pathologist

Introduction

A picturebook is text, illustrations, total design; an item of manufacture and commercial product; a social, cultural, historical document; and foremost, an experience for a child.

As an art form it hinges on the interdependence of pictures and words, on the simultaneous display of two facing pages, and on the drama of the turning of the page.

On its own terms its possibilities are limitless.

Barbara Bader, *American Picturebooks from Noah's Ark to the Beast Within.*
New York: Macmillan, 1976

Year after year, talented writers, artists, and publishing houses collaborate to contribute to a growing body of outstanding books for children. These books reflect changes in our society, including our knowledge about how children learn to read and write. Listening, speaking, reading, and writing are closely intertwined. The extent to which the development of these major life skills can be addressed through literature depends on the nature of the book and the ability of educators (and parents) to use it to meet the individual needs of children. Exposing children to books, enhancing the language that a particular work of literature generates, and facilitating interaction to build language learning, speech production, and literacy have been the goal of *Books Are for Talking, Too!* since its first printing.

It is well established that picture books are excellent resources and materials for providing instruction, facilitating communication, and engaging children in conversation for a wide range of objectives. Like the children's book genre, the study of language development and literacy continues to grow, and *Books Are for Talking, Too!* is revised once again to provide its readers with a resource that reflects both the best in current literature and advancements in the fields of language and literacy learning. This introduction provides various ways that the reader can use the resource and highlights new aspects of this third edition.

What Kinds of Children's Books Will I Find in *Books Are for Talking, Too!* (Third Edition)?

The anthology of children's literature contains three catalogs of books divided by grade level and gathered from all sections of the library. Wordless picture books, storybooks, classic tales, informational texts, and poetry can be found within these pages. They are classified as easy readers, juvenile fiction, nonfiction, folklore, and poetry and are available in most school libraries and bookstores and at online providers. Although these books span a wide range of language complexity, interests, and genres, they have several common characteristics.

One commonality is a quality text that is minimal in length. (The exceptions are wordless picture books and a few books with longer texts that are included because of their longstanding popularity with children and their excellent potential for facilitating particular objectives.) A minimal-length text allows for maximum interaction in a shortened time frame, which is preferable when intervention sessions are relatively brief and the focus is on the individual's performance and practice. Many quality children's books contain a small amount of text, but the words are rich with language possibilities. These books are mined for their ability to bring about the language experience; many contain a miraculous vein that can be tapped for an array of speech, language, and literacy objectives.

Another characteristic that most of these books share is that of visual images. *Books Are for Talking, Too!* (Third Edition) continues to draw on the unique properties of the picture book and the artist's conveyance of the message in providing material for speech, language learning, and literacy. Many of these images are powerful, reflecting our cultures, the times in which we live, and the times and cultures in which others once lived. They reflect many different forms of art, from collage to oil and watercolors, and even to the capabilities of the high-tech world. Talented, gifted, and truly great artists create art so that children can experience the world through their ability to extract a quality or essence or experience a particular aspect of life. Artists mesmerize, fascinate, and help hold an attraction for the story—not only for children but for adults, too. They can enhance the meaning of the words, add a new dimension to the story, or tell a story by themselves. They should not be covered up or thought of as juvenile but seen as an integral part of a medium that makes them vehicles for learning, experiencing, feeling—and talking, too!

Who Can Benefit from This Resource?

Books Are for Talking, Too! (Third Edition) offers professionals working with children a resource for promoting communication by using the picture book genre of children's literature. It can be used in interaction with an individual child, groups of children, and a whole classroom of children—from preschoolers to preadolescents and adolescents. Professionals can use the resource to plan sessions, select literature, and facilitate language learning and literacy, among many other objectives. It provides many specific strategies for the varied aspects of language, literacy, and speaking, and it can also be used creatively to open up avenues of conversation and communication with many diverse learners. Any adult who works with children, whether as a parent or as a professional, can benefit from the information presented in this book.

What Is the Best Way To Use This Resource?

The book is divided into five primary sections: Sections 1 through 3 contain researched information on the uses of books, suggestions for looking for more books, and extensive catalogs of books; Section 4 contains reproducible parent handouts; and Section 5 contains indexes. Two indexes, the Topic Explorations and Skills indexes, are cross-referenced with the books in the catalogs. Two additional indexes provide book listings by author and title.The catalogs, indexes, and other sections are tabbed so that they can be used interchangeably for easy reference and planning.

➤ **Catalogs:** Sections 1 through 3 contain catalogs where collections of literature are presented by grade and interest level. There are catalogs in sections designated for the following:

- Children in Preschool and Kindergarten,
- Children in Grades 1 Through 5, and
- Preadolescents and Adolescents in Grades 6 Through 12.

Good books are rarely confined to one category or age group and can overlap in many ways—many of the books are listed in more than one catalog, and many more can be used across all age groups. It is important when looking for books to search the indexes and peruse each of the catalogs for suitability when making selections.

Each book in the catalogs contains (a) publication information, (b) suggested grade and interest levels, (c) a synopsis, (d) a sample of the skills the book can be used to address, and (e) methods for developing a wide range of language learning, literacy, and speech production skills. Many books also list topics or themes that the book can be used to explore and an extended activities section designed to extend the concept of the book to other disciplines and learning experiences.

The components of the methods section are organized to reflect the way proficient readers spontaneously and purposefully generate questions during their independent reading. Suggestions for questions and discussions are planned so that interaction can take place before, during, and after the book's presentation. Activities are designed to target a wide range of speech- and language-related objectives while underscoring some of the fundamental processes of achieving literacy.

☛ **Parent Handouts.** Section 4 contains reproducible handouts that provide sound advice on ways that parents and caregivers can engage children in meaningful communication to develop literacy, language learning, and skills in good speech production. Handouts cover such topics as how to use children's literature interactively to learn the meanings of words; develop grammar usage, such as present and past tense; sequence story parts; and develop storytelling skills. Handouts of suggested read-alouds are also included. The following are some ideas on how to use the handouts:

- Include handouts in any helpful material on home carryover activities for speech, language, and literacy development.
- Make handouts available at back-to-school night.
- Present handouts during a PTA meeting or preschool parent gathering on literacy and language learning.
- Include handouts in communication sent home to parents, such as newsletters.
- Include handouts in materials presented to parents during May-Is-Better-Speech-and-Hearing Month.
- Offer handouts at Individualized Education Program meetings, interdisciplinary team meetings, and parent conferences.
- Give handouts to other professionals during curriculum meetings.

☛ **Indexes.** Section 5 contains four indexes. Two indexes are cross-referenced with the books in the catalogs. They include the following:

- **Topic Explorations.** This index groups the books in all the catalogs into different thematic units. Examples include such themes as American, Hispanic, and Japanese Culture and History; Famous People; Seasons of the Year; Weather; and a host of others. For those looking for books that tie into a classroom theme on Native Americans, for example, a list of books pertaining to the study can be found in this section. Users can learn more about the books in the catalog section. Professionals coordinating activities with special education and classroom teachers can use this section as a resource for locating books that relate to a theme of interest.

  Using a thematic approach to literature not only creates continuity to learning; it also provides a contextual framework within which to learn language. The thematic approach to teaching language also creates opportunities to generate more vocabulary and language learning because of the topic being explored.

- **Skills.** This index groups books according to the goal areas listed under "Skill Builders" in the book entries of the catalogs. First, search the index for a skill you want to develop (e.g., Prepositions) and find the titles of books that can be used to target that aspect of language. (To the right of the book's title is a code designating the library section in which the book is most likely to be shelved and the catalog(s) in this manual in which the book is listed.) Then find the books in the catalog(s) and select those you deem appropriate or readily accessible in your school or local library, bookstore, or online provider.

  Please note that this index is provided as a guide, not a prescription. As you read and reread the books cataloged here, you will undoubtedly think of many creative ways to use them to address skills other than the ones for which they are recommended.

☛ Two additional indexes in Section 5 include

- **Author.** This index lists the children's books referred to throughout the book alphabetically by author.
- **Title.** This index lists the children's books alphabeticaly by title.

What's New in This Third Edition?

- **Pragmatic Language Activities.** Many recently published books focus on the social uses of language and the appropriateness of conversational skills and manners. Snow, Burns, and Griffin (1998) state that "one avenue for introducing and refining new pragmatic functions is through experience with books and other literacy activities" (p. 49). Children beginning preschool become interested in stories with themes that center on the rules of relationships, which can be effective in building language pragmatics. Later, children become interested in stories in which characters use language to deceive and pretend. Books that incorporate the aspect of language pragmatics are found throughout all the catalogs of this resource.

- **Higher-Level Concepts.** The acquisition of concepts is a major linguistic and cognitive achievement during preadolescence and adolescence. Higher-level concepts are especially important to address in language intervention because the secondary school curriculum is based on knowledge of many concepts (Larson & McKinley, 1995). Books that clearly identify concepts and are of interest to the preadolescent and adolescent population are included in the Grades 6 through 12 catalog.

- **Morphological Awareness.** More books that provide opportunities for teaching morphological units in words (such as prefixes and suffixes) are listed in the Pre-K and Grades 1 through 5 catalogs. Awareness of these meaningful word parts can benefit the acquisition of literacy (Moats, 2000). Evidence suggests that meaningful connections between words (i.e., word networks) may be established through an awareness of the morphological relationships among words. Exposure to print along with a sensitivity to the word and phoneme structures of language are thought to be factors in the acquisition of these derivational forms. For children with language disabilities, maturation and exposure to literature may not be enough to achieve word decoding and comprehension. Direct instruction similar to phonological awareness instruction is indicated for these children (Moats, 2000; Moats & Smith, 1992). New language games for teaching morphological units are included in *Books Are for Talking, Too!* (Third Edition) to further address language learning and literacy.

- **Phonological Awareness (PA) Games.** Picture books provide an ideal medium in which to teach children how to attend to the sounds of words. The third edition of *Books Are for Talking, Too!* includes a series of phonological awareness games for a select group of books using the words of the text and the illustrations. These games are designed for systematic and cumulative instruction. Adams, Foorman, Lundberg, and Beeler (1998) state that unfamiliar words are difficult for children to focus on phonologically, particularly in their phonemic makeup. Stanovich (1993) and Snow et al. (1998) also address the importance of understanding the meanings of words used in phonological awareness training. Based on these findings, the PA games are presented so that vocabulary comprehension can first be addressed in the context of the literature, understood and used in the child's own production of language, and then used again in the games that follow. For these reasons, it seems both natural and imperative to develop a means of using as many different kinds of literature in as many ways possible when facilitating phonological awareness training.

The American Speech-Language-Hearing Association's (ASHA, 2001) position statement and guidelines focused widespread attention on the role of speech–language pathologists in the development of literacy, including phonological awareness. Phonological awareness (PA) is (a) the conscious awareness that words are made up of sounds and (b) the ability to attend to the sounds in a hierarchical series of finite skills. Children need to become aware of these small elements of sound and the sequences of sounds in words during the early literacy period.

Understanding this system is the key to understanding the alphabetic principle (Snow et al., 1998). Several decades of extensive research have consistently yielded the same information: There is a strong correlation between the acquisition of phonological awareness and the ability to learn to read (Adams, 1990; Lundberg, Frost, & Peterson, 1988; Snow et al., 1998; Stanovich, Cunningham, & Freeman, 1984). Phonological awareness has been shown to be a stronger predictor of reading achievement than IQ (Stanovich, 1993) and perceptual abilities (Adams, 1990; Snider, 1997). Children who do not read well usually demonstrate weaknesses in PA (Moats, 2000). Children in the early grades with weak PA abilities do not achieve the level of decoding skills that good readers achieve in the later grades (Juel, 1988).

Another correlation is shown to exist between children's level of PA and their level of early oral language development, including semantic, syntactic, and morphological abilities (Catts, Fey, Zhang, & Tomblin, 2001). Catts and Kamhi (1999) further underscore these findings, stating that "research indicates that 50 percent or more of children with LI [language impairments] in preschool or kindergarten go on to have reading disabilities in primary or secondary grades" (p. 108). Rather than outgrowing a language delay, many children who exit speech and language services later exhibit reading disabilities caused by deficits in an underlying ability to process symbolic systems (Brown, Aylward, & Keogh, 1996). These findings indicate that basic language proficiency is a key prerequisite in the acquisition of literacy (Snow et al., 1998).

Because of the high correlation of early spoken language delay and subsequent delay in learning to read, PA training has come to the critical attention of those involved with early childhood education and early language intervention. Despite the risk of reading failure, research shows that children with language delay who receive instruction in PA can make significant gains in literacy achievement as well as speech production (articulation) skills (Gillon, 2000). Speech–language pathologists can play an important role in facilitating this development of PA in young children. Their role may include direct work with children as well as forming partnerships with other professionals concerned with children and literacy learning (ASHA, 2001; Catts et al., 2001).

How Do I Use Picture Books for Phonological Awareness Training?

Because PA is not one unitary skill but rather a complex system of increasing awareness levels (listening, memory, word, syllable, and phoneme tasks), it would not be adequate to present only a few activities within this spectrum in the methods section of some of the books, nor would it demonstrate the potential of picture books to address so many of these subskills. Therefore, the PA activities included in selected book entries are various games from a cumulative set of games that have been devised to address a wide spectrum of skills (see Tables 1 and 2 for a complete listing of the games). Activities begin in the Pre-K section, where they are played mostly at the word and syllable level. Some of the games conclude at that point, especially if a book is listed only in the Pre-K catalog. However, many of the games in books listed in the Pre-K section continue in the same books listed in the Grades 1 through 5 section, offering even more activities on the PA spectrum. Users of this book are encouraged to select the entry level that is most appropriate for the learner and begin with games in that catalog section regardless of the child's chronological age.

For example, a 6-year-old child in the first grade has been assessed as having PA skills at the word level but demonstrates difficulty identifying syllables within words. After first locating Phonemic Awareness in the Skills index and selecting the book, *The Adventures of Taxi Dog*, one would begin by locating the book in the Pre-K catalog—even though the child is in the first grade—because typically that is where syllable-level games will be listed.

The adult then reads the book aloud, spending time before, during, and after the reading familiarizing the child with the meanings of the words in the text. The level at which the child would enter in the PA games might begin with an early syllable game, such as Clap-and-Count. The adult presents a word such as *taxi, city,* or *backseat* and demonstrates how to clap and count each part until the child can do it on his or her own.

Similarly, a 5-year-old kindergartner who has progressed to the phoneme level of awareness would begin playing a game from *The Adventures of Taxi Dog* that is found in the Grades 1 through 5 catalog. The adult would select the game at the appropriately determined level, such as Say-It-Until-You-Hear-It, and present one-syllable words such as *ride, sit,* and *roam,* divided into onset and rime for the child to synthesize, or blend the parts until he or she can hear the word on his or her own.

TABLE 1
Phonological Awareness Games Typically Found in the Pre-K Catalog

Listening Awareness Level

Can-You-Hear-It? Children listen for sounds in the environment or the sounds that words make.

Word Awareness Level

Word-Count. Children count words from progressively longer portions of text, either by counting or by moving the corresponding number of manipulables.

Stand-Up-to-the-Word. Children demonstrate word awareness by standing up when the word to which they have been assigned (in the title of a story or recognizable line of text) is called.

Which-Word-Is-Missing? Children select a word from a word string that has been omitted from the previously given word string.

Rearrange-It. Children rearrange, in correct word order, a scrambled phrase or short sentence from the text.

Initial Sound Awareness Level—Alliteration

Same-Sound. Children identify whether two words (or three-word strings) selected from the text begin with the same sound (e.g., Do *sail* and *sea* start with same sound?).

Odd-One-Out. Children select from a string of alliterative words the one that does not belong based on its beginning sound (e.g., Say *sail, sea, land.* Which one doesn't belong?).

Word-Search. Children search for a word in an illustration from the book or recall a word from the text that begins with the same sound as a target sound or target word.

Say-the-Sound. Children listen to a series of words taken from the text and produce the initial sound common to each word.

Rhyming Awareness Level

Finish-the-Rhyme. Children supply the rhyming word left out at the end of a familiar verse.

Rhyme-It-Again. Children identify the rhyming word heard after a rhyming set is given.

Do-They-Rhyme? Children identify whether word pairs rhyme.

Which-One-Rhymes? Children select a rhyming word from a word string that matches the target word presented.

Make-a-Rhyme. Children supply another rhyming word, either after a rhyming word from the story is presented or after a set of two rhyming words is presented.

Rhyming-Ings. Children rhyme root words with *–ing* suffixes.

Syllable (and Compound Word) Awareness Level

Clap-and-Count. Children clap to, and then count, the number of syllables in a word.

What's-the-Word? Children synthesize syllables or little words into words or compound words (e.g., Playground. Guess what word I said.)

Find-the-Little-Words. Children analyze words to hear each element in a compound or two-syllable word (e.g., What little words do you hear in *playground*? [play, ground]).

Leave-It-Out. Children delete a little word within a compound word or a syllable within a two-syllable word to create a new, smaller word (e.g., Say *snowman*, but leave out *man*. What little word is left? [snow]).

Add-It-On. Children add two syllables or two little words together to make a bigger word (e.g., Say *sail*, and then add *boat*. What new word can you make? [sailboat]).

Turn-It-Around. Children reverse the parts of the compound or two-syllable word that they have previously synthesized and analyzed (e.g., Using the word *pancake*—Say *pan* and then add *cake*. What word can you make? [pancake] Now turn it around and say *cake* and then add *pan*. What word can you make? [cakepan]).

Switch-It. Children exchange part of a compound or two-syllable word with a new part to make another word or words (e.g., Say *cobweb*, then take out *cob* and put in *spider*. What do you have now? [spider, web]).

TABLE 2
Phonological Awareness Games Typically Found in the Grades 1 Through 5 Catalog

Initial Sound Awareness Level

Odd-One-Out. A review of earlier levels. Children select from a string of alliterative words the one that does not belong.

Word-Search. Children search an illustrated page for a word that begins with the same sound as a target word. For example, "I'm thinking of a word in the story that starts with *sh*. Search for the word."

Say-the-Sound (initial). Children identify the beginning phoneme they hear in word pairs by saying the sound. For example: What's the beginning sound in *sea* and *sail*?

Final Sound Awareness Level

Same-Sound. Children identify whether word pairs end with the same sound. For example, "Say *ship, stop*. Do they end in the same sound?"

Odd-One-Out. Children select from a string of words ending in the same sound the one that does not belong. For example, "*eat, bite, plate, dog*. Which one doesn't belong?"

Word-Search. Children search an illustrated page for a word that ends with the same sound or target word given. For example, "I'm thinking of a word in the story that starts (or ends) with *sh*."

Say-the-Sound (final). Children listen to a series of words taken from the text and produce the final sound that is common to each word.

Middle Sound Awareness Level

Odd-One-Out. Children select from a string of words with the same middle sound the one that does not belong. For example, "*cake, rain, feet*. Which one doesn't belong?"

Synthesis—Onset-Rime

Say-It-Until-You-Hear-It. Children synthesize one-syllable words divided into onset-rime. Activities begin with onset parts that are continuous, single sounds (*f, l, m, n, r, s, v, y,* and *z*), as in *mmm . . . ap*, and proceed to single stop sounds (*b, c, d, g, h, j, k, p, q,* and *x*), as in *c . . .-ap*.

A second stage follows that contains onsets with two-consonant clusters, such as *ffffllll . . .-ap*. Onset clusters begin with two continuant sounds and proceed to one continuant sound, as in *clllll–ap*.

Synthesis—Phonemes

Roll-It-Out. Children synthesize a consonant–vowel–consonant (C-V-C) word by blending each of its phonemes until they can identify the word. For example, what is the word: *s–u–n.* Response: *ssss . . . uuuu . . . nnnn* is the word *sun*.

Analysis—Phonemes

Break-It-Up. Children analyze a one-syllable, three-sound C-V-C word in three stages: identifying the beginning, middle, and ending sounds. A last stage follows that requires children to identify all the sounds in the word. For example, what are all the sounds in the word *sail*?

Manipulation—Phonemes

Delete-It. Children omit the first sound in one-syllable words from the text. First three-sound words are presented, then four-sound words. Children then delete initial sounds in a series of words, such as the title of the book or familiar, high-impact words of the text. For example, delete the *m* in *mice* to get *ice* or delete the *p* in *sheep* to get *she.*

Add-To-It. Children insert a new sound into a word to make a new word. For example, *sip* becomes *slip*.

Switch-It. Children delete the initial sound of the word and replace it with a new sound to make another word. Activities begin at the single word level and add in word length for games with a series of words, such as the title of the book or a familiar, high-impact line of text. For example, *Sheep on a Ship* becomes *Bleep on a Blip*.

Games can be played simultaneously with both of the children from these examples when the facilitator is familiar with the various games and uses the list of words provided in the methods section for each game, directing different activities to each child. This individualized instruction is facilitated in much the same way as articulation and language games are played with small groups of children.

Where Can the PA Games Be Found?

A listing of all the games in *Books Are for Talking, Too!* (Third Edition) is found in Tables 1 and 2. However, not all games appear for each book that addresses phonological awareness; the games that appear in the book entries have been cumulatively designed for the unique text, illustrations, and format of each book.

There are 40 books with PA games listed in the catalogs. Twenty-four books begin at the early levels in the Pre-K catalog and continue to advanced levels in the Grades 1 through 5 catalog. Ten books containing PA games begin at the early levels and are found only in the Pre-K catalog. There are 5 books that are found only in the Grades 1 through 5 catalog, most of which include PA games beginning at the early stages and progressing through the later levels of PA.

It's easy! Users of this book looking for PA activities can find a listing of all the books that address PA skills in the Skills index. Users can also thumb through the pages of each catalog and quickly locate the games because they are visually set apart in a shaded presentation. Once users are familiar with the cumulative set of games listed in Tables 1 and 2, beginning at the appropriate level is as easy as reviewing the method, finding the book, and beginning to read.

How Have the Phonological Awareness Games Been Designed?

Each phonological awareness activity in *Books Are for Talking, Too!* (Third Edition) has been given a name for easy identification. The activities are called "games" because of their fun nature and use with popular children's books. Calling the games by their names also helps children identify the task of each activity. The objective of each game appears after the name of the game, and the wording can easily be adapted for Individualized Education Program (IEP) objectives. Materials are not necessary; however, using manipulables (e.g., blocks, buttons, or felt squares) for some of the games can be beneficial for many children. The use of a puppet can also be a charming feature in demonstrating syllable production and in continuing the theme of the book because the puppet takes on a character from the story.

The games follow several key principals in Snider's (1995) primer on phonological awareness. The following is a description of how the games adhere to those principals:

• **Systematic and Cumulative.** Activities are designed for the scope and sequence of PA levels. Although research has provided consistent information about the ages at which specific awareness is typically acquired, the exact progression in the instruction of these subskills is not consistent in the literature. Uhry (1999) has reviewed a significant number of commercial PA programs and states that the elements in all of the programs follow a hierarchical sequence of activities similar to that of Adams's (1990) research. In her seminal work, *Beginning to Read: Thinking and Learning About Print,* Adams lists skills in the following order:

- Knowledge of nursery rhymes
- Oddity tasks (e.g., detecting rhyme or alliteration)
- Syllable splitting and blending
- Phoneme synthesis and analysis
- Phoneme manipulation (add, delete, or move individual phonemes in the word)

• **Onset-Rime Activities—The Middle Step.** Onset-rime activities are added as an important intermediate step between syllable-level activities and phoneme blending and segmenting. Adams et al. (1998); Chard and Dickson (1999); Moats (2000); O'Connor, Jenkins, Leicester, and Slocom (1993); O'Connor, Notari-

Syverson, and Vadasy (1998); Snider (1995); and others note that awareness of onsets and rimes is the intermediate step between blending syllables and blending phonemes. For this reason, *all* books listed in the Grades 1 through 5 catalog provide this activity in the game Say-It-Until-You-Hear-It.

• **Modeled Activities.** Sample language for demonstrating an activity is included in most games. Snider (1995) states, "It is essential to provide sufficient instruction before providing practice activities" (p. 448). Users of this book should familiarize themselves with the differences between language used in demonstration and language used in practice.

• **Explicit Instruction.** Games in this book begin with demonstration because the most explicit instruction has been shown to produce the strongest growth (Torgesen et al., 1999). Continuing to scaffold skills for children who are developing PA is critical (O'Connor et al., 1998). Users need to explicitly teach every game, gradually eliminating support as the child finds success in frequent and repeated practice. Language is built into the games for the purpose of showing children strategies for achieving success. It may be necessary for the user to continue to find ways to fully and clearly express and demonstrate these tasks.

• **Continuous Sounds Before Stops.** Onset-rime activities and phoneme blending and segmenting games present word lists beginning with continuous sounds before word lists beginning with stop sounds. Continuous sounds are those that can be stretched out, such as *f, l, m, n, r, s, v, w, y*, and *z*. Stop sounds, such as *b, c, d, g, h, j, k, p, m, q*, and *x*, cannot be stretched out, so they are harder to use in blending activities and should be used when children are able to synthesize word parts more easily.

• **Smaller Units Before Larger Units.** At the onset-rime and phoneme level, synthesis and analysis activities begin with words containing fewer sounds, such as one-syllable consonant–vowel–consonants words, and continue to words containing more sounds, such as initial blends and two-syllable, four-sound words. Snow et al. (1998) note that children find it initially difficult to split blends and perceive the first sound in *play*, for example, to be *pl* rather than *p*. Moats (2000) shows the skill developing until age 8 years. For this reason, the second stage of onset-rime activities involves an onset composed of an initial two-consonant blend, blended and segmented, leaving the consonant cluster intact.

• **Synthesis Before Analysis.** Synthesis activities (blending) begin before analysis activities (segmenting). According to research, these are the skills that correlate most highly with beginning reading acquisition (Snider, 1997; Snow et al., 1998).

Although the games in *Books Are for Talking, Too!* (Third Edition) are presented for the purpose of developing PA, they are meant to be used as additional instruction to complete curricula, including materials such as the following:

Ladders to Literacy: A Kindergarten Activity Book (O'Connor et al., 1998)

The Lindamood Phoneme Sequencing (LiPS) Program for Reading, Spelling, and Speech (Lindamood & Lindamood, 1998)

Phonological Awareness Skills Program (Rosner, 1999)

Phonological Awareness Training for Reading (Torgeson & Bryant, 1993)

Phonemic Awareness in Young Children: A Classroom Curriculum (Adams et al., 1998) adapted from the study by Lundberg and associates (Lundberg et al., 1988)

Reading Mastery (Engelmann et al., 1995)

Sounds and Letters for Readers and Spellers: Phonemic Awareness Drills for Teachers and Speech-Language Pathologists (Greene, 1995)

Sourcebook of Phonological Awareness Activities: Children's Classic Literature (Goldsworthy, 1998)

You Are the Creative Force and Energy That Facilitates Learning

Children's picture books and the possibilities for their use are truly endless. As a facilitator of language, you are the key element in facilitating the language and literacy experience. Whether you use books to facilitate vocabulary development, teach strategies for the development of narratives, provide phonological awareness training, or remediate the misarticulation of speech sounds, you are the creative force that enables the use of the picture book to address intended objectives and, ultimately, the enjoyment of good literature.

If some of your favorite books are not listed in this edition, look through the catalogs for ideas, methods, and activities that you can adapt to the books you love. The suggested activities may also trigger ideas for entirely new and exciting activities.

Planning to meet the needs of diverse learners can be rewarding when you achieve results. *Books Are for Talking, Too!* is designed to help make planning easier, more efficient in providing for diverse learners, more time efficient, more inspiring in creating new methods for presenting books, and more enjoyable when using children's picture books for talking, too!

Section 1

Books Are for Talking with Children in Preschool and Kindergarten

- ❧ Using Picture Books To Build Oral Communication Skills and Emergent Literacy

- ❧ Looking for Books That Help Build Communication Skills and Emergent Literacy

- ❧ Suggestions for Book Talk with Preschool and Kindergarten Children

- ❧ A Catalog of Picture Books for Children in Preschool and Kindergarten

Using Picture Books

To Build Oral Communication Skills and Emergent Literacy

The talk is the site of learning; the book reading
is important because it is the site of the talk.

—Snow (1994, p. 270)

In designing the successful prekindergarten and kindergarten StaR program, Karweit (1994) envisioned storybooks as "perfect vehicles" for bringing about children's language use through meaningful activities (p. 55). Her research in the use of picture books and numerous studies during the past few decades conclude that joint picture book reading—whether conducted by parents at home, day-care providers, interventionists, or teachers in the classroom—contributes to strong language growth and emerging literacy in young children.

Spoken Language

With careful selection, planning, and facilitation, the use of picture books can address almost any of the components of spoken language, including the following:

- Vocabulary: To acquire words, especially different kinds of words, such as nouns, verbs, prepositions, pronouns, and so on.
- Phonetics: To produce speech sounds.
- Phonology: To learn how to change the structure of sounds in words and learn how sounds are distributed and changed when changing one word into another (as discussed under phonological awareness).
- Morphology and syntax: To learn the rules for arranging words in sentences and to learn the meaningful parts that make up words.
- Semantics: To learn the meanings of words, including concepts, words with multiple meanings, synonyms, antonyms, and figurative language.
- Pragmatics: To learn how to engage in an interchange of language for social purposes.

Emergent Literacy

Emergent literacy refers to the time during which children acquire rudimentary knowledge and awareness about print structures before formal reading instruction begins (Neuman, Copple, & Bredekamp, 2000).

During this time, children develop print awareness (e.g., knowing that writing moves from left to right), strong language systems to support later reading development, use in the forms of print (e.g., writing their names), and a conscious awareness of the sounds of spoken language (phonological awareness) (Whitehurst et al., 1999). During this time, children also learn the concept of story, the ability to retell a story, how to describe people and happenings in a story, and how to relate a story to their own experiences (Moats, 2000).

The link between children and their unique genre of literature is key to laying the groundwork for emergent literacy and eventual reading success. However, it is the strategies in facilitating this awareness that can enhance, and in some instances be ever critical to, achievement in emergent literacy. By carefully selecting a work of literature and planning for its use based on features inherent in its design, strategies emerge that enable adults to assist children in developing a number of aspects of emergent literacy, including the following:

Developing a range of discourse abilities. A growing body of evidence supports that when young children participate in the language of stories read aloud, they increasingly build a higher level of linguistic skills (Adams, 1990; Arnold & Whitehurst, 1994; Hoffman, Norris, & Monjure, 1990; Karweit, 1994; Whitehurst et al., 1988). They begin by talking about objects in the illustrations and continue to use language in more complex and abstract ways. "The child's ability to produce and comprehend complex sentences . . . then enables him or her to discuss abstract ideas ('What if . . . ?'), absent objects, and past events" (Snow et al., 1998, p. 49).

Talking about stories while using the language of stories enables children to rely less on the immediate context in their language expression. In doing so, they establish a bridge that ultimately leads to the use of decontextualized language, the kind of language used in school (Westby, 1985).

Reading and talking about picture books can produce increasingly complex informational exchanges between an adult and a child, including the following:

- Description: To describe a story illustration.
- Action sequences: To organize and report events of the story in logical, temporal, and causal sequences.
- Relating personal experiences: To report previously experienced events in logical order.
- Storytelling: To tell a story with the components of setting, initiating event, response, plan, attempt, consequence, and ending.

  Note: Children with poor narrative abilities may be unable to attend to a story if the content and structure of the story are above their ability level. Although they may have acquired semantic and syntactic skills at the word and sentence levels, they may experience difficulty participating in verbal interactive tasks that are part of larger units of discourse (Westby, 1990).

Reading and talking about picture books can help children develop a literate language style or language literacy. Children who interact with adults by using the information contained in literature learn how to ask questions about the literature. This process and informational exchange—especially the kinds of thoughtful answers children receive to their questions—help them develop conceptual knowledge and thinking skills (Kamhi & Catts, 1999). These are the same skills they will use later when comprehending text as thoughtful readers and when talking and writing about the text. These skills include the following:

- Predicting outcomes: To state what might happen next in the story, based on evidence or familiarity of experience.
- Identifying cause-and-effect relationships: To state the events that have led to a problem and to state what caused the problem to occur (e.g., *Rosie's Walk* and *The Thing That Bothered Farmer Brown* are books that require understanding of cause-and-effect relationships).

- Problem solving: To state facts about a problem, think of ways to solve the problem, and provide evidence to defend potential solutions to the problem. To comprehend and retell a goal-based story, children must be able to identify the problem and the attempts the character or characters make in responding to it (e.g., *One Fine Day, King Bidgood's in the Bathtub*, and *Click, Clack Moo: Cows That Type* are books that require an understanding of the problem and the characters' attempts to solve it).

Developing a sufficient lexicon base. Building a strong vocabulary is crucial for eventual reading success. More than simply relying on the context of the word, skilled readers are able to decode "when the meaning of the word is adequately established in memory" (Stanovich, 1993, p. 283). Other research substantiates that vocabulary size contributes more to early reading ability than does age or general developmental level and that an insufficient vocabulary base can impede the development of phonological awareness (Snow et al., 1998). Vocabulary size includes not only *quantity* of words but also *kinds* of words, such as nouns, verbs, articles, and prepositions. Discussing words during shared activities based on picture book reading is an excellent way to develop vocabulary acquisition and establish words in children's memories. It also may be necessary before children can thoroughly achieve phonological awareness.

Developing metalinguistic awareness. Linguistic knowledge, or the ability to speak a language, is an unconscious process that does not require speakers to define what they know about the act of speaking. Metalinguistic knowledge, on the other hand, is conscious knowledge about and insights into language itself. Children's metalinguistic skills in all of the spoken language components begin during the preschool years as they grow to think about, analyze, and manipulate language. "Indeed, literacy growth, at every level, depends on learning to treat language as an object of thought, in and of itself" (Snow et al., 1998, p. 45).

Snow et al. (1998) further report that semantic and syntactic skills in children are highly correlated to performance of phonological tasks. "These findings indicate that the development of phonological awareness (and other metalinguistic skills) is closely intertwined with growth in basic language proficiency during the preschool years" (p. 53).

Awareness of each of the following language components unfolds over time at varying rates and can be facilitated through the use of selected works of children's literature:

- Semantic awareness: To develop an understanding of a word and to understand that words are distinct from their referents. Ways to think about words include the introduction of synonyms, antonyms, multiple meanings, thematic associations, idioms, and other forms of figurative language. "Deep, rich knowledge of words and varied experiences with their uses are necessary for proficient reading and writing" (Moats, 2000, p. 128). For example, *A Cache of Jewels and Other Collective Nouns*, by Ruth Heller, explains how one word can be used for a collection or group of things. *A Hole Is to Dig: A First Book of Definitions*, by Ruth Krauss, and *Exactly the Opposite*, by Tana Hoban, are other examples of books that help children think about the semantic aspect of language.

- Phonological awareness: To develop an appreciation and sensitivity to the sounds of words as distinct from their meanings. The term *phonological awareness* is used to define a spectrum of skills that culminates at the level of *phonemic* awareness, that is, "the understanding that words are made up of individual sounds or *phonemes* and the ability to manipulate these *phonemes*, either by segmenting, blending or changing individual phonemes within words to create new words" (Chard & Dickson, 1999, p. 262).

- Scientific research substantiates that achievement in phonological awareness levels is the best predictor—including IQ (Stanovich, 1993) and perceptual skills (Adams, 1990)—of early reading success. Preschool- through kindergarten-aged children typically master these skills up to the syllable level. Research suggests that children should be able to demonstrate some degree of phonemic blending and segmentation by the end of kindergarten (Chard & Dickson, 1999). The continuum of phonological awareness includes the following activities listed in order of their complexity:

- Appreciating rhymes and alliteration
- Reciting rhyme and making rhyming words
- Sentence segmentation: Using the portions of the text to count words
- Syllable segmentation and blending: Using words of the text to segment and blend syllables into words
- Onset-rime, blending, and segmentation
- Blending and segmenting individual phonemes: Identifying and pronouncing each separate phoneme in a single-syllable word
- Manipulating phonemes: Adding, deleting, or substituting phonemes to generate a word from the remainder

Children's picture books can be ideal material with which to develop carefully planned, systematic instruction in the hierarchical levels of phonological awareness. Recently published picture books abound with the elements of sounds in their text and titles. Examples include *Click, Clack, Moo: Cows That Type; Sing, Sophie!; Zin! Zin! Zin! A Violin; Gabriella's Song;* alliterative titles such as *Mouse Mess, Counting Crocodiles,* and *Piggie Pie;* and a host books with rhyming texts such as *The Adventures of Taxi Dog* and *The Thing That Bothered Farmer Brown.*

- Morphological awareness: Phonological awareness facilitates morphological awareness in young children, and both are closely linked in intervention (Carlisle & Normanbhoy, 1993; Moats, 2000; Moats & Smith, 1992). Young children begin to sense word derivations and to think about how words are built from other words. For example, the words *swim* and *Swimmy,* the name of the fish in Leo Lionni's picture book by the same name, are seen as related. *Things That Are Most in the World,* by Judi Barrett, is another instance of a picture book designed to help children focus on the morphological aspects of language.

- Syntactical awareness: To develop an awareness of word order in sentences and that variations in syntax affect the meaning of a message. Five-year-old children begin to develop the rudimentary ability to correct syntactic errors (Ely, 2001). Young children also become aware of syntactic structure in their ability to identify the subject of a sentence (Ferreira & Morrison, 1994). Books such as *Jabberwocky,* by Lewis Carroll, can be used to develop children's awareness of sentence subjects even when nonsense words are used as text. Other examples of picture books that capture the essence of parts of speech include those in Ruth Heller's language series, such as *Kites Sail High: A Book About Verbs* and *Merry-Go-Round: A Book About Nouns.*

- Pragmatic awareness: To develop an awareness of the relationship between language and the social context in which it is used—including the ability to explain with specificity the rules of social language—whether or not behavior demonstrates adherence to those rules (Ely, 2001). *Chimps Don't Wear Glasses,* by Laura Numeroff, and *The Rat and the Tiger,* by Keiko Kasza, are examples of books that can teach the various uses of language.

Speech Production

With a bit of planning and preparation, a carefully chosen picture book can also help to achieve almost any objective in the area of speech–sound production, including the following:

To Improve Articulation

- To discriminate the target sound. Before reading, the text and illustrations can be used for auditory bombardment to stimulate target sounds. Throughout the reading, attention can be drawn to target sounds in the text by stressing their production.

- To produce the target sound in words and structured phrases and sentences. After stressing target sounds within the text and before turning each page, the reader can pause to have the child

  - repeat words in the story that contain the target sound,
  - say a carrier phrase appropriate to the story, or
  - answer a question that elicits a word or words from the text.

- To produce the target sound in conversation. After reading, the story's events can be discussed in language that contains the target sound.

To Speak Fluently

Metrical verses help children learn the natural rhythm of speech. Books that call for a rhythmic, melodic, or singsong type of response are beneficial.

Many alphabet and counting books are also excellent for this purpose (e.g., *Ten, Nine, Eight*, by Molly Bang). They can be used creatively to help a child maintain airflow in responses that increase in length from a single word, to a short phrase, to a full sentence.

Keep in mind that, while using a picture book to systematically increase the length of fluent responses, book talk can also incorporate other objectives, such as improving eye contact and communication appearance.

To Improve Vocal Quality and Minimize Vocal Abuse

Adults can use books for shaping children's vocal quality as well as for fluency by having the child use the optimal voice in progressively longer responses. Some stories make reference to the characters' voices. *Cuckoo: A Mexican Folktale*, by Lois Ehlert, and *The Three Billy Goats Gruff*, by Peter Asbjornsen, are examples of stories with characters whose voices are described as "golden" and "raspy" or "hoarse" and "loud." They can be used to draw a young child's awareness to vocal quality and intensity and to model various manners of vocal production to add further meaning and to generalize knowledge about the uses of voice in other contexts.

Regardless of the objectives in teaching communication skills and early literacy training, they undoubtedly can be facilitated through thoughtful planning and careful selection of a picture book from within the immense domain of children's literature.

Looking for Books

That Help Build Communication Skills and Emergent Literacy

Searching for the right books—picture books that hold potential for interaction and facilitate a variety of specific communication and literacy skills—takes time. The Catalog of Picture Books in this section and the Skills index were created to save you time. You will undoubtedly add to your collection of favorites. When making additional selections for young children, keep in mind the following:

Find the books that you love. The value of sharing your love and enthusiasm for the literature is perhaps the foremost prescription for helping children to build language and early literacy skills.

Find the books that you think _children_ will love. Capturing a child's interest and imagination is the first step in inspiring him or her to respond to the literature. Snow (1994) reminds us that, ultimately, the child judges the quality of the book.

Choose predictable books. Young children love knowing what comes next in a story. Therefore, choose books with words and actions that appear over and over again. Predictable books have

- repetition, rhyme, and verse;
- sequenced events; and
- allow for both spoken and imitated speech.

Examples of predictable books are _Chicken Soup with Rice_, by Maurice Sendak; _The Napping House_, by Audrey Wood; and _The Thing That Bothered Farmer Brown_, by Teri Sloat.

Pictures are important. Be sure the book's text is supported by good illustrations. The best illustrations are representational, easily interpreted, and appealing. To assist children in focusing on the oral language of the text, look for books in which

- each line of text has pictures to illustrate its meaning, and
- the pictures provide more language opportunities than the text alone.

Examples of such books are _Goodnight Moon_, by Margaret Wise Brown, and _The Thing That Bothered Farmer Brown_, by Teri Sloat.

Be sure the story is relevant. The text and illustrations are most effective when

- they reflect the child's surrounding culture,
- they make sense to the child, and
- the child can relate to them from personal experience.

Look for award winners. Not all of the books that are ideal for promoting language and literacy win awards, but lists of award-winning books can help you begin your search. Lists of Caldecott Medal winners, Children's Notables, and other award-winning books are available online, including the following Web sites:

- Association for Library Service to Children (ALSC): www.ala.org
- MacKin Library Media: www.mackin.com
- Booksellers such as Amazon.com (www.amazon.com) and Barnes & Noble (www.bn.com)

Make books a topic of conversation. Adults love to talk about and share good children's books. Ask friends, colleagues, librarians, and parents for titles of books they have enjoyed reading aloud.

Suggestions
for Book Talk
with Preschool and Kindergarten Children

Talking about storybook reading helps young children to link stories to their everyday lives. Taking about reading enhances meaning and language learning, and it also promotes early literacy. Here are some useful guidelines to follow when sharing a picture book:

Introduce the book. Before beginning to read, do the following:

- Ask children what they know about the book's topic
- Find out what questions children may have before you begin to read
- Give background information, if necessary
- Talk about other books that relate to the same topic
- Read the title and give the names of the author and illustrator

Pause to ask questions. Modify story reading to encourage children's active participation in the following ways:

- Ask prediction questions about the story
- Ask open-ended questions about the story
- Elicit picture descriptions and action sequences

Elaborate on the language

- Relate the story to the children's experiences and interests
- Assist children in expressing their ideas with the use of scaffolding
- Follow a child's lead. By following the child's interests and talking about what he or she points out, the adult can help the child learn more readily and enhance language even more (Arnold & Whitehurst, 1994).

Give feedback. In addition to the question-and-answer format, Fey (2001) suggests the following ways to give feedback to children:

- Request clarification of a child's utterances
- Recast the child's sentences
- Recast and recap the story content

Reread the story. Rereading enables children to become familiar with predictable language and thereby better acquire the concepts and gain an understanding of the story (Neuman et al., 2000). When children can anticipate what is coming next in a story or line of verse, they begin to have a sense of mastery over books (Cullinan & Bagert, 1996). Fey (2001) suggests several ways to allow children to participate, including the following:

- Fill in the blanks during cloze activities (I know an old lady who swallowed a _____)
- Recite words in unison (choral reading)
- Retell the story (with and without the aid of pictures)

Stay with the book-related activities. Continue to use the book for various language and literacy activities for more than one day or one session. Catherine E. Snow (1994), a leading authority in reading research, writes that

> the learning that occurs in book reading can build from repeated exposures to books. . . .
> A second or third reading of a story gives a chance for deeper processing, more probing and reflecting. It provides for the active engagement that is crucial to mature uses of literacy. (p. 272)

Suggestions for multiple sessions include the following:

- Introduce the book, its topic, and read it through on the first reading
- Reread the book, pausing to ask comprehension questions and engage in discussions
- Do a picture walk-through and retell the story
- Engage in phonological awareness activities with the words of the story
- Do an extended activity (e.g., collect objects featured in the story, make class murals of the story's setting, or dramatize the tale or nursery rhyme)

Collaborate with others. Special educators can coordinate books and topics to be covered with other educators. The American Speech-Language-Hearing Association (ASHA, 2001) has guidelines on collaborating with teachers, speech–language pathologists, and special educators so that language- and literacy-based activities are relevant to the classroom curriculum and individualized intervention programs.

A Catalog of Picture Books for Children in Preschool and Kindergarten

The Adventures of Taxi Dog

by Debra Barracca and Sal Barracca
New York: Dial Books for Young Readers, 1990

Suggested Grade and Interest Level: Pre-K

Topic Explorations: Animals, Dogs; Cities, New York City; Careers; Community; Transportation

Skill Builders:

Vocabulary	**Language literacy**
Idioms	Relating personal experiences
Similes and metaphors	Sequencing
Grammar and syntax	Discussion
Two- and three-word utterances	**Phonological awareness**
Noun–verb agreement	
Tenses, present and past	

Synopsis: In delightful rhyming verse, Maxi tells the story of how he came to belong to taxi-driver Jim. No longer a stray avoiding the pound, he now rides around New York City all day long. The story is based on the authors' experience of a New York City taxi ride with a driver and his dog that sat next to him in the front seat. Maxi, like the real taxi dog, travels with Jim to any number of different places. Follow them around, from airport to theater to hospital, and meet the characters Maxi meets, from all walks of life and in all sorts of circumstances.

Method: Before the read-aloud, elicit the children's background knowledge of taxicabs and big cities such as New York. If children have been to a big city, encourage them to relate their experiences. Explain what a taxicab is and how it is used.

During the read-aloud, allow children to experience of the story so that they hear the flow of the text—the rhythm and rhyme—without interruption. Use a dog puppet as you read to give children a sense that the dog is telling the story.

After the read-aloud, allow the children to ask questions of the dog puppet as if it were Maxi. Then reread the story, pausing after each page to increase vocabulary skills, utterance length, and story comprehension. Discuss the following vocabulary words:

roam	building
avoid	fare

Discuss the following idioms:

Cleaned the plate	Broke into a song
Start life anew	Put on a show

Talk about the following similes and what each might mean:

Like lightning we flew	It's just like a dream

Describe the colorful characters that get into the taxi. Recall their occupations. Point out the activity in the city and have children describe the action depicted in the illustrations. Model and shape grammatical structures. Then see if children can find the black cat that is hiding on every page.

Have children sequence the beginning parts of the story. What happened at the beginning of the story? (e.g., Jim found Maxi.) What happened next? (e.g., Jim took Maxi home, fed him, etc.) Then encourage children to continue the sequence as they recall one event that Jim and Maxi experienced when giving people rides in the city.

Hold a discussion about the importance of being kind to animals. What might have happened to Maxi had Jim never found him? Do you think that dogs respond differently when people are nice to them than when they are mean and angry toward them?

For phonological awareness training, reread the text, then play the games beginning at the appropriate developmental level for the child.

PLAY **Word-Count.**

Children count the number of words in a short line from the text. Demonstrate by assigning one word to one finger as you (or a dog puppet named Maxi) say(s) the words. For example, say

> Maxi

as you hold up one finger for the one word. Continue counting words until you have an entire line, as in

> My name is Maxi
> How many words did Maxi say?

for a four-finger count. Or repeat

> next to Jim

from the line "I sit next to Jim" for a three-finger count. Gradually allow the children to do the counting by themselves.

If children don't have one-to-one correspondence, give each child a collection of manipulables (i.e., blocks, felt squares, buttons, etc.) to use for representing words. Demonstrate by saying (or use the Maxi puppet to say) the words from the story that you want the children to count. Repeat them again as you (or the puppet) move out one item (blocks, square, button) for each corresponding word stated. Then you (or the puppet) count out loud the number of blocks moved to get the word count. Gradually allow the children to do the counting by themselves. Use words directly from a page of text arranged in hierarchical order, such as

I	My head
I sit	He patted
Next to	He patted my
I sit next to	Patted my head
I sit next to Jim	He patted my head

PLAY **Which-Word-Is-Missing?**

Children select a word from a word string that has been omitted from the previously given string. Choose two to four words from the text to present in the word strings. You or the puppet can repeat the words, leaving one out for the children to identify. For example, say

(continues on next page)

(PLAY) **Which-Word-Is-Missing?** *Continued*

> dog, city, taxi, pound
> dog, city, pound
> Which word is missing? (taxi)

If necessary, begin with two-word strings. When the child is successful, increase to three words, then four. Additional word strings include

dirt, food, dark, roam	park, taxi, lost, man	home, food, ride, tire
plate, kiss, scarf, head	love, care, true, good	streets, lights, building, people
fare, show, lady, sing	wife, sick, lightning, night	planes, stand, slow, line

(PLAY) **The Same-Sound game.**

Children identify whether word pairs or three-word strings begin with the same sound. For example, say

> Maxi, man
> Do they start with the same sound? (Yes)

To make an unmatched pair, exchange one word with another word from the story. Additional word pairs and three-word strings include

taxi, town	city, sing	line, lost, look
pound, park	roam, ruff	dog, dirt, dark
lost, look	home, hungry	taxi, town, take
		ride, ruff, roam
		Jim, joy, jog

(PLAY) **Odd-One-Out.**

Children select the word that does not belong from a string of words beginning with the same sound. Stress initial consonant sounds if necessary. For example, say

> Maxi, man, dog
> Which word doesn't belong? (dog)
> That's right. *Dog* is the odd one out.

Use the words provided in the Same-Sound game. Insert a one-syllable word from the story with a different initial sound for the children to identify, such as

> take, town, Jim
> food, lost, look
> roam, look, ruff
> pound, park, line

and so on, gradually increasing to four-word strings.

PLAY **Finish-the-Rhyme.**

Children supply the rhyming word left out at the end of a verse that you or the puppet reads aloud. Teach children to use the meaningful clues in the pictures as well as the meter of the verse to rhyme the word. If necessary, prompt with picture cues and with the initial phoneme, then gradually remove the scaffolding. For example, say

> "My name is Maxi
> I ride in a (t) _____
> I sit next to Jim
> I belong to (h) _____
> He came over and said
> As he patted my (h) _____"

PLAY **Rhyme-It-Again.**

Children identify the rhyming word heard after a rhyming set is given. Give initial consonant cues if needed. For example, say

> *Maxi* rhymes with (t) _____.
> *Said* rhymes with (h) _____.

PLAY **Make-a-Rhyme.**

Children supply another rhyming word after a rhyming word from the story is read aloud by you or the puppet. Give initial phoneme cues if needed. Accept any nonsense word. For example, ask

> What word rhymes with *Maxi*? T . . . (taxi)
> That's right. *Maxi* and *taxi* rhyme.

Some rhyming words from the story include

him (Jim)	way (day, pay)	dark (park)
red (head)	roam (home)	eat (seat)
down (town)	Sadie (lady)	ride (side)

PLAY **Rhyming-Ings.**

Children rhyme root words with added *–ing* suffixes using words in the text (root + added suffix, if necessary). Give initial phoneme cues if needed. Accept any rhyming nonsense word. For example, say

> Maxi is looking out the window. (Stress *looking* and show the picture)
> What word rhymes with *looking*? C . . . (*cooking, hooking, booking,* and nonsense words such as *mooking, tooking,* and *nooking*)

Practice with the following words, giving initial phoneme cues if necessary:

> looking (cooking, hooking, booking)
> sitting (hitting, fitting, knitting)

(continues on next page)

PLAY Rhyming-Ings. *Continued*

riding (hiding, siding)
patting (batting, chatting)
roaming (combing, foaming)
kissing (missing, hissing)
singing (ringing, winging, bringing, slinging, swinging)
eating (meeting, seating, beating, cheating)
sharing (caring, daring, tearing, glaring, staring)
wagging (sagging, lagging, nagging, tagging)

PLAY Clap-and-Count.

Children clap to, then count, the number of syllables heard in words from the text. Demonstrate by clapping to a word and then asking children how many parts they heard. For example, say and clap

city
How many parts in the word? Clap it out. (two)
Ci–ty. One, two.

Maxi, or the dog puppet, can also demonstrate by opening and closing its mouth to indicate syllables. Begin with two-syllable words and proceed in length. Stress and elongate syllables when presenting words such as

ta-xi (pronounced *tack-see*)	back-seat	hos-pi-tal	a-round
bis-cuit	air-port	pass-en-gers	hot-dog
sur-prise	light-ning	ev-ry-where	

PLAY What's-the-Word?

Children synthesize syllables into words from the pictures and text. You or the puppet say the syllables, inserting a clear pause between them, and have the children say the syllables quickly and repeatedly until they identify the word. Demonstrate first, for example,

tack–see
What's the word?
Say it until you hear it. Tack–see. Tack-see. Taxi.
Taxi is the word.

Continue with the two-syllable words provided in Clap-and-Count.

PLAY Find-the-Little-Words.

Children listen for "little" words within two-syllable words in the text. You or the puppet stress the separate parts when presenting the word. For example, say

back-seat
Can you find any little words in *backseat*?
That's right. *Back* is a little word in *back*seat.
Seat is another little word in *backseat*.

(continues on next page)

PLAY Find-the-Little-Words. *Continued*

Additional compound words

up-town (up, town)	a-round (a, round)	al-ways (all, way, ways)
air-port (air, port)	hot-dog (hot, dog)	

Then present two-syllable words, changing the stress as necessary so the children can hear all the "little" words, such as

tax-i (tack, see)	ci-ty (sit, tea)	sur-prise (sir, prize)
light-ning (light)	ri-ding (ride)	buil-ding (bill, ding, build)

PLAY Leave-It-Out.

Children say a compound or two-syllable word, then leave out the beginning or final part to create a smaller word. For example, say

> Say *backseat*, but leave out *seat*.
> What little word is left? (back)

Continue using the compound and two-syllable words provided.

PLAY Add-It-On.

Children put two words together to make a compound word or two syllables together to make a two-syllable word. Say part of the word and have the child supply the rest. For example, say

> Say *back* and then add on *seat*.
> What new word can you make? (backseat)
> That's right. *Back. Seat. Backseat.*

Continue using the compound and two-syllable words provided.

PLAY Turn-It-Around.

Children reverse the parts of some of the compound words to make nonsense words. Children then switch the parts back again to make the word what it was before they reversed it. For example,

> Put the word *seat* at the beginning of *back*.
> What funny word can you make? (seatback)
> What was it before you turned it around? (backseat)

Use the following compound words to make nonsense words: *uptown* to make *townup*, *airport* to make *portair*, and *hotdog* to make *doghot*.

☛ See the catalog for Grades 1 through 5 for continuing activities in the hierarchy of phonological awareness.

Read also *Maxi, the Hero; Maxi, the Star;* and *A Taxi Dog Christmas.*
Note: This book is also available in a Spanish version, titled *Las Aventuras de Maxi: El Perro Taxista.*

Airport

by Byron Barton
New York: Crowell, 1982

Suggested Grade and Interest Level: Pre-K

Topic Explorations: Careers; Transportation

Skill Builders:

Vocabulary	Grammar and syntax	Language literacy
Categories	Two- and three-word utterances	Relating personal experiences
	Noun–verb agreement	Sequencing
	Present tense	

Synopsis: Bold, colorful pictures and simple text explain in detail the things that take place during air travel, from the time passengers arrive at the airport until the plane is in the air.

Method: Before the read-aloud, lead into the story by presenting the cover and asking children what they know about airports. Encourage the children who have traveled to relate their personal experiences. Ask what types of jobs people do at airports.

During the read-aloud, pause to define words like *security checkpoints, rolling stairs, fuel trucks,* and so on. Also, talk about the various jobs people perform, such as pilot, flight attendant, and maintenance worker. For early utterances and noun–verb agreement, structure the text for the repetition of word combinations, such as

Workers clean.	The boy waits.	They find their seats.
People wait.	The boy finds his seat.	

Present-tense structure sentences might include

The mechanics are checking the engines.
The boy is standing at the ticket line.
They are putting luggage in the overhead bins.

After the read-aloud, ask children to tell a story about what happens at an airport by sequencing the events as they are shown in the illustrations. Assist with scaffolding as needed. Categorize different jobs and vehicles, including different types of airplanes.

Aldo

by John Burningham
New York: Crown, 1991

Suggested Grade and Interest Level: Pre-K

Topic Explorations: Feelings; Friendship

Skill Builders:

Grammar and syntax	Language literacy
Personal and possessive pronouns	Relating personal experiences
Tenses, present and past	Drawing inferences
	Discussion

Synopsis: A little girl describes the comforts—especially during difficult times—of having an imaginary friend. The sparse text with many wordless pages is ideal for encouraging children to interject language.

Method: Before the read-aloud, talk about the different types of people who can be our friends (e.g., neighbors, class-mates, and siblings). Talk about how special things—such as teddy bears and blankets—can also be our friends. Ask children to share stories about some of their special friends. Introduce the book as a story about a girl with a special friend.

During the read-aloud, pause to draw inferences about the meaning of the story.

Is Aldo real? What makes you think so?
What does "imaginary" mean?
How does the girl feel as she eats her ice cream sundae and watches the other children in the restaurant playing? Shape and model productions of target structures, such as present tense and pronouns.

After the read-aloud, recall times when the girl needed Aldo, such as when other children wouldn't play with her or when she awoke in the dark. Talk about times in the children's own lives when they would have liked to have had a special friend, whether real or imaginary. Ask, What are the good things that friends do for us?

Alfie Gets in First

by Shirley Hughes
New York: Lothrop, Lee & Shepard Books, 1981, 1987

Suggested Grade and Interest Level: Pre-K

Topic Explorations: Careers; Community; Family relationships

Skill Builders:
    Language literacy

Relating personal experiences	Problem solving
Predicting	Verbal expression
Storytelling	

Synopsis: Alfie, his mom, and his sister Annie Rose are coming home from shopping. Alfie runs ahead and, in a race to get home first, accidentally locks them out of the house. Alone inside, with his mom and Annie Rose outside, Alfie can't reach the latch to let them in. One by one, neighbors try to help solve the problem.

Method: For verbal expression, pause to allow children to tell, in their own words, what is happening. Encourage them to give more details about the story by interpreting the illustrations.

For predicting, have children make use of the clues in the story to guess what might happen next. For example, when the picture shows Alfie getting a chair and bringing it to the door, ask what will happen next.

For relating personal experiences, talk about what happens when we do things without first thinking. Some-times, things happen that we don't intend. Share a time when you did something without first thinking—for example, going to the grocery store without a list and forgetting to buy milk.

For problem solving, talk about what Alfie forgot to think about when he closed the door. How did Alfie solve his own problem? Encourage children to tell about times they thought of their own solutions to problems, just like Alfie did.

For storytelling, reread the pages and ask questions about story grammar elements to scaffold the retelling of events, such as

Where does the story take place?

What can you tell about how Alfie feels from looking at his expression?

Alligators All Around: An Alphabet

by Maurice Sendak
New York: Harper & Row, 1962; HarperCollins, 1991

Suggested Grade and Interest Level: Pre-K

Topic Exploration: Alphabet

Skill Builders:
   Grammar and syntax
   Two- and three-word utterances   Noun–verb agreement   Present tense

Synopsis: Alligators doing all kinds of absurd things in this little alphabet book make for lots of fun and plenty of language stimulation.

Method: Before the read-aloud, ask the children what they know about alligators. Explain that the book is an alligator alphabet book and lead into the story with predictions about what the alligators might do.

For early utterances, encourage children to repeat two or three words of the text after you read them. Some examples include

   Getting giggles
   Never napping
   Ordering oatmeal

Also, shape and model word combinations based on the action shown in each picture:

   Pop balloon
   Juggle jellybeans
   Push boy

For present tense, expand the text into utterances such as the following:

   He is popping the balloon
   He is juggling jellybeans
   He is washing dishes
   He is drying dishes

Extended Activity: Play an imaginary game. Have the group or class suppose that the helpful alligators are all around your room. What would they be doing? Some ideas include

   Turning on lights
   Hanging up coats
   Telling stories
   Never pushing

Animalia

by Graeme Base
New York: Abrams, 1986, 1987

Suggested Grade and Interest Level: Pre-K

Topic Exploration: Alphabet; Animals; Animals, Zoo

Skill Builders:

Vocabulary	Articulation, general	Voice
Phonological awareness	Fluency	

Synopsis: This extraordinary alphabet picture book presents an amazing array of animal and object illustrations beginning with a particular letter along with an alliterative sentence.

Method: Before the read-aloud, talk about the boy in the striped shirt hidden within the pages that illustrate words beginning with a letter sound. Encourage the children to hunt for him among the objects and animals depicted.

During the read-aloud, have children seek out and name as many objects and animals as possible whose names begin with the alphabet letter named. Use the book to teach new vocabulary words and put them into sentences. For example, using the letter *F* pages, read the phrase, "Four fat frogs fishing for frightened fish." Find other target words hidden in the illustration, including *fox, Frankenstein, fork, fire, fan, flue, floodlight, fish, falcon, fairy, flamingo,* and *fuchsia.* Demonstrate the new word by using the words of the text, such as "Four fat frogs are fishing near the pink flamingo."

For phonological awareness training, you can continue through the various activities using the same page, use a different page for the different activities, or use a variety of pages for the different activities. Allow children to search for the words in the illustrations after you've completed each game.

PLAY   **Word-Count.**

Use part of the alliterative text from each page. For example, the text for the alphabet letter *B* reads, "Beautiful blue butterflies basking by a babbling brook." Demonstrate by assigning one word to one finger as you say

> Blue butterflies
> How many words did I say? (two)

Then say

> Beautiful blue butterflies

for a three-finger count.

If children don't have one-to-one correspondence, give each child a collection of manipulables (i.e., blocks, felt squares, buttons, etc.) to use for representing each of the stated words. Demonstrate by saying (or use a puppet to say) the words from a page of text that you want the children to count. Repeat them again as you (or a puppet) move out one item at a time to correspond to your stated word. Then you (or a puppet) count out loud the number of blocks moved to get the word count. Gradually allow the children to do the counting by themselves. Use words directly form a page of text in hierarchical order to the desired word length. (It is easy to select from word sources on each page.)

(PLAY) Which-Word-Is-Missing?

Children identify the word in a word string that has been omitted from a previously given string. Choose two to four words from the illustration and text to make up a string. Repeat the words, leaving one out for the children to identify. For example, using the page for alphabet letter *D*, say

> doughnut, dice, dictionary, dragon
> dice, dictionary, dragon
> Which word is missing? (doughnut)

If necessary, begin with one-syllable words in two-word strings. When the child is successful, increase to three words, then four. You can easily choose words from a multitude illustrated on each page.

(PLAY) The Same-Sound game.

Children identify whether word pairs or three-word strings begin with the same sound. For example, for the page with pictures showing the initial alphabet letter *C*, say

> cap, cat
> Do they start with the same sound? (Yes)

Children can find a multitude of words on every page that begin with the same sound. Have them say aloud two words that they find and listen to whether they begin with the same sound.

(PLAY) Odd-One-Out.

Children select one word that does not belong from a string of words that begin with the same sound. For an example, using the *C* page, say

> cat, cow, dog
> Which word doesn't belong? (dog)
> That's right. *Dog* is the odd one out.

First, use one-syllable words that are illustrated on each alphabet letter page. Insert a word with a different initial sound for the children to identify, such as

> comb, can, boy
> cork, pot, card

More one-syllable words from the *C* page for three-word strings include

> cap, coin   cake, cup
> car, cage   cook, cone
> cane, Coke

Increase to four-word strings with two-, three-, and four-syllable words, such as

> camel, cauldron, camera   candle, canoe, coffee
> castle, canon, collar   carcass, cabin, Concorde (jet)
> canary, carefully, cucumber   calculator, caterpillar, candelabra

PLAY **Word-Search.**

Children search the picture for the word you are thinking of that begins with the same sound as a given word. For example, say

> I see something in this picture that starts with the same sound as *cat.*
> What other word starts with *c*? (Give phoneme/sound only.)
> Search for the word.
> That's right. *Cat* and *camera* start with *c.*

Word sources are abundant on every page.

PLAY **Clap-and-Count (syllables).**

Children clap to, then count, the number of syllables heard in selected words from the illustration and accompanying text. Demonstrate by clapping to a word and asking children how many parts they heard. For example, using the page for the letter *E*, say and clap

> eggs
> How many parts in the word? Clap it out. (one)

An *Animalia* puppet can also demonstrate by opening and closing its mouth to indicate syllables. Stress and elongate syllables when presenting words such as

> ear-ring
> el-e-phant
> E-liz-a-beth

Word sources are abundant on each page.

PLAY **What's-the-Word?**

Children synthesize syllables into words using words from the pictures in the book. Present the syllables, inserting a clear pause between them, and have the children say them quickly and repeatedly until they identify the word. Demonstrate by saying

> li–zard
> What's the word?
> Say it until you hear it. *Liiiii-zard. Liii-zard. Lizard.*
> *Lizard* is the word.

Word sources are abundant on each page.

PLAY **Find-the-Little-Words.**

Children listen for and find "little" words within two- and three-syllable words of the pictures and text. Change the stress as necessary so the children can hear all the "little" words. Use the names of things found in the illustrations. For example, when using the letter *F*, say

(continues on next page)

PLAY Find-the-Little-Words. *Continued*

> flamingo
> Can you hear any little words in *flamingo*? (go)
> fla-min-go
> That's right. *Go* is a little word in *flamingo.*

Additional words include

> fairy (fair)
> fishing (fish)
> forest (for, rest)
> frighten (fry, fright, ten)
> floodlight (flood, light)
> Frankenstein (frank)

Word sources are abundant on each letter page.

PLAY Leave-It-Out.

Children say a compound or two-syllable word, then leave out the beginning or final part to create a smaller word. For example, using the page for the letter *G,* say

> Say *greenhouse.*
> Now say *greenhouse* but leave out *house.*
> What little word is left? (green)

Then say

> Now say *greenhouse* but leave out *green.*
> What little word is left? (house)

Some two-syllable words from the *G* page include

> growing (grow)
> guitar (tar)
> goblet (gob, let)
> garden (gard [guard])

Word sources are abundant on each page.

PLAY Add-It-On.

Children put two words or two syllables together to make a compound or two-syllable word. For example, using the page for the letter *H,* say

> Say *lady.*
> Now say *lady* and add *bug.*
> What bigger word can you make? (ladybug)
> That's right. *Lady. Bug. Ladybug.*

(continues on next page)

PLAY **Add-It-On.** *Continued*

More words include

> hump—hump, tea (Humpty)
> ham—ham, ick (hammock)
> ham—ham, burger (hamburger)
> hand—hand, bag (handbag)

(*Hint:* Handbag is behind the branch that the ladybug is on in the foreground.)

More word sources are abundant on each page.

☞ See the catalog for Grades 1 through 5 for continuing activities in the hierarchy of phonological awareness.

Annie and the Wild Animals

by Jan Brett
Boston: Houghton Mifflin, 1985, 1989

Suggested Grade and Interest Level: Pre-K

Topic Explorations: Animals, Cats; Forest; Feelings; Pets; Seasons, Winter

Skill Builders:

Grammar and syntax	**Language literacy**	**Articulation,** *F* **and** *K*
Noun–verb agreement	Relating personal experiences	
Tenses, present and past	Predicting	
	Verbal expression	

Synopsis: Against the backdrop of a wintry forest, a little girl fears that her cat, Taffy, is lost. She sets out corn cakes each night, hoping to find a new pet. Every morning, a different (and unsuitable) animal appears, creating drama. Pictures around the borders of the illustrations show that Taffy is having kittens. The border pictures also help children form predictions about which animal will appear next.

Method: Before the read-aloud, talk about the word *litter* (in the sense of a brood of babies) and how cats have litters in different hidden places, often far from people.

During the read-aloud, enhance verbal expression and use of grammar and syntax skills by encouraging children to participate in the story. Ask them to describe each action in complete sentences (e.g., The moose is walking in the snow, and The wildcat is chasing the bird.).

For predicting, pause after reading several pages. As the children begin to realize that the border pictures give clues to the animal that will appear next, ask questions such as, "Do you think Annie will find a suitable pet when she wakes up in the morning? What makes you think so?"

After the read-aloud, have children relate personal experiences. Ask them what they do when they have no one to play with. How do they feel? What do they do? Discuss children's experiences of losing pets. Talk about how people feel when their pets disappear. Is it similar to how Annie felt? Discuss ways children have attempted to get their pets back. Ask, "If you were Annie, what would you do to find a new pet? Why was it a good thing Annie didn't find one? What might have happened if she had?"

For articulation, encourage the child's use of high-frequency words such as *Taffy* and *corn cakes* when pausing for interaction. Other *K* words include

> cat
> curled
> come
> like
> look
> looked

Other *F* words include

> find
> friend
> food
> furry
> family
> wolf

and the words in the phrase "soft and friendly like Taffy."

Arthur's Nose

by Marc Brown
Boston: Little, Brown, 1976, 1986

Suggested Grade and Interest Level: K

Topic Explorations: Careers; Friendship; Self-esteem

Skill Builders:

Grammar and syntax	Language literacy
Possessive nouns	Storytelling
Pronouns—personal, possessive, and reflexive	

Synopsis: Arthur is an aardvark whose family loves him, including his nose, which Arthur happens to detest. Even his schoolmates laugh at it. So Arthur visits the rhinologist to find a new one while his associates wait anxiously outside. When he comes out, everyone is surprised. Arthur's nose hasn't changed a bit. "I'm just not me without my nose!" he exclaims.

Method: Before the read-aloud, ask children what they know about anteaters and have the children describe them. What are their special characteristics? What do they do with their long noses and long tongues? Then make story predictions based on the book's cover.

Throughout the read-aloud, model grammar and syntax structures directly from the text, such as "Arthur's house," "Arthur's family," "Arthur's friends," and so on. Shape responses, such as the following:

> *He* didn't like *his* nose.
> *She* thought *his* nose was funny.
> *She* wanted to change *her* seat.
> *He* wasn't *himself* without *his* nose.
> Arthur liked *himself.*

For storytelling, encourage children to retell the story of Arthur's nose, using story grammar elements to provide scaffolding. Use the pictures as visual prompts. Discuss Arthur's problem and how he learned to solve it by himself.

Note: Read also *Arthur's Eyes, Arthur's First Sleepover, Arthur's New Puppy, Arthur's Tooth, Arthur's Pet Business,* and other books in this series.

At the Beach

by Anne Rockwell
New York: Macmillan, 1987, 1991

Suggested Grade and Interest Level: Pre-K

Topic Exploration: Sea and the seashore

Skill Builders:
Vocabulary	**Language literacy**
Grammar and syntax	Relating personal experiences
Two- and three-word utterances	Sequencing
Noun–verb agreement	
Present tense	

Synopsis: Bold and striking illustrations of seashore activities are accompanied by simple text written in the first person. The story is a nice lead-in to discussing children's own activities at a beach, lake, or picnic.

Method: Before the read-aloud, talk about going to the beach. Use words associated with the beach, such as *sand, seashore,* and *ocean.* What do children do at the beach? If children have been on an outing to the beach, encourage them to relate their experiences.

During the read-aloud, help build children's vocabulary by pausing to discuss some of these words:

shovel	pail	aluminum foil
beach umbrella	sandpipers	footprints

Use the words in sentences and relate each word as much as possible to the children's own lives. For grammar and syntax, pause to model and shape two- and three-word utterances, noun–verb agreement, and present tense using the text and illustrations. Suggestions include

At the beach	The girl swims
Collect shells	She is building sand castles
Bucket of sand	

After the read-aloud, help children sequence the events of going to the beach.

How do you get there?
What's the first thing you do when you arrive?
What do you do for play?
What do you do when it's time to go home?

Include elements of setting up an umbrella, laying out a towel, swimming in the water, building sand castles, eating lunch, resting, and looking for seashells.

The Baby Beebee Bird

by Diane Redfield Massie
New York: HarperCollins, 2000

Suggested Grade and Interest Level: Pre-K

Topic Explorations: Animals, Zoo; Birds; Nighttime; Zoos

Skill Builders:

Phonological awareness	**Articulation, B**
	Oral motor exercises

Synopsis: A tiny baby beebee bird keeps the zoo animals up at night because, as he explains, he's not tired. His continual *beebeebobbibobbi* sounds annoy the tiger, giraffe, bear, elephant, rhinoceros, snake, and eagle—until they think of an idea. They all *beebeebobbibobbi* throughout baby beebee's naptime, and the baby beebee bird can't sleep. Then, when nighttime comes, all is finally quiet as the exhausted animals fall asleep—including the baby beebee bird, nestled tightly inside a little linden tree leaf.

Method: Before the read-aloud, ask children if they can produce a baby's vocalizations to direct their listening skills to sound awareness. What kinds of sounds would a baby bird make? What kinds of sounds would other baby zoo animals make?

During the read-aloud, pause to use the *beebeebobbibobbi* sounds to enhance oral motor exercises, lip closure, and production of *B*. Encourage children to repeat after you the sounds the baby bird makes.

After the read-aloud, use the zoo animal sounds to help develop children's beginning phonological awareness skills of memory and attention to sequences of sounds. Produce the sounds that some of the animals make for the children to identify. Once they can identify a single sound, present a sequence of sounds, such as the hiss of a snake and the *beebeebobbibobbi* sound of the baby bird. Have children identify the sequence of sounds by naming, in order, the animals that made them.

Barn Dance!

by Bill Martin Jr. and John Archambault
New York: Henry Holt, 1986

Suggested Grade and Interest Level: Pre-K

Topic Explorations: Animals, Farm; Country life; Music, musicians, and musical instruments; Nighttime; Owls; Seasons, Autumn; Sounds and listening

Skill Builders:

Vocabulary	**Language literacy**	**Phonological awareness**
Categories	Verbal expression	**Articulation, K**
Attributes		

Synopsis: Late at night, with the moon shining bright, everything seems quiet out by the old barn. Or is it? As a boy listens to the sounds of the night from his bedroom window, an owl comes to lead him out across the fields and into the barn. There he sees a scarecrow hosting some mighty fine, western-style dancin'. This book is great for tapping out rhythms and is perfect for autumnal reading.

Method: Before the read-aloud, ask children what they know about barn dances. Discuss harvest festivals and how farmers celebrated finishing their work of harvesting corn and picking pumpkins off the vines with music and dancing in the barn. Show the cover with the scarecrow and his fiddle and a boy crawling through the rails of a fence in the moonlight. Have children predict what the story will be about.

During the read-aloud, demonstrate the rhythm of the text by tapping it out with your foot or by playing it on a small instrument as you read the lines. Encourage children to join in. For vocabulary, pause to talk about the fiddle and the type of music the scarecrow is playing on it. Discuss how barn dancing differs from other kinds of dancing. Other words include

kin	shadow
hound dog	wonderment
partner	curtsey

For verbal expression, pause in the reading to discuss the story. When the boy arrives at the barn, let the children find where he is hiding. Ask what the boy sees from his perspective. Point out the autumnal details, including scarecrows, apples in a barrel, pumpkins, and dried corn.

After the read-aloud, list attributes to describe the barn dance, such as *lively, active,* and *happy.*

For categories, recall the items mentioned or shown in the story that can be found on a farm. Then divide these items into categories, such as farm animals (cows, chickens, and pigs), produce (corn, pumpkins, apples, and wheat), and structures (barn, fence, house, loft, and silo).

For phonological awareness training, reread the text. Play the following games, beginning at the appropriate level for the child.

PLAY **Word-Count.**

Children count words presented from a line of text read aloud. Demonstrate by assigning one word to one finger as you say the words. For example, say

> Barn dance

as you hold up one finger for each word until two fingers are showing. Ask

> How many words did I say?

Or repeat

> "Full moon shinin'"

for a three-finger word count. Shorten text as necessary. For example, say

> "pushin' back shadows"

from the longer text,

> "Pushin' back the shadows, holdin' back the night."

(continues on next page)

PLAY **Word-Count.** *Continued*

If children don't have one-to-one correspondence, give each child a collection of manipulables (i.e., blocks, felt squares, buttons, etc.) to use for representing each of the stated words. Demonstrate by saying (or use a puppet to say) the words from a page of text that you want the children to count. Repeat them again as you (or a puppet) count out one item at a time to correspond to your stated word. Then you (or a puppet) count out loud the number of blocks moved to get the word count. Gradually allow the children to do the counting by themselves. Use words from a page of text in any desired combination and word length, such as

> Full moon
> Full moon shinin'
> Shinin' big
> Shinin' big and bright
> Full moon shinin' big and bright
> Whisper
> Just the whisper
> Whisper of leaves
> Just the whisper of leaves

PLAY **Which-Word-Is-Missing?**

Choose two to four words of the text and create a word string. Repeat the words, leaving one out for the children to identify. For example, in a four-word string, say

> moon, boy, dance, barn
> moon, dance, barn
> Which one is missing? (boy)

If necessary, begin with two-word strings. When the child is successful, increase to three words, then four. Additional word strings include

> fence, moon, barn, tree   fiddle, strings, music, night
> dance, square, barn, cow   cow, rabbit, chicken, pig
> tree, quiet, barn, sleep   scarecrow, skinny, partner, kid
> bed, owl, rabbit, dog   barrel, pigs, sky, owl
> bright, shining, leaves, tree

PLAY **Rearrange-It.**

Children rearrange, in correct word order, a scrambled phrase or sentence from a portion of the text. For example, say

> Dance barn
> Can you help me say those words in the right order?
> That's right. *Dance barn* should really be *Barn dance*.

> **PLAY**   **Rearrange-It.** *Continued*
>
> More words to rearrange include
>
> > Glasses wear
> > Moon full
> > Old dog hound
> > Rabbits after dreaming
> > Questions his in head
> > The owl night said
> > Closer a little come
> > Coming the corn field from
> > The kid skinny
> > Saw no one the kid skinny

> **PLAY**   **The Same-Sound game.**
>
> Children identify whether alliterative word pairs begin with the same sound. For example, say
>
> > barn, back
> > Do they start with the same sound? (Yes)
>
> Intersperse nonalliterative words into the following sets to make odd pairs, such as *barn, dance.*
> More word sets include
>
> | | | |
> |---|---|---|
> | corn, kid | night, noise | back, bow (as in take a bow) |
> | kin, kid | fiddle, fence | dance, donkey |
> | shining, shadows | listen, leaves | faint, fiddle |

> **PLAY**   **Odd-One-Out.**
>
> Children select the one word that does not belong from a string of alliterative words. For example, say
>
> > barn, back, night
> > Which word has a different beginning sound? (night)
> > That's right. *Night* is the odd one out.
>
> Using the words provided in the Same-Sound game, insert a word from the story with a different initial sound for the children to identify, such as
>
> > corn, kid, *moon*
> > night, *barn*, noise
>
> and so on.

> **PLAY**   **Finish-the-Rhyme.**
>
> Children supply the rhyming word left out at the end of a verse. Teach children to use the meaningful clues in the pictures as well as the meter of the verse to rhyme the word. If necessary, prompt with a picture cue and with the initial phoneme, then gradually remove the scaffolding. For example, say
>
> *(continues on next page)*

PLAY **Finish-the-Rhyme.** *Continued*

> *"Right hand! Left hand! Around you go!*
> Now back-to-back your partner in a do-si-_____." (*do*, sounds like *doe*)
> "Mules to the center for a curtsey an' a bow!
> An' hey there, skinny kid! Show the old cow _____." (how)
> "Out came the skinny kid, a-tickin' an' a-tockin'
> An' a hummin' an' a-yeein' an' a-rockin' an' a-sockin'.
> An' he danced his little toe through a hole in his (st)_____!" (stockin')

PLAY **Rhyme-It-Again.**

Children identify the rhyming word heard after a rhyming set is given. Prompt with auditory and visual cues as needed. For example, say

> *Rockin'* rhymes with (st)_____. (stockin')

PLAY **Do-They-Rhyme?**

Children identify whether word pairs rhyme. For example, say

> head, bed
> Do they rhyme? (Yes)

Insert nonrhyming words from the text into the following rhyming pairs:

> head, bed
> low, so
> chin, kin
> bow, how
> go, do (sounds like *doe*)
> day, say
> eye, by
> bright, night
> low, crow
> twenty, plenty

PLAY **Make-a-Rhyme.**

Children supply another rhyming word after a rhyming word from the story is presented. Accept any nonsense rhyming words. For example, ask

> What rhymes with rockin'?
> Rockin' (stockin', talkin', walkin')
> That's right. *Rockin'* and *stockin'* rhyme.

Continue with the rhyming sets provided.

PLAY   Clap-and-Count.

Children clap to, then count, the number of syllables heard in words from the text. Demonstrate by clapping to a word and then asking children how many parts they heard. For example, say and clap

> scarecrow
> How many parts in the word? Clap it out. (two)
> Scare–crow. One, two.

A puppet can also demonstrate by opening and closing its mouth to indicate syllables. Begin with two-syllable words and proceed in length (or demonstrate with one-syllable words if needed). Stress and elongate syllables when presenting compound and one- and two-syllable words such as

hoe-down	ski-nny	part-ner
barn-yard	mu-sic	un-der-neath
tip-toe	fi-ddle	won-der-ment
farm-house	curt-sey	co-tton-wood

PLAY   What's-the-Word?

Children synthesize syllables into words from the pictures and text. Say the syllables with a clear pause between them, and have the children say the syllables quickly and repeatedly until they identify the word. Demonstrate by saying

> scare–crow
> What word did I say?
> Say it until you hear it. *Scarrrrre—crow. Scarre-crow. Scarecrow.*
> *Scarecrow* is the word.

Continue using the two-syllable words provided in Clap-and-Count.

PLAY   Find-the-Little-Words.

Children find and say the "little" words within the compound words and the two- and three-syllable words in the pictures and text. For example, stress and elongate the syllables when saying the following:

> skinny
> Can you hear any little words in *skinny*.
> Ski-neee. Ski-nnee.
> That's right. *Knee* is a little word in *skinny*.

Then, change the stress pattern. Say

> Let's try in a different way.
> Skinn-ee.
> That's right. *Skin* is another little word in *skinny*.

PLAY Find-the-Little-Words. *Continued*

Using these additional words, change the stress as necessary so the children can hear all the "little" words.

barnyard (barn, yard)	whisper (*per,* sounds like "purr")	closer (close, sir)
tiptoe (tip, toe)	partner (part)	chatter (chat)
farmhouse (farm, house)	pumpkin (pump, kin)	shin-ing (or shinin' [shine])
hoedown (hoe, down)	humming (or hummin' [hum])	ticking (tick, ing)
	fifteen (teen)	farmer (farm, arm)

PLAY Leave-It-Out.

Children say a compound or two-syllable word, then leave out a part to create a smaller word. Demonstrate first, saying

> Say *barnyard.*
> Now say *barnyard,* but leave out *yard.*
> What little word is left? (barn)
> That's right. *Barn* is the only word left.
> *Barnyard. Barn.*

Then, children leave out the other part. For example, say

> Now say *barnyard,* but leave out *barn.*
> What little word is left? (yard)

Continue with the compound words and two-syllable words provided in Find-the-Little-Words.

PLAY Add-It-On.

Children put two words or two syllables together to make a compound or two-syllable word. For example, say

> Say *tip.*
> Now, say *tip* and add *toe.*
> What new word can you make? (tiptoe)
> That's right. *Tip. Toe. Tiptoe.*

Continue with the words provided in Find-the-Little-Words.

PLAY Turn-It-Around.

Children reverse the parts of previously learned compound words, and analyze and synthesize them according to their parts. For example, say

> Put the word *toe* at the beginning of *tip.*
> What word do you have? (toetip)
> What was it before you turned it around? (tiptoe)

Continue with the compound words provided in Find-the-Little-Words.

☞   For a continuation of phonological awareness activities, see this book entry in the Grades 1 through 5 catalog.

For *K* articulation therapy, use the words in the text and the illustrations to elicit the target sound. Phoneme *K* words from the text and pictures include *kid, kids, cottonwood, country, quiet, questions, come, curtsey, cow, kitchen, curtains, except, plunkin', tickin', tockin', stockin, punkins', rocket, welcome, turkey, seek, magic, back, pink,* and *blink.*

Phoneme *k* blends include *skinny, scarecrow, closer, critters,* and *sky.*

Extended Activity: Have a fall feast, country style. Bake hot biscuits and pumpkin pie, drink apple cider, and decorate tables with scarecrows, corncobs, and gourds. Play country music and have children clap along with the beat. If possible, play a game of horseshoes. Ask all the children to share what they like best about the fall season. Have them pretend that they are in a barn for the feast. What kinds of things would they see and hear? What would they use for music? Who would play?

Bear Noel

by Olivier Dunrea
New York: Farrar, Straus & Giroux, 2000

Suggested Grade and Interest Level: Pre-K

Topic Explorations: Animals; Bears; Holidays, Christmas; Seasons, Winter; Sounds and listening

Skill Builders:

Vocabulary	**Grammar and syntax**
Similes and metaphors	Present tense
	Question structures

Synopsis: A lovely book for the holiday season and ideal for encouraging children's participation at story time. The quiet story—with its breathtaking, snowy scenes—is set in the north woods on Christmas Eve. Wolf, Hare, Fox, Boar, Hedgehog, Possum, Owl, and Mole listen in anticipation for Bear Noel (a clever pun on "Pere Noel," the French Father Christmas). "This is the night when all creatures may come together without fear," declares the big, jovial bear. The repetitive text is an accumulation of what each animal hears Bear Noel doing as he comes closer and closer. When Bear Noel appears, he brings a feast for them to share as they put away their quarrels and find joy in celebrating the season together.

Method: Before the read-aloud, set the stage and prepare children to listen to the sounds of Bear Noel, just like the animals in the forest do. Talk about the quietness of snow falling and little sounds that can be heard in the silent forest. When all is quiet, what can the animals hear? Then show the first few pages and invite children to describe the snowy scenes with their own words.

During the read-aloud, encourage children to participate in saying the repetitive, cumulative verse. Pause occasionally to briefly define a word or point out a detail. Shape present-progressive tense by having children repeat the lines of the story, such as

> He is laughing
> He is singing
> He is tramping through the snow
> He is jingling his bells
> He is getting nearer
> He is bringing something wonderful
> He is coming

Have children who are working on question structures repeat the predictable lines of the text after the words, "He is coming," whispers Hare. Children ask, "Who is coming?"

After the read-aloud, go back through the pictures to review the vocabulary in context. Phrases to discuss include the following:

"Snow *blankets* the forest."
Explain how metaphors use words in a comparison, but they don't use *like* or *as*. In this example, the author describes what the snow in the forest is like without using many words. Another way to say the sentence using a simile is that "The snow looks *like* a white blanket across the ground in the forest."

"Wolf *lopes* toward him (Hare)."
Have children guess at what the word *lopes* means. Does it mean to move fast or slow? What other animal in the story might lope? Have children construct sentences with the word or demonstrate the wolf's stride.

"Into the *clearing* strides Bear Noel."
Talk about the forest behind Bear Noel and go back to the first pages of the book to give the children a sense of where he has just been in the thick trees. Then ask children to describe a "clearing" (i.e., land that contains no trees or bushes). Have children construct simple sentences about Bear Noel using the word *clearing* in relation to where he is standing in the picture.

"His furry feet *sweep a broad path* through the snow."
Ask children if they can hear what Bear Noel sounds like when he comes into the clearing. Is it a quiet sound? A "whooshing" sound? What other words do the children have for it? Ask what the snowy ground looked like after Bear Noel walked on it to enable children to use all or part of the words, "a broad path in the snow."

". . . his bells *faintly* ringing in the quiet night."
Have children guess at what the word *faintly* means. Do the bells sound loud or soft? Far away or near? Have children construct sentences with the word.

Extended Activity: Hold a reader's theater with children taking the parts of the animals and saying their lines. When Owl asks, "Who is coming?" the other children in the audience can say, "Bear Noel!" adding whatever embellishments they want to create and add to the text.

Berlioz the Bear

by Jan Brett
New York: Putnam, 1991; Scholastic, 1992

Suggested Grade and Interest Level: Pre-K

Topic Explorations: Bears; Careers; Community; Music, musicians, and musical instruments

Skill Builders:

Vocabulary	Grammar and syntax	Language literacy
Categories	Present tense	Cause-and-effect relationships
	Pronouns, personal and	Problem solving
	possessive	Verbal expression

Synopsis: Berlioz has been practicing his double bass for weeks. When the day comes for the orchestra to play at the village ball, the musicians load into the bandwagon (border pictures show the animals of the town making preparations for the feast). But the wagon is detained when the mule decides to stall. Will the musicians get to the ball in time? Various animals try to help. At last, a strange phenomenon coming from Berlioz's bass gets them to the ball on time.

Method: Before the read-aloud, discuss the book's cover and have children make predictions about the story. Elicit prior knowledge about the instruments on the cover.

During the read-aloud, pause to elicit verbal expression by interacting with children about the story and its characters. Talk about what a border is and point out the story within the book's border. Ask the children to describe the preparations for the ball that are depicted in the border. Shape and model target grammatical and syntactic structures within the context of the story.

For problem solving and identifying cause-and-effect relationships, pause during the story and ask the children to define each of the problems. The first problem arises when Berlioz can't get the bee out of his bass. The second problem arises when the mule does not budge. For each problem, brainstorm possible solutions. See whether the children can explain how the problems are related.

After the read-aloud, discuss what might have happened if the bee had not stung the mule (which then took the musicians to the party in time) and solved both problems. What effect would arriving late for the ball have on the story? Have the children recount different ways the musicians could get to the party. How else might the musicians have gotten to the party? Could they have done something else to solve the problem? Which solution do the children think is best?

Extended Activity: Play a recording of Rimsky-Korsakov's *The Flight of the Bumblebee*. Talk about how the members of the symphony orchestra are like the musicians in *Berlioz the Bear*. Turn to one of the last pages in the book to identify and categorize the musical instruments, including the bass, violin, French horn, oboe, drum, and trombone. Talk about how *The Flight of the Bumblebee* tells a story—not in words, but with musical notes. See whether the children can identify any of the musical instruments in the recording. Ask children to describe the music. What words can they think of to describe the sounds of the bumblebee? Where is the bumblebee? What might the bumblebee want to do? How might the bumblebee feel?

Big Pumpkin

by Erica Silverman
New York: Scholastic, 1992

Suggested Grade and Interest Level: Pre-K

Topic Exploration: Holidays, Halloween

Skill Builders:

Vocabulary	Language literacy
Associations	Predicting
	Sequencing
	Drawing inferences

Synopsis: A witch wants to make pumpkin pie, so she plants a pumpkin seed. It grows to be such a big pumpkin that she cannot pull it out of the ground. "Drat," says the witch. First a ghost tries to help, with no success. Then a vampire tries but cannot budge the pumpkin either. The mummy tries, too, but to no avail. It isn't until the bat comes along and pulls on the mummy, who pulls on the vampire, who pulls on the ghost, who pulls on the witch, that the big old pumpkin finally gives way. Then everyone shares a pumpkin pie until it is time to go. "Drat," says the witch.

Method: Before the read-aloud, talk about planting some vegetables that are harvested in the fall, such as corn, squash, and pumpkins, and ask children to name items associated with planting. Suggestions include a shovel, trowel, watering can, hose, seeds, and bulbs. Show the dedication page that has a shovel, watering can, and seeds on it and ask the children if the items they named can be found there. Show the book's cover with the witch holding the shovel and ask children to predict what the story will be about.

During the read-aloud, encourage children to predict what will happen next. After the ghost can't pull out the pumpkin, what do they think will happen next? Continue to ask prediction questions at predictable moments in the text.

After the read-aloud, help children develop sequencing skills. First, sequence the steps in growing a pumpkin from seed. Include preparing the soil, digging the hole, watering, weeding, and waiting for it to sprout, then have children sequence the events of the story, using the illustrations to help recall the events. Who came along first? What did he do? Who came next? What did he do? and so on. Help children use the words *first, then, next,* and *at last,* so they can express the sequences within the continuity of a story.

Big Red Barn

by Margaret Wise Brown
New York: William R. Scott, 1956; HarperCollins, 1989 (rev. ed.); HarperCollins, 1991

Suggested Grade and Interest Level: Pre-K

Topic Explorations: Animals, Farm; Colors

Skill Builders:

Vocabulary	Grammar and syntax	Language literacy
Adjectives	Tenses, present and past	Verbal expression

Synopsis: A charming classic about all the animals that live on a farm, the noises they make, and what they do from sunrise to sunset—all written in rhyming text.

Method: Before the read-aloud, have the children brainstorm all the animals that live on a farm. Make a list, then read the story, pausing at appropriate places to ask questions and shape responses (e.g., "The horses stomped in the hay" and "The little black bats flew away."). After the read-aloud, have children recall the animals that lived in the story's big red barn (with as many of the adjectives as they can remember). See how the list grows!

Extended Activities: Using the list of animals the class has brainstormed, create a bulletin-board scene of a farm and a big red barn (complete with cornfields and a scarecrow). Have each of the children draw and then cut out one of the animals from the list and then place the animal anywhere in the scene. Ask each child to describe the animal, make its sound, and tell where the animal is and explain what it likes to do on the farm.

This is a good story for a flannel or felt board because it encourages even the most reluctant child to participate. It is well worth the time to cut out the animal shapes, especially because they can be used every year. Cut out pieces of felt or flannel for the barn and for all the animals, each in a different color. Have the children press the pieces onto a felt- or flannel-covered board as they name the colors of the animals and tell the story of the big red barn.

Note: This book is also available in a Spanish translation, titled *El gran granero rojo.*

Brown Bear, Brown Bear, What Do You See?

by Bill Martin Jr.
Orlando, FL: Holt, Rinehart & Winston, 1967, 1983

Suggested Grade and Interest Level: Pre-K

Topic Explorations: Animals; Colors

Skill Builders:

Vocabulary	Grammar and syntax	Fluency
Categories	Two- and three-word utterances	
Adjectives	Question structures	

Synopsis: The sing-song text asks and answers what a series of brightly colored animals see looking at them.

Method: Encourage children to join in reciting the repetitive text. Label all of the animals on the last page, then go back through the pages and have the children predict which animal will appear next.

Build fluency through the repetition of the verse "Brown Bear, Brown Bear, what do you see?" and through the responses to the questions "I see a _____ looking at me."

Extended Activities: Play "Sea horse, sea horse, what do you see?" having children fill in animal names from the category of ocean creatures. Play with other categories of animals, such as birds—"Hummingbird, hummingbird, what do you see?" "Penguin, penguin, what do you see?" "Toucan, toucan, what do you see?"

Make enough tagboard templates of the animals in the story to be evenly distributed among the children. (*Note:* You can trace the animal outlines from the illustrations or project the images onto tagboard using an overhead projector.) You or the children can place each template against the inside of a paper plate and draw around it with a magic marker. Make puppets to represent characters in the book by having children color in and cut out the animal shapes. Glue a craft stick to the paper plate for a handle, then reread the story, having the children participate by raising their puppets when the corresponding animal name is mentioned and reciting what their animal sees. For example, green frogs would respond by holding up their puppets and saying, "I see a purple cat looking at me."

A Cache of Jewels and Other Collective Nouns

by Ruth Heller
New York: Grosset & Dunlap, 1987

Suggested Grade and Interest Level: Pre-K

Skill Builders:

Vocabulary
  Categories

Synopsis: Brilliant use of rich design, rhyming text, and the "collection" concept makes this book a real treasure as a language experience.

Method: Present the book and talk about animals, flowers, objects, or ideas associated with the pictures and text. Introduce categories by asking children questions, such as, Into which category would one put a pea pod? and Into which category would one put the kittens? (both are pictured on the same page). Ask if the children can name things one might find in the ocean besides oysters, or items of jewelry one might find in a jewelry box besides a string of beads. Reinforce unfamiliar words by asking questions (e.g., What do we call a secret stash of jewels?) to elicit the response, "A *cache* of jewels."

Extended Activities: Make collections of things. Invite children to bring in and share their own collections of stuffed animals, rocks, shells, jewelry, baseball cards, and so on. Go for a walk to gather collections of rocks, twigs, leaves, and insects. (Allow each child or group of children to collect something different.) When you return, allow the children to take turns presenting their collections to the class.

Pass around several bags full of items such as buttons, twigs, rocks, and bottle caps. Have children choose several items from each bag to make up their own collections. Mount the items on paper. Help children label their pictures with collective nouns, such as "a group of rocks," "a bunch of shells," "a pile of twigs," or "a collection of junk."

Note: See also *Kites Sail High: A Book About Verbs* and other books in Ruth Heller's language series.

Caps for Sale: A Tale of a Peddler, Some Monkeys and Their Monkey Business

by Esphyr Slobodkina
New York: Harper & Row, 1940, 1947, 1968; Scholastic, 1987

Suggested Grade and Interest Level: Pre-K

Topic Explorations: Clothing, Hats; Colors

Skill Builders:

Vocabulary	**Language literacy**	**Articulation,** *K*
Categories	Predicting	**Fluency**
Prepositions	Sequencing	
	Phonological awareness	

Synopsis: An unusual peddler carries his wares on his head, calling, "Caps! Caps for sale! Fifty cents a cap!" When he falls asleep under a tree, monkeys in the tree do what monkeys do—monkey business, of course! Kids love to imitate the peddler as he tries to retrieve his caps in this all-time favorite.

Method: During the read-aloud, pause to briefly discuss vocabulary words such as *peddler* and *refreshed* and words with multiple meanings, including *wares, upset,* and *checked.*

Model prepositions from the text, such as "He looked *in back* of him," "He looked *behind* the tree," and "He pulled *off* his cap." Also, pause to structure phrases based on the illustrations, such as "on his head," "in the tree," "under the tree," "up in the sky," and "beside the pond."

For predicting, ask children what the monkeys will do when the peddler shakes his fist, throws his cap on the ground, and does other predictable events.

After the read-aloud, children can practice sequencing skills by describing how the peddler puts the caps on his head: first his own checked cap, then the gray caps, then the blue caps, and so on, as shown in the text and pictures.

For phonological awareness training, use the book to play sound games with the words.

PLAY **Word-Count.**

Children identify the words in part or all of a sentence from the text. For example, demonstrate by holding up one finger for each word as you say

> "Caps for sale."
> How many words did I say? (three)

(continues on next page)

PLAY **Word-Count.** *Continued*

Gradually allow the children to do the counting by themselves.

If children don't have one-to-one correspondence, give each child a collection of manipulables (i.e., blocks, felt squares, buttons, etc.) to use for representing each of the stated words. Demonstrate by saying (or use a puppet to say) the words from a page of text that you want the children to count. Repeat them again as you (or a puppet) move out one item at a time to correspond to your stated word. Then you (or a puppet) count out loud the number of blocks moved to get the word count. Gradually allow the children to do the counting by themselves. Use words directly from a page of text in hierarchical order to the desired word length. Some of the words in the text to count include

Fifty cents	My caps
Fifty cents a cap	Give me my caps
You monkeys	Give me back my caps
You monkeys you	You give me back my caps

PLAY **Which-Word-Is-Missing?**

Children identify the word in a word string that has been omitted from a previously given string. Choose up to four words from the text to present, then repeat the words, leaving out one for the children to identify. For example, say

caps, sale, head, tree
caps, sale, tree
Which word is missing? (head)
That's right. *Head* is the word that's missing.

At early levels, begin with one-syllable words in two-word strings. When the child is successful, increase to three words, then four. Some word from the text include

tree, trunk, caps, sleep	lunch, hungry, sell, caps
sun, checked, walk, rest	hand, awoke, felt, back
blue, brown, red, gray	flying, threw, pulled, ground
town, street, tree, country	looked, into, behind, checked
	angry, peddler, monkey, morning

PLAY **Rearrange-It.**

Children rearrange, in correct word order, a scrambled phrase or sentence from a portion of the text. For example, say

Sale for caps
Can you help me say those words in the right order?
That's right. *Sale for caps* should really be *Caps for sale.*

More words to rearrange include

For caps sale	Cap a cents fifty	Right he to the looked
Cents fifty	He sleep to went	Me give back
Cents fifty a cap	He right to the looked	Me back give my caps

PLAY The Same-Sound game.

Children identify whether word pairs begin with the same sound. For example, say

> sale, cents
> Do they start with the same sound? (Yes)

To make an unmatched pair, exchange one of the following words with another word from the text, such as *sale, caps.*

sell, sale	fort, fork	slow, sleep
cap, cat	red, rest	tree, trunk
felt, feel	left, leaves	
woke, wore	slow, sleep	

PLAY Clap-and-Count.

Children clap to, then count, the number of syllables heard in selected words from the illustrations and text. Demonstrate by clapping to a word and then asking children how many parts they heard. For example, clap and say

> key
> How many parts in the word? Clap it out. (one)
> Key. One.

Clap and say

> monkey
> How many parts in the word? Clap it out. (two)
> Mon–key. One, two.

A monkey (or any kind of puppet) can also demonstrate by opening and closing its mouth to indicate syllables. Stress and elongate syllables when presenting and clapping to words such as

ca-lling	be-hind	ca-rry-ing
coun-try (sounds like *tree*)	sha-king	an-gri-ly
res-ted	a-way	or-din-ar-y
stan-ding	fly-ing	

PLAY What's-the-Word?

Children synthesize two syllables into a word. Use pictures in the book as cues if needed. Present the syllables, inserting a clear pause between them, and have children say them quickly and repeatedly until they identify the word. Demonstrate first, for example

> mon–key
> What's the word?
> Say it until you hear it. Monnn-key. Monn-key. Monkey.
> *Monkey* is the word.

Stretch out word parts at first if necessary. Continue with the words listed in Clap-and-Count.

PLAY Find-the-Little-Words.

Children listen for and find the "little" words within the compound words and two- and three-syllable words in the pictures and text. For example, stress and elongate the syllables when saying

> monkey
> Can you hear any little words in *monkey*? (key)
> That's right. *Key* is a little word in *monkey*.

In presenting the following additional words, change the stress pattern as necessary so children can hear the "little" words.

coun-try (tree)	res-ted (rest, Ted)	a-way (a, way)
be-hind (be)	sha-king (shake, king)	or-din-ar-y (or, air)
fly-ing (fly)	stan-ding (stand, ding)	

PLAY Leave-It-Out.

Children say a two-syllable word, then leave out the beginning or final part to create a smaller word. For example, say

> Say *slowly*.
> Now, say *slowly*, but leave out *–ly*.
> What little word is left? (slow)
> That's right. *Slowly. Slow.*

Then say

> Now, say *slowly*, but leave out *slow*.
> What little word is left? (*–ly*, pronounced *lee*)
> That's right. *Slowly. Lee.*

Continue with the two-syllable words provided in Find-the-Little-Words.

PLAY Add-It-On.

Children put two syllables together to make two-syllable word. For example, say

> Say *slow*.
> Now, say *slow*, and add *–ly*.
> What bigger word can you make? (slowly)
> That's right. *Slow. Slowly.*

Continue with the two-syllable words provided in Find-the-Little-Words.

☞ For continued phonological awareness activities, see the catalog for Grades 1 through 5.

For articulation of *K*, read each page, stressing the target sound. At the end of the page, ask a short question to elicit a response heavily loaded with the target sound. Also, have children repeat the predictable words of the text.

For fluency, have a child take the part of the peddler, maintaining airflow while repeating the dialogue from the story: "Caps! Caps for sale! Fifty cents a cap!" and "You monkeys, you! You give me back my caps." Have the child list the colors of the caps in the order on which the peddler places them on his head, increasing the length of utterance produced with uninterrupted airflow as the peddler piles the caps back on his head.

Note: A Spanish version of this book is available, titled *Sevenden corras: La historia de un vendedor ambulante, unos monos y sus travesuras.*

The Carrot Seed

by Ruth Krauss
New York: Harper & Row, 1945, 1989; Scholastic, 1993

Suggested Grade and Interest Level: Pre-K

Topic Explorations: Growing cycles and planting; Vegetables

Skill Builders:

Grammar and syntax	Language literacy	Articulation, *K*
Tenses, present and past	Relating personal experiences	
	Sequencing	

Synopsis: The classic story of a boy tending his seed illustrates the process of growing a carrot—in this case, an extraordinary carrot! This is an ideal book for modeling and eliciting sentences.

Method: Before the read-aloud, talk about where vegetables and other foods come from and the children's experiences with planting, caring for, and watching something grow.

Use the text directly to elicit past tense, for example,
    "A little boy planted a carrot seed."
    "Every day the little boy pulled up the weeds . . .
    . . . and sprinkled the ground with water."

Or structure your own "is-verbing" sentences, such as
    The boy is planting
    The boy is watering
    The boy is pulling the weeds

For articulation of *K,* read each page, stressing the target sound. At the end of each page, ask a question to elicit a short response using the word *carrot*. Also, have children repeat the predictable words of the text.

Extended Activities: Assign four children to play the parts of the characters, then reread the story. Have children pantomime the actions while you prompt them to repeat the text (e.g., "I'm afraid it won't come up."). Interact with the audience as well (e.g., ask, "What did the boy's father say?") so that all the children can repeat the words.

Play a sequencing game. Designate four children to be actors. As the audience tells each part in the sequence of planting and caring for the carrot, the actors perform the described action (planting the seed, waiting, pulling weeds, etc.).

Chicka Chicka Boom Boom

by Bill Martin Jr. and John Archambault
New York: Simon & Schuster Books for Young Readers, 1989

Suggested Grade and Interest Level:	Pre-K
Topic Exploration:	Alphabet

Skill Builders:

Phonological awareness	**Articulation, *K***

Synopsis: This is a clever alphabet rhyme about all of the alphabet letters trying to climb up a coconut tree. As they come down, they become personified as children, with names such as "skinned-knee D and stubbed-toe E."

Method: Read and reread this clever rhyme. For phonological awareness training, use the book to play sound games with the words.

PLAY > **Which-Word-Is-Missing?**

Children identify the word omitted from a previously given word string. For example, say

> tree, top, room, more
> top, room, more
> Which word is missing? (tree)

If necessary, begin with two-word strings. When the children are successful, increase to three-word strings, then four. Additional word strings include

chicka, chicka, boom, boom	skit, skat, skoodle, doot	flip, flop, flee, tree
uncles, aunts, dears, pants	help, pile, knee, toe	breath, tangle, cry, knot
loop, stoop, twist, knee	tooth, eye, knee, look	sun, tree, moon, bed
dare, tree, catch, moon	coconut, boom, tree, double	

PLAY > **Rearrange-It.**

Children rearrange, in correct word order, a scrambled phrase or sentence from a portion of the text. For example, say

> Chicka boom boom chicka
> Can you help me say the words of the title in the right order?
> That's right. *Chicka boom boom chicka* should really be *Chicka chicka boom boom.*

More words to rearrange include

I'll you meet	Who's coming look	Sun the down goes
He here comes	Breath out of all	The alphabet whole
Tree the up	I'll you beat	Full moon a there's
Way on their		

PLAY The Same-Sound game.

Children identify whether two words selected from the text begin with the same sound. For example, say

> chicka, chicka
> Do the words begin with the same sound? (Yes)

To make an unmatched pair, exchange one of the following words with another word from the text, such as *chicka, tree*. More word sets include

pants, pile	boom, bed	flip, flop
top, tooth	dear, dust	flop, flee
tip, top		skit, sat

PLAY Odd-One-Out.

Children select from a string of alliterative words the one word that has a different beginning sound. For example, using a line of text, say

> skit, skat, skoodle, doot
> Which word has a different beginning sound? (doot)
> That's right. *Doot* is the odd one out.

Using another line of text, say

> flip, flop, flee, tree
> Which is the odd one out?

Use the words listed in the Same-Sound game. Add a word from the story that does not belong to the list, such as

> loop, look, boom

so that the odd one can come out. Then add another same-initial sound word to vary the length of the word string.

PLAY Finish-the-Rhyme.

Children supply the rhyming word left out at the end of a verse. Teach children to use the meaningful clues in the pictures as well as the meter of the verse to rhyme the word. If necessary, prompt with picture cues and with the initial phoneme, then gradually remove the scaffolding. For example, say

> "A told B
> and B told C
> 'I'll meet you at the top
> of the coconut (tr) _____.'" (tree)

> "Chicka chicka boom boom!
> Will there be enough (r) _____?" (room)

(continues on next page)

PLAY **Finish-the-Rhyme.** *Continued*

"Look who's coming!
It's black-eyed P,
Q R S,
And loose-toothed _____." (T, as in the word *tee*.)

PLAY **Rhyme-It-Again.**

Children identify the rhyming word after you read each set. Provide initial phoneme cues as needed. For example, say

"P rhymes with _____." (T, as in the word *tee*)

PLAY **Do-They-Rhyme?**

Children identify whether word pairs rhyme. For example, say

boom, room
Do they rhyme? (Yes)

Insert nonrhyming words from the text into the following sets of rhyming words to make an unmatched set:

tree/flee	aunts/pants	cry/tie
looped/stooped	free/tree	me/tree
C/D	whee/tree	

PLAY **Make-a-Rhyme.**

Children supply another rhyming word after a set of words is presented. Give initial phoneme cues if needed. Accept any rhyming nonsense verse. For example, ask

What word rhymes with *tree*? *Tree, flee, (m)* _____. (me)

Practice with the following words, giving initial phoneme cues: *see, bee, C, D, G, P, T, V, Z, fee, flee, free, knee,* and *wee.*

Then continue with the rhyming sets provided in Do-They-Rhyme?

PLAY **Clap-and-Count.**

Children clap to, then count, the syllables heard in selected words from the illustrations and text. Demonstrate by clapping to a word and then asking children how many parts they heard. For example, clap and say

pile
How many parts are in the word? Clap it out. (one)

(continues on next page)

PLAY Clap-and-Count. *Continued*

Clap and say

> pileup
> How many parts are in that word? Clap it out. (two)
> Pile–up. One, two.

A puppet can also demonstrate by opening and closing its mouth to indicate syllables, stressing and elongating them when presenting words, such as

chi-cka	ru-nning	a-lley-oop
co-ming	ji-ggle	co-co-nut
wi-ggle	kno-tted	al-pha-bet

PLAY Find-the-Little-Words.

Children listen for the "little" words within the two-syllable words of the text. For example, say

> wiggle (changing the stress to wigg-le and drawing out the word)
> Can you hear any little words in *wiggle*? (wig)
> That's right. *Wig* is a little word in *wiggle*.

Present the list of two- and three-syllable words provided in Clap-and-Count, and find the little words within the larger words, changing the stress pattern as necessary so children can hear all the "little" words.

PLAY Leave-It-Out.

Children say a two-syllable word, then leave out the beginning or final part to create a smaller word. For example, say

> Say *pileup* but leave out *up*.
> What little word is left? (pile)
> That's right. *Pileup. Pile.*

Continue using the two-syllable words provided in Clap-and-Count.

PLAY Add-It-On.

Children put two words together to make a compound word, or two syllables together to make a two-syllable word. For example, say

> Say *pile*.
> Now say *pile*, and add *up*.
> What larger word can you make? (pileup)
> *Pile. Up. Pileup.*

Continue with the two-syllable words provided in Clap-and-Count.

PLAY **Say-It-Until-You-Hear-It.**

Children synthesize one-syllable words divided into onset-rime. Start with words that begin with a continuous, single-consonant sound. Demonstrate by presenting each part of the word separately. Show children how to elongate the onset part and to blend the two parts together, saying them a little quicker each time until they are readily identified. For example, say

> Put these two sounds together: *m-eet*
> Say it until you hear it. *Mmmmm—eet. Mmm-eet. Meet.*

Words beginning with a single consonant and divided into onset-rime include

f-ull	r-oom	b-eat
m-ore	s-un	t-ie
m-oon	h-ug	t-op

Continue with these consonant–vowel–consonant (C–V–C) words from the text beginning with a single sound.

tr-ee (tree)	br-eath (breath)	sk-at (skat)
fl-ee (flee)	fl-op (flop)	sk-in (skin)
fl-ip (flip)	sk-it (skit)	st-ubbed (stubbed)

For *K* articulation therapy, use the recurring words *chicka chicka* and *coconut* to practice the target sound, first with auditory bombardment, then in unison, then in single production, then in cloze activities, and so on. Other *K* and *K* blend words from the text and pictures include *comes, coming, cried, skinned, K* (the letter), *look*, and *catch.*

Chicken Soup with Rice

by Maurice Sendak
New York: Harper & Row, 1962; Scholastic, 1986, 1991

Suggested Grade and Interest Level: Pre-K

Topic Explorations: Months of the year; Seasons

Skill Builders:

Grammar and syntax	**Phonological awareness**
Present tense	**Fluency**

Synopsis: The repetition and rhyming in this whimsical collection of verses lend themselves nicely to speaking in unison. Each picture depicts a different action, scene, and verse about a month of the year. Ideal for modeling sentence structures or sound production, this book will become a favorite that you'll use again and again.

Method: Before the read-aloud, talk about different kinds of soups the children like to eat and ask children to tell about when they like to eat soup.

During the read-aloud, pause to model or structure present tense, such as

> He is riding an elephant (and dreaming about soup)
> He is pouring soup (on the roses)
> He is sprinkling the roses (with the soup)
> He is pepping up the roses (with the soup)
> The whale is spouting (hot soup)

> The wind is blowing (down the door)
> He is paddling ("down the chicken soupy Nile")

After the read-aloud, children can practice sequencing the months of the year and the seasons as you show the illustrations.

For phonological awareness training, use the book to play sound games with the words.

PLAY **Word-Count.**

Children count the number of words in a short line from the text. Demonstrate by assigning one word to one finger as you say the words. For example, say

> chicken

as you hold up one finger. Ask,

> How many words did I say?

Then progress until you have added all the words of the title

> Chicken soup with rice

for a four-finger count. Gradually allow the children to do the counting by themselves.

If children don't have one-to-one correspondence, give each child a collection of manipulables (i.e., blocks, felt squares, buttons, etc.) to use for representing each of the stated words. Demonstrate by saying (or use a puppet to say) the words from a page of text that you want the children to count. Repeat them again as you (or a puppet) move out one item at a time to correspond to your stated word. Then you (or a puppet) count out loud the number of blocks moved to get the word count. Gradually allow the children to do the counting by themselves. Use words directly from a page of text in hierarchical order to the desired word length. Also use the refrain in each verse, as in

> Sipping once
> Sipping soup
> Sipping chicken soup
> Sipping chicken soup with rice

PLAY **Which-Word-Is-Missing?**

Children identify the word in a word string that has been omitted from a previously given string. Choose two to four words from the illustration and text to make up a string. Repeat the words, leaving one out for the children to identify, as in

> sip, soup, peep, whale
> sip, soup, peep
> Which word is missing? (whale)
> That's right. *Whale* is the word that is missing.

(continues on next page)

PLAY **Which-Word-Is-Missing?** *Continued*

Words from the text include

> pep, soup, rice, pot
> ice, soup, once, cake
> hot, Nile, witches, toast
> nest, once, think, robin
> happy, March, floor, spill
> cheap, chicken, soup, November
> dream, twice, April, soup
> once, twice, sliding, chicken
> roses, pepped, droop, group

PLAY **Rearrange-It.**

Children rearrange, in correct word order, a scrambled phrase or sentence from a portion of the text. For example, say

> soup chicken
> Can you help me say the words in the right order?
> That's right. *Soup chicken* should be *chicken soup.*

More words to rearrange include

> Soup chicken rice with
> Once sipping
> Once sipping, twice sipping
> Soup chicken sprinkle
> I them up pepped
> I will crocodile a ride
> I will tail my flop
> Once told you I
> Told you I twice

PLAY **The Same-Sound game.**

Children identify whether word pairs begin with the same sound. For example, say

> sip, soup
> Do they start with the same sound? (Yes)

Intersperse words ending in a different sound from the story into the following sets to make odd pairs. To make an unmatched pair, exchange one of the following words with another word from the text, such as *soup, rice.* Present one-syllable words first.

sip, soup	pot, peep	cheap, chicken
door, down	ride, rice	gusty, gale
rose, rice	robin, rice	skate, scarf
pep, peep		baubled, bangled

PLAY **Finish-the-Rhyme.**

Children supply the rhyming word left out at the end of a familiar verse. Provide the initial phoneme cue and prompt by pointing to the illustration, if needed. For example, read

> "In January/ it's so nice
> while slipping/ on the sliding _____ (ice)
> to sip hot chicken soup/ with _____ . (rice)"

PLAY **Rhyme-It-Again.**

Children identify the rhyming word after each set is given. For example, say

> *Ice* rhymes with (r) _____ . (rice)

PLAY **Do-They-Rhyme?**

Children identify whether word pairs rhyme. For example, say

> ice, rice.
> Do they rhyme? (Yes)

Intersperse the following rhyming words from the text with nonrhyming words

ice, rice	pot, hot	nice, rice
more, floor	best, nest	nest, rest
peep, cheap	host, ghost	me, tree
away, bombay		

PLAY **Make-a-Rhyme.**

Children supply another rhyming word after a set of two is presented. Give initial phoneme cues if needed. Accept any nonsense rhyming word. For example, ask

> What word rhymes with *rice*? *Rice, nice,* (m) _____ (mice)

Continue with the rhyming sets provided in Do-They-Rhyme?

PLAY **Rhyming-Ings.**

Children rhyme root words with added *-ing* suffixes using words in the text (root + added suffix, if necessary). Give initial phoneme or cluster cues and picture prompts if needed. For example, say

> Listen to how I can rhyme a word ending in *-ing*
> rowing, sewing
> Now you do one.
> What word rhymes with *rowing*?
> *rowing, sewing* (*mowing, going,* and nonsense words that also rhyme)

(continues on next page)

PLAY Rhyming-Ings. *Continued*

Practice with the following words, giving initial phoneme cues as needed. Accept any nonsense word that rhymes.

> sipping (dipping, nipping, ripping, tipping, whipping, yipping, slipping, dripping, flipping)
> eating (meeting, seating, beating, heating, bleating)
> selling (smelling, shelling, yelling, swelling)
> cooking (booking, looking, hooking)
> blowing (rowing, sewing, towing, showing, flowing, glowing, lowing, mowing, knowing)

PLAY Clap-and-Count.

Children clap to, then count, the number of syllables heard in selected words from the illustrations and text. Demonstrate by clapping to a word and then asking children how many parts they heard. For example, clap and say

> chick
> How many parts in the word? Clap it out. (one)

Clap and say

> chicken
> How many parts in that word? Clap it out. (two)
> Chi-cken. One, two.

A puppet can also demonstrate by opening and closing its mouth to indicate each syllable, stressing and elongating them in words such as

sea-sons	con-coc-ting	croc-o-dile
snow-man	Oc-to-ber	ann-i-ver-sa-ry
spout-ing	No-vem-ber	
be-come	De-cem-ber	

PLAY What's-the-Word?

Children synthesize syllables into words using the words and pictures of the book. Present the syllables with a clear pause between them, and have the children say them quickly and repeatedly until they can identify the word. Demonstrate by saying

> chi–cken
> What word did I say?
> Say it until you hear it. *Chiii–cken. Chiiii-ken. Chicken.*
> *Chicken* is the word.

Continue using the two-syllable words. Intersperse some of the *-ing* words of the text listed above as well.

PLAY   **Find-the-Little-Words.**

Children listen for the "little" words within two-syllable words of the text. Stress and elongate syllables when presenting the word. For example, say

> chicken
> Can you hear any little words in *chicken*? (chick)
> Yes, *chick* is a little word in *chicken*.
> *Chicken. Chick.*

Continue with two-syllable words, changing the stress as necessary so children hear all the "little" words.

snowman (snow, man)	seasons (sea)	spouting (spout)
cooking (cook, king)	selling (sell)	become (be, come)
inside (in, side)	charming (charm)	paddle (pad)

PLAY   **Leave-It-Out.**

Children say a compound word or two-syllable word and then leave out the beginning or final part to create a smaller word. For example,

> Say *snowman.*
> Now say *snowman* but leave out *man.*
> What little word is left? (snow)
> Yes. *Snowman. Snow.*

Then say

> Now, say *snowman* but leave out *snow.*
> What little word is left? (man)
> Yes. *Snowman. Man.*

Continue with the two-syllable words provided in Find-the-Little-Words.

PLAY   **Add-It-On.**

Children put two syllables together to make two-syllable words. For example,

> Say *snow.*
> Now, say *snow* and add *man.*
> What bigger word can you make? (snowman)
> Yes. *Snow. Man. Snowman.*

Continue with the two-syllable words provided in Find-the-Little-Words.

☞See the catalog for Grades 1 through 5 for continuing activities in the hierarchy of phonological awareness.

For fluency, use the repetitive phrase

> ". . . going once
> going twice
> going chicken soup with rice"

to practice maintaining airflow during phonation.

Chimps Don't Wear Glasses

by Laura Numeroff
New York: Scholastic, 1995

Suggested Grade and Interest Level: Pre-K

Topic Explorations: Animals; Imagination

Skills Builders:

Grammar and syntax	**Phonological awareness**
Noun–verb agreement	**Articulation, *M* and *K***
Present tense	
Negative structures	
Question structures	

Synopsis: A series of animals are illustrated doing outrageously silly acts, while the text, in short rhyming verse, refutes their actions.

Method: Before the read-aloud, read the title, *Chimps Don't Wear Glasses,* and ask children to describe what's happening on the book's cover. (Children will describe animals—two of which are chimps wearing crazy sunglasses—driving cars on the freeway.) You might reply, "Hmmm, let's discover what this book is all about."

During the read-aloud, pause at natural intervals for interaction about the text and pictures. Rhyming verses often are completed on a two-page spread and, with the pictures depicting the text, make for a natural pause in the reading. This gives children an opportunity to observe and talk about what's going on in the illustrations.

For teaching negative structures, read and have the children repeat a line of text (e.g., "Chimps don't wear glasses."). After the line is repeated, ask, "They don't? But what's happening here?" to elicit picture descriptions of chimps performing in a rock band wearing wild and crazy glasses.

After the read-aloud, play a fun game in the spirit of the book by using the illustrations to teach question structures. Go back over the pages and demonstrate how to change the text from a statement to a question. You or the rest of the class must answer the question. For example, on a two-page spread, the text reads

> "And zebras don't cook
> And you won't see a kangaroo reading a book."

Prompt children to look at the illustration of a zebra cooking, and ask, "Do zebras cook?" to which the class responds, "Yes, zebras cook!" then ask, "Does a kangaroo read a book?" to which the class answers, "Yes, a kangaroo reads a book!" Turn the page and read, "Horses don't hang glide." Prompt a child to ask, "Do horses hang glide?" to which the class responds, "Yes, horses hang glide!" Once children get the hang of it, they can expand on their answer.

Note that the question-and-answer format also teaches noun–verb agreement, depending on the way the question is stated. Take a cue from the illustration whether the question should be stated with a singular or plural noun. For example, if a picture shows giraffes driving, ask, "Do giraffes drive?" and receive the response, "Yes, giraffes drive." Or, "Does a llama shop?" "Yes, a llama shops."

After reading the text "Reindeer don't square dance," have children respond to the contrary, as illustrated in the book (e.g., "But the reindeer are square dancing."). Other examples include

But the chimps <u>are</u> wearing glasses.
But the kangaroo <u>is</u> reading a book.
But the horses <u>are</u> hang gliding.
But the llama <u>is</u> shopping.

For phonological awareness training, use the book to play sound games with the words.

(PLAY) Word-Count.

Children count the number of words in a short line from the text. Demonstrate by assigning one word to one finger as you say the words. For example, say

>   Camels sing

as you hold up one finger for each word until two fingers are showing. Ask

>   How many words did I say?

Then say

>   Camels don't sing.

for a three-finger count. Gradually allow the children to do the counting by themselves.

If children don't have one-to-one correspondence, give each child a collection of manipulables (i.e., blocks, felt squares, buttons, etc.) to use for representing each of the stated words. Demonstrate by saying (or use a puppet to say) the words from a page of text that you want the children to count. Repeat them again as you (or a puppet) move out one item at a time to correspond to your stated word. Then you (or a puppet) count out loud the number of blocks moved to get the word count. Gradually allow the children to do the counting themselves. Use words directly from a page of text in hierarchical order to the desired word length. Shorten the text as necessary, as in the stimulus

>   Weasels don't travel.

from the longer line of verse, "Weasels don't travel to see all the sights."

(PLAY) Which-Word-Is-Missing?

Choose two to four words from the text to present in word strings. Repeat the string, leaving out one word for the children to identify. For example, say

>   chimps, glasses, play, guitar
>   chimps, play, guitar
>   Which one is missing?
>   That's right. *Glasses* is missing.

Some word lists from the text include

zebra, cook, kitchen, book	horse, hang, mountain, glide
jar, giraffe, penny, car	llama, shop, hat, ring
dance, square, barn, deer	king, chipmunk, lion, crown
tiger, ice, wolf, mug	juggle, lion, paw, egg
lizard, quilt, sew, how	

PLAY **Rearrange-It.**

Children rearrange, in correct word order, a scrambled phrase or sentence from a portion of the text. For example, say

> Cook don't zebras
> Can you help me say the words in the right order?
> That's right. *Cook don't zebras* should really be *Zebras don't cook.*

More words to rearrange include

Glasses wear	Clean hamsters don't	Quilts sew lizards
Book read	Sing don't camels	Fly kites seals don't
Shop llamas	Boats on hippos	All sights the see

PLAY **The Same-Sound game.**

Children identify whether word pairs begin with the same sound. For example, say

> horse, hang
> Do they start with the same sound? (Yes)

To make an unmatched pair, exchange one of the following words with another word from the text, such as *horse, cook.* Present one-syllable words first.

chimp, cheer	lion, lizard	piglet, penny
mice, march	tiger, tutu	turtles, taste
panda, pole	puppet, pug	kangaroo, cook

PLAY **Odd-One-Out.**

Children select the word that does not belong from a string of alliterative words. For example, say

> chimps, cheer, lion
> Which word has a different beginning sound? (lion)
> That's right. *Lion* is the odd one out.

Continue with the words provided in the Same-Sound game, introducing a word with a different sound so that the "odd one" can come out. Then add another same-initial sound to make a four-word string.

PLAY **Word-Search.**

Children search the picture for the word you are thinking of that begins with a given sound. For example, show the illustration with the text, "Giraffes don't drive cars" and say

> I see something in this picture that starts with the same sound as *piglet.*
> What other word starts with *p*? (Give phoneme/sound only.)
> That's right. *Pennies* is a word that starts with *p.*

Continue with initial *p* words (*purse, pink*). Children can search for other words with different initial sounds on each page of the story.

PLAY **Finish-the-Rhyme.**

Children supply the rhyming word left out at the end of a verse. Teach children to use the meaningful clues in the pictures as well as the meter of the verse to rhyme the word. If necessary, prompt with picture cues and with the initial phoneme, then gradually remove the scaffolding. For example, say

> "Giraffes don't drive cars
> And you won't see a piglet
> saving pennies in _____. (jars)"

PLAY **Rhyme-It-Again.**

Children identify the rhyming word you read after each set. Provide initial phoneme cues and picture prompts if needed. For example, say

> "*Cars* rhymes with (j) _____." (jars)

PLAY **Do-They-Rhyme?**

Children identify whether word pairs rhyme. For example, say

> cook, book
> Do they rhyme? (Yes)

Intersperse a word from the text that doesn't rhyme into the following word sets to make an unmatched set.

> cars, jars   sing, king   boats, floats
> shop, mop   mugs, pugs   stilts, quilts
> kites, sights

PLAY **Make-a-Rhyme.**

Children supply another rhyming word to a set of two rhyming words. Give initial phoneme and picture cues if needed. Accept any nonsense rhyming word. For example, ask

> What word rhymes with *cook*? (and starts with *b*?) (book)
> That's right. *Book* starts with *b*.

Other words to rhyme include *hook, look, nook, took, shook, crook,* and any nonsense word.

Continue using the rhyming sets in Make-a-Rhyme.

PLAY **Clap-and-Count.**

Children clap to, then count, the number of syllables heard in selected words from the story. Demonstrate by clapping to a word and then asking children how many parts they heard. For example, clap and say

> chip
> How many parts in the word? Clap it out. (one)

(continues on next page)

PLAY **Clap-and-Count.** *Continued*

Clap and say

> chipmunk
> How many parts in that word? Clap it out. (two)
> Chip–munk. One, two.

A puppet can also demonstrate by opening and closing its mouth to indicate syllables. Stress and elongate syllables when presenting words, such as

pig-let	ham-ster	pe-nnies
rein-deer	wea-sels	pu-ppet
sur-prise	hand-made	

PLAY **What's-the-Word?**

Children synthesize two syllables into a word. Use pictures in the book as cues, if needed. Present the syllables, inserting a clear pause between them, and have children say them quickly and repeatedly until they identify the word. Demonstrate first, as in

> ham–ster
> What's the word?
> Say it until you hear it. *Hammmmm–ster. Hammm-ster. Hamster.*
> *Hamster* is the word.

Continue with the two-syllable words *pennies, reindeer, weasels,* and *surprise.*

PLAY **Find-the-Little-Words.**

Children listen for "little" words within two-syllable words of the text. Stress and elongate syllables when presenting the word. For example, say

> chipmunk
> Can you hear any little words in *chipmunk*? (chip, monk)
> That's right. *Chip* is a little word in *chipmunk*.

Continue with two-syllable words, changing the stress pattern as necessary so children hear the "little" words.

> hand-made (hand, made)
> ham-ster (ham)
> pe-nnies (pen, sounds like *knees*)
> rein-deer (sounds like *rain*, deer)
> wea-sels (sounds like *we*)
> pu-ppet (pup, pet)
> sur-prise (sir, sounds like *prize*)

PLAY **Leave-It-Out.**

Children say a compound word or two-syllable word then leave out the beginning or final part to create a smaller word. For example,

> Say *chipmunk.*
> Now say *chipmunk* but leave out *munk.*
> What little word is left? (chip)
> That's right. *Chipmunk. Chip.*

Then say

> Now say *chipmunk* but leave out *chip.*
> What little word is left? (munk)
> That's right. *Chipmunk. Monk.*

Continue with the compound and two-syllable words provided in Find-the-Little-Words.

PLAY **Add-It-On.**

Children put two parts or syllables together to make compound or two-syllable words. For example, say

> Say *hand.*
> Now say *hand,* and add *made.*
> What bigger word can you make? (handmade)
> That's right. *Hand. Made. Handmade.* The quilt is *handmade.*

Continue with the two-syllable words provided in Find-the-Little-Words.

☞See the catalog for Grades 1 through 5 for continuing activities in the hierarchy of phonological awareness.

For *K* articulation therapy, use the words of the text and illustrations to elicit the target sound. Also, for the *k* sound, reread the book, changing *don't* to *can't.* For example, Chimps can't wear glasses, Zebras can't cook, and You can't see a kangaroo reading a book.

Then, do a picture walk-through and label each illustration with what the animal *can* do. For example, Chimps *can* wear glasses, Zebras *can* cook, and so on.

Phoneme *K* words from the text and pictures include *cook, book, kangaroo, kite, camel, chipmunk,* and *clean.*

Phoneme *m* words from the text and illustrations include *music, mess, mop, mice, mugs, jam, broom,* and *hamster.*

Note: Read also *Dogs Don't Wear Sneakers,* by the same author and illustrator.

Click, Clack, Moo: Cows That Type

by Doreen Cronin
New York: Simon & Schuster Books for Young Readers, 2000

Suggested Grade and Interest Level: Pre-K

Topic Explorations: Animals; Farm, Farms; Literacy; Sounds and listening

Skills to Build:

Vocabulary	**Language literacy**	**Phonological awareness**
Grammar and syntax	Relating personal experiences	**Articulation,** *K*
Two- and three-word utterances	Problem solving	
	Verbal expression	

Synopsis: Typing cows turn life on Farmer Brown's farm upside down when their demand note is tacked up in the barn. They want better working conditions in the form of electric blankets. When the farmer doesn't budge, they go on strike and refuse to give milk. Duck, the neutral party, waddles over to deliver the farmer's ultimatum to the cows. A mutually agreeable solution is achieved, but wait—all does not end here. Word spreads, and soon "click, clack, moo" turns to "click, clack, quack." Look what the cows have started! What a great way to show the rewards of literacy— and compromise! A Caldecott Medal award winner.

Method: Before the read-aloud, ask children to predict what they think the story will be about based on the title. Talk about what a typewriter is and have children share their experiences, if any.

Read and enjoy the book, pausing to let the children join in with the "click, clack, moo" refrain. Clarify meaning where necessary.

After the read-aloud, build vocabulary skills by talking more about words children may not have heard, such as *demand, ultimatum,* and *neutral.* Use the words in the context of the story and in real-life contexts. Add the word *compromise.*

Ask the children to identify the problem. Discuss whether the animals and the farmer did the right thing by compromising. Encourage verbal expression and problem-solving skills by asking children to decide whether it was a fair agreement. Do the children have other ideas about how Farmer Brown could have solved the problem? What would have happened if the farmer and the cows had not compromised?

Children can relate personal experiences of having resolved issues by compromising. When might they have had to agree on doing something differently than the way they expected? Talk about classroom events that have happened as examples.

For two- and three-word utterances, encourage children to repeat the lines of the text, such as "click, clack, moo," "no milk today," and others.

For phonological awareness training, first ask children to describe what cows typing on a typewriter might sound like. (Although typewriters may not be highly visible today, computer keyboards make a similar click-clack sound.)

PLAY **Word-Count.**

Children count the number of words in a short line from the text. Demonstrate by assigning one word to one finger as you say the words of the title. For example, say

> click, clack, moo

as you hold up one finger for each word until three fingers are showing. Ask,

> How many words did I say?

If children don't have one-to-one correspondence, give each child a collection of manipulables (i.e., blocks, felt squares, buttons, etc.) to use for representing each of the stated words. Demonstrate by saying (or use a puppet to say) the words from a page of text that you want the children to count. Repeat them again as you (or a puppet) move out one item at a time to correspond to your stated word. Then you (or a puppet) count out loud the number of blocks moved to get the word count. Gradually allow the children to do the counting by themselves. Use words directly from a page of text in hierarchical order to the desired word length. Some words from the text to count include

Dear Farmer Brown,	We would like some blankets.	We are closed.
The barn is very cold.	Sincerely, The Cows.	No milk today.
We want blankets.	Sorry.	

PLAY **Which-Word-Is-Missing?**

Choose two to four words from the text to present in word strings. Repeat the words, leaving one out for the children to identify. For example, say

> cows, moo, type, click
> cows, type, click
> Which word is missing? (moo)
> That's right. *Moo* is missing.

Additional words from the text include

moo, cow, duck, farmer	milk, blankets, barn, cold	clack, click, type, moo
farmer, cold, type, duck	milk, hens, electric, type	

PLAY **Rearrange-It.**

Children rearrange, in correct word order, a scrambled phrase or sentence from a portion of the text. For example, say

> moo, click, clack
> Can you help me say the words in the right order?
> That's right. *Moo, click, clack* should be *Click, clack, moo.*

More words to rearrange include

Farmer, dear, Brown	Sorry, closed, we're
Today milk no	The barn cold is very

PLAY **The Same-Sound game.**

Children identify whether word pairs begin with the same sound. For example, say

> cow, cold
> Do they start with the same sound? (Yes)

Intersperse nonalliterative words into sets to make odd pairs, such as *cow, type.* Some word sets include

cow, cold	duck, day
milk, moo	click, clack
closed, clack	farm, fun
type, talk	hen, house
note, night	

PLAY **Odd-One-Out.**

Children select from a string of alliterative words the one that does not belong. For example, say

> click, clack, moo
> Which word has a different beginning sound? (moo)
> That's right. *Moo* is the odd one out.

Use the words provided in the Same-Sound game. Intersperse an additional word from the story with a different initial sound for the children to identify, such as *cow, cold, type,* and so on.

PLAY **Rhyming-Ings.**

Children rhyme root words with added *-ing* suffixes using words in the text (root + added suffix, if necessary). Give initial phoneme or cluster cues and picture prompts if needed. For example, say

> Listen to how I can rhyme a word from the story ending in *-ing.*
> Typing. Wiping. Griping.
> Now you rhyme the *-ing.* Typing. Wi . . . (wiping)
> Good. Now here's another one:
> What word rhymes with *meeting*?
> Meeting. Gr . . . (eeting)

Demonstrate with *cheating, beating,* and *bleating,* and then have children supply other nonsense words that rhyme.

Other words from the text to rhyme with words or nonsense words include

> walking (talking)
> growing (blowing, towing, flowing, sewing)
> working (lurking, perking)
> diving (striving)
> waiting (baiting, dating, mating)
> boring (snoring, pouring)

PLAY **Clap-and-Count.**

Children clap to, then count, the syllables heard in selected words from the story. Demonstrate by clapping to a word and then asking children how many parts they heard. For example, clap and say

> back

Ask

> How many parts in the word? Clap it out. (one)

Clap and say

> background
> How many parts in that word? Clap it out. (two)
> Back. Ground. One, two.

A puppet can also demonstrate by opening and closing its mouth to indicate each syllable. Stress and elongate syllables when presenting the following words from the text:

out-side	neu-tral	un-der-stand
be-lieve	an-swer	fur-i-ous
ty-ping	prob-lem	im-pa-tient
de-mand	ex-change	im-po-ssi-ble
blan-ket	sin-cere-ly	ul-ti-ma-tum

PLAY **What's-the-Word?**

Children synthesize two little words into a compound word and then two syllables into a two-syllable word. Use pictures in the book as cues, if needed. First, present the little words, inserting a clear pause between them, and have children say them quickly and repeatedly until they recognize the word. Demonstrate first, such as

> be-lieve
> What's the word?
> Say it until you hear it. *Beeeeeeee–llllieeeeve. Beee-lllieve. Believe.*
> *Believe* is the word.

Continue with the compound and two-syllable words.

PLAY **Find-the-Little-Words.**

Children listen for "little" words within two-syllable words of the text. Stress and elongate syllables when presenting the word. For example, say

> background
> Can you find any little words in *background*?
> That's right. *Back* is a little word in *background*.
> *Ground* is another little word in *background*.

(continues on next page)

PLAY Find-the-Little-Words. *Continued*

Continue with these words:

out-side (out, side)
be-lieve (be, leave)
ty-ping (tie, ping [also stressed differently to hear *type*])
an-swer (an, sir)
neu-tral (new)
ex-change (change)
un-der-stand (under, stand)

PLAY Leave-It-Out.

Children say a compound word or two-syllable word, then leave out the beginning or final part to create a smaller word. For example, say

Say *background*.

Then say

Now say *background* but leave out *ground*.
What little word is left? (back)

Then say

Now say *background* but leave out *back*.
What little word is left? (ground)

Continue with the compound word *outside* and two-syllable words *believe, typing,* and *answer.*

PLAY Add-It-On.

Children put two syllables together to make two-syllable words. For example, say

Say *back*.
Then say

Now say *back* and add *ground*.
What bigger word can you make? (background)

Continue with the compound word *outside* and two-syllable words *believe, typing,* and *answer.*

☛ See the catalog for Grades 1 through 5 for continuing activities in phonological awareness training.

For *K* articulation therapy, use the words of the text that are heavily loaded with the *K* sound in various constructions. Words include

cow	cold	duck
milk	electric	blanket
click	clack	closed

Corduroy

by Don Freeman
New York: Viking Press, 1968, 1993

Suggested Grade and Interest Level: Pre-K

Topic Explorations: Bears; Careers; Family relationships; Money

Skill Builders:

Vocabulary	**Language literacy**
Categories	Relating personal experiences
Prepositions	Storytelling
Grammar and syntax	**Articulation,** *K*
Pronouns, personal and possessive	
Tenses, present and past	

Synopsis: When a girl shows interest in a teddy bear on a department store shelf, her mother points out that it is missing a button on its overalls. That night, the teddy bear goes to the furniture section to look for a button, but the night watchman finds him and returns him to the shelf. The next day the girl returns for him, and the bear finds a home with someone who loves him—with or without a button.

Method: Before the read-aloud, ask children to bring in and share their favorite stuffed animals. Compare features of the different stuffed animals and encourage children to relate their histories.

During the read-aloud, pause to clarify meaning and teach prepositions by talking about where Corduroy is (on the shelf, beside the bunny), where he goes (up and down the escalator), where the girl and mother go, where the night watchman shines his flashlight (under the beds), and so on.

After the read-aloud, do a picture walk-through so that children can tell the story. Ask questions to provide scaffolding and elicit responses containing target structures. Also, ask children to relate their personal experiences about wanting something and paying for it with their own money.

Teach categories by naming sections commonly found in a department store. Name various items for children to place in the section in which they are most likely to be found.

For articulation, pose questions so that the responses include *Corduroy* and other target words.

Extended Activities: Provide a class teddy bear, and keep it in a basket with the book and a class journal. Tell children they will each have a chance to take the bear home for a weekend stay. Prepare a short letter to parents introducing the bear and asking them to read the story to their child and record in the journal the child's dictated sentences about the bear's overnight experiences. When the child returns with the basket, read the journal entry to the class and ask the child to elaborate on his or her experiences with the bear.

Counting Crocodiles

by Judy Sierra
New York: Scholastic, 1997

Suggested Grade and Interest Level: Pre-K

Topic Explorations: Folklore, Pan Asian; Number concepts; Trickster tales

Skill Builders:

Vocabulary	**Language literacy**
Grammar and syntax	Sequencing
Tenses, present and past	Drawing inferences

Synopsis: A monkey on an island in the Sillabobble Sea spies another island close by. Seeing a sweet stack of bananas on a tree, he wants to take a trip across the sea. But how will he get there? Cleverly. The monkey tricks the crocodiles into forming a bridge across the water under the pretext of counting them. Written in rhyming verse, the whimsical illustrations show every crocodile (or group of crocodiles) engaged in an activity or sporting interesting items of clothing. There are plenty of descriptions and lots of possibilities from which to spin off language activities.

Method: Before the read-aloud, ask children to predict where the story takes place. Talk about islands and their special features.

Read the story aloud, pausing briefly to define vocabulary words, to state the monkey's goal, and to discuss the way in which he tricked the crocodiles.

After the story, review the illustrations and allow the children to describe what is happening. Slightly reshape the text to match the illustration, recasting the text to elicit target syntactic structures. For example,
> Two crocs are resting on rocks.
> Three crocs are rocking in a box.
> Four crocs are building with blocks.
> Five crocs are tickling a fox.

Use the activities taking place in the pictures to further describe the characters' actions. For example, from "nine crocks with chicken pox,"
> A nurse is looking in one croc's ear.
> Crocs are using back scratchers to itch themselves.
> The monkey is pouring calamine lotion over one croc's head.
> One croc is reading a story to another croc eating soup in bed.

There's a fox living on the island with the monkey, who assists the clever character in his attempt to get across the sea. Review the pages to describe what the fox was doing all along to help. Use past tense for these structures, such as
> He brought the monkey lemonade.
> He tossed a lemon into the air.
> He caught the crocodiles' attention.
> He dove into the water.
> He wrote on the crocodile's tummy.
> He carried the bananas back home.
> He put a stake in the ground that labeled the lemon tree a "banana" tree.

For sequencing, ask children to retell the events of how the monkey and the fox got across the sea with connector words, such as *first, and, then,* and *next.* Provide scaffolding by repeating some of the lines of text. For example,
> First, they climbed onto one croc's back.
> Then, they jumped onto the "crocs resting on rocks."
> Next, they hopped onto "three crocs rocking on a box."
> (Any variation of the text is acceptable.)

For drawing inferences, ask the students to infer what the monkey really meant when he asked aloud, "I wonder, are there more crocodiles in the sea, or monkeys on the shore?" Infer what the crocodiles really meant when they asked, "Will you count us, please?"

What does the monkey really want?
What do the crocodiles want?
After the monkey got to the island, what did it really mean when it said, "Line up now, crocodiles! I need to count you *one more time.*"

Once the text has been read several times, use the familiar words for phonological awareness training, beginning at the child's developmental skill level.

(PLAY) Word-Count.

Children count the number of words in a short line from the text. Demonstrate by assigning one word to one finger as you say the words. For example, say

> Two crocs

as you hold up one finger for each word until two fingers are showing. Ask

> How many words did I say?

Gradually allow the children to do the counting by themselves.

If children don't have one-to-one correspondence, give each child a collection of manipulables (i.e., blocks, felt squares, buttons, etc.) to use for representing each of the stated words. Demonstrate by saying (or use a puppet to say) the words from a page of text that you want the children to count. Repeat them again as you (or a puppet) move out one item at a time to correspond to your stated word. Then you (or a puppet) count out loud the number of blocks moved to get the word count. Gradually allow the children to do the counting by themselves. Use words directly from a page of text in hierarchical order to the desired word length.

> Two crocs
> Two crocs resting
> Two crocks resting on rocks

(PLAY) Rearrange-It.

Children rearrange, in correct word order, a scrambled phrase or sentence from a portion of the text. For example, say

> Crocodiles counting
> Is that right? Are the crocodiles counting? (No)
> Can you help me say the words of the title in the right order?
> That's right. *Crocodiles counting* should be *Counting crocodiles.*

More words to rearrange include

> Resting two crocs
> Building crocs four
> A fox tickling
> Five crocs a fox tickling
> Clocks juggling seven crocs
> Crocs nine with pox chicken

PLAY **The Same-Sound game.**

Children identify whether word pairs begin with the same sound. For example, say

> rest, rock
> Do the words start with the same sound? (Yes)

Intersperse words from the text with different beginning sounds into the following matched sets to make odd pairs. Present one-syllable words first.

count, cool	side, sea	socks, side
pool, pox	pan, pool	back, box
fox, fool	fox, find	

PLAY **Odd-One-Out.**

Children select a word that does not belong from a string of words containing the same beginning sounds. For example, say

> rest, fox, ride
> Which word has a different beginning sound? (fox)
> That's right. *Fox* is the odd one out.

Use the words provided in the Same-Sound game. Insert an additional word with a different initial sound from the story for the children to identify.

The words of the text are ideal to practice rhyming because the rhyming words come close together in each short couplet.

PLAY **Finish-the-Rhyme.**

Children supply the rhyming word left out at the end of a verse. Teach children to use the meaningful clues in the pictures as well as the meter of the verse to rhyme the word. If necessary, prompt with picture cues and with the initial phoneme, then gradually remove the scaffolding. For example,

> "She ate lemons boiled and fried,
> steamed, sauteed, pureed and dr _____.
> She ate lemons till she cried,
> 'I'm all puckered up ins _____.'
> Then across the sea so wide,
> A banana tree she sp _____."

PLAY **Rhyme-It-Again.**

After each rhyming set, ask students to identify the rhyming word. For example,

> *fried* rhymes with _____ (dried)
> *wide* rhymes with in _____ (side)

PLAY Do-They-Rhyme?

Children identify whether word pairs rhyme. For example, say

> cool, pool
> Do they rhyme? (Yes)

Intersperse a nonrhyming word into the following pairs of rhyming words to make an unmatched set:

more, shore	hunch, bunch	blocks, fox
rocks, box	lunch, bunch	clocks, sox
pox, locks		

PLAY Make-a-Rhyme.

Children supply another rhyming word to a two-word set. Give initial phoneme cues if needed. Accept any non-sense rhyming word. For example, ask

> What word rhymes with *cool? cool, pool (t)* _____
> (Also, *rule, school, drool, cruel,* etc.)

Continue with the provided rhyming sets.

PLAY Clap-and-Count.

Count the number of syllables in words and illustrations of the book. For example,

> How many parts in the word *island*? (as in *eye*-land) (two)
> That's right. Island. One, two.

A puppet can also demonstrate by opening and closing its mouth to indicate each syllable as you stress and elongate the parts. Other two-syllable words include

mon-key	Mo-hawk	coun-ting
sal-ty	le-mons	ga-lore
tick-ling	jugg-ling	

Three-syllable words include

cro-co-dile	de-li-cious	ba-na-na
su-spi-cious	de-li-cious	ca-vor-ting

PLAY What's-the-Word?

Children synthesize syllables into words using words from the pictures in the book. Present the syllables with a clear pause between them, and have the children say them quickly and repeatedly until they can identify the word. Demonstrate by saying

> is–land
> What word did I say?

(continues on next page)

PLAY **What's-the-Word?** *Continued*

> Say it until you hear it. *Illll(s)–land. Il(s)-land. Island.*
> *Island* is the word.

Continue with the provided list of two-syllable words.

PLAY **Leave-It-Out.**

Children say a two-syllable word, then leave out the beginning or final part to create a smaller word. Demonstrate by saying

> Say *Mohawk.*
> Now say *Mohawk* but leave out *hawk.*
> What little word is left? (mo) (as in *mow* the lawn)
> That's right. *Mohawk. Mo.*

Then say

> Now say *Mohawk* but leave out *mo.*
> What little word is left? (hawk)
> That's right. *Mohawk. Hawk.*

Continue with the list of two-syllable words presented in Clap-and-Count.

PLAY **Add-It-On.**

Children put two syllables together to make two-syllable words. Demonstrate by saying

> Say *mo.*
> Now say *mo* and add *hawk.*
> What bigger word can you make? (Mohawk)
> That's right. *Mo. Hawk. Mohawk.*

Continue with the two-syllable words provided in Clap-and-Count.

☛ See the catalog for Grades 1 through 5 for continuing activities in the hierarchy of phonological awareness.

Cucú: Un cuento folklórico mexicano/ Cuckoo: A Mexican Folktale

by Lois Ehlert
San Diego: Harcourt Brace, 1997

Suggested Grade and Interest Level: Pre-K

Topic Explorations: Birds; Folklore, Mexican

Skill Builders:

Vocabulary	Language literacy	Pragmatic language
Attributes	Sequencing	Articulation, *K*
Proverbs	Cause-and-effect relationships	Voice
	Drawing inferences	

Synopsis: An adaptation of a lovely Mayan Indian tale is presented with illustrations inspired by Mexican crafts and folk art, including cut-paper fiesta banners, a "tree of life" candelabra, and wooden toys. Spanish and English languages are printed on each page. A cuckoo bird, recognized among the other animals for her beauty and her golden voice, isn't appreciated when she doesn't do her share of work. Because of her selfishness, the others tire of her melodious voice. One night, she discovers a nearby field on fire. She undertakes a heroic deed, carrying seeds, one by one, back and forth through the smoky sky and placing them down a mole's hole. When the animals wake and see the blackened fields, they fear their food will be gone. They hear an unfamiliar, raspy voice, but they don't recognize Cuckoo at first. When they see the scorched bird above, they learn a lesson: Real beauty is within, and character cannot be judged by "looking at its feathers."

Method: Begin by introducing children to the concept of character. Talk about things that people do—such as being kind to their neighbors and showing respect to living creatures—and how their actions demonstrate their characters.

During the read-aloud, pause at natural intervals for interaction about the text and pictures. Clarify words such as *singed* and *scorched* to add meaning to the story. Shape present-progressive tense by having children occasionally repeat short portions of the text.

After the read-aloud, discuss the concept of character again. What was Cuckoo like before the fire? Generate attributes such as *lazy* and *selfish*, then ask children to generate the attributes Cuckoo displayed during and after the fire, such as *brave, courageous, helpful,* and *kind.* Did Cuckoo change, or did she possess those attributes all along? Help children gain understanding of the words in proverbs, such as, "You can't judge a bird by looking at its feathers." What did the storytellers who handed this story down for many generations mean by the words? Correlate it to the proverb "you can't tell a book by its cover."

Later, or on another day, do a picture walk-through and have children retell the story, developing sequencing skills and expressing cause-and-effect relationships. Focus on the text that relates to Cuckoo flying back and forth through the fire, then ask children to state why Cuckoo has a raspy voice and why her feathers are blackened and scorched. Prompt retelling with words such as *then, so,* and *because.*

To increase vocabulary skills, have children use the words of the story, such as *singed, scorched,* and *raspy,* in their own sentences. Relate the words to their own experiences.

For pragmatic language, talk about the rules of relationships and working together. Discuss ways the other animals in the story could have used words in an acceptable way to ask Cuckoo to do her fair share of work. Begin with "I" messages and polite requests. Talk about the importance of taking turns in conversation rather than having one person do all the talking or "singing."

For articulation of *K,* initiate auditory bombardment of the sound before the read-aloud. Stress the target sound when reading and talking about the bird. Pause throughout the story to have children imitate words and repeat phrases. After the reading, use the bird's name, Cuckoo (Cucú), to practice *K* in short phrases and in carrier phrases to increase production of the phoneme at the sentence level.

For voice, use the words of the text that describe Cuckoo's voice after the fire. Bring awareness of the different sounds of voices (*golden* and *raspy*) by imitating their sounds. Use other words to describe the sounds of a voice. Talk about what can happen to a person's (or an animal's "voice") if the individual is not careful.

Note: You may want to alter the story and make predictions that Cuckoo will get her beautiful voice back after some "voice rest" and carefully learning how to reuse it.

Daddy Makes the Best Spaghetti

by Anna Grossnickle Hines
New York: Clarion Books, 1986, 1988

Suggested Grade and Interest Level: Pre-K

Topic Explorations: Daily activities; Family relationships

Skill Builders:
   Language literacy
   Relating personal experiences
   Sequencing

Synopsis: A book of everyday routines made into joyful, loving games. Follow Corey's day from the time Daddy picks him up from day-care to Mom and Dad's goodnight kiss.

Method: Before the read-aloud, ask children to talk about the things they like to do with different family members. For example, What do you like to do with your dad? With your mom? Who brings you to school? To day-care? Who makes breakfast? Lead into the book by reading the title, showing the cover, and then having children make predictions about the story based on this information.

During the read-aloud, briefly pause and allow children to interject descriptions of their own daily routines. How are Corey's daily routines like theirs?

After the read-aloud, review the events and sequence the story using the pictures. Use the book to help children sequence their own daily routines.

A Dark, Dark Tale

by Ruth Brown
New York: Dial Books for Young Readers, 1981, 1984

Suggested Grade and Interest Level: Pre-K

Topic Exploration: Holidays, Halloween

Skill Builders:

Vocabulary	**Language literacy**	**Articulation, *K***
Adjectives	Sequencing	**Fluency**
Prepositions		

Synopsis: This spooky tale leads the reader to a house, through the door, up the stairs, down the passage, and on and on until the surprise ending. The repetition in this "dark tale" adds to the suspense and models how to add adjectives to simple sentences. The sequence of events is ideal for retelling.

Method: Before the read-aloud, show the cover and share predictions about where the story will take place and what the story will be about.

During the read-aloud, shape or model appropriate structures from the text and illustrations. Capitalize on the numerous opportunities to describe locations, such as "around the corner," "up the stairs," and "through the hall."

After the read-aloud, help children sequence the events of the story by retracing the steps taken in the spooky tale. Have children think of other adjectives to describe the house, the stairs, the passage, and the cat.

For articulation of *K*, pause to ask questions that elicit words containing the target sound or to allow children to echo the text, including *dark, spooky,* and *black cat.*

For fluency, use the short words and phrases of the text to practice maintaining airflow during phonation.

Extended Activity: Mark a path around the room with tape leading to a cupboard or other location where you have hidden a Halloween treat. Mark stopping places on the tape in red. Have children take turns acting out the part of the cat as they follow the path around the room. As the child stops at each red mark, other children can describe the child's journey (e.g., going under the table, beside the chairs, along the bulletin boards, etc.) until the child reaches the cupboard and finds the reward.

Dinosaurs, Dinosaurs

by Byron Barton
New York: Thomas Y. Crowell, 1989

Suggested Grade and Interest Level: Pre-K

Topic Exploration: Dinosaurs

Skill Builders:

Vocabulary	Grammar and syntax
Adjectives	Two- and three-word utterances
Attributes	

Synopsis: This award winner is a favorite among young children. Lots of adjectives in simple sentences describe dinosaurs. The pages are illustrated in nonthreatening, colorful images—similar to a child's artwork. The inside cover labels many kinds of dinosaurs with an easy pronunciation guide.

Method: Before the read-aloud, elicit children's background knowledge of dinosaurs. What names of dinosaurs can the children recall? Talk about the word *extinct* and how dinosaurs lived so long ago that all that is left of them today are their bones that have been buried for millions of years. Ask children if they have seen skeletons of dinosaurs in museums.

During the read-aloud, talk about the different characteristics that dinosaurs depicted in the text and illustrations have, such as horns, spikes, clubs, and armored plates. Model and structure two- and three-word utterances from the text using adjectives, such as *sharp claws, long sharp claws,* and *long tails.*

Extended Activity: Follow up by having each child draw a picture of a dinosaur that has one of the special features mentioned in the book. Have children dictate labels for their drawings that name the special features (e.g., "spikes," "sharp claws," or "a club on its tail").

Don't Fidget a Feather!

by Erica Silverman
New York: Simon & Schuster Books for Young Readers, 1994

Suggested Grade and Interest Level: Pre-K

Skill Builders:
Language literacy   Articulation—*F, K,* and *G*
Relating personal experiences
Predicting

Synopsis: Duck and Gander learn a lesson about winning when their contest to see who won't "fidget a feather" leads them straight to the fox's hole to be his supper. The story has become a favorite among many children.

Before the read-aloud, talk about children's games, such as Tag, You're It. Introduce children to the story by showing the book's cover and making story predictions. Discuss the meaning of the word *fidget* and predict what game the Duck and Gander will play. Practice target phonemes with selected words from the title and the following text.

Throughout the read-aloud, pause to ask prediction questions, clarify meaning, and practice production of target sounds, as outlined in the following articulation paragraphs.

After the read-aloud, ask children what they think the author is saying. What is important to remember about games and winning? Ask children to relate their own experiences about contests and playing games. Scaffold with words such as *once, and then,* and *finally.*

For *F, K,* and *G* articulation therapy, use the multiple reference to the characters' names—Duck, Gander, and Fox—to practice target sounds. Use the high-frequency words, "Don't fidget a feather," to practice *F* in initial position. Practice characters' names and the "fidget" phrase in single production before the reading, then in repetition, unison, and cloze activities throughout the reading. Practice again in retelling.

Other *F* and *F* blend words from the text to practice before the reading include *fast, faster, fastened, fly, flew, freeze,* and *fluttered.* Other *K* and *K* blend words from the text to practice include *lake, caw, cawed, cluster of crows, quack, luck, corner, sack, cook, pick, knocked,* and *clouds.* Other *G* and *G* blend words include *greetings, zigzagged, leapfrogged, gusted, grove, dragged, garlic,* and *go.*

Don't Forget the Bacon

by Pat Hutchins
New York: Greenwillow Books, 1976

Suggested Grade and Interest Level: Pre-K

Topic Explorations: Humor; Memory and remembering

Skill Builders:
Vocabulary   **Language literacy**   **Articulation,** *F*
                             Relating personal experiences
                             Sequencing

Synopsis: A little boy leaves for the store after his mother tells him what she needs (and reminds him not to forget the bacon), but as he passes various neighborhood sites, he forgets the items. As he tries to remember, the sites around him help him to recall the items. Oops! Everything but the bacon.

Method: Present the book by talking about what it is like to be forgetful and how sometimes it's hard to remember things. Relate one of your own experiences of forgetting something.

During the read-aloud, pause occasionally throughout the story to ask the children whether they can recall what the boy in the story is forgetting.

After the read-aloud, discuss what the word *memory* means, and talk about remembering and forgetting to do things. For relating personal experiences, ask children to share times when they forgot to do something. To start, you might ask, Has your mother ever told you to do something, and then you forgot? Talk about strategies for remembering things. What helped the boy in the story to remember what he needed to buy?

For sequencing, do a picture walk-through of the pages of the story, and then assist children in telling the events of the boy's trip to the store and back in temporal order. Help them add details about his forgetfulness along the way.

For articulation, read and pause to allow the children to echo the last phrase on every page, "And don't forget the bacon." Do the same with other phrases in the text that contain the *F* sound, including "six farm eggs," "six fat legs," and "a flight of stairs."

Each Peach Pear Plum

by Janet Ahlberg and Allan Ahlberg
New York: Viking Kestrel, 1978, 1992

Suggested Grade and Interest Level: Pre-K

Topic Explorations: Fairy tales and nursery rhymes

Skill Builders:

Vocabulary	**Grammar and syntax**
Prepositions	Personal pronouns
	Present tense

Synopsis: This book contains a sequence of wonderfully illustrated scenes, each containing a hidden nursery-rhyme character. It's filled with other subjects and activities for continued language expansion. Children can actively partic-ipate by playing the game I Spy.

Method: Before the read-aloud, introduce the children to the game I Spy and the meaning of the word *spy*.

During the read-aloud, have the children point to ("spy") the referent of each verse, then model a sentence con-taining the target structure. For example, you might read aloud

> "Tom Thumb in the cupboard
> I spy Mother Hubbard.
> Mother Hubbard down the cellar
> I spy Cinderella."

When the children find Cinderella hidden in the picture, model or elicit, "She is dusting the shelf."

Note: You may wish to modify the text to include the copula in order to syntactically model sentences (e.g., Tom Thumb *is* in the cupboard. Mother Hubbard *is* down in the cellar.).

Emma's Pet

by David McPhail
New York: E. P. Dutton, 1985, 1988

Suggested Grade and Interest Level: Pre-K

Topic Explorations: Bears; Pets

Skill Builders:
  Vocabulary
  Categories
  Adjectives
  Grammar and syntax
  Pronouns, personal and possessive
  Present tense
  Language literacy
  Relating personal experiences

Synopsis: An affectionate story nicely illustrated for language stimulation. A little teddy bear wants a soft, cuddly pet, and nothing seems to satisfy her. However, her search ends in the arms of her loving father, the cuddliest thing of all.

Method: Sentences for modeling or shaping present tense include

She is watching a bug.	The snake is licking her face.
She is holding a mouse.	Emma is crying.
She is fishing.	He is hugging.
A bird is flying.	She is hugging.
A frog is jumping.	

For teaching adjectives, talk about how different things must feel to Emma, such as a wet, slippery fish and a soft, cuddly bear.

Categorize the pets in the book into types of animals, and have the children add more animals to the groups.

For relating personal experiences, ask children to describe how they acquired their family pet. Did they find it in a pet store? At the pound? How did they decide which one to take home? Many families have interesting stories about how they came to adopt their pets. If possible, relate one of your own experiences.

The Empty Pot

by Demi
New York: Henry Holt & Company, 1990; Owlet, 1996

Suggested Grade and Interest Level: Pre-K

Topic Explorations: Feelings; Folklore, Chinese; Growing cycles and planting; Honesty; Self-esteem

Skill Builders:

Vocabulary	**Language literacy**
Morphological units	Relating personal experiences
	Sequencing

Synopsis: In a far-away land, a boy named Ping grows beautiful flowers. When the emperor wants to name a successor, he invites all the children of the kingdom to grow a flower from one of his seeds. Whoever grows the best flower will then succeed him to the throne. To Ping's disappointment, however, his seed does not sprout. His decision to face the emperor with his empty pot (his best effort) is rewarded for its honesty, and he is named as the successor. Children relate to this simple story of excitement, disappointment, honesty, and doing one's best. An American Bookseller "Pick of the Lists" and an International Reading Association's Children's Choice book.

Method: Before the read-aloud, show the book and make predictions based on its title and cover. Elicit background knowledge about the setting and culture. To increase vocabulary and story comprehension, discuss such words as *emperor* and *successor.* Explain that in some countries, kings are leaders, and in other countries, emperors or presidents lead. Discuss what it means to be the next in line to hold a job or a title. Who might be the next to hold a job in the classroom? Who might be the next president? The person who comes next in line, or *succeeds* the person before him (or her), is called a *successor.*

During the read-aloud, pause to discuss other vocabulary, such as *honesty, courage, empty, sprout,* and *seed.*

After the read-aloud, discuss the feelings of the characters. How do you think the boy feels when he

> hears about the emperor's news?
> can't grow his seed?
> faces the emperor in front of the other children?
> sees the other children's flowers?
> hears the emperor declare him the successor?

For relating personal experiences, cite examples of honesty and courage that the children have shown. Have the children tell stories about when they, like the boy in the story, showed courage and told the truth about something they didn't want to admit.

For sequencing story elements, use questions as scaffolding to assist children in retelling the events. For younger children, break down parts of the story into smaller units. For example,

> Q: What happened when the boy took the seed home? First he . . .
> A: Put the seed into the pot.
> Q: Then he . . .
> A: Watered it.
> Q: And . . .
> A: It didn't come up.
> Q: Then he . . .
> A: Put the seed into a bigger pot.
> Q: And . . .
> A: He watered it, but it still didn't sprout.

Have the children generate their own sentences using the words. For example, "Honesty is when . . ." or "Courage is when. . . ."

For morphological units, capitalize on the frequency of the word *best,* as in

> "Whoever can show me their best in a year's time."
> "All the children put on their best clothes to greet the Emperor."
> "You did your best. Your best is good enough."

Put in sentence form other comparative forms, using them in sentences generated from the story, if possible. Some examples include

> good, better, best (e.g., their best clothes; the boy's best effort)
> big, bigger, biggest (e.g., the bigger pot)
> large, larger, largest
> happy, happier, happiest (e.g., the boy growing his flowers, learning of the seed, becoming the successor)
> pretty, prettier, prettiest (e.g., flowers coming into bloom)
> small, smaller, smallest (e.g., the smaller pot)

Exactly the Opposite

by Tana Hoban
New York: Greenwillow Books, 1990

Suggested Grade and Interest Level: Pre-K

Skill Builders:
   Vocabulary
   Synonyms
   Antonyms

Synopsis: Tana Hoban's photographic works have been exhibited in many museums around the world, including the Museum of Modern Art in New York. She has been the recipient of many awards for her work. Here, her exceptionally fine color photographs of natural life occurrences are arranged to illustrate opposite concepts. No text accompanies them; therefore, viewers must come up with their own words to describe the concepts.

Method: View the pages and name the opposites shown. There may be more than one opposite concept for some of the pictures. For example, a sunflower faces forward and backward, east and west, front and back. The bicyclist on the road is near and far, close and distant, here and there.

How many synonyms can the children think of for each of the opposite words? For example, the cactus is prickly, sharp, pointed, spiny, and spiked. The fire is hot, warm, flaming, burning, glowing, and fiery.

Extended Activity: The children can act out the concepts. For example, children can open and close their hands; zip and unzip a jacket; and tie and untie shoes, jacket strings, and hair ribbons. Children can face forward and backward, like a sunflower. Also, children can stand near and far from each other, the door, or other referents in the room while explaining the opposite concept.

Note: Read also *Is It Larger? Is It Smaller?* (listed in this catalog); *Is It Rough, Is It Smooth, Is It Shiny?; Over, Shapes, Shapes, Shapes; So Many Circles, So Many Squares;* and *Under, Through and Other Spatial Concepts* by Tana Hoban.

Farmer Duck

by Martin Waddell
Cambridge, MA: Candlewick Press, 1992

Suggested Grade and Interest Level: Pre-K

Topic Explorations: Animals, Farm; Feelings; Humor; Speaking and communicating

Skill Builders:

Vocabulary	**Language literacy**
Prepositions	Storytelling
Grammar and syntax	Problem solving
Two- and three-word utterances	Drawing inferences
Noun–verb agreement	**Articulation—*K*, *F*, and *H***
Tenses, present and past	**Voice**

Synopsis: A humorous tale of a lazy farmer who makes his duck do all the work so he can stay in bed. The other animals decide to take matters into their own hands and do something about the injustice. A jewel in your repertoire of read-alouds, you'll pull this one out again and again.

Method: Before the read-aloud, talk about the word *lazy* and elicit children's background knowledge by asking them to give examples of what it means to be lazy.

During the read-aloud, have children describe the duck's chores and make the quacking response. Shape responses to elicit target structures and sounds.

After the read-aloud, discuss the problem in the story. Talk about how the other characters felt about the duck having to do all the work. Discuss what the "quack" of the duck might mean and what the rest of the animals might be saying. What did they do to solve the problem? Discuss the story elements and take turns retelling the story.

Reread the book with greater class participation. Have one side of the class repeat the text and the other side repeat the duck's quack. Let the children decide what the duck might say about the work if he could speak. Use the dialog to elaborate the response (e.g., Quack. There sure is a lot of work. Quack. I'm getting awfully tired. Quack. Can't keep up with it. Quack. Can't talk now.).

For articulation, initiate auditory bombardment of speech sounds before reading aloud. Then read and pause to ask questions that elicit answers containing the target sound.

Words containing *K* include *duck, cow, candy, box, cap, cluck, quack,* and *rake.*

Words containing *F* include *farmer, farm, fat,* and *food.*

Words containing *H* include *hen, house, hard* (work), *hall, whole* (story), and *hill.*

For voice, have children initiate the repetitive sentence, "How goes the work?" with an easy onset.

The Foolish Tortoise

by Richard Buckley
Saxonville, MA: Picture Book Studio, 1985

Suggested Grade and Interest Level: Pre-K

Topic Explorations: Self-esteem

Skill Builders:
    Language literacy
    Sequencing
    Storytelling
    Discussion

Synopsis: Written in rhyme, the story tells of a tortoise who laments that things would be better if only it didn't have a shell. It takes off the shell, only to encounter a scary series of events that make it glad to be what it is—a tortoise.

Method: Allow the children to talk about what is happening in the pictures as you pause at appropriate places in the text. After the read-aloud, use questions as scaffolding to assist children in retelling the events. Ask what the tortoise wanted to do. How did it feel? What did it want to do because of this? Use connective words such as *and, then, so,* and *because* to demonstrate temporal and causal relationships.

Extended Activity: Discuss the meaning of the word *unique* and that all creatures, including boys and girls, are unique. Talk about what a tortoise has that makes it unique, and then have children think of other animals and encourage them to say what makes each of them unique. For example,

> What is unique about a giraffe? (It has a long neck.)
> What if a giraffe didn't like its long neck?
> What might happen if it didn't have its long neck anymore?

> What is unique about a dog? (It barks.)
> What if a dog didn't like its bark?
> What might happen if it didn't bark anymore?

Then ask children what is unique about each of them. Encourage children to talk about their special qualities. Offer suggestions only if necessary. Initiate a discussion about "Why I wouldn't change me." Follow up with self-portraits in which children show and tell about their unique qualities.

For Laughing Outloud: Poems To Tickle Your Funnybone

Compiled by Jack Prelutsky
New York: Knopf, 1991

Suggested Grade and Interest Level:	Pre-K
Topic Exploration:	Humor

Skill Builders:

Phonological awareness	**Articulation**—*B, P, M, N, K, G, F,* and *V*
	Fluency

Synopsis: Jack Prelutsky's selection of crazy poems—many from authors you will recognize—are sure to delight both reader and listener.

Method: Before the read-aloud, introduce the title of the book and talk about what the word *funnybone* means. Introduce the book by telling children that playing with sounds of words can be fun.

For phonological awareness training, use the many poems in the book to play the sound games.

PLAY **Rearrange-It.**

Children rearrange, in correct word order, a scrambled phrase or sentence from a portion of the text. For example, using the sentence, "Never Take a Pig to Lunch," say

> Take a never pig
> Can you help me say the words in the right order?

Continue to add more words until children can rearrange a scrambled title. For more word strings, take short phrases from various poems and rearrange the word order for the children to untangle.

PLAY **The Same-Sound game.**

Children identify whether word pairs begin with the same sound. An example from "The Pancake Collector" follows:

Reread the poem and discuss the meanings of words, if necessary. Then select words with the same initial sound and put them into pairs, such as

> bag, box
> Do they start with the same sound? (Yes)

To make an unmatched pair, exchange one of the following words with another word from the text, such as *boxes, hooks.* Some one- and two-syllable words from the example include

> hangers, hooks   coated, covered   flaky, fluffy

PLAY **Finish-the-Rhyme.**

Children supply the rhyming word left out at the end of a verse. Teach children to use the meaningful clues in the pictures as well as the meter of the verse to rhyme the word. If necessary, prompt with picture cues and initial phonemes, then gradually remove the scaffolding. An example from "Be Glad Your Nose Is On Your Face" follows:

> "Be glad your nose is on your face,
> Not pasted on some other (pl) _____, (place)
> For if it were where it is not,
> You might dislike your nose a (l) _____ (lot)."

PLAY **Rhyme-It-Again.**

Children identify the rhyming word heard after a rhyming set is given. For example,

> *Not* rhymes with (*l*) _____ (lot).

PLAY **Do-They-Rhyme?**

Children identify whether word pairs rhyme. Intersperse some unmatched sets within rhyming word pairs from the text, as in

> not, lot   not, nose

PLAY **Make-a-Rhyme.**

Children supply another rhyming word after a set of two is presented. Accept any nonsense rhyming word. For example, ask

> What rhymes with *not? Not, lot . . .*
> (cot, got, jot, shot, rot, sought, taught, fought, bought)

PLAY **Clap-and-Count.**

Children clap to, then count, the number of syllables heard in selected words from the illustrations and text. Demonstrate by clapping to a word and then asking children how many parts they heard. For example, using "The Pancake Collector," say and clap

> pan
> How many parts in the word? Clap it out. (one)

Clap and say

> pancake
> How many parts in that word? Clap it out. (two)
> Pan–cake. One, two.

Stress and elongate syllables when presenting compound and two-syllable words, such as

your-self	mi-tten	ba-tter
con-ceal	car-pet	flu-ffy

PLAY **Find-the-Little-Words.**

Children listen for "little" words within two-syllable words of the text. Stress and elongate syllables when presenting the word. For example,

> pancake
> Can you hear any little words in *pancake*? (pan, cake)
> That's right. *Pan* is a little word in *pancake*.
> *Cake* is another little word in *pancake*.

Continue with the following compound and two-syllable words, changing the stress pattern as necessary so children can find all the "little" words.

yourself (your, self)	conceal (seal)	mitten (mitt)
carpet (car, pet)	batter (bat)	fluffy (fluff, fee)

PLAY **What's-the-Word?**

Children synthesize two syllables into a word using the words and pictures in the book as cues. Present the syllables, inserting a clear pause between them, and have children say them quickly and repeatedly until they identify the word. Demonstrate first, as in

(continues on next page)

What's-the-Word? *Continued*

> flu-ffy
> What's the word?
> Say it until you hear it. *FFFluu-fffy. FFlu-ffy. Fluffy.*
> *Fluffy* is the word.

Continue with the two-syllable words provided in Clap-and-Count.

 Leave-It-Out.

Children say a compound or two-syllable word, then leave out the beginning or final part to create a smaller word. For example, say

> Say *pancake.*
> Now say *pancake,* but leave out *cake.*
> What little word is left? (pan)
> That's right. *Pancake. Pan.*

Then say

> Now say *pancake* but leave out *pan.*
> What little word is left? (cake)
> That's right. *Pancake. Cake.*

Continue with the words provided in Clap-and-Count.

 Add-It-On.

Children put two syllables together to make a two-syllable word. For example, say

> Say *pan.*
> Now say *pan,* and add *cake.*
> What bigger word can you make? (pancake)

Continue with the words provided in Clap-and-Count.

 Turn-It-Around.

Children reverse the parts of the compound words they previously analyzed and synthesized, such as

> Put the word *cake* at the beginning of *pan.*
> What word do you have? (cakepan)
> What was it before we turned it around? (pancake)

➡ See the catalog for Grades 1 through 5 for continuing activities in the hierarchy of phonological awareness.

For articulation, search the Title index of this book of poems for a list of poems heavily loaded with any sound you wish to target. A few selections include

> "A Big Bare Bear"
> "Bananananananananana"

"The Giggles"
"Friendly Fredrick Fuddlestone"

For fluency, use the target words on a page of illustrations to practice sustaining airflow during the production of words, phrases, and sentences.

Fortunately

by Remy Charlip
New York: Parents Magazine Press, 1964; Aladdin, 1993

Suggested Grade and Interest Level: K

Topic Exploration: Journeys

Skill Builders:

Vocabulary	**Language literacy**
Adverbs	Relating personal experiences
Antonyms	Predicting
Morphological units	Verbal expression
Grammar and syntax	**Phonological awareness**
Past tense	**Articulation, *F***

Synopsis: Through a series of fortunes and misfortunes, Ned arrives at a surprise party, which turns out to be for him!

> "Fortunately a friend loaned him an airplane
> Unfortunately the motor exploded
> Fortunately there was a parachute in the airplane
> Unfortunately there was a hole in the parachute . . ."

Method: Before the read-aloud, explain the meaning of the word *fortunately* and use it in a sentence. Discuss how sometimes our experiences can at first seem unfortunate but later turn out to be fortunate.

For verbal expression, ask what is good about Ned's parachute breaking (he can land on the haystack). Then ask what will be the bad thing about Ned falling into the haystack. (He will fall on the pitchfork.) Build grammar and syntax skills by modeling appropriate structures from the text.

For morphological endings, play phonological awareness games using the systematic, structured approach in a hierarchy of levels.

Note: The following activities may be enhanced by beginning with the Extended Activity, described later in this section.

First, talk about the meaning of the root word *fortune* and encourage children to generate sentences using the word. Some examples include the following:

> Did Ned have good fortune? Why do you think so?
> Did Ned have bad fortune? Why do you think so?
> What kind of fortune did Ned have at the end of the story?
> Have you ever had good fortune? What happened?

PLAY Clap-and-Count.

Children clap to, and then count, the number of syllables heard in the word. Demonstrate by clapping to a word and then asking children how many parts they heard. For example, clap and say

> for

Ask

> How many parts in the word? Clap it out. (one)

Continue building on the word, asking

> How many parts in the word *fortune*?
> How many parts in the word *fortunate*?
> How many parts in the word *fortunately*.
> How many parts in the word *unfortunately*?

PLAY Find-the-Little-Words.

Children listen for "little" words within two-syllable words of the text. Stress and elongate syllables when presenting the word. For example, say

> fortune
> Can you find any little words in *fortune*? (for)
> That's right. *For* is a little word in *fortune*.

PLAY Sentence-It.

Help children generate a sentence using the words *fortune, fortunate, fortunately,* and *unfortunately.* For example,

> Ned had good fortune. (He found his way to the party.)
> Ned was fortunate (that the party was for him).
> Fortunately, there was a party.
> Unfortunately, the party was far away.

Note: More advanced phonological awareness activities using the root word *fortunate* can be found in the catalog for Grades 1 through 5.

For articulation of *F,* ask children to make up sentences based on experiences similar to Ned's (e.g., "Unfortunately I missed the bus. Fortunately my dad could bring me to school.").

Extended Activity: Begin by discussing shared unfortunate or fortunate experiences, and help children put them into sentences. An example from one kindergarten class follows: "Unfortunately, I fell in the river. Fortunately, my mom saved me." Then demonstrate with an example of how to draw a picture of these experiences. Fold a large sheet of paper in half. Draw a picture of the unfortunate experience on one side of the paper (simple marking pen drawings turn out best). Show the experience turning out to be fortunate on the other side of the paper. Have children dictate a brief story underneath. Title the project, "My Story." Have each child present the story to the class as you provide scaffolding and elaboration as needed.

Note: The methods for teaching morphological units correspond nicely to those of *Suddenly!,* by Colin McNaughton, listed in the catalog for Grades 1 through 5.

Frederick

by Leo Lionni
New York: Knopf, 1967; Dragonfly Books, 1995

Suggested Grade and Interest Level: Pre-K

Topic Explorations: Creativity; Seasons; Self-esteem

Skill Builders:

Vocabulary	Language literacy	Phonological awareness
	Cause-and-effect relationships	
	Discussion	

Synopsis: Just because Frederick sits quietly collecting words and colors in his thoughts while his family works hard gathering food doesn't mean Frederick is lazy. He is simply artistic and imaginative, qualities that also are important in life. When winter comes, the food the family has gathered sustains them at first but eventually runs out. Frederick's memories of the colors and sights of spring, shaped into poems and stories, take the others' minds off their troubles and get them through winter. The story of Frederick reminds us of the importance of nurturing the creative spirit. It is just as powerful—and popular—today as it was in 1967, when this classic was first published.

Method: Before the read-aloud, play the Imagine game. Talk about what happens when you imagine. Have children close their eyes and imagine *warm*. What pictures do they see in their minds? What are some words to describe the pictures? (A toasty fire? A cat in your lap?) Now imagine *cold*. What do they see in their minds? What words can they use to describe *cold*? (Snow? Running water from a hose?)

Then show the book's cover and tell children they will hear a story about a family gathering supplies for the winter. Talk about the meaning of the word *supplies*. Give examples, such as paints, paintbrushes, and paper for a making a picture or bread, tuna, potato chips, plastic wrap, and paper sacks for packing a lunch. Make predictions about what supplies a family of mice might need during the winter.

During the read-aloud, increase vocabulary and story comprehension by briefly pausing to talk about the words of the text. In addition to words already noted, discuss the meanings of the following in context:

stones (stone wall)	graze (cows grazed)	chatty (a chatty family)
abandoned (an abandoned barn)	granary	hideout
except	reproachfully	memory

After the read-aloud, reinforce the learning of new vocabulary. Explain expressions of speech and the meaning of the words *stood empty, take their hideout in the stones,* and *the corn was only a memory.*

For cause-and-effect relationships, and to promote discussion, ask the students questions such as

> What happened when winter came?
> What caused the family not to chatter?
> How did Frederick's family feel when he entertained them with his poem?
> What effect did gathering words and colors of spring have on the family?
> How does one "gather" words?
> How does one "gather" colors?
> Where did Frederick put the words and colors he gathered?

Recall your earlier discussion about supplies. If you were Frederick, what would you say if your family asked you, "What about your supplies, Frederick?"

What words would you gather about spring or summer?

For phonological awareness training, use the familiar words of the text to play phonological games, beginning at the child's development skill level.

PLAY **Word-Count.**

Children can count the number of words in a short line from Frederick's poem. Demonstrate by assigning one word to one finger as you say the words. For example, say

> Who lights?

as you hold up one finger for each word until two fingers are showing. Ask

> How many words did I say?

Then progress until you have

> Who lights the moon?

for a four-finger count. Gradually allow the children to do the counting by themselves.

If children don't have one-to-one correspondence, give each child a collection of manipulables (i.e., blocks, felt squares, buttons, etc.) to use for representing each of the stated words. Demonstrate by saying (or use a puppet to say) the words from a page of text that you want the children to count. Repeat them again as you (or a puppet) move out one item at a time to correspond to your stated word. Then you (or a puppet) count out loud the number of blocks moved to get the word count. Gradually allow the children to do the counting by themselves. Use words directly from a page of text in hierarchical order to the desired word length. Words to Frederick's poem are located at the end of the book.

PLAY **The Same-Sound game.**

Children identify whether alliterative words begin with the same sound. For example, say

> dim, day
> Do they start with the same sound? (Yes)

Intersperse nonalliterative words into the following two- and three-word sets to make odd pairs, such as *dim, moon*. Present one-syllable words first.

four, field	snap, snack	cold, cough, color
wind, word	hide, hand	she, shiver, shake
mice, moon	snow, spoil	wind, winter, weather

PLAY **Finish-the-Rhyme** (with the words of Frederick's poem).

Children supply the rhyming left out at the end of a verse. Provide the initial phoneme cue and picture prompts if needed. For example, say

> Who scatters snowflakes?   Who spoils the weather?
> Who melts the ice?   Who makes it (n) _____? (nice)

PLAY **Rhyme-It-Again.**

Children identify whether the rhyming word heard after a rhyming set is read. For example, say

> ice, nice
> Do they rhyme?
> Yes. *Ice* and *nice* rhyme.

More words include

June, moon	shy, I	showers, flowers
wheat, feet	four, more	

PLAY **Make-a-Rhyme.**

Children supply another rhyming word after a set of two is presented. For example, say

> What other word rhymes with *ice* and *nice*?

Prompt, if necessary, with a cue, such as

> Frederick belonged to a family of _____? (mice)

PLAY **Clap-and-Count.**

Children clap to, and then count, the number of syllables heard in compound words and two- and three-syllable words from the illustrations and text. For example, clap and say

> snow
> How many parts in the word? Clap it out. (one)

Clap and say

> snowflake
> How many parts in that word? Clap it out. (two)
> Snowflake. One, two.

Stress and elongate syllables when presenting compound words, such as

hide-out	day-dream	snow-drift
snow-ball	snow-fall	day-time
sun-shine	af-ter-noon	frost-bite

And one- and two-syllable words, such as *win-ter*, *cha-tty*, and *ga-ther-ing*.

PLAY **What's-the-Word?**

Children synthesize syllables into words using words from the pictures in the book. Present the syllables with a clear pause between them and have the children say them quickly and repeatedly until they identify the word. Say

(*continues on next page*)

PLAY **What's-the-Word?** *Continued*

win-ter
What word did I say?
Say it until you hear it. *Winnn-ter. Winn-ter. Winter.*
Winter is the word.

More two-syllable words from the text include

mea-dow	ga-ther	shi-ver
po-et	show-ers	sca-tter
wea-ther	flow-ers	
clo-ver	sea-son	

PLAY **Find-the-Little-Words.**

Children listen for "little" words within the compound words found in the text. Stress and elongate syllables when presenting the word. For example, say

snowflake
Can you hear the little words in *snowflake*? (snow, flake)
That's right. *Snow* is a little word in *snowflake*.
Flake is another little word in *snowflake*.

Continue with compound words presented in Clap-and-Count.

PLAY **Leave-It-Out.**

Children say a compound word, then leave out the beginning or final part to create a smaller word. For example, say

Say *snowflake.*
Now say *snowflake,* but leave out *flake.*
What little word is left? (snow)

Then say

Now say *snowflake,* but leave out *snow.*
What little word is left? (flake)

Continue with the compound words provided in Clap-and-Count.

PLAY **Add-It-On.**

Children put two little words together to make a compound word. For example, say

Say *hide.*
Now say *hide,* and add *out.*
What bigger word can you make? (hideout)
Hide. Out. Hideout (where Frederick and his family lived in the winter).

Continue with the compound words provided in Clap-and-Count.

➤ See the catalog for Grades 1 through 5 for continuing activities in phonological awareness.

Extended Activities: For further generalization and understanding of the concepts of the story, have children act out the role of Frederick (or Frederika) by sitting very still, daydreaming, and gathering thoughts in his or her mind. Give each child different, vividly colored pieces of construction paper. Have the children go to workstations and tear the paper into shapes of mouse body parts to make a brightly colored collage mouse. When the children are finished, have them gather around, pretending (if necessary) it is a cold, winter day. After you reread Frederick's poem, let children take turns "warming the class" with their mouse and the different words used to describe it and its colors. Remember to have the rest of the children give positive feedback after they have been warmed.

Note: Be sure to check the inside of the cover of the paperback edition by Dragonfly Books for more activities and interesting facts. Here's one: Do you know where the word *mouse* came from? A Sanskrit word meaning *thief*.

Also Note: This book is available in a Spanish version under the same title.

Freight Train

by Donald Crews
New York: Greenwillow Books, 1978; Morrow, 1992 (paperback)

Suggested Grade and Interest Level: Pre-K

Topic Explorations: Colors; Trains; Transportation

Skill Builders:

Vocabulary	Grammar and syntax	Language literacy
Categories	Two- and three-word utterances	Compare and contrast
Prepositions	Tenses, present and past	

Synopsis: A freight train, with cars identified from the engine to the caboose (including a hopper car, gondola car, and cattle car), races to its destination in a colorful display of motion.

Method: Before the read-aloud, ask children to tell what they know about trains. Where do trains go? What do they carry? Talk about the word *freight* and what it means, leading into the cover and title.

During the read-aloud, pause to model and shape target structures. Prepositions from the text include *through, by, across,* and *over.* You can add more, and ask children what they think each car carries. For example, ask

What goes inside a cattle car? A gondola car? (coal) A hopper car? (grain, gravel, and cement).

Who needs and uses these materials?
Where are they going?
Where did they come from?
What if you were riding in this train? Where would you like to be? Why?

For categories, ask what other transportation vehicles can be identified. What other vehicles carry a load? What are some of the materials and products that make up a load? What is a load called on board a ship? On an airplane?

Compare and contrast a train to a boat. How is a boat like an airplane? Like a truck? How it is different?

Extended Activities: Have children brainstorm ideas for their own freight train. What will it carry? Where is it going? Cut long black strips of construction paper for railroad ties and short black strips for connecting pieces between cars.

Cut brown circles for wheels and different-colored rectangles for the cars (see the book's simple illustrations for a model). Have students paste the rectangles in sequence to create the train, then connect the cars and finish with other pieces. Have them dictate one or two names of the freight cars, which you can write on the cars.

Make a class freight train named Room _____'s Freight Train. Have the children decide what they would like it to carry to other students in the school. Have each child make one of the cars and sign his or her name on it. Connect all the cars on the bulletin board. Cut pictures of products out of magazines to serve as the train's freight. Tuck the products partially inside the rectangles so that the cars appear to be carrying them. Label the contents and have each child sign his or her name on the appropriate car.

Gabriella's Song

by Candace Fleming
New York: Simon & Schuster, 1997; Aladdin Paperbacks, 2001

Suggested Grade and Interest Level: Pre-K

Topic Explorations: Boats; Careers; Community; Music, musicians, and musical instruments; Sounds and listening

Skill Builders:

Vocabulary	Grammar and syntax
Categories	Two- and three-word utterances
Idioms	Tenses, present and past
Homonyms	**Phonological awareness**

Synopsis: A young girl finds delight in all the sounds around her as she walks around her hometown of Venice, Italy. With sounds in her head and joy in her heart, she mingles them together and turns them into a song. Singing her song as she walks through the city, she delights her neighbors, one of whom is a composer who is so inspired that he writes a symphony. A heartwarming story that teaches children not only to listen to the beauty of sounds around them, but also how songs are born.

Method: Before the read-aloud, introduce the book by talking about far-away places in other countries, some of which are very unique and beautiful. Introduce the city of Venice, and explain that it was once called "the city of music" because opera was first performed there. Explain how it was built on small, close-together islands and how people today use the waterways, or canals, to get from one island (part of the city) to another. Show the cover of the book and describe the boats called *gondolas* that the people travel in.

During the read-aloud, pause to briefly talk about words that give meaning of the story. The beginning page will set the stage:

"Ah, Venice. The Piazza San Marco. The Grand Canal. St. Mark's Cathedral."

Vocabulary words include

gondolas	gondoliers	composer
marketplace	tethered	
symphony	canals	

For grammar and syntax, encourage children to repeat some of the characters' words in prompting two- and three-word utterances, such as

> Hot pie
> Sweet, sweet cream
> Fresh, fresh fish

After the read-aloud, go back for a picture walk-through of the book. Describe what is happening on the pages, shaping present and past tense and other grammatical structures.

Talk about idioms, or expressions of speech, to gain greater meaning from the story. What did the baker mean when he said, "It makes my heart light and my feet feel like dancing"? Can feet really feel like dancing? Elicit children's interpretations on the meaning. Explain that it is the author's way of saying that the baker felt his troubles go away and he felt so good that he wanted to dance when he heard Gabriella's song.

For homonyms, talk about what the baker meant when he said, "It makes my heart light." Explain that the word *light* can mean cheerful, or happy, as in *lighthearted*. Talk about other homonyms that can be used with examples from the story. For example,

> **road, rowed**—A *road* is something you travel on. In our story, the roads in Venice are really water roads. *Rowed* sounds just like it and means that someone rowed a boat, much like the gondoliers did in the story when they paddled, or rowed, the gondolas.

> **flour, flower**—*Flour* is what the baker needed for bread. Another word that sounds just like it is *flower*, which is often sold at flower stands in Venice.

> **bow, bow**—A *bow* is the front part of a boat. Another word that sounds just like it is *bow*, which is what an actor, conductor, or composer—like Giuseppi in our story—does when they acknowledge applause from the audience.

> **story, story**—A *story* is what we just heard; it is told or written down, like it was in this book. A word that sounds just like it is *story*, the level or floor of the building on which Gabriella lived.

> **hear, here**—*Hear* is what you do when you listen to someone or listen to the sounds of the city, as Gabriella did. *Here* can also mean "come here" or "come home," like what Gabriella's mother wanted her to do.

For developing categories, categorize types of music—such as rock, rap, country western, and classical—like the music of the composer in the story. Categorize places to hear music (including on the car radio) and musical instruments. Use all of the people in the story to categorize jobs that people hold in their communities. Also, categorize different types of stores in a mall and compare them to a marketplace, where everything is sold in one place.

Gabriella made up her own song that touched the lives of her neighbors. To enhance phonological awareness, go back and reread some of the pages that describe the sounds that Gabriella hears. Talk about the words used to describe the sounds, such as

> "Flap, flap slap of the clothes hanging on the line
> Ting-a-ling, ling of the church bells.
> The rhythm of the tethered boats thumping against the canal walls."

Ask children to imagine such sounds. Then make songs out of the words (especially the Italian words) of the story. Play with words such as *gondola* and *gondolier*, elongating the vowels and counting the syllables. Ask how many parts, or syllables, can be heard in each one's song.

Ask the children how Gabriella's mother might have called her name down the streets of Venice, where canals of water run between the old buildings where people live. Elongate the syllables of Gabriella. *Gaaaa-breeee-elllll-aaaa*. Have children say the word as Gabriella's mother might have. Then have students call their own names, prolonging the syllables. (If students have only one-syllable names, change the pitch of your voice while saying their name to give them a sense of their name's song.)

Extended Activities: The author of *Gabriella's Song* believes that music can be heard in everyday noises. Prove this by taking a community walk. Listen to the sounds and identify them as you meander along. Upon returning, make a list of what was happening, and in another column, list the noises that can be recalled from the activities. Intersperse the words of the activity with the words (especially rhyming and alliterative words, although they don't need to be) that describe the sound, and make a poem. For example,

> Bing, zing-zing, ding,
> The cash machines sing
>
> Zoom, zum, zizz, stop
> Cars come into the parking lot
>
> Tweet, chirp, peep
> Birds greet

Each child can be a composer. Write down the children's words, have each child draw a picture of the words, and make a class book, called *Our Song*.

Play a favorite classroom song, a child's favorites CD, or one of your favorites that you want to share with the children. Ask the children how it makes them feel. Is it a happy song? Recall how Gabriella's song made the baker feel like dancing.

Geraldine's Blanket

by Holly Keller
New York: Greenwillow Books, 1984; Morrow, 1988

Suggested Grade and Interest Level: Pre-K

Topic Exploration: Growing up

Skill Builders:

Vocabulary	**Language literacy**
Prepositions	Relating personal experiences
Grammar and syntax	
Pronouns—personal, possessive,	
and reflexive	
Present tense	

Synopsis: Geraldine the pig refuses to give up her outworn and outgrown blanket until she comes up with her own solution to the problem.

Method: Before the read-aloud, discuss items that are important to people and make them feel good. Encourage children to tell about the things that are special to them.

The pictures and text lend themselves nicely to interaction. Pause to model or shape sentences, such as

She is stamping her foot.	She is loving her blanket.
She is hiding the blanket.	She is hugging her new doll.
She is cutting the blanket.	She is sewing.
She is making a dress.	

After children have mastered personal pronouns in subject position, introduce possessive pronouns in phrases or sentences, such as these:

> She is stamping *her* foot.
> She is hugging *her* new doll.
> She is cutting *her* blanket.

Then, introduce the reflexive pronoun, *herself.*

> She made the dress herself.
> She gave up the blanket by herself.

Extended Activity: Invite children to bring a possession to share with the class the following day. When they share, ask them to tell how they got their special object and what they like most about it. Reinforce possessive nouns by asking the audience to whom each object belongs.

Give each child a doll and a blanket for a hands-on experience (use small plastic dolls that come in large quantities in toy stores, and use pinking shears to precut pieces of cloth to make blankets). Have children wrap their babies in the blankets. To reinforce prepositions, have children put the blankets over the babies, under the babies, and beside the babies, just as Geraldine would have done.

Good Night, Gorilla

by Peggy Rathmann
New York: Putnam, 1994

Suggested Grade and Interest Level: Pre-K

Topic Explorations: Animals, Zoo; Gorillas; Nighttime; Zoos

Skill Builders:

Vocabulary	**Language literacy**
Morphological units	Sequencing
Grammar and syntax	**Articulation,** *G*
Two- and three-word utterances	**Fluency**
Noun–verb agreement	**Voice**
Personal pronouns	

Synopsis: "Good night, Gorilla," bids the night watchman as he prepares to leave the zoo for home. But unbeknownst to him, the impish gorilla reaches into his back pocket and removes the key to the cages. A sequence of unlocked cages leads to a parade of animals following the night watchman home, all the way into his bedroom. When he says good night to his wife, she wakes up to find a gorilla in her bed. She calmly marches them back to the zoo, climbs into bed, and says, "Good night, dear." The story is told mostly through the illustrations that even the youngest of children can relate to. As its sales record shows, this book is a hit with children.

Method: Present the book's cover—which shows the gorilla stealing the key and signaling "shhh"—and encourage children to verbalize what the story will be about.

During the read-aloud, read the sparse dialog, consisting of the good night phrases, and have the children express what is happening on each page of the story. Increase grammar and syntax skills by shaping target structures, depending on the language level of the child. Some suggestions for two- and three-word utterances include

good night
good night gorilla
steals key
good night lion
leave the zoo
go home
go to sleep
back to zoo
balloon goes up
ate banana

Some suggestions for noun-verb agreement, pronouns, and present progressive tense include

He leaves.
They leave. They are leaving the zoo.
He goes home. He is going home.
They go out the gate. They are going out the gate.
They follow. They are following him home.
He gets home. He is getting home.
He goes to bed. He is going to bed.
They go to bed. They are going to bed.
She wakes up. She is waking up.
She goes back. She is leading them back to the zoo.
They go back. They are going back to the zoo.
She comes home. She is getting home.
She says good night. She is saying good night.

For sequencing events, go back through the pages and talk about the series of events illustrated on each page. The children can take turns telling the story, or one child can sequence the actions at the zoo, another child can sequence what happened at home, and another child can sequence the trip back to the zoo. Look for details to point out, like the mouse carrying a banana on a string on every page.

For increasing understanding and usage of the morphological ending -er, have children keep track of the progress of the balloon released from the gorilla's cage throughout the story, using words such as *higher and higher, smaller and smaller,* and *farther and farther.*

For articulation, pause to have the child repeat the phrase, "Good night, gorilla" (and the other animal names). After the reading, shape progressively longer phrases and sentences using the *good night* and *gorilla* theme.

Goodnight Moon

by Margaret Wise Brown
New York: Harper & Row, 1947; HarperCollins, 1977; Scholastic, 1993

Suggested Grade and Interest Level: Pre-K

Topic Exploration: Nighttime

Skill Builders:

Vocabulary	Grammar and syntax	Articulation, *G*
	Two- and three-word utterances	
	Noun-verb agreement	
	Present tense	

Synopsis: Here's a classic that remains one of the best books to stimulate language in young children. Because so much is left unsaid in the text, children can supply their own words for what they see in the illustrations. The same nursery-room scene appears on every other page. The author skillfully weaves a story in rhyming verse around a little bunny going to bed and saying goodnight to all the things in his room—incongruous things, such as a telephone, a red balloon, and a mouse going unnoticed by cats.

Method: Look for all the subtle changes in the illustrations and talk about them as you turn the pages. In addition, ask the children to find the mouse in each green room scene.

Use the short text to model two-word utterances. Use the illustrations to shape sentences at appropriate intervals. Some examples include

> The fire is burning.
> The moon is rising.
> The cow is jumping over the moon.
> The bunny is turning around.
> He is saying goodnight.
> He is hugging his knees
> The old lady is rocking.

For noun-verb agreement, include

The fire burns.	The moon rises.	The cats play.
The bunny turns around.	The bunny says "goodnight."	The old lady rocks.

Note: A French version of this book is available, as well as a Spanish version titled *Buenas noches, luna.*

Good-Night, Owl!

by Pat Hutchins
New York: Macmillan, 1972; Aladdin, 1990

Suggested Grade and Interest Level: Pre-K

Topic Explorations: Nighttime; Owls

Skill Builders:

Vocabulary	Grammar and syntax	Language literacy
Categories	Past tense	Storytelling
		Drawing inferences
		Discussion

Synopsis: With bees buzzing, squirrels cracking nuts, and crows croaking, how can a night owl ever get any sleep? The repetition of "Owl tried to sleep" on each page provides consistency for structuring language. After all the animals have finished with their noisemaking, the complete text—every sentence—is repeated on the last page, which is great for reinforcement. Then, when night falls and all is silent, guess what? SCREECH!

Method: The text is all you'll need to model sentences in past tense. Ask children to tell a simple story about how an owl was kept up all day by noisy animals. Be sure children can infer what kept the owl awake. Discuss owls and their sleeping habits. Brainstorm names of other animals that sleep during the day, such as bats, leopards, opossums, and raccoons.

Extended Activities: Have each child create a puppet representing one of the noisy animals that kept the owl awake. Draw the outline of each animal on a paper bag or paper plate for the children to color in. Affix a craft stick to the paper plate. Reread the story in a circle as children participate with their puppets. Each child can repeat the lines of the text that relate to his or her puppet and make the appropriate noises while holding up the puppet. For example, read, "The bees buzzed. Buzz buzz," then have the child or children with bee puppets repeat the lines and make the noises. Encourage the whole class to echo the repeated line, "And Owl tried to sleep."

This is also a good story to act out with a flannel or felt board because it encourages even the most reluctant child to participate. It is well worth the time you spend cutting out the pieces because they can be used year after year. Cut out felt or flannel pieces to represent the owl, the tree, and several animals in the tree (it's not necessary to include every one in the story). Have the children press the animal pieces one by one on a felt- or flannel-covered board as they tell what sound the animal made. And what did Owl try to do?

Grandfather Twilight

by Barbara Berger
New York: Philomel Books, 1984; Putnam, 1990

Suggested Grade and Interest Level: Pre-K

Topic Explorations: Animals, Forest; Nighttime

Skill Builders:

Vocabulary	Grammar and syntax	Language literacy
	Tenses, present and past	Sequencing
		Verbal expression
		Articulation, *G*

Synopsis: This is a magnificent book you'll want to recommend to parents for a bedtime story. An almost surreal quality to the illustrations evokes serenity and gentleness. At day's end, Grandfather Twilight puts down his reading glasses, takes a pearl from a chest, and walks through the forest. As he walks, the pearl becomes larger, and the sky becomes darker. When he reaches the ocean shore, he gently hands the shiny orb to the sky, and nighttime descends.

Method: Before reading, ask children what they know about twilight. At what time of day does it occur? Explain that the length of twilight varies, depending on where on the earth one is. In the Northwest, for example, twilight is especially long and beautiful in the summer.

During the read-aloud, model or shape target structures. The short text and many wordless pages of illustrations are ideal for encouraging verbal expression. Ask children to interpret how the animals feel toward Grandfather Twilight.

After the read-aloud, do a picture walk-through while children sequence the events that happen at twilight. Close the book and ask questions such as, What happens outside? What happens inside? How does the story say twilight happens?

For articulation, use the *goodnight* phrases for auditory bombardment and repetition.

The Grouchy Ladybug

by Eric Carle
New York: Harper & Row, 1977; HarperCollins, 1986

Suggested Grade and Interest Level: Pre-K

Topic Explorations: Insects and spiders; Sharing

Skill Builders:

Vocabulary	Language literacy	Pragmatic language
Categories	Sequencing	Articulation, *F*
Attributes	Compare and contrast	
Morphological units		

Synopsis: A grouchy ladybug encounters a sweet, friendly ladybug who doesn't want to share some tasty aphids on a leaf. When the friendly ladybug suggests that the grouch pick on someone bigger, it does just that. Look how many big creatures it finds along its way.

Method: Before the read-aloud, talk about the word *grouchy*. Be sure to read the short foreword that describes and illustrates aphids and ladybugs. Talk about what aphids are and how they are food for insects like ladybugs.

Then go through the increasingly bigger pages of increasingly bigger animals, reviewing and labeling as you go. Use the morphological ending *–er,* pausing to reflect as the bad-tempered bug becomes nicer, happier, and kinder. Point out the clock on the pages and use it to teach the concept of time, as the changing colors of the illustrations reflect the early warmth of day and the coolness of the night.

After the read-aloud, talk about the category of insects. Name other insects, such as fireflies, crickets, grasshoppers, bees, beetles, and butterflies. Describe how aphids and ladybugs are alike (e.g., both are bugs, they're small, they're found on plants, and they have six legs). Ask how they are different (e.g., color, diet, and markings).

Review the 14 other animals and their distinguishing characteristics. Give attributes for the animals.

Discuss the grouchy ladybug's way of talking to the other animals. Ask children to suggest another way that the ladybug could greet her friends. Discuss manners and social behavior—treating others with respect and using kind words instead of grouchy words.

For articulation of *F*, use words in the text for auditory bombardment before reading aloud, then pause throughout the story to have the child imitate words and repeated phrases, such as "want to fight?" "oh, you're not big enough," and "and flew off." Words in the text for stimulating *F* include

fireflies	aphids
friendly	flew
off	breakfast
flight	itself
enough	

Note: This book is also available in a Japanese translation, and in a Spanish translation titled *La mariquita malhumorada.*

Growing Vegetable Soup

by Lois Ehlert
New York: Harcourt Brace Jovanovich, 1987

Suggested Grade and Interest Level: Pre-K

Topic Explorations: Cooking; Growing cycles and planting; Vegetables

Skill Builders:
Vocabulary
Categories
Language literacy
Sequencing

Synopsis: A father and child share the joys of planting, watering, and watching seeds grow in order to grow vegetables for a delicious bowl of soup.

Method: Before the read-aloud, discuss how comforting it is to sip hot soup on a chilly day. Brainstorm different kinds of soups. What ingredients do many soups share? Discuss the importance of vegetables. Tap any prior knowledge students may have about growing vegetables.

During the read-aloud, encourage children to recall the names of seeds and sprouts. Have them think of other vegetables besides the ones planted. Talk about how each step in the growing process is important to the plant's life cycle.

After reading, recall the different tools and gardening equipment needed to grow the plants. Then recall the different seeds and sprouts shown to classify vegetables. For sequencing, ask what's necessary for the seeds to grow. Recall the steps for growing vegetables.

Extended Activity: Make a vegetable soup collage. Cut triangles of orange construction paper for carrots and red triangles for tomato wedges. Cut green rectangles for beans, green circles for peas, and yellow half circles for corn. Use the illustration on the last page of the book as a guide. On a large piece of construction paper, place a large circle for the bowl and paste the vegetable pieces into the center for the soup. Ask the children to decide which vegetable the shape represents, then label the pieces for the children just as they are labeled in the book.

Also, make vegetable soup as a class project. Bring in vegetables, pretending that they have just been picked from your garden. Now it is time to wash them, cut them, and put them in a pot. Share the soup with the whole class.

Also, grow seeds as a class project. All you need is a sunny window, containers, dirt, and seeds. Assign one or two students to tend to the seeds each day. When they start to sprout, reread the story and relate it to the classroom experience.

Note: This book is also available in a Spanish language translation, titled *A sembrar sopa de verduraso.*

The Hallo-wiener

by Dav Pilkey
New York: Scholastic, 1995

Suggested Grade and Interest Level: K

Topic Explorations: Animals, Dogs; Holidays, Halloween

Skill Builders:

Vocabulary	**Grammar and syntax**
Beginning concepts	Pronouns, personal and possessive
Prepositions	Tenses, present and past
Homonyms	

Synopsis: Oscar the Wiener Dog, "half-a-dog tall and one-and-a-half dogs long," didn't like it when the other dogs made fun of him. Even his mother called him her little Vienna sausage. When Halloween came, Oscar was looking forward to all the fun, especially dressing up for trick-or-treating. Excitedly he opened the box in which his mother had put his costume and discovered a giant hotdog bun with a big yellow ribbon of mustard down the center. Not wishing to hurt his mother's feelings, he wore the silly costume and was made fun of most of the night until he rescued the other dogs from some masquerading cats. That's when the other dogs changed his nickname to Hero Sandwich. This is a delightful Halloween book that children will thoroughly enjoy.

Method: Before the read-aloud, lead into the story with discussions of Halloween activities. Then present the book's cover with the illustration of the dachshund inside a giant hotdog looking glum while other dogs are laughing. Infer what the story is about.

During the read-aloud, pause briefly to point out details in the illustrations, like the trick-or-treat bag dangling from Oscar's tail when he shows up on Halloween night. Use humor to elicit and shape grammar and syntax structures from the children's responses. For example, at doggy school, one pupil writes on the board, "I will not sniff my neighbor." Ask the children to explain why he is writing on the chalkboard. (He was sniffing dogs.) Talk about the picture of Oscar on the wall at his house and ask why it was framed in three parts, with the longest part in the middle (Oscar is too long to fit into one picture). Talk about what it was about the monster that gave it away (Oscar saw the cat paws).

For prepositions, point out the locator words (such as *inside, beside, along, within, by*, etc.) in the text and illustrations, and encourage children to use them in their constructions.

After the read-aloud, revisit the pages that use the puns in the text to develop vocabulary and comprehension of homonyms. For instance, when Oscar shows up in his Halloween costume, the text reads, "Then Oscar showed up, looking quite frank." Ask children to explain why the words are funny. Discuss the meaning of the word *frankfurter.* Also, discuss why Oscar's name was changed to Hero Sandwich. What is a hero? What is a hero sandwich? Why is it funny to change his name?

For developing concepts of size and shape, continue to discuss what Oscar looked like. Talk about other things that are short and long.

Hattie and the Fox

by Mem Fox
New York: Bradbury Press, 1987, 1992

Suggested Grade and Interest Level: Pre-K

Topic Explorations: Animals, Farm

Skill Builders:

Vocabulary	**Articulation—H, K, and G**
Idioms	**Fluency**
Language literacy	**Voice**
Predicting	
Drawing inferences	

Summary: Hattie the hen discovers a fox in the bushes and runs to tell her neighbors. The nonchalant reactions from various farm animals make a repetitive, sequential text that's fun to dramatize.

Method: During the read-aloud, encourage children to predict what might happen after the cow says, "What next?" Once they can recall the order of the animal's comments, encourage them to join in as you read the repetitive text.

For teaching idiomatic language, ask the children to interpret the animal's responses. Also, ask what Hattie is trying to do by telling the animals what she sees in the bushes. Is her plan working? Why not?

At the end of the story, ask the children to infer why the animals didn't say anything. How might they have felt? Why do the children think so?

For articulation of *K* and *G*, reinforce target words during interaction, capitalizing on the many target sounds in the expressions, such as "Good gracious me," and "'Good grief,' said the goose."

For fluency, have the child say more and more of the animals' lines, maintaining uninterrupted airflow throughout the utterances.

For voice and articulation of *H*, have children practice initiating the airstream prior to phonation of the word *Hattie*, especially in response to questions such as, Who saw the fox? and Who don't the animals believe?

Hey! Get Off Our Train

by John Burningham
New York: Crown, 1989, 1990

Suggested Grade and Interest Level: Pre-K

Topic Explorations: Animals, Endangered; Conservation; Journeys; Trains; Transportation

Skill Builders:

Vocabulary	**Language literacy**
Categories	Predicting
Grammar and syntax	**Articulation, *G***
Tenses, present and future	

Synopsis: At bedtime, a young boy takes a trip on board his train and rescues many endangered animals. The repetitive pattern of animals wanting to come on board enables good use of prediction skills.

Method: Before the read-aloud, ask children to say what they know about endangered animals. What does *endangered* mean? Ask whether they can name any animals they know are endangered. Present the book's cover and suggest that they will soon discover more.

For tenses, pause to model or structure target structures. Many of the wordless pages contain illustrations depicting actions. Interact by asking questions that require responses in the present and future tenses. Also, ask students to rephrase each animal's explanation of why it wants to board the train (e.g., a hunter will shoot the polar bear for its fur; people will pollute the water, so the seal will have nothing left to eat).

Elicit predictions about the next animal that will want to come aboard. After the characters yell, "Hey! Get off our train," elicit predictions about why the animal wants to get on. After the animal explains its endangered status, make predictions about what will happen next. Will the other characters let it on board? Why do you think so?

Categorize these and other animals by their endangered status, by their habitat, and by their species.

For articulation of *G*, pause in the reading to repeat the words, "Hey, get off our train."

A Hole Is To Dig: A First Book of First Definitions

by Ruth Krauss
New York: Harper, 1952, 1989

Suggested Grade and Interest Level: Pre-K

Skill Builders:
Vocabulary	**Language literacy**
Grammar and syntax	Verbal expression
Noun-verb agreement	

Synopsis: The author got the material for this book by letting children think up their own definitions for familiar words and by coming up with some definitions of her own in the same style. Maurice Sendak's whimsical illustrations help rank this book among the classics. Shows boys and girls

jumping in the mud	rolling in the snow
doing dishes	dancing in the snow
hugging	curtsying
wiggling their ears	sucking their toes

Method: For noun-verb agreement, structure the words of the text for repetition. For example, the text reads, "Mud is to jump in and slide in and yell doodleedoodleedoo." After children have fun with the doodle word, point out the illustration and restructure the text as, "Kids jump." "He jumps." "She jumps." Or read the text, "Dogs are to kiss people." As you point to the picture, restructure the text into, "Dogs kiss. Dogs lick."

To improve vocabulary and verbal expression skills, ask children to make up original definitions following the author's model. Try out some of your own definitions to see whether the children agree with them. For example, read, "Dogs are to kiss people."

Ask what else dogs are for. Here are a few ideas to try out:

A dog is to . . .
. . . greet you when you come home.
. . . bark.
. . . sleep on your bed.
. . . take for walks.

Then vary the format. Turn the page and, before reading the text, ask, for example, what a face is for. See what the children come up with independently. Then read the text and find out what the author wrote.

Whether the definitions are pragmatic or based on emotions or fantasy, this exercise is great fun and loaded with possibilities for language expansion.

I Know an Old Lady Who Swallowed a Fly

Illustrated by Stephen Gulbis
New York: Scholastic, 2001

Suggested Grade and Interest Level: Pre-K

Topic Explorations: Humor; Insects and spiders

Skill Builders:

Grammar and syntax	**Phonological awareness**
Tenses, present and past	**Fluency**
Language literacy	**Voice**
Sequencing	
Cause-and-effect relationships	

Synopsis: This is the familiar, wacky tale (and song) about an old woman who gulps down animals to pursue those she has already swallowed! This version is hands on, encouraging more involvement with the story. Each page has a wheel for the children to spin, representing the old lady's tummy. The fly is joined by a spider, a bird, a cat, a goat, and a cow; as the wheel gets bigger and bigger, the old lady gets larger and larger. Very visual and very charming.

Method: After the read-aloud, go back over the illustrations and sequence what this silly lady did. Help children sequence events by using connecting words, such as *and then* and *next* as they review the events from the illustrations.

For comprehension and expression of cause-and-effect relationships, show the illustrations, asking why the old lady swallowed the last stated animal and what happened as a result. For example, why did she swallow the cat? (To catch the bird.) What happened? (She got bigger and bigger.) Then close the book and make a game of remembering the chain of causality.

Opposite the page with the "tummy wheel" is a picture showing the old lady in pursuit of each animal. Ask children to describe what's happening in the pictures to shape present-tense responses. Actions show the old lady

> Climbing a ladder in search of the spider
> Flying in a balloon with a butterfly net to catch the bird
> Casting a shadow over the doghouse to catch the dog
> Driving a bulldozer in pursuit of the cow (catch the pun)
> Whirling a lasso in pursuit of the horse

Children can express language in past tense with picture descriptions as well as with the repetition of text, as in, "She swallowed the dog."

Once the text has been read several times, use the familiar words for phonological awareness training, beginning at the child's developmental skill level.

> **PLAY** **Word-Count.**
>
> Children count the number of words in a short line from the text. Demonstrate by assigning one word to one finger as you say the words. For example, say
>
> > old lady
>
> *(continues on next page)*

PLAY **Word-Count.** *Continued*

as you hold up one finger for each word until two fingers are showing. Ask

How many words did I say?

Gradually build to "I know an old lady," then allow the children to do the counting by themselves. Present progressively longer word arrangements from the text for children to count.

If children don't have one-to-one correspondence, give each child a collection of manipulables (i.e., blocks, felt squares, buttons, etc.) to use for representing each of the stated words. Demonstrate by saying (or use a puppet to say) the words from a page of text that you want the children to count. Repeat them again as you (or a puppet) move out one item at a time to correspond to your stated word. Then you (or a puppet) count out loud the number of blocks moved to get the word count. Gradually allow the children to do the counting by themselves. Use words directly from a page of the text in hierarchical order to the desired word length.

PLAY **Rearrange-It.**

Children rearrange, in correct word order, a scrambled phrase or sentence from a portion of the text.

For example, say

Lady old
Is that right? Can you help me say the words in the right order?
That's right. *Lady old* should really be *Old lady.*

More words to rearrange include

Fly swallowed a	Fly a swallowed who	Lady I know an old
Die she'll perhaps	Who spider a swallowed	

PLAY **The Same-Sound game.**

Children identify whether alliterative word pairs begin with the same sound. For example, say

bone, buzz
Do they start with the same sound? (Yes)

To make an unmatched pair, exchange one of the following words with another word from the text, such as *bone, ghost*. Present one-syllable words first.

bird, bug	cat, course	dog, die
hog, horse	house, home	lady, ladder

PLAY **Finish-the-Rhyme.**

Children supply the rhyming word left out at the end of a verse. Provide the initial phoneme cue and picture prompt if needed. For example, say

"I know an old lady who swallowed a spider
It wiggled and wiggled and tickled in . . . _____." (prompt with, "Where?")

PLAY Rhyme-It-Again.

Children identify the rhyming word heard after each set. For example, say

> *That* rhymes with _____ . (cat)

PLAY Do-They-Rhyme?

Children identify whether word pairs rhyme. Intersperse nonrhyming words into the following rhyming sets:

that, cat	goat, throat	how, cow
horse, course	why, die	wiggle, jiggle

PLAY Clap-and-Count.

Children clap to, and then count, the number of syllables heard in selected words from the illustrations and text. Demonstrate by clapping to a word and then asking children how many parts they heard. For example, clap and say

> tickle
> How many parts in the word? Clap it out. (two)
> That's right. Ti–ckle. One, two.

Stress and elongate syllables when presenting words, such as

la-dy	spi-der	swa-llow
wi-ggle	ba-lloon	o-pen
la-sso	ji-ggle	per-haps

PLAY What's-the-Word?

Children synthesize syllables into words using words from the pictures in the book. Present the syllables with a clear pause between them and have the children say them quickly and repeatedly until they can identify the word. Demonstrate by saying

> la–dy
> What word did I say?
> Say it until you hear it. *Laaaa–dy. Laa-dy. Lady.*
> *Lady* is the word.

Continue with the two-syllable words provided in Clap-and-Count, or any two-syllable word from the story.

PLAY Find-the-Little-Words.

Children listen for "little" words within the two-syllable words of the text. Stress and elongate syllables when presenting the word. For example, say

> Swallow. (The old lady wanted to *swallow* a fly.)
> Can you find any little words in *swa-llow*? (low)
> That's right. *Low* is a little word in *swallow.*

Continue with the two-syllable words *lady* (lay), *spider* (spy), *wiggle* (wig), *balloon* (loon), *lasso* (so), and *perhaps* (purr).

PLAY Leave-It-Out.

Children say a two-syllable word, then leave out the beginning or final part to create a smaller word. For example, say

> Say *lady.*
> Now, say *lady,* but leave out *–dy.*
> What little word is left? (lay)

Continue with the two-syllable words provided in Clap-and-Count.

PLAY Add-It-On.

Children put two syllables together to make two-syllable words. For example, say

> Say *lay.*
> Now say *lay* and add *dee.*
> What new word can you make? (lady)

Continue with the two-syllable words provided in Clap-and-Count.

☞ See the catalog for Grades 1 through 5 for continuing activities in the hierarchy of phonological awareness activities.

For fluency and voice, use the cumulative, repetitive text to improve fluency and vocal quality as you shape words into progressively longer phrases and sentences. Talk about how the old lady's voice must sound, mimicking hoarseness and stridency.

I Went Walking

by Sue Williams
New York: Gulliver Books, 1989, 1991, 1992

Suggested Grade and Interest Level: Pre-K

Topic Explorations: Animals, Farm; Colors

Skill Builders:

Grammar and syntax	Language literacy	Articulation, *K* and *G*
Two- and three-word utterances	Predicting	
Past tense	Verbal expression	
Question structures		

Synopsis: A little boy goes walking and sees a variety of animals on the way. A partial view of the animal gives a clue as to what is illustrated on the following page. The repetitive, questioning text creates nice opportunities for interaction.

Method: Before the read-aloud, present words containing *K* and *G* from the text for auditory bombardment of speech sounds. Words containing *K* include

walking	looking	cat
basket	black	cow
duck	pink	lick

Words for articulation of *G* include

logs	bag	dog
pig	grass	

For verbal expression and predicting, read and interact about what is happening on the pages. Invite children to predict what animal the boy will see next.

For question structures, divide the group in half. Reread the text, then have one side repeat the statement ("I went walking") and the other side ask, "What did you see?" Have the first side answer according to the text (e.g., "I saw a pink pig looking at me."). Also select one child to be the main character in the story, saying the words, "I went walking" while the group asks, "What did you see?" Repeat the process so that each child has a chance to play the main character.

I Wish I Were a Butterfly

by James Howe
San Diego, CA: Harcourt Brace Jovanovich, 1987

Suggested Grade and Interest Level: K

Topic Explorations: Feelings; Friendship; Insects and spiders; Self-esteem

Skill Builders:

Vocabulary	**Language literacy**
Attributes	Predicting
Antonyms	Cause-and-effect relationships
	Problem solving
	Drawing inferences

Synopsis: The author acknowledges a group of Ohio schoolchildren for the beginning of this tale. A cricket who believes he is ugly wants to be a beautiful butterfly. With the help of a wise spider he learns where beauty comes from. Only then does he begin to love himself and others and come to know how special he is.

Method: Before the read-aloud, ask children what they know about crickets. Elicit many descriptions and stories about different experiences.

During the read-aloud, pause to identify the problem. What facts can be stated about it (e.g., The cricket doesn't want to make music. He doesn't want to be a cricket.)? How does the cricket try to solve his problem? What ideas do the children have about how the cricket might feel better about himself?

For cause-and-effect relationships, pause to ask what happened to the cricket because of how he felt about himself. What happened that finally caused him to feel good? What effect did the spider's friendship with the cricket have on the cricket?

For drawing inferences, talk about how the cricket feels based on his thoughts and actions. Talk about the frog who told the cricket he was an ugly creature. What might have caused the frog to say that? When the spider told him he was beautiful and he looked at his reflection, "his ugliness began to fade away." What does this mean? Who has the most influence on the way we feel about ourselves?

For attributes and antonyms, have children describe the different insects presented in the pictures. What words can they use to describe the dragonfly? The glowworm? The ladybug? Can they think of antonyms for these words (e.g., *beautiful/ugly, colorful/dull, quiet/loud, melodic/monotonous*)?

If You Give a Mouse a Cookie

by Laura Numeroff
New York: Harper & Row, 1985

Suggested Grade and Interest Level: Pre-K

Skill Builders:

Vocabulary	**Grammar and syntax**	**Language literacy**
Associations	Tenses—present, past, and future	Sequencing
		Predicting
		Storytelling

Synopsis: Children love this story about a demanding little mouse who makes a series of requests after a boy gives him a cookie. In fact, Californians voted it one of their favorites, for which it won the Young Reader's Medal.

Method: Before the read-aloud, ask children to think of something that goes with a cookie (e.g., Cookies and _____ go together). Some possibilities are *milk, napkin, plate, cookie jar,* and *ice cream.* Continue to string associations together, building on the associations the children offer. For example,

> What goes with milk? (a straw)
> What goes with a straw? (blowing bubbles)

Introduce the book as a story about how one thing leads to another and how it all starts with a cookie.

During the reading, interact with the children using present-progressive tense to discuss what the mouse is doing. Then review the story and model or shape future-tense structures. For example,

> Q: What will he do when you give him the milk?
> A: He'll ask for a straw.
> Q: What will he do when he looks in the mirror?
> A: He'll ask for some scissors.

For sequencing, do a picture walk-through and have the child tell the order of events, then close the book and see whether the child can remember some of the events that resulted from giving the mouse a cookie.

Extended Activity: Have children make up their own stories using the same format. For example, "If you give an opossum a flower, she'll . . ." or "If you give a hippo a suitcase he'll . . ." or any other creative starters you or the children may offer.

Note: Read also, *If You Give a Moose a Muffin, If You Give a Pig a Pancake,* and *If You Take a Mouse to the Movies,* by Laura Numeroff.

This book is also available in a Chinese version, as well as a Spanish version titled *Si le das una galletita a un raton,* along with *Si llevas un raton al cine.*

In the Haunted House

by Eve Bunting
New York: Clarion Books, 1990

Suggested Grade and Interest Level: K

Topic Exploration: Holidays, Halloween

Skill Builders:

Vocabulary	**Language literacy**
Prepositions	Sequencing
Grammar and syntax	**Phonological awareness**
Past tense	

Synopsis: A walk inside a haunted house reveals all sorts of scary features and creatures. At the end of the story, a girl and her father come out of what is then recognized as a Halloween House. The text is in a fun, quick-paced rhyming verse.

Method: Before the read-aloud, have children relate personal experiences about Halloween houses. What kinds of things occur?

During the read-aloud, allow children to experience the story without interruption so that the flow of the text, the rhythm and rhyme, are not interrupted.

After the read-aloud, go back over the text and ask children to tell the story by walking through the Halloween House, just as the girl and her father did. Use their feet, which are shown in each illustration, for sequencing the sights they saw. Include connecting words, such as *then they, next they,* and *so they.* For grammar and syntax, especially past tense, shape responses to form target structures. Use the illustrations to construct prepositional phrases. Some examples include

Inside the house	Up the stairs
Behind the door	Inside the box
On top of the box	Behind the box (the tell-tale sign of the can of paint)
Through the door	Under the floor boards

For phonological awareness training, reread the story, stressing some of the featured words, such as *house, bats, ghosts, witches, coffin, mummy,* and so on. Then play a series of phonological games, depending on the level of each student's development in the hierarchy of skills.

> **PLAY** **Word-Count.**
>
> Children count the number of words in a short line from the text. Demonstrate by assigning one word to one finger as you say the words. For example, say
>
> three witches
>
> as you hold up one finger for each word until two fingers are showing. Ask
>
> How many words did I say?
>
> Then say
>
> three witches appear
>
> for a three-finger count. Gradually allow the children to do the counting by themselves.
>
> If children don't have one-to-one correspondence, give each child a collection of manipulables (i.e., blocks, felt squares, buttons, etc.) to use for representing each of the stated words. Demonstrate by saying (or use a puppet
>
> *(continues on next page)*

PLAY Word-Count. *Continued*

to say) the words from a page of text that you want the children to count. Repeat them again as you (or a puppet) move out one item at a time to correspond to your stated word. Then you (or a puppet) count out loud the number of blocks moved to get the word count. Gradually allow the children to do the counting by themselves. Use words directly from a page of the text in hierarchical order to the desired word length. Some words from the text to count include

"Do not lift."   "Stay close to me."   "It might be a spook."
"Winking at me"   "Dark as a tomb"
"Dead as can be"   "I don't want to look."

PLAY Which-One-Is-Missing?

In a word string, children select a word that has been omitted from the previously given string. For example, say

house, bat, witch, ghost
house, witch, ghost
Which one is missing? (bat)
That's right. *Bat* is the word that is missing.

Some words from the text include

stay, lift, lid, box   hang, dark, wall, face   door, light, lock, crack
jump, tub, smile, sleep   ghost, scary, door, fun

PLAY Rearrange-It.

Children place, in correct order, scrambled phrase or sentence from a portion of the text. For example, say

House in the haunted
Is that right? Can you help me say it in the right order?
That's right. *House in the haunted* should really be *In the haunted house.*

More words to rearrange include

Winking me at (winking at me)
Dead as be can (dead as can be)
Close stay to me (stay close to me)
Tomb as a dark (dark as a tomb)
Look I to don't want (I don't want to look)
Might spook it a be (It might be a spook)

PLAY Finish-the-Rhyme.

Children supply the rhyming word at the end of a verse. Provide initial phoneme cue, if needed. For example,

"It's playing and playing, but nobody's (th) _____." (there)

Also, prompt with a context cue, such as asking, "Where?"

PLAY **Rhyme-It-Again.**

Children identify the rhyming word you read after each set. For example, say

Air rhymes with _____. (there)

PLAY **Do-They-Rhyme?**

Children identify whether word pairs rhyme. Use the following rhyming words from the text and intersperse with unmatched sets:

ice, rice	wings, things	sun, fun
creep, sleep	ghost, toast	deep, sleep
shout, out	tub, scrub	ladder, madder

PLAY **Clap-and-Count.**

Children clap to, and then count, the number of syllables heard in selected words from the illustrations and text. Demonstrate by clapping to a word and then asking children how many parts they heard. For example, clap and say

hall
How many parts in the word? Clap it out. (one)

Clap and say

hallway
How many parts in that word? Clap it out. (two)
That's right. Hall–way. One, two.

Stress and elongate syllables when presenting words, such as

cob-web	sca-ry	mu-mmy
vam-pire	cree-ping	Hall-o-ween
craw-ling	or-gan	chan-de-lier
in-side	were-wolf	fu-ner-al

PLAY **What's-the-Word?**

Children synthesize syllables into words using words from the pictures in the book. Present the syllables with a clear pause between them and have the children say them quickly and repeatedly, until they identify the word. Demonstrate by saying

la–dder
What word did I say?
Say it until you hear it. *Laaaaa–dder. Laaa–dder. Ladder.*
Ladder is the word.

Continue with the two-syllable words presented in Clap-and-Count.

PLAY **Find-the-Little-Words.**

Children listen for the "little" words within compound words in the text. Stress and elongate syllables when presenting the words. For example, say

> hallway
> Can you hear any little words in *hallway*? (hall, way)
> That's right. *Hall* is a little word in *hallway*.
> *Way* is another little word in *hallway*.

Continue with the following words:

inside	nobody
someone	cobweb
werewolf	

When presenting the following two-syllable words from the text, change the stress pattern so children can hear the "little" words.

scar-y (scare)	soft-ly (soft)
creep-ing (creep)	wash-ing (wash)
or-gan (or)	mumm-y (*me*)
crawl-ing (crawl)	coff-in (*cough*, in)

PLAY **Leave-It-Out.**

Children say a compound word or two-syllable word, then leave out the beginning or final part to create a smaller word. For example, say

> Say *cobweb*.
> Now, say *cobweb*, but leave out *web*.
> What little word is left? (cob)

Then say

> Now, say *cobweb*, but leave out *cob*.
> What little word is left? (web)

Continue with the compound and two-syllable words provided in Find-the-Little-Words.

PLAY **Add-It-On.**

Children put two syllables together to make two-syllable words. For example, say

> Say *cob*.
> Now say *cob* and add *web*.
> What bigger word can you make? (cobweb)

Continue with the list of words provided in Find-the-Little-Words.

(PLAY) Switch-It.

Children delete part of a compound or two-syllable word and exchange it with a new part to make another compound word. Prompt with cues as necessary. For example, say

> Say *hallway*.
> Now say *hallway*, only take out *hall* and put in *path*.
> What new word can you make? (pathway)

Some word exchanges include

> Say *cobweb*, only take out *cob* and put in *spider*. (two words: spider web)
> Say *inside*, only take out *in* and put in *out*. (outside)
> Say *nobody*, only take out *no* and put in *some*. (somebody)
> Say *someone*, only take out *some* and put in *no*. (two words: no, one)
> Say *someone*, only take out *one* and put in *thing*. (something)

Some syllable exchanges include

> Say *spider*, only take out *spy* and put in *sigh*. (cider)
> Say *monster*, only take out *mon* and put in *sis*. (sister)
> Say *mummy*, only take out *ee* and put in *bull*. (mumble)
> Say *crawling*, only take out *crawl* and put in *creep*. (creeping)
> Say *frighten*, only take out *ten* and put in *ning*. (frightening [pronounce "fright-ning"])

☛ See the catalog for Grades 1 through 5 for continuing activities in the hierarchy of phonological awareness activities.

The Important Book

by Margaret Wise Brown
New York: Harper & Row, 1949

Suggested Grade and Interest Level: Pre-K

Topic Exploration: Self-esteem

Skill Builders:

Vocabulary	Language literacy
Categories	Relating personal experiences
Associations	Verbal expression

Synopsis: Here's a classic that teaches children how to describe a familiar word from the world of the senses. For example, "The important thing about a shoe is that you put your foot in it. You walk in it, and you take it off at night and it's warm when you take it off. But the important thing about a shoe is that you put your foot in it."

Method: Read and interact about the idea presented. Talk about the child's own experiences, and ask the children to make up their own definitions. For example, Is there anything else important about a shoe? Then use the same format to define additional words. What's the important thing about a hamburger? A book? Roller skates? A leprechaun?

Introduce categories by naming types of shoes or things that go on your foot (e.g., sandals, slippers, boots, etc.). Do the same for other words that are defined (e.g., An apple is a fruit. What other kinds of fruit are there?).

For associations, ask children to think of things that go with each pictured item. For example, what goes with an apple (e.g., tree, teacher, worm, etc.)?

Is It Larger? Is It Smaller?

by Tana Hoban
New York: Greenwillow Books, 1985, 1997

Suggested Grade and Interest Level: Pre-K

Topic Exploration: Shapes and visual images

Skill Builders:

Vocabulary	**Grammar and syntax**
Categories	Singular and plural nouns
Morphological units	

Synopsis: A series of color photographs without text depicts the concept of size in relation to leaves, pigs, bears, boats, hands, and more.

Method: Use the photographs as visual stimuli to elicit language and target comparatives and superlatives. For example, say

> Look at these two umbrellas.
> Which is bigger? Which is smaller?
> Now tell me about that one.

To teach morphological units, explain that *–er,* when attached to the end of a word, makes that word comparative (e.g., One umbrella is bigg*er.* One umbrella is small*er.*). Give examples and demonstrate visually with objects, such as

> small, smaller
> big, bigger
> low, lower
> bright, brighter

Encourage children to use the words in sentences.

Play the Suffix game.

> Put *–er* after *loud.* What word is it now? (louder)
> Put *–er* after of *tall.* What word is it now? (taller)

More words include

soft	plain	quiet
happy	sad	dry
wet	smooth	

Capitalize on the realism in the photographs when teaching categories and verbal naming. Can the children think of other types of leaves? Another kind of bear? Other boats, body parts, and so on?

Extended Activity: Play the game with things around the room (e.g., Which is larger, the book or the chair?), then go outside and observe things in nature (e.g., Which is smaller, a blade of grass or the leaf of a maple tree?).

Note: Read also *Exactly the Opposite* (listed in this catalog); *Is It Rough, Is It Smooth, Is It Shiny?; Shapes, Shapes, Shapes; So Many Circles, So Many Squares;* and *Over, Under, Through and Other Spatial Concepts* by Tana Hoban.

Is Your Mama a Llama?

by Deborah Guarino
New York: Scholastic, 1989, 1991, 1992

Suggested Grade and Interest Level: Pre-K

Topic Explorations: Animals, Zoo; Family relationships

Skill Builders:

Vocabulary	Grammar and syntax	Articulation, *M* and *L*
Attributes	Negative structures	
	Question structures	

Synopsis: A baby llama learns about life as it questions its friends about whether their mamas are llamas. In rhyming verse, the friends describe what their mothers do and the baby llama learns that all mothers are different.

Method: Pause at appropriate places in the text to model and shape target structures.

To teach attributes, play an animal guessing game. Recall which animals the baby llama encountered in the story. Then describe each animal. What does it look like? What does it do? Describe other animals, too.

For articulation, reinforce target phonemes by using the text for auditory bombardment and by encouraging children to recite the repetitive text, as well as other target words.

Note: In Spanish, *ll* is pronounced as *y*. Therefore, the book may not be appropriate for *L* remediation with certain students.

It Looked Like Spilt Milk

by Charles G. Shaw
New York: Harper & Row, 1947, 1988

Suggested Grade and Interest Level: Pre-K

Topic Explorations: Clouds; Shapes and visual images

Skill Builders:

Grammar and syntax	Language literacy
Two- and three-word utterances	Verbal expression
Past tense	
Negative structures	

Synopsis: A familiar silhouette, such as an ice cream cone, is presented against a blue background on each page. The form continues to change on each page, eluding identification. The child is repeatedly invited to guess the form until its identity is finally revealed—a cloud!

Method: Before the read-aloud, introduce the book by reading the title and presenting the book's cover. Ask children to describe what spilt milk looks like. See if they can identify any of the white images shown on the cover.

Read the story, pausing to encourage verbal expression by talking about how each object on a page is relevant to the children's lives. For two- and three-word utterances, model or shape constructions based on the simple text or illustrations, such as, "Like a bird," "That's a bird," and "White bird." For past tense, encourage repetition of the text, "It looked like. . . ." For negatives, repeat the last line of text on each page (e.g., But it wasn't an ice cream cone.), or model a simplified negative (e.g., Not ice cream.).

After the read-aloud, talk about other forms a cloud might take.

Extended Activity: Children can make their own interesting cloud images. Give them each one sheet of dark blue or black construction paper and one sheet of white construction paper. Demonstrate how to tear the white paper around the perimeter to make a shape, then look at the shape. What does it look like? An ice cream cone? A dog? A pair of pajamas? Or spilt milk? Once the children have all decided, have them glue the images onto the dark sheet of paper. Children can dictate a label or title for their picture.

Note: Read also *Dreams* by Peter Spier.

It's a Spoon, Not a Shovel

by Caralyn Buehner
New York: Dial Books for Young Readers, 1995

Suggested Grade and Interest Level: K

Topic Exploration: Manners and etiquette

Skill Builders:
   Pragmatic language   **Phonological awareness**

Synopsis: This "manners" book in quiz format is a great way to have fun. The text escorts children through a series of social situations, humorously depicted by the vivid illustrations. Children select from the appropriate and not-so-appropriate (in some cases, downright rude) behavior by selecting the correct letter. The answers are obvious, but after all, shouldn't manners be, too? To double-check the answer, children will find the correct letter selection hidden within each page—and other little creatures, too.

Method: This is an ideal book to use for language pragmatics, making use of the lighthearted vein, which is nonetheless effective. Before the read-aloud, ask children to recall some rules about behaving in appropriate ways, then let go and prepare for laughs.

During the read-aloud, read the text and present the quiz without interruption, such as "Marty Mouse has been saving crumbs for weeks to give to Elmer Elephant for his birthday. Elmer exclaims (a) 'Your whiskers are twitching.' (b) 'Rats! That's not what I wanted!' (c) 'Thank you, Marty!'" The location of the correct answer, *c,* is found inside the elephant's eye. For a list of locations of all answers, see the back of the book.

After the read-aloud, continue to address language pragmatics. Go back to a few preselected pictures and ask children to express, in their own words, which good manners should be used by the characters in the situation. For example, ask, "When Karla Kangaroo played hide-and-seek in the bushes and didn't see Harold Hyena, what should she have said when she accidentally hopped right on top of him?" Ask the children what the consequences might have been if she'd said one of the other incorrect selections.

For increasing phonological awareness, play the following games with the names of the characters in the book beginning at the child's developmental skill level.

PLAY **The Same-Sound game.**

Children identify whether the characters' names begin with the same sound. The cast includes

Victor Vulture	Sam Buzzard (first name supplied)
Marty Mouse	Elmer Elephant
Karla Kangaroo	Harold Hyena
Arvin Anteater	Wolfgang Smith (last name supplied)
Lilly Crocodile (first name supplied)	Trevor Tarantula
Mama Tarantula	Tiny Tarantula
Walter Warthog	Larry Lion
Sheila Lion (first name supplied)	Melissa Mandrill
Timmy Snaptooth	Cory Cobra
Buster Bunny	Lettuce Breat

PLAY **Clap-and-Count.**

Children clap to, and then count, the number of syllables heard in selected words from the illustrations and text. Demonstrate by clapping to a word and then asking children how many parts they heard. For example, clap and say

> Victor
> How many parts do you hear in the name? Clap it out. (two)
> That's right. Vic-tor. One, two.

Clap and say

> Vulture
> How many parts do you hear in the name? Clap it out. (two)
> That's right. Vul-ture. One, two.

Then ask

> How many parts do you hear in the whole name of Victor Vulture? (four)
> That's right. Vic-tor-Vul-ture. One, two, three, four.

Stress and elongate syllables when presenting the list of names.

PLAY **What's-the-Word?**

Children synthesize syllables into words using words from the pictures in the book. Present the syllables with a clear pause between them and have the children say them quickly and repeatedly until they can identify the word. Demonstrate by saying

> vul-ture
> What word did I say?
> Say it until you hear it. *Vullll-ture. Vull-ture. Vulture.*
> *Vulture* is the word.

Continue with the two-syllable names listed in the Same-Sound game.

PLAY **Find-the-Little-Words.**

Children listen for "little" words within compound words. Stress and elongate syllables when presenting the word. For example, say

anteater
Can you hear any little words in *anteater*? (ant, eat, eater)
That's right. *Ant* is a little word in *anteater*.
And *eat* is another little word in *anteater*.
Eater is another little word in *anteater*.

Other compound words include

Warthog	Snaptooth	Wolfgang

Names with little words in two-syllable words include the following (change the stress pattern as necessary):

Sam Buzzard (buzz)   Harold Hyena (hi)
Larry Lion (lie)   Karla Kangaroo (Karl)
Melissa Mandrill (drill)   Lettuce Breath (let)
Elmer Elephant (elm)   Tina Tarantula (teen, ran)
   (Hint: It's the name of a tree.)

PLAY **Leave-It-Out.**

Children say a compound or two-syllable word, then leave out the beginning or final part to create a smaller word. For example, say

Say *warthog.*
Now say *warthog* but leave out *hog.*
What little word is left? (wart)

Then say

Now say *warthog* but leave out *wart.*
What little word is left? (hog)

Continue with the words provided in Find-the-Little-Words.

PLAY **Add-It-On.**

Children put word parts together to make compound and two-syllable words. For example, say

Say *hi.*

Then say

Now say *hi* and add *ena.*
Whose name can you make? (hyena, as in Harold Hyena)

Continue with the list of names provided in Find-the-Little-Words, first presenting only the target word. Once the word is synthesized, then include the full name of the character.

(**PLAY**) **Turn-It-Around.**

Children reverse the parts of a word they have previously analyzed and synthesized, such as

> Put the word *hog* at the beginning of *wart*.
> What word do you have? (hogwart)
> What was it before we turned it around? (warthog)

Continue with the list of compound word names and two-syllable names provided in Find-the-Little-Words.

(**PLAY**) **Exchange-It.**

Children delete a part in a compound or two-syllable word and exchange it with another word, syllable, or little word. Prompt with first syllable cue as needed. For example, say

> Say *warthog*.
> Now say *warthog*, only take out *wart* and put in *ground*.
> What new word can you make? (gr) _____. (groundhog)

Some word exchanges include

> Say *vulture*, only take out *vul* and put in *cap*. (capture)
> Say *inside*, only take out *in* and put in *out*. (outside)
> Say *buzzard*, only take out *buzz* and put in *must*. (mustard)
> Say *Marty*, only take out *ee* and put in *tian*. (Martian)
> Say *Karla*, only take out *la* and put in *ton*. (carton)
> Say *Arvin*, only take out *vin* and put in *thur*. (Arthur)

☛ See the catalog for Grades 1 through 5 for continuing activities in the hierarchy of phonological awareness activities.

It's the Bear!

by Jez Alborough
Cambridge, MA: Candlewick Press, 1994

Suggested Grade and Interest Level: Pre-K

Topic Explorations: Bears; Food; Woods

Skill Builders:

Vocabulary	Grammar and syntax	Language literacy
Categories	Two- and three-word utterances	Drawing inferences
Prepositions	Noun–verb agreement	**Phonological awareness**
	Pronouns, personal and possessive	
	Present tense	

Synopsis: The sequel to the popular *Where's My Teddy?* gets even better. Eddie, having been scared by a bear in the woods once before, doesn't want to return for a picnic with his mom. His mom insists there are no bears, and he reluctantly goes along. Mom has to leave to get the forgotten blueberry pie, and once again Eddie finds himself alone in the forest. When he hears the bear, he hides in the picnic basket. Upon mom's return, they both are confronted by the big bear in a hilarious sequence of actions. The rhyming, quick-paced text and humorous illustrations are a delight, providing lots of ideas for language stimulation.

Method: Before the read-aloud, lead into the story with a discussion about picnics. Ask what kinds of things are packed in a picnic basket and elicit children's background experience. If children have been exposed to *Where's My Teddy?* ask if anyone can recall the story and tell it to the class. Make predictions about the current story based on the cover illustration.

Then, read the rhyming text, showing the pictures without pausing for interaction (in this way, children enjoy the illustrations and hear the words without a break in the rhythm and flow of the verse).

After the read-aloud, do a picture walk-through, having children sequence the parts of the story. Model and shape target grammar and syntax structures appropriate to each page of the story. Some two- and three-word utterances include

It's the bear!	Eddie is scared	Great big bear
Eddie hides	Huge bear	Bear sat down
The bear munched		

Examples of noun–verb agreement include

Eddie walks.	The bear sits on the basket.	They both yell.
Eddie and Mom walk.	The bear's teddy sits.	Mom comes.
He hears bear.	They both sit.	Eddie points.
He cuddles his teddy.	The bear opens the basket.	Mom yells.
Eddie and his teddy hide.	Eddie yells.	They run.
The bear steps out of the trees.	The bear yells.	The bear runs.

For possessive pronouns, elicit target structures as you share in talking about the action in the illustration. For personal pronouns, change the names in the following sample sentences to *he, she,* and *they.* Suggestions include

Mom has *her* basket.
Mom is wearing *her* hat.
Eddie has *his* teddy.
Mom forgot *her* pie.
The bear has *his* teddy.
They both have *their* teddies.
The boy cuddles *his* teddy.
The bear sits on *his* (Eddie's) basket.
The bear eats *their* (Eddie and Mom's) food.
Mom loses *her* hat.
The bear eats *their* blueberry pie.

Also use the illustrations to teach prepositions, such as

along the path
through the forest
through the trees
inside the picnic basket
on top of the picnic basket
in front of the bear
under his arm (location of the bear's teddy)

For developing skills in the area of categories, ask children to name the things Mom took out of the picnic basket and ask which ones belong in the food category. Suggested items include

cookies	napkins
crusty brown bread	hard-boiled eggs
cups	chips
blanket	forks
cream cheese spread	orange juice

Then ask children to brainstorm items that would fall into the picnic category.

Also talk about types of toys. Different toys fall under different categories, such as vehicles, board games, pull-toys, dolls, and stuffed animals. Ask if children can come up with other categories of toys, then name types of toys that belong in the stuffed animal category (e.g., teddy bears, beanie babies, snurfs, etc.).

To use the words of the text for phonological awareness training, first reread the story, then play a series of games, based on each student's level of phonological sensitivity.

PLAY Word-Count.

Children count the number of words in a short line from the text. Demonstrate by assigning one word to one finger as you say the words. For example, say

>   It's the bear

as you hold up one finger for each word until three fingers are showing. Ask

>   How many words did I say?

Start at a one- or two-word count and gradually increase the number. Allow the children to do the counting by themselves. Some words of the text to count include

>   "I can smell food!"
>   "Where can I hide?"
>   "I want my Mom!"

If children don't have one-to-one correspondence, give each child a collection of manipulables (i.e., blocks, felt squares, buttons, etc.) to use for representing each of the stated words. Demonstrate by saying (or use a puppet to say) the words from a page of text that you want the children to count. Repeat them again as you (or a puppet) move out one item at a time to correspond to your stated word. Then you (or a puppet) count out loud the number of blocks moved to get the word count. Gradually allow the children to do the counting by themselves. Use words directly from a page of the text in hierarchical order to the desired word length.

PLAY Which-One-Is-Missing?

Children select a word from a word string that has been omitted from the previously given string. For example, say

>   Mom, Eddie, picnic, woods
>   Mom, Eddie, woods

(continues on next page)

PLAY **Which-One-Is-Missing?** *Continued*

> Which one is missing?
> That's right. *Picnic* is the word that is missing.

Some word lists from the text include

Teddy, big, bear, scared	woods, forest, path, tree	path, mom, basket, hat
blanket, chips, bread, pie	bear, trees, hide, inside	sit, yell, run, hide

PLAY **Rearrange-It.**

Children rearrange, in correct word order, a scrambled phrase or sentence from a portion of the text. For example, say

> The bear it's
> Is that right? Can you help me say the words in the right order?
> That's right. *The bear it's* should really be *It's the bear.*

More words to rearrange include

> Scared I'm (I'm scared)
> Can I where hide? (Where can I hide?)
> Don't him let come (Don't let him come)
> My Mom I want (I want my Mom)
> Sat lid on the down (Sat down on the lid)

PLAY **Finish-the-Rhyme.**

Children supply the rhyming word left out at the end of a verse. Provide the initial phoneme cue and prompt by pointing to the illustration, if needed. For example, say

> "The bear munched
> and he crunched.
> He chomped and he chewed,
> and greedily gobbled up
> all of the ____."

PLAY **Rhyme-It-Again.**

Children identify the rhyming word heard after a rhyming set is given. For example, say

> *Chewed* rhymes with (f) ____. (food)

PLAY **Do-They-Rhyme?**

Children identify whether word pairs rhyme. Intersperse an unrhymed word into the following rhyming sets to make unmatched sets:

(continues on next page)

PLAY Do-They-Rhyme? *Continued*

chewed, food	Freddie, ready
Eddie, teddy	huddle, cuddle
munched, crunched	hurt, dessert

PLAY Rhyming-Ings.

Children rhyme root words with added –*ing* suffixes using words of the text (root + added suffix, if necessary). Give initial phoneme or cluster cues if needed. Accept any rhyming nonsense word. For example,

eating (meeting, seating, beating, cheating)
munching (crunching, lunching)
chewing (mooing, stewing)
sitting (hitting, fitting)
hiding (riding, siding)
walking (talking, shocking, gawking)
running (sunning, funning, cunning, stunning)
yelling (smelling, telling, selling)
licking (kicking, picking, ticking, sticking)
chomping (romping, stomping)

PLAY Clap-and-Count.

Children clap to, and then count, the number of syllables heard in selected words from the illustrations and text. Demonstrate by clapping to a word and then asking children how many parts they heard. For example, clap and say

Ted
How many parts in the word? Clap it out. (one)

Clap and say

Teddy
How many parts in that word? Clap it out. (two)
That's right. Tedd–y. One, two.

Stress and elongate syllables when presenting words, such as

le-ttuce	coo-kies
bas-ket	near-by
clamb-ered	in-side
li-cking	sni-ffing
be-llow	whis-per
cu-ddle	hu-ddle
go-bbled	de-ssert
to-ma-toes	blue-be-rry

PRE-K–K

PLAY **What's-the-Word?**

Children synthesize syllables into words found in the pictures and text of the book. Present the syllables with a clear pause between them and have the children say them quickly and repeatedly until they can identify the word. Demonstrate first, saying

> bas–ket
> What word did I say?
> Say it until you hear it. *Basssss–ket. Bass–ket. Basket.*
> *Basket* is the word.

Continue with the two-syllable words provided in Clap-and-Count.

PLAY **Find-the-Little-Words.**

Children listen for "little" words within the compound words of the text. Stress and elongate syllables when presenting the words, such as

> nearby
> Can you find any little words in *nearby*? (near, by)
> That's right. *Near* is a little word in *nearby.*
> *By* is another little word in *nearby.*

More compound words include

> inside (in, side)   blueberry (blue, bear, berry)

Children then listen for little words within the two-syllable words of the text. For example,

> pic-nic (pick)
> coo-kies (keys)
> li-cking (king)
> sniff-ing (sniff)
> com-ing (come)
> be-llow (low) (and bell-ow for bell)

PLAY **Leave-It-Out.**

Children say a compound word or two-syllable word, then leave out the beginning or final part to create a smaller word. For example, say

> Say *nearby.*
> Now, say *nearby,* but leave out *by.*
> What little word is left? (near)

Then say

> Now, say *nearby,* but leave out *near.*
> What little word is left? (by)

Continue with the words provided in Find-the-Little-Words.

PLAY **Add-It-On.**

Children put two little words or two syllables together to make new words. For example, say

> Say *blue*.

Then say

> Now, say *blue*, and add *berry*.
> What bigger word can you make? (blueberry)

Continue with the two-syllable words provided in Find-the-Little-Words.

➥ See the catalog for Grades 1 through 5 for continuing activities in the hierarchy of phonological awareness activities.

Note: See also *Where's My Teddy?* by the same author featured in this catalog section.

The Itsy Bitsy Spider

by Iza Trapani
Boston: Whispering Coyote Press, 1993

Suggested Grade and Interest Level: Pre-K

Topic Exploration: Insects and spiders

Skill Builders:

Vocabulary	**Language literacy**
Adjectives	Cause-and-effect relationships
Prepositions	
Grammar and syntax	
Past tense	

Synopsis: The famous little spider who struggles up the waterspout is back for further adventures. Follow her up a kitchen wall, a yellow pail, a green rocker, and finally, a maple tree, where she decides to give it one more try. At last, her web is spun, and oh, how sweet it is! Play the game of finding the spider in each beautiful picture, rendered from the perspective of an itsy bitsy being.

Method: When each mishap happens, pause to talk about what caused the spider to fall down the wall, off the pail, and so on. Encourage use of words such as *because* and *since* to place information in meaningful temporal relationships.

Encourage use of prepositions to describe the spider's direction or position in the pictures. Elaborate descriptions with adjectives that describe the color, shape, and size of the spider and the objects in the story.

For training in past tense, pause to have children repeat and use in a sentence the verbs of the text, including

wove	spun
climbed	slipped
plopped	knocked
fell	flicked

Jamberry

by Bruce Degen
New York: Harper & Row, 1983; Scholastic, 1990, 1992

Suggested Grade and Interest Level: Pre-K

Topic Explorations: Bears; Food

Skill Builders:

Vocabulary	**Grammar and syntax**
Categories	Two- and three-word utterances
Prepositions	

Synopsis: Follow the bear and its friends on a journey through jamberry land for a mouth-watering experience.

Method: The illustrations have plenty of action to describe and words to label. Look for other foods to identify in the pictures, such as marshmallows on reeds, crackers posing as lily pads, and slices of bread hanging from the trees. Vocabulary includes

waterfall	fiddle
streamers	brass band
ice skating rink	jelly rolls
hot air balloons	

Use the text and pictures to model and shape early word combinations. For prepositions, ask where the berries are in the pictures and model or structure various prepositional phrases.

For categories, have children name all the kinds of fruit they can recall from the story and to which of the food groups they belong.

Extended Activity: Improvise new *berry* phrases, such as

pianoberry
musicberry
sing me a songberry
teacherberry
childberry
we all love to learnberry
katieberry
joshberry
I'm glad you're here at school berry

Jesse Bear, What Will You Wear?

by Nancy White Carlstrom
New York: Macmillan, 1986

Suggested Grade and Interest Level: Pre-K

Topic Explorations: Bears; Daily activities; Family relationships

Skill Builders:

Grammar and syntax   **Articulation, *K* and *G***

Two- and three-word utterances
Pronouns—personal, possessive, and reflexive
Tenses, present and future
Question structures

Synopsis: This rhyming romp through Jesse Bear's daily routine is as full of delight as the pictures.

Method: During the read-aloud, encourage children to chime in, if they can. Then go back over the illustrations and have children describe the actions. Structure sentences to target noun–verb agreement (Jesse swings), present tense (Jesse is blowing bubbles), future tense (Jesse will wear his red shirt), or pronouns (Jesse gets dressed by *himself*).

For articulation remediation, use the target sounds found in the text and illustrations for auditory bombardment and sound production. Words with *K* include

comb	catch	call, calls
comes	carrots	cup
stuck	cookies	cook
clock	suitcase	

Extended Activity: Following the pattern of the text, call on a child, using the child's name with *bear*. For example, "Jackie Bear, what will you wear? What will you wear to school?" Ask children what they would like to wear tonight, tomorrow, to the fair, to the park, or to other places. Here are a few examples:

He'll wear his hat
Then we'll give him a pat
That's what he'll wear to the park.
She'll wear cowboy boots
Boots and a smile
That's what she'll wear to the fair.

King Bidgood's in the Bathtub

by Audrey Wood
San Diego, CA: Harcourt Brace Jovanovich, 1985, 1993

Suggested Grade and Interest Level: Pre-K

Topic Exploration: Long ago and far away

Skill Builders:

Language literacy   **Articulation, *K* and *G***

Predicting
Sequencing
Problem solving

Synopsis: A fun-loving king refuses to get out of his bathtub. Everyone in the court tries a different strategy, but it's the page who finally comes up with the obvious.

Method: Before the read-aloud, ask children to tell what they know about kings and queens and where they live. Elicit background knowledge about castles.

During the read-aloud, invite children to predict what might be tried next to get the king out of his bathtub. For articulation, pause to interact about the story, having the children use the text that is heavily loaded with target phonemes.

After the read-aloud, have children retell the story of the king who wouldn't get out of his bathtub, recalling the problem in the story and how the others tried to get him out. Provide scaffolding as necessary. For articulation, read the text, eliciting target sounds.

Extended Activity: Stage a creative dramatization of the story. A few props—such as a large cardboard box for the bathtub; some toy boats and soldiers; and plates, cups, and saucers for the lunch—can enhance children's participation.

Decide who will play the various parts, including King Bidgood, the queen, duke, knight, and page. As the king acts out playing in his bathtub, ask the other children what King Bidgood might be saying in order to prompt the king's dialog. Encourage the page to repeat the lines of the text, leading the audience in the lines of "Help, help. King Bidgood's in the bathtub. . . ." Prompt the other characters to give their solutions to the problem using the dialog in the text to act out the story.

Lilly's Purple Plastic Purse

by Kevin Henkes
New York: Greenwillow Books, 1996

Suggested Grade and Interest Level: K

Topic Exploration: School activities

Skill Builders:

Vocabulary	Language literacy
Adjectives	Cause-and-effect relationships
Grammar and syntax	Problem solving
Possessive nouns and pronouns	Drawing inferences
Past tense	**Phonological awareness**

Synopsis: Lilly loves going to school and wearing her red cowboy boots with stars. She wants to be a teacher when she grows up, just like her adored Mr. Slinger. But when Mr. Slinger asks Lilly to wait until the appropriate time to share her new movie star sunglasses with the glittery diamonds and her purple plastic purse that plays music, Lilly becomes impatient. When she is reprimanded, she writes her teacher an unkind note, for which she is very sorry later. Then she, her parents, and Mr. Slinger must work to resolve the problem.

Method: Before reading what may be a familiar story to the children, obtain their background knowledge about the characters and events in the book. Ask who the story is about, where it takes place, what happens to start the story off, and what the major events are in the story.

During the read-aloud, briefly pause to allow the children to elaborate on the meaning and expand on the descriptions and actions. Ask children to interpret the feelings of Lilly based on the text and illustrations and state what precipitated them. Model, shape, and recast target structures of grammar and syntax such as past tense.

Use Lilly's cherished red cowgirl boots, movie star sunglasses, and purple plastic purse to elicit possessive forms of nouns and pronouns. Use the many adjectives in the text when describing her special articles of clothing. Also, pause to allow the children to use the story's many adjectives in sentences of their own.

After the story, talk about what Lilly learned from her experience. Work on problem identification and problem-solving skills by asking children to state the problem in the story. When Lilly couldn't wait and interrupted Mr. Slinger's lesson, what happened? What are some of the things Mr. Slinger did in response to her problem? Talk about the way Lilly felt because of the problem. What things did she do to handle her problem? Draw inferences about how Lilly came to decide upon these solutions. What did Lilly do with her parents that helped solve the problem? What was the result? What did Mr. Slinger do?

For cause-and-effect relationships, ask children to state what caused Lilly to write the unkind note that she sneaked into Mr. Slinger's bag.

> What effect did the note have on Lilly's relationship with Mr. Slinger?
> What effect did Mr. Slinger's note and the snack that he placed in her purple plastic purse have upon Lilly? What did this cause her to do?
> What was the effect upon her teacher of her freshly baked snacks and note of apology? Upon her?

As children respond to these questions, use scaffolding in helping them structure their responses with words such as *then*, *because, resulted in, caused, since,* and *the reason.*

Play the following phonological awareness games, beginning at the child's developmental level.

PLAY   The Same-Sound game.

Children identify whether two words (or three-word strings) selected from the text begin with the same sound. For example, say

> boots, bag
> Do they start with the same sound? (Yes)

To make an unmatched pair, replace one of the following words with another word from the text or list.

boots, bag	bus, born, best	desk, day
wow, way	week, wink	wait, want
tie, take	lab, long	last, look
say, sad, said	now, note, nice	gone, got
purse, point	heart, hand, hard	chalk, cheese, choice
time, tune	wrote, ride	

PLAY   Odd-One-Out.

Children select from a string of words that begin with the same sound the one that does not belong. For example, say

> wow, wink, milk

(continues on next page)

PLAY **Odd-One-Out.** *Continued*

Ask

Which word has a different beginning sound? (milk)
That's right. *Milk* is the odd one out.

Use the words provided in the Same-Sound game. Insert an additional unmatched word from the story that has a different initial sound for the children to identify, such as

boots, bag, purse

and so on.

PLAY **Say-the-Sound.**

Children produce the beginning sound they hear in a series of words that begin with the same sound. For example, ask

What sound do you hear at the beginning of *now, note,* and *nice*?
Hear it, make it. *Nnnnow, Nnnote. Nnnnnice.*
N is the sound.

Some word strings include

boots, bag, bus	bus, born, best	wow, way, week
lab, long, look	say, sad, said	now, note, nice
get, gone, got	purse, point, put	heart, hand, hard
chalk, cheese, choice	time, tune, told	wrote, ride, read
desk, day, done	week, wink, want	

PLAY **Clap-and-Count.**

Children clap to, and then count, the syllables heard in the compound words from the story. Demonstrate by clapping to a word and then asking children how many parts they heard. For example, clap and say

lunch
How many parts in the word? Clap it out. (one)
Lunch. One.

Clap and say

lunchroom
How many parts in that word? Clap it out. (two)
Lunch-room. One, two.

Use a puppet named Lilly to demonstrate the game by opening and closing its mouth to indicate the syllables. Stress and elongate the syllables when presenting the following compound words:

(continues on next page)

PLAY Clap-and-Count. *Continued*

lunchroom	classroom	sunglasses
classmates	hallways	lightbulb
became	everything	semicircle
hairdresser		

Then count syllables in longer words, such as

e-ra-ser	am-bu-lance	de-mon-stra-ted
fa-bu-lous	in-cre-di-ble	en-cy-clo-pe-di-as
gli-tter-y	con-si-der-ate	un-co-o-per-a-tive
ex-ce-llent		

PLAY Find-the-Little-Words.

Children listen for "little" words that make up the compound words of the text. Stress and elongate syllables when presenting the word. For example, say

sunglasses
Can you hear any little words in *sunglasses*? (sun, glass, glasses)
That's right. *Sun* is a little word in *sunglasses*.
Glasses is another little word in *sunglasses*.
And *glass* is another little word in *sunglasses*.

Continue with the first list of compound words, then proceed with the following two-syllable words, changing the stress pattern as necessary so children hear all the "little" words.

pur-ple (purr, pull)	plas-tic (tick)	tas-ty (taste, tea)
shi-ny (shy, knee)	squea-ky (squeak, key)	men-tion (men)
pic-tures (pick)	draw-ing (draw)	
de-light (light)	pen-cil (pen)	

PLAY What's-the-Word?

Children synthesize two syllables into a word. Use pictures in the book as cues, if needed. Present the syllables, inserting a clear pause between them, and have children say them quickly and repeatedly until they can recognize the word. Demonstrate first, as in

pur-ple
What's the word?
Say it until you hear it. *Purrrrr-ple. Purrr-ple. Purple.*
Purple is the word.

Continue first with the compound and then with the two-syllable words in Clap-and-Count.

PLAY **Leave-It-Out.**

Children say a compound or two-syllable word, then leave out the beginning or final part to create a smaller word. For example, say

> Say *lunchroom*.
> Now, say *lunchroom*, but leave out *room*.
> What little word is left? (lunch)

Then say

> Now, say *lunchroom*, but leave out *lunch*.
> What little word is left? (room)

Continue with the list of compound words provided.

PLAY **Add-It-On.**

Children put two syllables together to make two-syllable words. For example, say

> Say *sun*.
> Now, say *sun*, and add *glasses*.
> What bigger word can you make? (sunglasses)

Then reverse the order in which the words are presented. For example, say

> Put *glasses* at the end of *sun*. What word do you have? (sunglasses)

Continue with the list of compound words provided.

PLAY **Turn-It-Around.**

Children reverse the parts of the compound words previously analyzed and synthesized, as in

> Put the word *room* at the beginning of *lunch*.
> What word do you have? (roomlunch)
> What was it before we turned it around? (lunchroom)

Continue with the list of compound words provided.

PLAY **Switch-It.**

Children delete part of a compound or two-syllable word and exchange it with a new part to make another compound word. Prompt with cues as necessary. For example, say

> Say *sunglasses*.
> Now say *sunglasses*, only take out *sun* and put in *eye*.
> What new word can you make? (eyeglasses)

(continues on next page)

PLAY Switch-It. *Continued*

Some word switches include

> *Lunchroom.* Take out *lunch* and put in *class.* (classroom)
> *Classmates.* Take out *class* and put in *ship.* (shipmates)
> *Lightbulb.* Take out *bulb* and put in *house.* (lighthouse)
> *Became.* Take out *came* and put in *ware.* (beware)
> *Hairdresser.* Take out *dresser* and put in *cut.* (haircut)

➤ Phonological awareness games continue in the catalog for Grades 1 through 5.

Note: This book is also available in a French translation and Spanish translation, titled *Lily y su bolsa de plastico.*

Little Green

by Keith Baker
San Diego, CA: Harcourt, 2001

Suggested Grade and Interest Level: Pre-K

Topic Explorations: Birds; Creativity

Skill Builders:

Vocabulary	**Grammar and syntax**
Prepositions	Two- and three-word utterances
Morphological units	Noun–verb agreement
	Present tense

Synopsis: This is a lovely book for young children. A boy is fascinated by the flight of a hummingbird. He cleverly paints the flight of "Little Green" it as it zig-zags and loops around his garden. The rhyming text describes the hummingbird's journey in a few brief words that are ideal for language expansion. The illustrations are of cut-paper collage and are light and airy in strong primary colors.

Method: Before the read-aloud, lead children into the story by talking about hummingbirds and their special features. How is it that hummingbirds can stay in one place as they fly? Can you see their wings when they fly? What do they look like? How fast do you think their wings can move? How would you paint a hummingbird?

During the read-aloud, allow children to enjoy the pictures and words as you read the short, rhyming verse without interruption.

After the read-aloud, revisit the pages and encourage children to take part in the words of the story. Help build understanding and usage of prepositions by building on the words in the story, such as *in, between, around, up,* and *down.* Point out the positions of the hummingbird while constructing short phrases for repetition.

As you go back through the pages, find the tiny caterpillar on every two-page spread. Ask children to describe, from the caterpillar's point of view, what is happening on the pages. What does she see? The many action words on the page can easily be used to help structure two- and three-word utterances and sentences containing noun–verb agreement and present tense. For example, the text reads

"sip, sip, sipping"

Possible constructions include

He sips   He loops
He dips   Little Green hums
The boy paints   The boy watches

In another example, the text reads

"going, coming,
stopping, starting,
softly humming,
dashing, darting"

Possible constructions include

The bird is humming.
The bird is softly humming.
The little bird is softly humming beside the flower.
The bird is stopping.
He is stopping in front of the boy.

For developing morphological units, play Find-the-Little-Word. Present the text and illustration, "Sip, sip, sipping." Ask students to listen to the word *sipping*. Can they find the little word in *sipping*? Stress and elongate the syllables, then ask

What was the word before it became *sipping*? (root word *sip*)

Find more root words from words in the text.

| zipping | jigging | stopping | starting |
| jagging | dipping | dashing | darting |

For prompting, put the root word into the pattern used in the text (e.g., "zip, zip, zipping" and "jig, jig, jigging") so that children can hear the words in repetition and see how the morphological marker creates a new word.

Mama Cat Has Three Kittens

by Denise Fleming
New York: Henry Holt & Company, 1998

Suggested Grade and Interest Level: Pre-K

Topic Exploration: Animals, Cats

Skill Builders:
Vocabulary
Grammar and syntax   **Language literacy**
Two- and three-word utterances   Relating personal experiences
Noun–verb agreement   Predicting
Pronouns, personal
   and possessive

Synopsis: Fluffy, Skinny, and Boris are Mama cat's three kittens. When Mama engages in one activity (washing her paws, walking on the wall, sharpening her claws, etc.), Fluffy and Skinny do the same thing. But not Boris. He prefers to nap. Then, when Mama, Fluffy, and Skinny curl up to nap, guess who wakes up and wants to play? "An excellent choice for reading to groups," states *School Library Journal*.

Method: Read the book through once without a lot of interaction, so that the children can identify the pattern of the text. Then, reread the book, inviting children to help you tell the story.

For enhancing vocabulary skills, talk about what the words *fluffy* and *skinny* mean. Find other things to describe that are fluffy (e.g., soft pillows, grandma's hair) and skinny (e.g., little branches of trees, a crescent moon). Ask the children how they think the cats got their names.

For predicting, before a predictable moment (after the text tells and shows what Mama cat has done), ask children what Fluffy and Skinny will do next. What will Boris do?

For two- and three-word utterances, structure word combinations based on the words and the context of the illustrations. Encourage children to repeat the two or three words of the text as you read each page. For example,

Divide the children into two groups, or "voices." After reading the initial phrase

> "When Mama cat sharpens her claws"

have the first group say what happens next, using the words of the text as you supply the beginning, "Fluffy and Skinny . . . "

> First group: "Wash their paws" (or "Wash paws")

Then prompt the other group with the question and the illustration, "What does Boris do?" to which they respond

> Second group: "Boris naps."

Continue the interaction based on the pattern of the text.

For possessive pronouns, shape utterances with questions that require simple repetition of the text.

> Q: What does Mama cat wash?
> A: Her paws
> Q: What do Fluffy and Skinny wash?
> A: Their paws

For personal pronouns, shape other responses with the target structures *she, he,* and *they*.

She walks	They walk
He naps	She washes
They wash	He naps

For noun–verb agreement, shape responses to questions about what the characters do.

For relating personal experiences and generalizing the events of the story, talk about pet cats. Describe something your own cat does, if appropriate, such as rub against a chair or meow at the door. Ask children who have pet cats to describe what their cats do. Do they wash their paws like Fluffy and Skinny do? Curl up to nap like Boris? Chase leaves like Mama cat? What else?

Read also *In the Small, Small Pond* and *In the Tall, Tall Grass* by Denise Fleming.

Many Luscious Lollipops: A Book About Adjectives

by Ruth Heller
New York: Grosset and Dunlap, 1989, 1992

Suggested Grade and Interest Level: K

Skill Builders:

Vocabulary	**Grammar and syntax**
Categories	Two- and three-word utterances
Adjectives	
Morphological units	

Synopsis: This book about adjectives in Ruth Heller's entertaining language series captivates young ones with its imaginative designs and expressive words. It also teaches comparatives and superlatives (e.g., *taller* and *tallest*, *more* and *most*, *less* and *least*).

Method: Before the read-aloud, discuss how descriptive words can make what we say more interesting. Show the differences between two sentences, asking which sentence tells more. For example,

> That's my cat.
> That's my big, gray, soft, cuddly cat.

Define adjectives as "describing words" before introducing the book. Tell the children they will hear lots of information about these special words, but the important thing to remember is how nice they make our language sound.

Read aloud and practice expanding utterances using the adjectives presented. Talk about the meanings of the words presented, including the longer words, such as *asteroidial* and *universal*. Then encourage the children to use the words in sentences they create themselves.

Also, brainstorm other adjectives. For example, the text reads, "twelve, large, beautiful, blue, gorgeous butterflies." Ask the children what other words they can think of to describe butterflies (e.g., *colorful, fluttery, pretty, small*, and *delicate*). Continue to brainstorm other adjectives to describe the people, animals, objects, and ideas presented.

For categories, group objects shown in the book. For example, pause on the butterfly page and ask children if they can name some other pretty insects, such as ladybugs, grasshoppers, and moths.

Read also *A Cache of Jewels and Other Collective Nouns* and other books in the language series by Ruth Heller.

Mary Wore Her Red Dress and Henry Wore His Green Sneakers

by Merle Peek
New York: Clarion Books, 1985; Houghton Mifflin, 1991

Suggested Grade and Interest Level: Pre-K

Topic Explorations: Colors; Folk songs

Skill Builders:

Vocabulary
Prepositions
Grammar and syntax
Two- and three-word utterances
Pronouns, personal
  and possessive
Possessive nouns
Tenses, present and past

Language literacy
Relating personal experiences
Verbal expression

Synopsis: The text adopts an old Texas folk song about children coming to a party, each wearing a unique article of clothing in a different color.

Method: Don't miss this one! Not with all the opportunities it brings for language stimulation. Begin by asking children what they like to wear to parties. Obtain a variety of responses. (Ideal for reading on a child's birthday.)

For early utterances, encourage the child to join in at the repeated portions of the text ("all day long" or "red dress, red dress"). Pause to reinforce each utterance by asking a question that elicits the same response (e.g., What did Mary wear?).

For pronouns and possessive nouns, ask

> Whose red dress? (Mary's)
> Whose violet ribbons? (Stacy's)
> What did Henry wear? (His green shoes)
> What else did Ryan wear? (His star shirt)

For prepositions, ask questions, such as the following, based on the illustrations:

> Where's Mary's present? (Under her arm)
> Where's Henry's present? (Over his head)
> Where's Amanda's blindfold? (Around her head)
> Where are Katy's presents? (Beside her chair)
> Where is Henry sitting? (On top of the gazebo)

For verbal expression and relating personal experiences, go back over each page to discover what happened at Katy Bear's party. Talk about other parties children have attended. How were they like Katy Bear's?

Extended Activities: Expand on the idea of the bears' clothing and extend the verse to include children in the class. Ask the children to identify what they are wearing. Then respond with a verse about their clothing (e.g., "Josh wore his green sweatshirt, green sweatshirt, green sweatshirt . . ." or "Juanita wore her pink flowered corduroy overalls, her pink flowered corduroy overalls . . .").

Expand on the idea to target present and past tense. For example, say

> "Who slid down the slide, down the slide, down the slide?
> Who slid down the slide, all recess long?
> Juan slid down the slide, down . . ."
> "Who's looking ready to go to her desk,
> Ready to go to her desk,
> Ready to go to her desk,
> Who's looking ready to go to her desk, at this time?"

Note: Printed on the last page is music for the accompaniment.

May I Bring a Friend?

by Beatrice Schenk de Regniers
New York: Atheneum, 1964, 1971, 1989

Suggested Grade and Interest Level: Pre-K

Topic Explorations: Animals, Zoo; Friendship; Humor, Manners and etiquette

Skill Builders:

Vocabulary	**Language literacy**	**Pragmatic language**
Prepositions	Predicting	**Articulation,** *K*
Grammar and syntax		
Question structures		

Synopsis: A little boy responds to the king and queen's invitation to tea and brings his friends. The king and queen are indeed very gracious to receive an elephant, a giraffe, a rhinoceros, and everything else that comes through the castle doors. Written in repetitive, rhyming verse, with the refrain, "So I brought my friend."

Method: Before the read-aloud, elicit prediction questions with the book's cover. Ask children where they think the story will take place and who might be invited to see the king and queen.

During the read-aloud, pause to elicit question structures, such as "May I bring a friend?" Have children predict what might happen each time the king and queen invite the boy to tea. What type of friend do the children think the boy will invite this time? For language pragmatics, talk about the boy's use of language when asking the king and queen if he could bring a friend. What words did he use? Why is it always important to first ask? Why is politeness important?

After reading a page, elicit target words relating to activities in the illustrations.
For example,

> Q: Who invited him to tea?
> A: The king and queen
> Q: What did the queen do?
> A: Kissed him
> Q: Where did his friend sit?
> A: Next to him
> Q: What were they having on the elephant's back?
> A: Breakfast

After the story, talk about the events, and discuss the use of the boy's language. In what situations might the children need to ask permission to bring a friend? When going to a party? When they want to bring home another child from school? When leaving the classroom to go to the office? Have children practice throughout the day using the language "May I bring a friend?" For articulation, structure responses to target correct articulation of *K* in progressively longer utterances.

Mike Mulligan and His Steam Shovel

by Virginia Lee Burton
New York: Scholastic, 1939

Suggested Grade and Interest Level: Pre-K

Topic Explorations: Cities; Community; Construction and buildings

Skill Builders:

Vocabulary
Beginning concepts (spatial)
Categories
Prepositions
Morphological units

Grammar and syntax
Tenses, present and past
Phonological awareness

Synopsis: Mike and his steam shovel Mary Anne have had quite a history together, digging great canals through the mountains and excavating earth to erect big city skyscrapers. But with the end of the industrialization era comes the modernization of trucks and other heavy equipment, and Mike and his steam shovel are no longer needed. Finding themselves in the little town of Popperville, they make a bid to dig the cellar for a new town hall, promising the townspeople that if they can't dig it in just one day they'll accept no payment. Although they meet their deadline, they create a new problem: how to dig themselves out of the hole! It is the small boy in the crowd who comes up with the clever answer.

Methods: Before the read-aloud, talk about shovels and digging and how the roads we drive on and the houses we live in often need to be built first by moving dirt and digging holes in the ground. Elicit children's background knowledge about tractors, loaders, and earthmovers as you present the book's cover.

During the read-aloud, pause at times to explain the illustrations depicting the work that Mike and his steam shovel do. Build story meaning by discussing vocabulary, including

steam shovel	bulldozer
canal	cellar
diesel (motor)	rusty
junk	skyscrapers

After the read-aloud, use the text and illustrations for a lesson on prepositions and spatial concepts. Words from the text and illustrations include *through, under, beside, in,* and *along.* Use toys in the sandbox with phrases such as "digging deeper," "digging under," "going through," and so on to illustrate concepts and generalize the meaning of words.

For present and past tense, play word games with *dig, digging,* and *dug.*

Have the children fill in the missing word of your sentence. For example, say

Mike and his steam shovel did a lot of _____. (digging)
There were many deep holes that they _____. (dug)

PLAY I'll-Say-a-Word-That-Isn't-Right-and-You-Fix-It.

For example, say

"Mike's steam shovel _shimmed_ the great canals." (dug)
"Mike and Mary Anne _skinned_ through the mountains so the trains could get through." (dug)
"Mary Ann was a great steam shovel that _nugged_ many roads." (dug)
"Mike and Mary Anne are _wugging_ out the dirt for a new town hall." (digging)

For teaching morphological units, use the comparison words repeated throughout the story (e.g., *fast/faster, deep/deeper, better, low/lower, smooth/smoother, straight/straighter, tall/taller*) to teach the phonological marker -*er.* Some examples include

(continues on next page)

PLAY **I'll-Say-a-Word-That-Isn't-Right-and-You-Fix-It.** *Continued*

"Mike and Mary Anne dug fast. When people stood and watched, they dug even _____." (faster)

"They worked fast, but the new steam shovels could work _____." (faster)

"When the teacher called a long recess and the whole school came to watch, Mike Mulligan and Mary Anne dug still _____ and still _____." (faster, better)

"That skyscraper is tall, but this skyscraper is even _____." (taller)

Name other types of heavy equipment to increase children's skills in categorization. Some examples include tractors, backhoes, loaders, scrapers, excavators, dump trucks, and bulldozers. Ask, What are they all called? Use the words of the text to play phonological awareness games, beginning at the child's developmental level.

PLAY **Clap-and-Count.**

Children clap to, and then count, the number of syllables they hear. Demonstrate by clapping to a word, stressing and elongating the syllables, while the children count. For example, clap and say

air
How many parts in the word? Clap it out. (one)

Clap and say

airplane
How many parts in that word? Clap it out. (two)
Air–plane. One, two.

Use a puppet to demonstrate syllables by opening and closing its mouth to indicate the syllables. Continue with the following compound words from the text:

airplane	skyscraper	Booperville
railroad	steamshovel	Kopperville
sundown	newspaper	earthmover
postman	Popperville	bulldozer
milkman	Bangerville	everywhere

PLAY **Leave-It-Out.**

Children say a word, then leave out the beginning or final part to create a smaller word. For example, say

Say *airplane.*

Then say

Now, say *airplane*, but leave out *plane.*
What little word is left? (air)

(continues on next page)

PLAY **Leave-It-Out.** *Continued*

Then say

> Now, say *airplane*, but leave out *air*.
> What little word is left? (plane)

PLAY **Add-It-On.**

Children put two little words together to make a big word. For example, say

> Say *bull*.

Then say

> Now, say *bull*, and add *dozer*.
> What big word can you make? (bulldozer)

Then, reverse the order in which the words are presented. For example, say

> Put *dozer* at the end of *bull*. What word do you have? (bulldozer)

PLAY **Turn-It-Around.**

Children reverse the parts of a word they have previously analyzed and synthesized. For example, say

> Put the word *dozer* at the beginning of *man*.
> What word do you have? (dozerbull)
> What was it before we turned it around? (bulldozer)

PLAY **Switch-It.**

Children delete part of a compound word and switch it with a new part to make a new word. Prompt with cues if necessary. For example, say

> Say *airplane*.
> Now, say *airplane*, only take out *plane* and add *port*.
> What new word can you make? (airport)

Some word switches include

> *railroad* to *railcar*
> *sundown* to *sunup*
> *postman* to *postoffice*
> *milkman* to *milkcarton*
> *newspaper* to *newsstand*
> *Popperville* to *Rockerville*
> *Bangerville* to *Jumperville*

(continues on next page)

> **PLAY** ▷ **Switch-It.** *Continued*
>
> *Booperville* to *Superville*
> *everywhere* to *nowhere*
> *earthmover* to *dirtmover*

Note: For more than 60 years, this classic has continued to engage and delight the minds and hearts of the young. For its longstanding and endearing quality, it is included in this compendium of books that inspire and motivate children to talk. Because of the number of pages and words, language activities are recommended over an extended period of time.

Mr. Gumpy's Outing

by John Burningham
Orlando, FL: Holt, Rinehart & Winston, 1978, 1990

Suggested Grade and Interest Level: Pre-K

Topic Explorations: Animals, Farm; Boats; Country life; Journeys

Skill Builders:

Vocabulary	**Language literacy**
Grammar and syntax	Predicting
Possessive nouns	**Articulation, G**
Negative structures	
Question structures	

Synopsis: Mr. Gumpy goes for a ride on the river in his boat. As he paddles along, various animal friends ask to come. Mr. Gumpy agrees, but with the stipulation that they are not to cause a fuss. As the animals continue to accumulate in the boat, the inevitable happens.

Method: Before the read-aloud, introduce the book and ask children if they can explain the meaning of the word *outing*. Encourage them to give some examples and relate their experiences, such as when they may have gone for a ride. What are the various ways to "go for a ride?"

During the read-aloud, pause to elicit grammatical structures. For possessive nouns, ask whose boat the animals are in, whose house they are having tea at, and whose outing it was originally supposed to be. To practice question structures, ask the children to repeat the animals' requests to come along.

For negative structures, rephrase Mr. Gumpy's responses. For example, say

> He can't squabble
> He can't hop

Extended Activity: Make enough tagboard templates for the animals in the story so that they can be evenly distributed (the outlines can be traced from illustrations, or the illustrations can be projected onto tagboard using an overhead projector). Distribute the animals and allow the children to color them any color they wish. Affix a craft stick to each piece of tagboard as a handle, then reread the story. Children can participate by raising their puppets while reciting in unison what their animal says.

The Mitten: A Ukrainian Folktale

by Jan Brett
New York: Putnam, 1989, 1990

Suggested Grade and Interest Level: Pre-K

Topic Explorations: Animals, Forest; Folklore, Ukranian; Humor; Owls; Seasons, Winter

Skill Builders:

Vocabulary	Language literacy	
Attributes	Predicting	Drawing inferences
	Verbal expression	Discussion

Synopsis: Against her better judgment, Nicky's grandmother knits him white mittens. When Nicky leaves for the forest, one mitten falls on the snow and becomes home to an increasing number of animals. The border pictures build anticipation for the next approaching animal; they also show Nicky in the woods, unaware of his lost mitten. As an unbelievable number of increasingly larger animals share the cozy habitat, a surprising event reunites Nicky and his mitten—on the order of a big sneeze and a lucky catch!

Method: Before the read-aloud, elicit children's prior knowledge about forest animals, then introduce them to the names of the animals in the story. Ask what they know about hedgehogs. Talk about how hedgehogs' prickles are like those of porcupines. Ask children what they know about owls. Talk about owls having talons, just like eagles. Discuss badgers and their passion for digging.

During the read-aloud, pause to talk about the border pictures that show what is happening to Nicky in a different part of the forest as his mitten is filling up with animals. Once the pattern of the story is established, ask children whether they can predict, based on the border picture, which animal will come to the mitten next.

For drawing inferences, draw on prior knowledge to discuss the animals' reactions. Ask why the mole and rabbit didn't want to argue with anyone that had prickles. What was it about the owl's "glinty talons" that made the other animals quickly let him inside? Why did they offer the thumb of the mitten to the badger, after seeing his "diggers?"

For attributes, name the reasons the animals liked the mitten (e.g., it was white, good for camouflage, warm, soft, etc.).

Discuss the absurdities. What's funny about a mole and a rabbit being inside a boy's mitten? What's funny about a mole, a rabbit, and a hedgehog being inside a mitten? What about a mole, a rabbit, a hedgehog, and an owl inside a mitten? Also, ask what is funny about Nicky's grandmother's expression when she examines the stretched-out mitten. Do you think she knows what happened? Do you think she can figure it out?

The Mixed-Up Chameleon

by Eric Carle
New York: HarperCollins, 1975, 1984, 1988

Suggested Grade and Interest Level: Pre-K

Topic Explorations: Animals, Zoo; Colors; Humor; Part–whole relationships; Self-esteem

Skill Builders:

Vocabulary	**Language literacy**
Associations	Cause-and-effect
Attributes	relationships
Grammar and syntax	Compare and contrast
Possessive nouns	Verbal expression
	Discussion

Synopsis: Believing its life was not that exciting, a chameleon goes to a zoo. Wishing it were more like the animals it sees, the chameleon begins to adopt their characteristics. The chameleon becomes an increasingly hilarious, mixed-up mess of different animal parts, losing its identity. Finally (thankfully), it decides it likes itself better the way it is—a plain old chameleon.

Method: Begin by asking children what they know about chameleons. Discuss chameleons' characteristics and lead into the story by looking at the title and story predictions.

During the reading, pause for children to identify the colors the chameleon turns. Ask them to compare and contrast the animals by describing how the chameleon is like and unlike different things in the story.

For possessive nouns and attributes, pause to have children identify each animal part the chameleon acquires. As the chameleon adds more parts (reindeer's antlers, fish's fins, giraffe's neck, etc.), pause to recall from which animals they came. The tabs on the left show the original animals. For example, look at the polar bear tab to recall how the chameleon became big and white. Next, look at the flamingo tab and recall how the chameleon got pink wings and stilt-like legs. Continue in this way as you pause to tell the story of how the chameleon becomes so mixed up.

After the read-aloud, ask children to explain why the chameleon was so mixed up. What caused the chameleon to grow fins? What caused it to grow a giraffe's neck, and so on? Talk about what caused the chameleon to turn itself back into a chameleon. Then hold a discussion about the importance of liking yourself the way you are. Have all the children share something unique about themselves.

Extended Activities: Make felt animal parts to use on a felt board. Trace patterns for the different animal parts from the book's illustrations, then cut out different-colored felt pieces. Have children put the pieces on a felt board, labeling the parts and creating their own mixed-up chameleons.

Make a "collage chameleon." Trace the outline of the chameleon from one of the pages in the book. Transfer it to a stencil or onto paper for each child. Gather pipe cleaners for reindeer antlers, cotton balls for polar bear fur, red yarn for a fox tail, orange tissue paper for fish fins, and purple tissue paper for seal flippers. Have children paste these parts onto the outline to make their own mixed-up chameleon.

Note: This book is available in many different languages, including Arabic, Bengali, Chinese, Somali, Tamil, and Urdu.

Mouse Mess

by Linnea Riley
New York: Scholastic, 1997

Suggested Grade and Interest Level: Pre-K

Topic Explorations: Colors; Food; Messes; Shapes and visual images

Skill Builders:

Vocabulary	Grammar and syntax	Language literacy
Beginning concepts	Two- and three-word utterances	Sequencing
(sizes, colors, and shapes)	Noun–verb agreement	**Phonological awareness**
Categories	Present tense	Articulation—*F, M, K, B,* and *P*

Synopsis: A little mouse listens for the "all-clear" sign of human feet retreating up the stairs, then comes out of his cozy house for a midnight snack in the kitchen. Very shortly, Ritz crackers, Oreo cookies, and corn flakes spill about and clutter the counter, joining cheese, olives, peanut butter, and fruit in the messiest, jumbled-up kitchen counter you've ever seen. Short rhyming verse with plenty of "crunch-crunch, crackle-sweep" sound effects accompanies delectable pictures that take the reader through a sequence of rascally mouse actions. To finish his night's work, the mouse turns on the faucet, takes a bath in a teacup, and leaves for home just before the family (seen in silhouette) comes down for breakfast. This little sleeper is charming and rich with possibilities.

Method: Before the read-aloud, spend a few minutes identifying the mouse and all the different food items on the cover.

Read the story through without interruption while children connect with the pictures and the rhythm and flow of the short, rhyming text.

After the read-aloud, do a picture walk-through and pause at every page to describe the mouse's actions. Use the illustrations to elicit grammar and syntax constructions. Some possible constructions include

Mouse mess	Little mouse	Rakes corn flakes
Milk spills out	Pour and pat	Mouse is up
Time to eat	Mouse steps back	He looks around
Mouse climbs	Mouse rakes	Mouse tastes
Milk spills	Water flows	Food scatters
Mouse eats	Mouse sweeps	

Some possibilities for present-tense sentences (with optional prepositional phrases) include

> The mouse is building sandcastles with brown sugar.
> He is raking corn flakes into piles with a fork.
> He is jumping into the corn flakes.
> He is spreading peanut butter and jam onto the bread.
> He is popping the tops off the bottles.
> He is soaking the jam between his toes.
> He leaves the mess and goes into his little house.

While doing a picture walk-through, sequence the actions of the story—from the mouse sleeping in his little house, to him leaving the kitchen, to the mess he made, and then to him going back home to bed. Say, "Let's follow little mouse on this night and be the narrator, telling about what he does." Then have children take turns telling the action of the story, using the illustrations.

The vivid illustrations in large, eye-catching, cut-paper compositions are set against black backgrounds and framed in bright colors. Take the opportunity they provide to teach names of colors and various sizes and shapes (e.g., the round Ritz crackers, the round Oreo cookies, the curly corn flakes, the triangular cheese, the curved banana, the round oranges, the oval-shaped olives, the rectangular box, etc.).

For phonological awareness training, first reread the text, then play the series of games, depending on the level of students' phonological sensitivity.

PLAY **Word-Count.**

Children count the number of words in a short line from the text. Demonstrate by assigning one word to one finger as you say the words. For example, say

Mouse Mess

as you hold up one finger for each word until two fingers are showing. Ask

How many words did I say?

Gradually allow the children to do the counting by themselves.

If children don't have one-to-one correspondence, give each child a collection of manipulables (i.e., blocks, felt squares, buttons, etc.) to use for representing each of the stated words. Demonstrate by saying (or use a puppet to say) the words from a page of text that you want the children to count. Repeat them again as you (or a puppet) move out one item at a time to correspond to your stated word. Then you (or a puppet) count out loud the number of blocks moved to get the word count. Gradually allow the children to do the counting by themselves. Use words directly from a page of the text in hierarchical order to the desired word length. Some words from the text to count include

"On the stairs
The sound of feet
Mouse is up
It's time to eat!"
"Crunch-crunch
He wants a cracker
Munch-munch, a cookie snacker."

PLAY **Which-Word-Is-Missing?**

Children identify a word from a word string that has been omitted from the previously given string. For example, say

mouse, stairs, feet, eat
stairs, feet, eat
Which word is missing? (mouse)
That's right. *Mouse* is the word that is missing.

Here are some word strings. Present one-syllable word strings first.

milk, food, jam, bread
jump, pile, milk, cheese
rake, corn flakes, jump
cheese, milk, sniff, like
mess, pour, pat, wall
mess, believe, found, mouse
water, bubbles, toes, bath
cracker, munch, cookie, fork
olives, pickles, catsup, mustard

PLAY **Rearrange-It.**

Children rearrange, in correct word order, a scrambled phrase or sentence from a portion of the text.

For example, say

> *Mess Mouse*
> Is that the title of the book? Can you help me say it right?
> That's right. *Mess Mouse* should really be *Mouse Mess.*

More words to rearrange include

Wet it's	Around looks he
A mouse little	Steps mouse back
Mouse little hush	House inside his
Up is mouse	Cracker he wants a
He's taking out it	That's a castle not
A big mess he is making	Out milk the spills

PLAY **The Same-Sound game.**

Children identify whether word pairs begin with the same sound. For example, say

> mouse, mess
> Do they start with the same sound? (Yes)

Intersperse nonalliterative words into the following sets to make odd pairs, such as *mouse, feet.* Present one-syllable words first.

hush, house	food, feet
fed, found	fun, found
pour, pat	mess, make
jam, jump	pop, pickle
milk, mouse	pickles, peanuts
catsup, castle	gurgle, gooey
splish, splash	toes, top, taste

PLAY **Word-Search.**

Children search for a word found in an illustrated page from the book that begins with the same sound as a target word. For example, say

> I see something in this picture starts with the same sound as *pie.*
> What other word starts with *p?*
> That's right. *Pickle* starts with *p.*

Word sources are available on each page.

> **PLAY** **Finish-the-Rhyme.**

Children supply the rhyming word left out at the end of a verse. Provide the initial phoneme cue or prompt by pointing to the illustration, if needed. For example, say

> "Olives, pickles, catsup—fun!
> Pop the tops off, one by _____." (one)

> "Sticky-gooey, jam to spread
> with peanut butter smeared on _____." (bread)

> **PLAY** **Rhyme-It-Again.**

Children identify the rhyming word you read after each set. Give phoneme and picture cues as needed. For example, say

> "*Fun* rhymes with _____."
> "*Spread* rhymes with (br) _____."

> **PLAY** **Do-They-Rhyme?**

Children identify whether word pairs rhyme. Intersperse an unrhymed word into the following rhyming sets to make unmatched sets:

eat, feet	cheese, these	straw, paw
falls, walls	spread, bread	eat, treat
house, mouse	cracker, snacker	splash, flash
flows, toes	flakes, makes	sleep, leap
ted, bed		

> **PLAY** **Make-a-Rhyme.**

Children supply another rhyming word after a rhyming set is presented. Give initial phoneme cues, if needed. For example, ask

> What words rhymes with *eat*? *Eat, feet,* (m) _____
> (also *Pete, beat, neat, seat, wheat, sheet, cheat,* or any rhyming nonsense word)

> **PLAY** **Clap-and-Count.**

Children clap to, and then count, the number of syllables heard in the word. Demonstrate by clapping to a word and then asking children how many parts they heard. For example, clap and say

> crack
> How many parts in the word? Clap it out. (one)

(continues on next page)

PLAY **Clap-and-Count.** *Continued*

Clap and say

> cracker
> How many parts in that word? Clap it out. (two)
> That's right. Cra–cker. One, two.

A mouse puppet can also demonstrate by opening and closing its mouth to indicate the syllables. Stress and elongate the following words when presenting them:

sna-cker	coo-kie	be-lieve
a-sleep	pi-ckles	
in-side	a-round	

PLAY **What's-the-Word?**

Children synthesize syllables into words using words from the pictures in the book. Present the syllables with a clear pause between them and have the children say them quickly and repeatedly, until they can identify the word. For example, say

> pea–nut
> What's the word?
> Say it until you hear it. *Peeeeeea–nut. Peeea-nut. Peanut.*
> *Peanut* is the word.

Continue with the two-syllable words provided in Clap-and-Count.

PLAY **Find-the-Little-Words.**

Children listen for "little" words within the two-syllable words of the text. Stress and elongate syllables when presenting. For example, say

> asleep
> Can you find any little words in *asleep*. (a, sleep)
> That's right. *A* is a little word in *asleep*.
> *Sleep* is another little word in *asleep*.

Continue with the list of compound and two-syllable words given in Clap-and-Count.

PLAY **Leave-It-Out.**

Children say a compound or two-syllable word, then leave out the beginning or final part to create a smaller word. For example, say

> Say *asleep*.
> Now say *asleep* but leave out *sleep*.
> What little word is left? (a)

(continues on next page)

> **PLAY** **Leave-It-Out.** *Continued*
>
> Then say
>
>> Now say *asleep* but leave out *a*.
>> What little word is left? (sleep)
>
> Continue with the list of words provided in Clap-and-Count.

> **PLAY** **Add-It-On.**
>
> Children put little words and two syllables together to make a compound or two-syllable word. Demonstrate first, by saying
>
>> Say *a*.
>> Now, say *a* and add *sleep*.
>> What big word can you make? (asleep)
>> That's right. *A-sleep. Asleep.*
>
> Then reverse the order in which the word is presented. For example, say
>
>> Put *sleep* at the end of *a*.
>> What word do you have? (asleep)
>> That's right. *A-sleep. Asleep.*
>
> Continue with the words provided in Clap-and-Count.

☞ See the catalog for Grades 1 through 5 for continuing activities in the hierarchy of phonological awareness.

For articulation therapy, use the words of the text to elicit production at various levels.

For *F:* food, feet, falls, fun, found, fed, fork, off, knife, leaf, flag

For *M:* mouse, mess, milk, mustard, jam

For *K:* key, candle, kitchen, cracker, cookie, corn, milk, castle, catsup, pickles, cord, fork, soak(s), flake(s), rake(s), make(s), back

For *B:* bell, back, bubble, bath, bed, banana

For *P:* pile, peanut, pickles, pour, pat, pop, top, people, up, cup, apple, catsup, tip(ing), slip(ping)

The Napping House

by Audrey Wood
San Diego, CA: Harcourt Brace Jovanovich, 1984, 1991

Suggested Grade and Interest Level: Pre-K

Topic Exploration: Weather

Skill Builders:

Vocabulary	**Language literacy**
Adjectives	Predicting
Morphological units	Sequencing
Grammar and syntax	Cause-and-effect relationships
Present tense	

Synopsis: What happens in this house at naptime is most unusual. The inhabitants dream, doze, snore, snooze, and slumber—all stacked on top of one another! The littlest starts a chain reaction, causing them all to wake, one by one. Watch the dark, rainy sky change to a bright and sunny one, illustrating the passage of time.

Method: Before the read-aloud, introduce the story by talking about napping. See if children can think of other words that mean the same thing. Direct children to listen to see if they hear any of those words during the reading of the book.

During the read-aloud, read the cumulative text and pause to discuss the meanings of all the words used to denote sleeping. Continue to encourage children to think of other words and phrases, such as *rest* and *take a break*. Model or shape sentences with present tense by asking questions throughout the story. Direct children to the clues in the illustrations and ask them to predict what will happen next.

For morphological units, encourage children to talk about how the bed sags lower and lower, deeper and deeper. Continue to talk about how the bed gets heavier and heavier (which is the heaviest?), but the inhabitants get lighter and lighter, smaller and smaller, while the room gets darker and darker, then lighter and lighter, or brighter and brighter.

After the read-aloud, go back to find where the little mouse and the flea were located in each of the pictures. For sequencing and cause-and-effect relationships, ask children to take turns telling what happened after the granny fell asleep, after the boy climbed on top, and so on. Give children hints based on the sizes of the characters, then ask what happened when the flea landed on the mouse. What did the flea do? What happened because of this? Help children structure sentences using the conjunctions *because* and *so*.

Note: This book is also available in a Spanish translation, titled *La casa adormecida.*

Night in the Country

by Cynthia Rylant
New York: Bradbury Press, 1986; Macmillan, 1991

Suggested Grade and Interest Level: Pre-K

Topic Explorations: Country life; Nighttime; Sounds and listening

Skill Builders:

Grammar and syntax	**Language literacy**	**Phonological awareness**
Present tense	Verbal expression	

Synopsis: The quiet sounds of a night in the country are soothing and evoke restful images. Ideal for developing listening skills, calming a group, or lulling a young one to sleep.

Method: Before the read-aloud, encourage children to recall some of the sounds they hear at night. Snoring? Cars whizzing past? Clock ticking? The refrigerator motor running? Present the book and title, having children make predictions before you begin the story.

During the read-aloud, pause to encourage use of the verbs in the text, including *swoop, clink, patter,* and *nuzzle.*

After the read-aloud, recall all the sounds of a night in the country—owls hooting, frogs croaking, cats purring, screen doors creaking, the house squeaking, and so on. Then listen to sounds in the classroom. Is there any playground noise? Are there cars passing on the street? Bells ringing? Footsteps in the hall? Children's voices in the distance? Lights buzzing? Animals rustling in their cages?

Noisy Nora

by Rosemary Wells
New York: Dial Books for Young Readers, 1973, 1980; Puffin, 2000

Suggested Grade and Interest Level: Pre-K

Topic Exploration: Family relationships

Skill Builders:

Vocabulary	**Language literacy**
Morphological units	Relating personal experiences
Grammar and syntax	Storytelling
Noun–verb agreement	Drawing inferences
Present tense	

Synopsis: This story, in rhyming verse, tells about the naughty antics Nora uses to get attention while her mother tends to the other children. There's hardly a child who won't relate to Nora's situation with understanding.

Method: Before the read-aloud, talk about the word *noisy* and ask children to give examples of things that are noisy. Then introduce the story and its title, making predictions.

It is best to first read the verse in this short little book without pausing, then go back over the pictures and discuss what Nora is doing. Model or shape target structures.

For drawing inferences, ask the children why they think Nora was making all that noise. Why was everyone ignoring her? How do you think she felt? Was running away a good idea? Why not?

For relating personal experiences, encourage children to relate experiences of wanting attention when someone (mother, father, teacher, or baby-sitter) is too busy. What was the other person doing? Was Mommy on the phone? Was Daddy talking to Mommy? Was the family watching TV? How did you feel? Assist the children in formulating sentences that relate the inexperiences.

Extended Activity: Use role-playing to demonstrate appropriate ways to get attention. Have class members demonstrate appropriate ways to respond when they cannot get the teacher's attention. Talk about how hard it can be to wait for attention and the kinds of things children can do while waiting.

A Spanish version of text is available titled, *Julieta estate quieta.*

Noisy Poems

Collected by Jill Bennett
Oxford, England: Oxford University Press, 1987, 1989

Suggested Grade and Interest Level: Pre-K

Skill Builders:
Phonological awareness   **Articulation**
                               General articulation

Synopsis: A collection of humorous poems highlighting the versatility of how words make delightful sounds in English. Whimsical illustrations help to identify the sounds of the poems. This one is too good to miss!

Method: Poems like Spike Milligan's "Ning, Nang, Nong" demonstrate fun-loving wordplay, for example,

> "On the Ning Nang Nong
> Where the Cows go Bong!
> And the Monkeys all say Boo!
> There's a Nong Nang Ning
> Where the trees go Ping
> And the tea pots Jibber Jabber Joo."

Once children have heard the poem several times, the words are usually familiar enough for them to participate in the phonological awareness activities. The games provided are grouped under the poem selections.

For "Ning, Nang, Nong":

PLAY   **Word-Count.**

Children count the number of words in a short line from the text. Demonstrate by assigning one word to one finger as you say the words. For example, say

> Ning, nang

as you hold up one finger for each word until two fingers are showing. Ask

> How many words did I say?

Then say

> Ning, nang, nong

for a three-finger count. Gradually allow the children to do the counting by themselves.

If children don't have one-to-one correspondence, give each child a collection of manipulables (i.e., blocks, felt squares, buttons, etc.) to use for representing each of the stated words. Demonstrate by saying (or use a puppet to say) the words from a page of text that you want the children to count. Repeat them again as you (or a puppet) move out one item at a time to correspond to your stated word. Then you (or a puppet) count out loud the number of blocks moved to get the word count. Gradually allow the children to do the counting by themselves.

(continues on next page)

PLAY   **Word-Count.** *Continued*

Use words directly from a page of the text in hierarchical order to the desired word length. Some words from the text to count include

cows, go

cows, go, Bong

monkeys, all

monkeys, all, say

monkeys, all, say, Boo!

tea, pots

Jibber, Jabber

tea, pots, Jibber

tea, pots, Jibber, Jabber

PLAY   **Finish-the-Rhyme.**

Children supply the rhyming word left out at the end of a verse. Provide the initial phoneme cue and prompt by pointing to the illustration, if needed. For example, say

Help me say the words of this poem:

"On the Ning Nang _____

Where the cows go _____

And the monkeys all go Boo!

There's a Nong Nang _____

Where the trees go _____

And the tea pots Jibber Jabber _____."

Show the illustrations picturing, in cartoon style, cows uttering *bong*, trees declaring *ping*, monkeys hollering *boo*, and the successively smaller tea pots charmingly declaring *jibber, jabber,* and *joo.*

PLAY   **The Same-Sound game.**

Children identify whether alliterative word strings begin with the same sound. For example, say

ning, nang, nong

Do they start with the same sound? (Yes)

Some word strings with interspersed nonrhyming words include

ning, nang, bong

jibber, jabber, moo

ping, pong, doo

jibber, jabber, too

ting, tang, tong

jibber, jabber, joo

bang, bong, boo

ping, pong, poo

ping, pot, poo

For Elizabeth Coatworth's poem "Rhyme," the poem begins:

"I like to see a thunder storm

A dunder storm

A blunder storm

I like to see it, black and slow

Come stumbling down the hills."

PLAY **Word-Count.**

Use the illustration picturing the words for prompts. For example, ask

How many words are in _____?

I like to see
Thunder storm
I like to see it
Blunder storm
A thunder storm
Come stumbling down
Come stumbling down the hills

PLAY **Make-a-Rhyme.**

Children supply another rhyming word after a rhyming word is presented. Give initial phoneme cues, if needed. Accept any nonsense word. For example, ask

What word rhymes with *thunder*? *Thunder,* (bl) _____

More words:

plunder (thunder)   thunder (wonder)
dunder (plunder)   blunder (wonder)
wonder (thunder)

PLAY **Clap-and-Count.**

Children clap to, and then count, the number of syllables heard in selected words from the illustrations and text. Demonstrate by clapping to a word and then asking children how many parts they heard. For example, clap and say

plunder
How many parts in the word? Clap it out. (two)
Plun–der. One, two.

Stress and elongate syllables when presenting words, such as

plun-der   thun-der   dun-der
blun-der   won-der   stum-bling
hills   storm   storm-ing

For Jack Prelutsky's poem, "The Yak":
Some one- two- and three-syllable nonsense words include

yak   yackety   sliggildy
zag   sniggildy   zaggildy
yickity   snaggildy   scriffily

Have children make up more nonsense words. Some suggestions include *miggildy, maggildy, swiggildy, swaggildy, wickidy, wackidy, clackity, rackity.*

For "Song of the Train":
Play the Same-Sound and Clap-and-Count games with the words of the text.

For "Sampan" by Tao Lang Pee:
Play rhyming games with the words, including *lap, flap, clap, tap.*

For articulation, poems like Tao Lang Pee's "Sampan" offer *P, K,* and *T* phonemes.

Officer Buckle and Gloria

by Peggy Rathmann
New York: Putnam, 1995

Suggested Grade and Interest Level: Pre-K

Topic Explorations: Animals, Dogs; Careers; Safety; School activities

Skill Builders:

Grammar and syntax	**Language literacy**
Tenses, present and past	Predicting
Pronouns, personal and possessive	Sequencing
Negative structures	Cause-and-effect relationships
Question structures	

Synopsis: No one heeds Officer Buckle's safety rules he so earnestly presents to the neighboring schools until Gloria, the police dog, joins him onstage. The little dog is so extraordinarily entertaining that the children and teachers finally start observing the rules. Their performances become very popular, but when Office Buckle realizes that Gloria is the real attraction, he is downhearted and sends her to the next assembly by herself. Feeling lonely without Officer Buckle, Gloria gets stage fright. Without anything to say, she is a flop, and the teachers and students revert to their unsafe ways. A set of calamitous events ensues, which leads to Officer Buckle's return with the pronouncement of Safety Tip 101: Always stick with your buddy. The Caldecott Medal winner is hilarious, endearing, and a great way to present safety issues—which says a great deal about the ways that children learn best, doesn't it?

Method: Before the read-aloud, elicit background knowledge about the word *safety,* and have children recall some safety rules. Ask children to listen to whether Officer Buckle says any of the ones they remember.

During the read-aloud, keep interaction to a minimum, allowing the children to connect with the words and pictures of the story.

After the read-aloud, use the words and illustrations to help build grammar and syntax skills within the context of the story. For developing negative structures, use Officer Buckle's safety lessons to model for repetition. For example,

> "Never stand on a swivel chair."
> "Never take other people's medicine."
> "Never play with matches."
> "Nobody ever listens."

For developing present-progressive tense structures, model and shape portions of the text, as applicable. Pictures offer opportunities for describing Gloria's actions onstage. Read Officer Buckle's rules and have the children describe how Gloria demonstrates what happens when you don't follow the rules. For example,

Rule: Always wipe up spills before someone slips and falls.
Possible sentences: Gloria is slipping; Gloria is sliding on her nose (with her tail-end in the air).

Rule: Never leave a thumbtack where you could sit on it.
Possible sentence: Gloria is jumping up; she is grabbing her hind end.

Use opportunities in the illustrations to structure sentences using the pronouns *he, she,* and *they* for Officer Buckle, Gloria, and the children.

On many pages, there are illustrations of accidents about to happen. For producing question structures, have children play the part of Officer Buckle and ask questions, such as

"What could happen if _____?"

while another child uses prediction strategies to express a possible effect.

For developing sequencing skills and expressing cause-and-effect relationships, retell the series of calamitous events at the school after Officer Buckle didn't come for the safety lesson. For example, prompt:

It started when . . . (Someone left banana pudding on the floor [breaking a rule].)
What effect did that have? (It caused everyone to slide into Mrs. Toppel.)
What effect did that have? (She screamed and let go of the hammer.)
What effect did that have? (She fell off her chair.)
What was Mrs. Topple doing that caused that to happen? (She was standing on a swivel chair [breaking a rule].)

Oh, A-Hunting We Will Go

by John Langstaff
New York: Atheneum, 1974, 1991

Suggested Grade and Interest Level: Pre-K

Topic Exploration: Folk songs

Skill Builders:

Grammar and syntax	**Phonological awareness**
Two- and three-word utterances	**Fluency**
Future tense	

Synopsis: An old folk song inspired singer John Langstaff to make up a few extra verses and put them into this whimsical text. The verse and illustrations are a delight.

Method: Use the text to help children recall and chant the verse. Build fluency by allowing children to supply more and more of the verse using uninterrupted airflow. For example,

Clinician: "Oh, a-hunting we will go,
A-hunting we will go;
We'll catch a whale"

Child: "And put him in a pail,
And then we'll let him go!"

After you have read the text a few times, play the rhyming games for phonological awareness training. The rhyming words of the verse come close together, making them more memorable.

PLAY   **Finish-the-Rhyme.**

Children supply the rhyming word left out at the end of a verse. Teach children to use the meaningful clues in the pictures as well as the meter of the verse to rhyme the word. If necessary, prompt with picture cues and with the initial phoneme, then gradually remove the scaffolding. For example, say

"We'll catch a whale
And put him in a (p)_____" (pail)

PLAY   **Rhyme-It-Again.**

Children identify the rhyming word you read after each set. For example, say

Whale rhymes with _____. (pail)

PLAY   **Make-a-Rhyme.**

Children supply another rhyming word after a set of rhyming words is presented. Give initial phoneme cues if needed. Accept any nonsense word. For example, ask

What word rhymes with *whale*? *whale, pail,* _____ (*jail, mail, nail, pail, sail, tail,* and *trail*)

Extended Activity: Let children make up their own silly hunting songs about things around the room, things in their homes, or things outside. Let children walk around the room, a-hunting as they go, and label the things they see. Pause when they come to a word they can rhyme. Help them make up the verse and perform the actions, then continue the walk. For example, say

We'll catch a chair,
And take it to the fair,
and then we'll let it go.
We'll catch a flower,
And keep it for an hour,
And then we'll let it go.

Old MacDonald Had a Farm

by Colin Hawkins and Jacqui Hawkins
New York: Price, Stern, 1991

Suggested Grade and Interest Level: Pre-K

Topic Explorations: Animals, Farm; Farms; Folk songs

Skill Builders:

Phonological awareness	Fluency
Articulation, *F*	Voice

Synopsis: The familiar song is accompanied by entertaining illustrations.

Method: Read the book, having the children join in to help tell the story and become familiar with the tale.

After the read-aloud, use the familiar song to play phonological awareness games that help children identify beginning, middle, and ending sounds in words. Sing the melody, but change the lyrics. For example,

Singing: What's the sound that starts with these words: *dog, dime,* and *doughnut*?
Children's response: (*d* sound)

Singing: *d* is the sound that starts these words: *dog, dime,* and *doughnut*.
With a *d, d* here and a *d, d* there. Here a *d*, there a *d*, everywhere a *d, d* . . .

Singing: What's the sound in the middle of these words: *sheep, feel,* and *meat*?
Children's response: (long *ee* sound)

Singing: *ee* is the sound in the middle of these words . . .
Once children become familiar with the game, sing the song again. When you come to the line, "And on that farm he had a dog," change the lyrics to an object and identify its beginning sound. Finish the song in the same manner as above. For example, sing

" . . . and on that farm he had a comb. Ee-aye-ee-aye-oh. With a *k, k* here and a *k, k* there . . ."

For articulation and voice, encourage children to recite or sing the text, producing the target sound while engaging in a fun language experience. Use the cumulative, repetitive text, which is heavily loaded with vowel sounds, to improve fluency and voice.

One Fine Day

by Nonny Hogrogian
New York: Macmillan, 1971, 1974

Suggested Grade and Interest Level: Pre-K

Topic Exploration: Folklore, Armenian

Skill Builders:

Language literacy	Articulation, *F*
Sequencing	
Cause-and-effect relationships	
Problem solving	

Synopsis: This Caldecott winner is based on a folktale about a fox that is in a fine fix until it gets its tail back from the old woman who cut it off.

Method: To teach problem-solving skills, pause to ask children to identify the problem in the story. Throughout the story, pause to ask questions, such as

> What is the fox's problem?
> What does the fox have to do now?
> Why does the fox need a bead?
> How is the fox trying to solve his problem now?

See whether the children can predict what the fox will have to find next to bring the milk back to the old woman in order to recover his own tail.

For articulation, read the text and make use of all the words containing the target sound. Structure a phrase, such as, "She cut off the fox's tail," for repetition at appropriate pauses. Ask the child to retell the story, emphasizing production of *F*.

Extended Activity: To teach sequencing and cause-and-effect relationships, let the children act out the fox's quest to bring back the milk to the old lady. First, assign each child to portray a character in the story. Then, make simple puppets to represent the characters (include the old lady, the fox, the cow, the grass, the stream, the maiden, the peddler, the hen, and the miller). Children can paste precut construction paper outlines of their characters onto paper plates. Affix a craft stick to each plate for a handle. (*Note:* If necessary, several children can play the parts of the water and the grass.)

Begin by telling each segment, then have children act out and explain the effect this action produces. For example, begin the story by telling about the old lady gathering firewood and the fox that comes along and drinks from her pail of milk. Have the actors create the scene as they hold their puppets and make up dialog for their characters. Ask the audience what happened because the fox stole the milk. When the children in the audience tell how the woman cut off the fox's tail, have the characters act out the part, creating the dialog for their puppets. Continue to provide scaffolding and prompt the audience to show the causal relationships between events. Encourage the actors to act out the events and create dialog for their puppets. Prompt with questions such as

> What does the old lady want that the fox must find?
> What happens next?
> What does the cow need that the fox must find?
> What happens next?

Over in the Meadow

Illustrated by Ezra Jack Keats (Original text by Olive A. Wadsworth)
New York: Four Winds Press, 1971

Suggested Grade and Interest Level: Pre-K

Skill Builders:
> **Grammar and syntax**
> Singular and plural nouns
> Tenses, present and past

Synopsis: The activities of different animals in their natural habitats are beautifully illustrated to accompany a familiar counting rhyme. Keat's version is aesthetically appealing and provides lots of opportunities for interaction. The repetition of "over in the meadow" makes a nice immediately memorable phrase, rich with many language possibilities.

Method: Read the rhyming verse that accompanies each scene. For example,

"Over in the meadow, in the sand, in the sun,
Lived an old mother turtle and her little
turtle one.
'Dig,' said the mother.
'I dig,' said the one.
So he dug all day.
In the sand, in the sun."

Then, use the illustrations to model or shape appropriate language structures. For example,

The turtle is digging a hole.
He is digging in the sand.
He is digging in the sun.

The turtle dug a hole.
He dug all day.
He dug in the sand.
He dug in the sun.

Note: There are several versions of this book. If you don't find this one on the shelf, ask your librarian if a different version is available.

The Owl and the Pussycat

by Edward Lear
Illustrated by Jan Brett
New York: The Putnam and Grosset Group, 1996

Suggested Grade and Interest Level: Pre-K

Topic Explorations: Boats; Fairy tales and nursery rhymes; Folklore, English; Owls; Sea and the seashore

Skill Builders:

Vocabulary	Grammar and syntax	Phonological awareness
	Tenses, present and past	
	Pronouns, personal	
	and possessive	

Synopsis: This is a Calypso, Caribbean-style version of the fanciful old tale of the owl who courts the pussycat in a beautiful pea-green boat. Illustrations in this version are ideal for explaining some of the unusual words of the rhyme. Included are the dapper owl and glamorous pussycat, hibiscus flowers, exotic fish, sea turtles, sea coral, and tropical fruit of the lush, green island.

Method: Before the read-aloud, present the book's cover and elicit background knowledge about the nursery rhyme. See if children can recite portions of the rhyme and tell what the story is about. Introduce this version by talking about where the story takes place. Describe what the characters are wearing, what's in the boat, and the types of fish featured beneath the ocean.

During the read-aloud, pause to interact with children about the action taking place, shaping or modeling grammatical and syntactic structures at appropriate intervals throughout the rhyming text. Also, build vocabulary as you clarify the meanings of several words. Note that children love fun, different-sounding words. For example,

a runcible spoon (a fork-like utensil with wide prongs, shown in the illustration of this version);
a five-pound note (similar to a five-dollar bill) and shilling (coin);
tarried (stayed in one place; waited);
mince (meaning mincemeat, as shown in the illustration of this version); and
quince (a type of fruit, also shown in this version).

Define *elegant* and *charming* (mannerly, polite, and kind) by pointing out the characters in the illustrations.

After the reading, play phonological awareness games. The illustrations make this book especially suitable for rhyming activities because the rhyming words (such as *money* and *honey*) fall closely together in the text.

PLAY **Word-Count.**

Children identify the words from the text in part or all of a sentence. Demonstrate by holding up one finger for each word as you say

pea green
How many words did I say? (two)

Then say

pea green boat (three)

for a three-finger count. Gradually allow the children to do the counting by themselves and continue to the desired word length.

If children don't have one-to-one correspondence, give each child a collection of manipulables (i.e., blocks, felt squares, buttons, etc.) to use for representing each of the stated words. Demonstrate by saying (or use a puppet to say) the words from a page of text that you want the children to count. Repeat them again as you (or a puppet) move out one item at a time to correspond to your stated word. Then you (or a puppet) count out loud the number of blocks moved to get the word count. Gradually allow the children to do the counting by themselves. Use words directly from a page of the text in hierarchical order to the desired word length. Some words from the text to count include

Pussycat
Owl and pussycat
The owl and the pussycat
To sea
Went to sea
Some honey
Plenty of money
Five pound
Five pound note

Continue presenting portions of the text in progressively longer word strings.

PLAY **Stand-Up-to-the-Word.**

Choose five children and assign each child to one of the words in the title, *The Owl and the Pussycat*. Seat the children in a group. Begin by stating the first word of the title, *The*. The child assigned to the word then stands and repeats *The*. Follow by stating *Owl*, and have the child assigned to that word stand up and repeat *Owl*. Continue until all the designated children are standing. Then have each standing child say his or her word again, and repeat until the title is understood.

PLAY **The Same-Sound game.**

Children identify whether word pairs begin with the same sound. For example, say

> sea, sail
> Do they start with the same sound? (Yes)

Intersperse nonmatched pairs into the following list of matched pairs. To make an unmatched pair, exchange one of the following words with another word from the text.

sang, sea	love, look
hat, hand	ring, wrapped
fish, fowl	land, look
day, dined	danced, dined
moon, marry	

PLAY **Odd-One-Out.**

Children select from a string of alliterative words the one that does not belong based on its beginning sound.

> sea, sail, land
> Which one doesn't belong?
> That's right. *Land* is the odd one out.

Continue with the words from the Same-Sound game.

PLAY **Word-Search.**

Children search the picture for the word that begins with the sound of a given word. For example, say

> I see something in this picture that starts with the same sound as *boat*.
> What other word starts with *b*? (Give phoneme/sound only.)
> Search for the word.

(Other *b* words featured in this version include *basket, beads, banana,* and *beach*.) Then find words that match other beginning sounds. Word sources are available on every page.

PLAY **Finish-the-Rhyme.**

Children supply the rhyming word left out at the end of a verse. Teach children to use the meaningful clues in the pictures as well as the meter of the verse to rhyme the word. If necessary, prompt with picture cues and with the initial phoneme, then gradually remove the scaffolding. For example, say

> "They sailed away, for a year and a (d)_____,
> To the land where the bong-tree grows;
> And there in a wood a Piggy-wig stood,
> With a ring at the end of his (n)_____." (Picture prompt shows a pig with a ring in his nose.)

PLAY **Rhyme-It-Again.**

Children identify the rhyming word heard after a rhyming set is given. If necessary, prompt with the initial phoneme, then gradually remove the scaffolding. For example, say

> *grows* rhymes with (n)_____. (nose)

PLAY **Make-a-Rhyme.**

Children supply another rhyming word after a set of rhyming words from the text is presented. Give initial phoneme cues if needed. Accept any nonsense word. For example, ask

> What word rhymes with *nose? Nose, toes,* (b)_____
> What other words rhyme with *nose?* (*hose, blows, rows, goes, hoes, mows, pose, sews, woes, flows, throws, chose,* and any rhyming nonsense word.)

Then move to high-impact words of the text that were not rhymed. For example, say

> What word rhymes with *bong?* (*tong, gong, long, wrong, song,* and any other words or nonsense words that rhyme.)

PLAY **Rhyming-Ings.**

Children rhyme root words with added *–ing* suffixes using words of the text (root + added suffix, if necessary). Give initial phoneme or cluster cues and picture prompts if needed. For example, say

> What word rhymes with *rowing?* (*sewing, mowing, going,* and other nonsense words that rhyme.)

Other words with *–ings* include:

> sailing (mailing, jailing, bailing, wailing, nailing)
> playing (saying, neighing, laying, praying, staying, straying)
> eating (meeting, seating, beating, cheating)
> singing (bringing, ringing, winging, slinging, swinging)
> dancing (prancing, glancing)
> charming (farming)

PLAY **Clap-and-Count.**

Children clap to, and then count, the number of syllables heard in words from the illustrations and text. Demonstrate by clapping to a word and then asking children how many parts they heard. For example, demonstrate by clapping to the word

> pig
> How many parts in the word? Clap it out. (one)

(continues on next page)

PLAY **Clap-and-Count.** *Continued*

Clap and say

piggie
How many parts in that word? Clap it out. (two)
Pi–ggie. One, two.

A puppet from the land where Bong trees grow can demonstrate by opening and closing its mouth to indicate the syllables. Present words from the text with varying syllable lengths, stressing and elongating the syllables. Words include

One syllable:

owl	pea	
green	sea	wrapped

Two syllables:

money	honey	guitar
married	turkey	

Three syllables:

pussycat	piggy-wig	beautiful
charmingly	banana	

PLAY **What's-the-Word?**

Children synthesize syllables into words using the words and pictures of the book. For example, show children the picture of the owl and the pussycat in the pea-green boat. Present the syllables of a pictured word with a clear pause between them and have the children say them quickly and repeatedly until they can identify the word. For example, say

whis–ker
What's the word?
Say it until you hear it. *Whis–ker. Whis–ker. Whisker.*
Whisker is the word.

Continue with any clearly illustrated word, such as *fea-ther* and *pine-a-pple.* Also, use two-syllable words from lists in Clap-and-Count and Find-the-Little-Words.

PLAY **Find-the-Little-Words.**

Children listen for "little" words within two-syllable words of the text. Stress and elongate syllables when presenting the word. For example, say

pussycat
Can you hear any little words in *pussycat*? (pussy, cat)

(continues on next page)

PLAY Find-the-Little-Words. *Continued*

Continue with two-syllable words of the text, such as

pigg-y (pig)   tur-key (key)
mo-ney (knee)   plen-ty (tea)

More words from the pictures include

is-land (eye, I)   sail-ing (sail)   sing-ing (sing)

PLAY Leave-It-Out.

Children say a compound word or two-syllable word, then leave out the beginning or final part to create a smaller word. For example, say

Say *pussycat* without saying *pussy*.
What little word is left? (cat)

Reverse the order. For example, say

Say *pussycat* without saying *cat*.
What little word is left? (pussy)

Continue with the two-syllable words provided in Find-the-Little-Words.

PLAY Add-It-On.

Children put two little words and two syllables together to make two-syllable words. For example, say

Say *sail*.
Now, say *sail*, and add *boat*.
What bigger word do you have? (sailboat)

Then reverse the order in which the words are presented. For example, say

Put *boat* at the end of *sail*.
What word do you have? (sailboat)

Continue with the two-syllable words provided in Find-the-Little-Words.

PLAY Turn-It-Around.

Children reverse the parts of the compound word *sailboat* and other words they have previously analyzed and synthesized, such as

Put the word *boat* at the beginning of *sail*.
What word do you have? (boatsail)
What was it before we turned it around? (sailboat)

> **PLAY** **Switch-It.**
>
> Children delete part of a compound or two-syllable word and switch it with a new part to make another compound word. Prompt with cues as necessary. For example, say
>
> > Say *sailboat.*
> > Now say *sailboat,* only take out *sail* and put in *row.*
> > What new word can you make? (rowboat)
>
> Some word switches include
> > Say *turkey,* only take out *tur* and put in *mon* (sounds like mong). (monkey)
> > Say *piggie,* only take out *ee* and put in *let.* (piglet)
> > Say *island,* only take out *land* and put in *ball.* (eyeball)

☛ See the catalog for Grades 1 through 5 for continuing activities in the hierarchy of phonological awareness.

Note: There are several versions of this book. The poem may also be found in a collection of poems. If you can't find this version of the book, ask the librarian if another version is available.

Pancakes for Breakfast

by Tomie de Paola
New York: Harcourt Brace Jovanovich, 1978

Suggested Grade and Interest Level: Pre-K

Topic Exploration: Cooking

Skill Builders:

Grammar and syntax	**Language literacy**	**Articulation, K**
Pronouns—personal, possessive, and reflexive	Relating personal experiences	
Present tense	Sequencing	
	Storytelling	
	Problem solving	

Synopsis: A wordless book about a woman who awakens on a snowy day in the woods and wants pancakes for breakfast. The illustrations show her reaching for her recipe book and fetching the ingredients but being besieged by obstacles at every step. She must milk the cow, collect eggs from the hens, churn the butter, and go out to buy maple syrup from the woodsman. When she returns, all of her efforts are foiled by a terrible mishap. Nonetheless, she finds that there is a solution to her problem and ends up with a nice stack of pancakes for breakfast.

Method: Before the read-aloud, ask children what they know about pancakes. How are they made? How do the children like to eat them? How many can they eat? Have children relate their experiences.

During the read-aloud, have children tell the story from the pictures as you shape and model syntactic structures as needed. Stress the reflexive pronoun in shaping sentences, such as "She's making pancakes for herself," "She's going out to get the eggs by herself," and so on.

For sequencing, ask children what happened after the old lady woke up. What steps did she take in order to make her pancakes? Help children recall the order of events.

For building storytelling skills, see scaffolding techniques in the Grades 1 through 5 catalog.

For articulation of *K*, use the following words of the text for auditory bombardment of the target sound. Practice words at the one-word level before reading the story, then reinforce the production of the sound through interaction as you share in the storytelling and the children join in. Target words include

pancakes	cat	curtains
cookbook	baking soda	basket
bucket	milk	cow
clock	mix	stack
breakfast		

Peter's Chair

by Ezra Jack Keats
New York: Harper & Row, 1967, 1983

Suggested Grade and Interest Level: Pre-K

Topic Explorations: Family relationships; Growing up

Skill Builders:

Vocabulary
Adjectives
Grammar and syntax
Possessive nouns
Pronouns, personal
    and possessive
Tenses, present and past

Language literacy
Relating personal experiences
Drawing inferences
Critical thinking

Synopsis: This story about growing up with a new baby at home can arouse many thoughts and feelings in children. Warmly told with imaginative, colorful illustrations, it's little wonder this tale has become a classic.

Method: For adjectives, include the following words when talking about the story:

pink chair	new baby
little chair	tall building

Use the text and illustrations to shape or model other target structures at appropriate intervals.

For critical thinking, discuss the story with questions that underscore the story's meaning. For example,

Why do you think they painted Peter's crib pink?
How do you think Peter feels about that?
What reasons might he have had to run away?
Why do you think he took his baby pictures with him?
What is Peter doing when he puts his shoes under the curtain?
Why does he want to trick his mother?
What happened when he did?

For relating personal experiences, have children talk about younger brothers and sisters in their homes. Converse about how difficult it is to give up something you love but have outgrown.

Piggie Pie

by Margie Palatini
New York: Houghton Mifflin, 1995

Suggested Grade and Interest Level: K

Topic Explorations: Animals, Farm; Cooking; Holidays, Halloween

Skill Builders:

Vocabulary	**Language literacy**
Attributes	Sequencing
Prepositions	**Phonological awareness**
Grammar and syntax	
Pronouns, personal and possessive	
Present tense	

Synopsis: Here's a feast of delicious words with which to say and play. Trendy, high-powered Witch Gritch is in the mood for the most delicious meal ever—piggie pie. But when she goes to the shelf to pull out her *Hag Cookbook*— PROBLEM! She has no pigs. She flies on her broom to Old McDonald's farm, but not without first giving herself away. As she arrives, she writes "Surrender Piggies!" in the sky with her broom, giving her victims enough time to problem solve. They disguise themselves as geese, chickens, cows, and even Old MacDonald—so that when she arrives in pursuit of them, she can't find a single porker. The tie-in to familiar nursery rhymes gives additional laughs.

Method: Perfect fare for the Halloween season (or any time), and there is a lot to do with this one! Read it the first time without pausing, then do a picture walk-through. For developing expression with the use of attributes, children can have fun describing the witch, including her long green fingernails, warty face, big pointy hat, and gap-toothed grin. Encourage other descriptions such as hungry, greedy, and sneaky.

For grammar and syntax, use the text and illustrations to model and shape target structures. Some present-tense examples with pronouns and prepositions include

> She is pulling down her *Old Hag Cookbook.*
> She is looking up a recipe in her cookbook.
> Gritch is stomping her feet on the floor.
> Gritch is pacing the floor.
> She is flying up in the sky.
> The pigs are running around the farm.
> They are talking about the witch.
> They are putting on costumes.
> They are walking next to each other, arm in arm.

For sequencing story parts, children can tell the order of events that occurs when Gritch consults the disguised animal on MacDonald's farm. Children will have fun including the formula answer for each (e.g., "The duck quack-quacked here. It quack quacked there, and everywhere it quacked, no piggies," etc.). Encourage children to use the words *first, next,* and *then* as they relate each encounter in the sequence.

For phonological awareness training, reread the text. Begin at the appropriate developmental level of the child, using the continuum of activities at the word and syllable levels provided.

PLAY **The Same-Sound game.**

Children identify whether word pairs begin with the same sound. For example, say

pig, pie
Do they start with the same sound? (Yes)

Intersperse nonmatched pairs into the following list of matched pairs:

pink, pig	heap, hay
dizzy, duck	duck, dumb
hand, hogs	stew, stomp
boiled, buzzard	lumpy, looking
purple, pudding	piggie, pie, pink
boiled, buzzard	dumb, dizzy, duck
stew, stomp, steer	pull, pace, pork
feet, farm, find	

PLAY **Word-Search.**

Children search the picture for the word you select that begins with the sound of a given word. For example, say

I see something in this picture that starts with the same sound as *pork*.
What other word starts with *p*? (Give phoneme/sound only.)
Search for the word.
That's right. *Pig* starts with *p*.

Word sources are available on each page.

PLAY **Clap-and-Count.**

Children clap to, and then count, the number of syllables heard in selected words from the illustrations and text. Demonstrate by clapping to a word and then asking children how many parts they heard. For example, clap and say

broom
How many parts in the word? Clap it out. (one)
Broom. One.

Clap and say

broomstick
How many parts in that word? Clap it out. (two)
Broom–stick. One, two.

Stress and elongate parts when presenting the following compound words:

barn-yard	bird-brain
drum-stick	o-ver-head
fin-ger-nail	ev-ery-where

(continues on next page)

PLAY Clap-and-Count. *Continued*

Two-syllable words include

pro-blem	pan-try	grum-py
far-mer	qua-cker	grou-chy
go-ggles	wa-ddle	
pu-dding	por-ker	

PLAY What's-the-Word?

Children synthesize syllables into words using words from the book's text and pictures. Present the syllables, with a clear pause between them, and have the children say them quickly and repeatedly until they can identify the word. For example, say

> pan–try
> What's the word?
> Say it until you hear it. *Pannn-try. Pann-try. Pantry.*
> *Pantry* is the word.

Continue with the list of compound words and two-syllable words provided in Clap-and-Count.

PLAY Find-the-Little-Words.

Children listen for "little" words within the compound words and two-syllable words of the text. Stress and elongate syllables when presenting the word. For example, say

> broomstick
> Can you hear any little words in *broomstick*? (broom, stick)
> Yes. *Broom* is a little word in *broomstick*.
> *Stick* is another little word in *broomstick*.

Continue with the list of the compound words provided in Clap-and-Count. Then, present the two-syllable words, changing the stress as necessary so the children can learn the "little" words. Words include

pantry (pan, tree, pant)	piggies (pig)	lumpy (lump, pea)
dragon (drag, gun)	buzzard (buzz)	landing (land, ding)
chickens (chick)	looking (look, king)	
waddle (wad)	porker (pork)	

PLAY Leave-It-Out.

Children say a compound or two-syllable word, then leave out the beginning or final part to create a smaller word. For example, say

> Say *broomstick*.
> Now say *broomstick* but leave out *stick*.
> What little word is left? (broom)

(continues on next page)

Leave-It-Out. *Continued*

Then say

> Now say *broomstick* but leave out *broom.*
> What little word is left? (stick)

Continue with the compound words and two-syllable words provided in Clap-and-Count.

 Add-It-On.

Children put two little words and two syllables together to make new words. For example, say

> Say *pan.*
> Now, say *pan*, and add *tree.*
> What bigger word can you make? (pantry)

Then reverse the order in which the words are presented. For example, say

> Put *pan* at the end of *tree.* What word do you have? (treepan)

Continue with the compound words and two-syllable words provided above in Clap-and-Count.

 Turn-It-Around.

Children reverse the parts of words they have previously analyzed and synthesized, such as

> Put the word *stick* at the beginning of *broom.*
> What funny word can you make? (stickbroom)
> What was it before we turned it around? (broomstick)

Continue first with compound words and then with two-syllable words. For example,

> barn + yard (yard barn, barnyard)
> pan + try (said *treepan*) (pantry)
> bird + brain (brainbird, birdbrain)
> And so on.

 Switch-It.

Children delete a part in a compound or two-syllable word and switch it with another word or syllable. For example, say

> Say *barnyard.*
> Now, say *barnyard*, only take out *barn* and put in *farm.*
> What new word can you make? (farmyard)

(continues on next page)

PRE-K-K

> **PLAY** **Switch-It.** *Continued*
>
> More syllable exchanges include
>
> | | |
> |---|---|
> | *barnyard* to *backyard* | *broomstick* to *yardstick* |
> | *broomstick* to *drumstick* | *overhead* to *overdue* |
> | *piggies* to *piglet* | *purple* to *purpose* |

➤ Continued training activities are provided in the catalog for Grades 1 through 5.

Note: If you haven't gotten your fill, read *Zoom Broom* by the same author for even more fun.

Planting a Rainbow

by Lois Ehlert
New York: Harcourt Brace Jovanovich, 1988, 1992

Suggested Grade and Interest Level: Pre-K

Topic Explorations: Colors; Growing cycles and planting

Skill Builders:

Vocabulary	**Language literacy**
Categories	Relating personal experiences

Synopsis: A mother and child plant flowers in the family garden. The bulbs, seeds, and sprouts bloom in all the colors of the rainbow. There is a page of flowers for each color.

Method: For vocabulary, talk about the words presented in the book and encourage children to learn a fun new word that identifies a beautiful flower. Words in the text include

bulbs	seeds	seedlings
plants	sprout	rainbow
garden center	marigold	tiger lily
poppy	pansy	and other names for flowers

For sequencing, talk about the process of growing plants from seeds, bulbs, and sprouts. Recall the steps involved in the sequence, including digging a hole, pulling weeds, and watering. Sequence the steps. Discuss what it took for the seeds to grow.

For categories, brainstorm the names of flowers that are yellow, such as marigolds, daffodils, and daisies. Then, brainstorm flowers that are blue, such as morning glories, hyacinths, and cornflowers. Use the pictures of the book to help recall the names.

Extended Activity: Augment the text by bringing in flowers from your own garden and, if appropriate, having the children pick and bring in flowers to share. See whether the class can match some of the real flowers to pictures in the book in order to identify them.

Think about what you can plant in the classroom (planting can be a fun activity in fall or spring). Have each child participate in the caretaking process until the plant's growth cycle is completed. Have group discussions several times throughout the growing season so that children can relate what is taking place and their experiences of gardening.

Make a bulletin board for fall or spring, complete with a rainbow. Have each child choose a flower from the book to re-create out of colored tissue and construction paper. Encourage the child to learn all about the flower, including its name and color. On a separate piece of paper, write the name of the flower. Then, as each child places the flower and its label on the bulletin board scene (similar to the author's illustrations), have him or her tell about the flower, including the name, color, whether it comes from a bulb or a seed, and so on.

Note: Read also *The Carrot Seed* by Ruth Krauss (listed in this catalog).

Polar Bear, Polar Bear, What Do You Hear?

by Bill Martin Jr.
New York: Henry Holt, 1991; Scholastic, 1992 (big book, 1993)

Suggested Grade and Interest Level: Pre-K

Topic Explorations: Animals, Zoo; Sounds and listening; Zoos

Skill Builders:
    Grammar and syntax
    Two- and three-word utterances
    Question structures
    Fluency

Synopsis: In a sing-song text, a polar bear answers questions about the sounds he hears from other animals in the zoo. This book is good for encouraging children to participate.

Method: Read the story dramatically, inviting the children to make animal sounds as appropriate. Reread the story with increasing participation. Use the cumulative, repetitive, and rhythmic verse to improve fluency.

Extended Activities: Create your own class story based on the story pattern. You may begin, "Bumblebee, bumblebee, what do you hear?" on your travels around the school playground, or "Baby chick, baby chick, what do you hear?" on your walk around the farm. Have children contribute to the story by identifying an appropriate sound maker and fitting it to the words of the text.

Make puppets for the animals in the book (you can trace animal outlines from the illustrations or project the images onto tagboard using an overhead projector). As the children color the puppets, circulate among them, and demonstrate the sound each animal makes. When the children return to the story circle, instruct them to lift their puppets and make their animal's special sound when appropriate. For example, after the line, "I hear a lion roaring in my ear," prompt children with lion puppets to roar. Or ask students, "What did the polar bear hear?" to elicit the unison response, "a lion roaring in his ear." On the last page, pause after each line, allowing the children to interject their sounds.

Reinforce the story with a trip to the zoo. Ask children to note the animal sounds they hear. Recall the sounds as well as your experiences on your return.

Note: This book is available in Spanish translation, titled *Oso pardo, oso pardo, ¿qué ves ahi?*

Quick as a Cricket

by Don Wood
Swindon, England: Child's Play International, 1990

Suggested Grade and Interest Level: K

Topic Exploration: Animals

Skill Builders:
> **Vocabulary**
> Adjectives
> Similes and metaphors

Synopsis: A series of animals, brilliantly illustrated in Don Wood's exuberant style, are portrayed by their most salient characteristic. A short simile creates the simple text.

Method: Before the read-aloud, talk about the characteristics of different animals. How would the children describe an elephant? A giraffe? A bumblebee? Make up similes for each, then introduce the book, telling children how they can make their language more fun, colorful, and descriptive.

During the read-aloud, have children join in. Apply each simile to a real-life situation (e.g., "When Carlos is on the playground, he is as quick as a cricket." "When I get up in the morning, I'm as slow as a snail."). Then, give the first half of the sentence and let the children fill in the simile. Once you've established the pattern, see whether children can create their own phrases.

Extended Activity: Play a game of pantomime. First, express the ideas in the book's similes. Ask children, Can anyone act out or pretend to be as slow as a snail? Who can be as sad as a basset hound? Have the whole group join in the pantomime. Give a signal to indicate when it's time to stop and listen to the next simile, then have children think up a descriptive adjective to act out (e.g., What are some words to describe a butterfly? Graceful? Fluttery? Colorful?). Then, express the simile (e.g., As graceful as a butterfly. As fluttery as a butterfly.). Add closure by asking children how it felt to be a butterfly, a bear, a giraffe, or other animals.

Rain Makes Applesauce

by Julian Scheer and Marvin Bileck
New York: Holiday House, 1964

Suggested Grade and Interest Level: Pre-K

Topic Explorations: Food; Fruit; Growing cycles and planting; Seasons, Autumn; Weather; Weather, Rain

Skill Builders:
> **Grammar and syntax**   **Phonological awareness**
> Two- and three-word utterances
> Present tense
> **Language literacy**
> Sequencing

Synopsis: Nonsense verses join with the repeated phrase "rain makes applesauce" to make the text of this whimsical book. If there is only one choice for a picture book as a historical, cultural document, it must be this one. Published in the 1960s, it has remained in print for over 30 years, has been an award and honor recipient, and has been listed on the *New York Times* 10 Best Illustrated Bookslist. The words, although not making sense, encourage children to join in and make their own "silly talk." Look closely at the illustrations to discover the real story, cleverly hidden within. Great for the fall season.

Method: Before the read-aloud, talk about rain and the growing cycle. What's inside an apple? How do apples grow? How do we get apples from trees? What must happen for the seeds to grow? Once apples are harvested, what are some of the foods that can be made with them?

During the read-aloud, elaborate on the text and ask children to join in as you repeat the refrain, "rain makes applesauce," and the girl's response, "Oh, you're just talking silly talk." Allow children plenty of time to view the illustrations and make comments.

After the read-aloud, go back to the first page and point out within the illustration the two children buying seeds from a seed cart. If necessary, explain what the children are doing; then, on the next page, see if the children can discover the story on their own. If necessary, point out the boy with the shovel and ask the children to tell what is happening. Continue searching each page to discover what happens in the story, modeling and structuring two- and three-word utterances and present-tense constructions.

On another occasion, have children sequence the steps of making applesauce using the illustrations as a guide. For example,

> First they buy the seeds.
> Then they dig the hole and plant them.
> They discover the sprout.
> When the tree grows, it eventually blossoms.
> After awhile, apples appear.
> The children pick the apples.
> Then they carry them in a cart,
> cut them and stir them up with sugar in the kitchen,
> put them over a fire-burning stove,
> and finally, on the last page, eat the applesauce and
> ride in barrels on a sea of applesauce.

Use the words of the text to play phonological awareness games.

PLAY **Word-Count.**

Children count the number of words in a short line from the text. Demonstrate by assigning one word to one finger as you say the words. For example, say

> dancing

as you hold up one finger. Ask

> How many words did I say? (one)

(continues on next page)

PLAY Word-Count. *Continued*

Then say

> Dolls go dancing

for a three-finger count. Gradually allow the children to do the counting by themselves.

If children don't have one-to-one correspondence, give each child a collection of manipulables (i.e., blocks, felt squares, buttons, etc.) to use for representing each of the stated words. Demonstrate by saying (or use a puppet to say) the words from a page of text that you want the children to count. Repeat them again as you (or a puppet) move out one item at a time to correspond to your stated word. Then you (or a puppet) count out loud the number of blocks moved to get the word count. Gradually allow the children to do the counting by themselves. Use words directly from a page of the text in hierarchical order to the desired word length. Some words from the text to count include

> lemon juice
> stars are made
> stars are made of lemon juice
> I wear
> I wear my shoes
> I wear my shoes inside out
> clouds hide
> clouds hide in
> clouds hide in a hole
> clouds hide in a hole in the sky
> salmon slide
> salmon slide down
> salmon slide down hippo's hide
> tickle
> tickle tree
> on a tickle tree
> grow on a tickle tree
> elbows grow on a tickle tree

PLAY Which-Word-Is-Missing?

Children identify the word in a word string that has been omitted from a previously given string. Choose two to four words from the illustration and text to make up a string. Repeat the words, leaving one out for the children to identify, such as

> stars, juice, lemon, rain
> stars, juice, rain
> Which one is missing? (lemon)

Some word lists from the text include

> shoes, out, wear, rain
> day, house, walk, goes
> wind, long, blows, night
> eat, smoke, monkey, tiger
> salmon, hippo, bear, elbow

> tickle, tree, grow, sauce
> go, dolls, moon, dance
> jelly, bean, soap, candy
> clouds, hole, sky, hide

PLAY **Rearrange-It.**

Children rearrange, in correct word order, a scrambled phrase or sentence from a portion of the text. For example, say

> Applesauce makes rain
> Is that right? Can you help me say the words in the right order?
> That's right. *Applesauce makes rain* should really be *Rain makes applesauce.*

More words to rearrange include

> Makes applesauce rain
> Juice lemon
> Out inside
> Dancing go dolls
> The backwards blows wind
> Clouds hole in the hide
> My sings bear
> You're talking talk silly
> Silly talking you're talk

PLAY **The Same-Sound game.**

Children identify whether word pairs begin with the same sound. For example, say

> made, moon
> Do they start with the same sound? (Yes)

Intersperse nonmatched pairs into the following list of matched pairs:

soap, sauce	hide, hole	hole, hippo
dolls, dance	long, loud	monkeys, mumble
moon, makes	sings, silly	jelly, jungle
	wear, walk	

PLAY **Make-a-Rhyme.**

Children make silly talk of their own by rhyming the word that ends the first half of the compound sentence before the words, "and rain makes applesauce." For example, say

> "Tigers sleep on an elephant's snoot . . ."
> What word rhymes with *snoot*?

Provide phoneme cues if needed, as in (b) _____ for *boot*. (Other possibilities include *hoot, loot, shoot, root, toot, fruit,* and any nonsense rhyming word.)

Then say the new silly talk. For example, say

> Tigers sleep on an elephant's boot and rain makes applesauce.

(continues on next page)

PLAY **Make-a-Rhyme.** *Continued*

Some phrases with ending words to rhyme include

The stars are made of lemon *juice* (*moose, loose,* and any nonsense rhyming word)
I wear my shoes inside *out* (*pout, shout,* and any nonsense rhyming word)
My house goes walking every *day* (*may, way,* and any nonsense rhyming word)
Dolls go dancing on the *moon* (*soon, tune,* and any nonsense rhyming word)

PLAY **Clap-and-Count.**

Children clap to, and then count, the number of syllables heard in selected words from the illustrations
and text. Demonstrate by clapping to a word and then asking children how many parts they heard. For example,
clap and say

> apple
> How many parts in the word? Clap it out. (two)
> A-pple. One, two.

Clap and say

> applesauce
> How many parts in that word? Clap it out. (three)
> That's right. A-pple-sauce. One, two, three.

Stress and elongate syllables when presenting words, such as

back-wards	in-side
mon-key	can-dy
chim-ney	hi-ppo
dan-cing	wa-lking
te-ddy	ti-ckle
ta-lking	

 PLAY **Find-the-Little-Words.**

Children listen for "little" words within the compound words of the text. Stress and elongate syllables when
presenting the word. For example, say

> backwards
> Can you hear any little words in *backwards*? (back, word, words)
> That's right. *Back* is a little word in *backwards*.
> *Words* is another little word in *backwards*.

Continue with the compound words and two-syllable words provided in Clap-and-Count. Then present the
two-syllable words, changing the stress as necessary so the children can hear all the "little" words.

PLAY **Leave-It-Out.**

Children say a compound word, then leave out the beginning or final part to create a smaller word. For example, say

> Say *backwards*.
> Now, say *backwards*, but leave out *wards*.
> What little word is left? (back)

Then say

> Now, say *backwards*, but leave out *back*.
> What little word is left? (words)

Continue with the words provided in Clap-and-Count.

PLAY **Add-It-On.**

Children put two little words together to make a compound word. For example, say

> Say *back*.
> Now, say *back*, and add *wards*.
> What bigger word can you make? (backwards)

Then, reverse the order in which the words are presented. For example, say

> Put *wards* at the end of *back*. What word do you have? (backwards)

Continue with the words provided in Clap-and-Count.

PLAY **Turn-It-Around.**

Children reverse the word parts they have previously analyzed and synthesized. For example, say

> Put *wards* (sounds like *words*) at the beginning of *back*.
> What word do you have? (wordsback) What was it before we turned it around? (backwards)

Continue with the words provided in Clap-and-Count.

☛ See the catalog for Grades 1 through 5 for continuing activities in the hierarchy of phonological awareness.

The Rat and the Tiger

by Keiko Kasza
New York: Scholastic, 1993

Suggested Grade and Interest Level: Pre-K

Topic Explorations: Friendship; Manners and etiquette; Sharing

Skill Builders:
> **Language literacy**   **Pragmatic language**
> Problem solving
> Drawing inferences

Synopsis: An incongruous pair, Rat and Tiger are best of friends, playing cowboys and sharing meals. Tiger is bigger, naturally, so when it comes to playing cowboys, he gets to be the good guy; when they share doughnuts, he gets the bigger half; and when he wants a flower at the bottom of a cliff, he's entitled to push Rat off to get it for him. Rat says he's just a little rat and silently endures. One day, Rat builds a castle and Tiger angrily kicks it to pieces. That is the last straw for Rat, who declares Tiger "a big mean bully" and no longer his friend. The rest of the story finds them on a new playing field as Rat shows Tiger what it's like to be on the receiving end of a "bullyship," rather than a friendship.

Method: Before the read-aloud, introduce the book by asking children to share some of the rules of playing together, such as turn taking and sharing. Have children brainstorm ways to be kind to their friends. Introduce the story of two friends, Rat and Tiger, and then describe the cover illustration.

Read the story aloud, pausing to point out and interpret, if necessary, the expressions of the characters.

After the read-aloud, ask children to tell how they felt about the story. What did they think about the way Tiger and Rat behaved? Help children build inferencing skills by filling in what happened between the pictures and the text. For example, after Tiger pushes Rat off the cliff, the next picture shows Rat with bandages. Ask, How did Rat come to have bandages on his shoulder and knee? Help children infer meaning, by asking

> What did Rat mean when he said, "What could I say? I'm just a tiny little rat?"
> Why couldn't Rat tell Tiger how he felt?
> How did Rat feel when Tiger didn't play fair?
> What did Tiger learn?
> What did Rat learn?

For problem-solving skills, ask children to state the problem in the story.

> Why didn't Rat tell Tiger how he felt when Tiger was a bully?
> How did Rat solve his problem?
> How did Tiger solve his problem?
> Are there other ways they could have solved their problems?
> What could they have done in the first place to keep from almost ruining their friendship?

For improving pragmatic language skills, go over the ideas about playing with friends that the children brainstormed before the read-aloud and talk about how the ideas apply both to the characters and to the children in real life. Include the following ideas:

> make polite requests
> express your feelings
> say things that give the speaker feedback
> be a good listener
> take turns in conversations
> say you don't understand someone

Ride a Purple Pelican

by Jack Prelutsky
New York: Greenwillow Books, 1986

Suggested Grade and Interest Level: Pre-K

Topic Exploration: Fairy tales and nursery rhymes

Skill Builders:
   Articulation—*B, P, K,* and *G*

Synopsis: A collection of short, nonsense verses is a modern-day version of nursery rhymes. For example,

> "Jilliky, jolliky, jellicky, jee,
> Three little cooks on a coconut tree.
> One cooked a peanut and one cooked a pea.
> One brewed a thimble of cinnamon tea."

Method: For articulation, check the table of contents for titles that are heavily loaded with target phonemes, such as

> "Poor Potatoes"
> "Little Pink Pig"
> "Grandfather Gando"
> "Betty Ate a Butternut"
> "Kitty Caught a Caterpillar"

Select the words containing target phonemes for auditory bombardment before reading aloud. Ask children to listen for words with their target sound. Reread the rhyme, pausing to let children complete the line with the appropriate target word, or cue children to repeat the target words along with you.

Rosie's Walk

by Pat Hutchins
New York: Macmillan, 1968, 1971

Suggested Grade and Interest Level: Pre-K

Topic Exploration: Animals, Farm; Farms

Skill Builders:

Vocabulary	**Language literacy**
Prepositions	Sequencing
Grammar and syntax	Cause-and-effect relationships
Two- and three-word utterances	Drawing inferences
Tenses, present and past	**Articulation,** *K*

Synopsis: A hen's walk around the farmyard is undisturbed, despite the fox that trails her. The fox has a series of mishaps (portrayed solely through pictures) that enables the unsuspecting Rosie to strut safely home to her coop.

Method: Before the read-aloud, set the stage by explaining that the story takes place in a farmyard. Encourage children to relate their experiences with farms. Talk about the objects children can expect to see, such as a beehive and a mill, and what these things are for. Explain that one of the characters is a fox that hunts for birds.

Read aloud, modeling or shaping sentences based on events in the illustrations. Encourage the repetition of prepositional phrases as you read the text. Ask whether the hen knows the fox is trailing her. How can the children tell? Is the fox having a good day? How does the fox feel when it doesn't catch the hen?

For cause-and-effect relationships, pause after each of the fox's mishaps to ask, "Can the fox catch the hen?" "Why not?" Elicit responses such as, "Because he fell in the pond" or "Because he got hit with the rake."

After the read-aloud, assist the children in telling the sequence of events that comprises the story of Rosie's walk. Also, ask children whether they laughed when they saw the pictures in the story. What was funny about the story?

For articulation, use the text for auditory bombardment of *K*. Words include

walk	fox	across
pitchfork	haystack	cart
(sacks of) corn	back	

Ask the children to tell you what Rosie is doing in each illustration to elicit "Rosie is walking" or a similar phrase. Ask questions to elicit other phrases containing the target sound.

Extended Activity: Create a farmyard like Rosie's on butcher paper, complete with pond, mill, and beehives. Use the illustration on the book's opening pages as a guide. Pin the paper to the bulletin board. Make a fox and a hen from construction paper. Before pinning them to the scene, have the children take turns retelling the story, explaining what happened to the fox along the way as they move the characters around the farmyard.

Note: This activity can also be done using a felt board. Invest the time to cut out props of felt, including the pond, mill, beehives, chicken coup, and characters. You'll have great materials to use year after year.

Sail Away

by Donald Crews
New York: Greenwillow Books, 1995

Suggested Grade and Interest Level: Pre-K

Topic Explorations: Boats; Journeys; Transportation; Weather

Skill Builders:

Vocabulary	**Articulation**
Prepositions	Oral motor exercises
Grammar and syntax	
Two- and three-word utterances	

Synopsis: Sail away with a family on a bright, sunny day. Join them in a little dinghy as they leave the harbor and row out to where their sailboat is moored. Then experience a whole day (complete with a storm and a sunset) and return home to a vista of the harbor lights at night.

Method: Model these prepositions from the text or in structured conversation: *under, away, up, down, under,* and *past.*

Emphasize, define, and use the words in the text related to seafaring, including

> dinghy
> mooring
> swell
> lifejacket
> lighthouse
> bridge
> port

Use the "putt . . . putt . . . put . . ." words of the text as a segue into exercises for strengthening oral-motor skills by having the child supply the motor sounds.

Scary, Scary Halloween

by Eve Bunting
New York: Clarion Books, 1986

Suggested Grade and Interest Level: Pre-K

Topic Explorations: Holidays, Halloween; Seasons, Autumn

Skill Builders:

Vocabulary	Grammar and syntax	Language literacy
Categories	Present tense	Verbal expression
Attributes		Discussion

Synopsis: A Halloween favorite, complete with a vampire, werewolf, skeleton, and plenty of action-packed illustrations. The nonthreatening, rhyming text is ideal for eliciting a variety of language skills.

Method: Before the read-aloud, have children describe the book's cover and elicit predictions about the story.

During the read-aloud, pause only to elaborate on the meaning, if necessary, so as not to interrupt the flow of the rhyming text, thus allowing children to experience the mood of the story.

For categories and attributes, brainstorm all of the Halloween creatures that fall into the scary-creature category, then go back through the pages and give attributes to each. Read the text on the page to start the children off. For example, say

> "A vampire and a werewolf prowl.
> One growls a growl, one howls a howl. . ."

Discuss who is telling the story. Through whose eyes are we seeing Halloween night? Reread the first paragraph for a clue. Go through the rest of the pages to find where the cat and her kittens are hiding and whose green eyes are peering out from the dark beneath the stairs. Ask questions, such as

> What do you think the cats are thinking about Halloween?
> What else might cats see on Halloween?
> What do you think your cat (or the neighborhood cat) sees on your street on Halloween night?

For syntax, go back over the illustrations to describe the action. Shape and model present tense and other syntactic forms.

School Bus

by Donald Crews
New York: Puffin, 1984; Scholastic, 1991 (paperback)

Suggested Grade and Interest Level: Pre-K

Topic Explorations: School activities; Transportation

Skill Builders:

Vocabulary	Grammar and syntax	Language literacy
Categories	Two- and three-word utterances	Relating personal experiences
Antonyms	Noun-verb agreement	
	Singular and plural nouns	

Synopsis: A versatile book for the youngest ones, with short phrases and simple line drawings of yellow school buses. The story follows a bus across town as it picks up students, takes them back and forth to school, and returns to its origin.

Method: Use the text to model early word combinations and noun-verb agreement. Some examples include

bus stops	man walks	bus goes
people stop	girl waits	buses wait
truck goes	boy waits	mom hugs

Encourage repetition of the text, including the phrases

Going this way	Head for school
Going that way	Here we are
Here it comes	Right on time
Bus is coming	School's over
See you later	

Interject other similar phrases as you read, such as

Bus is coming	Wave goodbye
Kids are waiting	Wheels go round

Pause to talk about what is happening in the pictures. Expand on the text to talk about the story the pictures portray. Encourage children to relate their own experiences of riding the school bus.

To expand vocabulary, including singular and plural nouns, label the parts of the bus, including the lights, mirror, tires, windows, stop sign, and tail lights.

For categorization, name the vehicles on the road (e.g., garbage truck, car, taxi, truck). Name other vehicles, and ask what other vehicles one might see on the road.

For antonyms, pair words and use them in context, such as

empty, full	fast, slow
stop, go	comes, goes
large, small	off, on
red light, green light	

The Secret Birthday Message

by Eric Carle
New York: Thomas Y. Crowell, 1971, 1986

Suggested Grade and Interest Level: Pre-K

Topic Exploration: Shapes and visual images

Skill Builders:
Vocabulary	Language literacy
Prepositions	Sequencing

Synopsis: A message in code starts Tim off on an exciting treasure hunt through a dark cave, an underground tunnel, and other exotic places until, at the end of his journey, he finds a pleasant surprise.

Method: Name the shapes in the secret message, turn the different-sized pages, and re-create the journey from the last illustration. Arrows give closure to each step of the search and provide an opportunity to sequence the events.

Extended Activities: Play I Spy with geometric shapes. Be sure there are many shapes represented from around the room. You may want to place some obvious-colored shapes on the bulletin board or against the chalkboard rail. Show children examples, such as round ball, rectangular books, square box, and so on. The player looks around the room and decides on an object in clear view. The child gives the first clue, for example, "I see a triangle," and the group takes turns guessing what object the child has chosen. If no one guesses the object, more clues can be given, such as its color and location. The child who guesses correctly can be the next to choose a shape, or you can select a child to ensure that everyone gets a turn.

Give each child a piece of aluminum foil or paper to fold into various shapes. Demonstrate how to fold the material into a square, first, and then, after each child has folded the square, demonstrate how to fold the square diagonally into a triangle. Have children identify the shapes and try re-creating some of their own.

Seven Blind Mice

by Ed Young
New York: Philomel Books, 1992

Suggested Grade and Interest Level: Pre-K

Topic Explorations: Colors; Days of the week; Folklore, India; Part–whole relationships; Shapes and visual images

Skill Builders:
Vocabulary
Adjectives

Synopsis: Based on the ancient fable from India about blind men and an elephant, this is a tale of six mice that disagree on what they see. Not until the seventh mouse resolves the dilemma do they learn a valuable lesson: The whole is bigger than its parts. Paper collage illustrations by Caldecott Award winner Young are captivating.

Method: Before reading, review the names of the days of the week and present the idea of giving a color to each day. Also name the parts of some animals to see whether children can guess the whole. Talk about how sometimes when we look at only a part of something, we may not know what it is. We try to find out in many ways, by turning it around, upside down, picking it up, and so on.

Read the story, explaining the meaning of words such as *pillar, spear, cliff,* and *whole.* When turning to the page showing the object, ask children to identify the color. Present part of the elephant as shown and ask children to pretend they are mice. What are they looking at?

For learning the days of the week, encourage repetition. For example, when the text says the mouse went on Wednesday, have children recite the days of the week up to Wednesday, and then repeat when the next mouse ventures out on the next day, until the children are reciting the days of the week by the end of the story. Use the class calendar as a visual aid, if necessary.

After reading, ask children why the story is called *Seven Blind Mice.* Recall some of the things the mice thought they were seeing when they saw only part of the elephant, and then give adjectives to those parts.

Note: This book makes a nice sequel to *It Looks Like Spilt Milk, Quick as a Cricket, I Went Walking,* or any of Tana Hoban's concept books.

Shadows and Reflections

by Tana Hoban
New York: Greenwillow Books, 1990

Suggested Grade and Interest Level: K

Topic Explorations: Shadows; Shapes and visual images

Skill Builders:
   Vocabulary
   Adjectives
   Language literacy
   Relating personal experiences
   Verbal expression
   Compare and contrast

Synopsis: This photographer's wordless book shows images of shadows and reflections in city streets, zoos, and places by the waters.

Method: Before the read-aloud, discuss shadows and reflections. Talk about the qualities of each. Explain how sunlight causes objects or people to cast shadows and causes reflections on shiny surfaces. Then present the book, inviting children to guess whether the photograph is of a reflection or a shadow. What makes it a shadow or a reflection? How are a shadow and reflection alike? How are they different? Brainstorm other places one may see shadows or reflections, such as on a mirror or on one's shoes or boots.

Extended Activities: Stand outside the school at different times of the day and note how the shadows change—how they point in one direction in the morning, are small at noon, and point in the opposite direction in the afternoon. Then have children draw pictures of a shadow they saw cast by an object or person. Let the children share their drawings, describing what they saw.

Go for a walk around the school or community and observe shadows and reflections. Take photographs. Put them in a book and let the children use it to share the experiences of their walk.

Sheep on a Ship

by Nancy Shaw
Boston: Houghton Mifflin, 1989, 1991

Suggested Grade and Interest Level: Pre-K

Topic Explorations: Animals; Boats; Sheep; Weather, Storms

Skill Builders:

Vocabulary	**Language literacy**
Grammar and syntax	Problem solving
Two- and three-word utterances	**Phonological awareness**
Noun–verb agreement	
Singular and plural nouns	
Tenses, present and past	

Synopsis: Short, playful text tells of sailing sheep that fall asleep before an oncoming storm. In the midst of a ship-wreck, they chop down the mast and make a raft that carries them safely (well, almost) into port.

Methods: Before the read-aloud, elicit story predictions based on the book's cover.

During the read-aloud, pause only to elaborate on the meaning, if necessary, so as not to interrupt the flow of the rhyming text. Then do a picture walk-through and talk about what happens in the story. To increase vocabulary, discuss the words of the text and their meanings, including

deep-sea	collide
deck	mast
drift	float
port	dock

To build grammar and syntax skills and increase utterance length, share talk using the grammatical forms of the text (e.g., "sheep sail," "sheep wake up," "sheep slip," and "sheep slide"). Or use your own noun–verb phrases to tell what happens in the story (e.g., "Sheep nap, sheep fall."). For tenses, rephrase and reshape the short text into sentences for repetition (e.g., "The sheep are napping." "The sheep napped."). For regular and irregular plural forms, contrast the words "sheep on a ship" with similar stories about "monkeys on a ship," "elephants on a ship," "mice on a ship," and so on.

Build language literacy skills by talking about the problem the characters had and what they did to solve it. Use the illustrations to help answer the questions, if necessary.

> Q: How did the sheep get into trouble? (They fell asleep.)
> Q: What did they do about it? (They chopped the mast.)
> Q: Was it a good idea to chop down the mast? Why? (Yes. They made it into a raft.)
> Q: How did they get back to port? (They floated on the raft until they saw land.)
> Q: What are some good words to describe how the raft moved in the water? (floated, bobbed up and down, meandered)
> Q: What did the sheep load on board at the beginning of the story? (The treasure chest)
> Q: Why did they take it with them on the raft? (They didn't want the treasure chest to sink with the ship.)

Increase phonological awareness with the words of the text. First do a picture walk-through to review the story.

PLAY **Can-You-Hear-It?**

Children imagine as you talk about the words that sound like what they describe, for example,

> Listen to the sound of the word *lap*.
> The story says, "waves lap."
> What sound does lapping waves make? Can you hear it?
> What else makes a lapping sound? (e.g., A kitten laps milk.)

More onomatopoeic words include

> *slosh*—"waves slosh" (e.g., A pig sloshes in mud.)
> *flap*—"sails flap" (e.g., Flags flap in the wind.)

PLAY **Word-Count.**

Children count the number of words in a short line from the text. Demonstrate by assigning one word to one finger as you say the words. For example, say

> On a ship

as you hold up one finger for each word until three fingers are showing. Ask

> How many words did I say? (three)

Then say

> Sheep on a ship

for a four-finger count. Gradually allow the children to do the counting by themselves.

If children don't have one-to-one correspondence, give each child a collection of manipulables (i.e., blocks, felt squares, buttons, etc.) to use for representing each of the stated words. Demonstrate by saying (or use a puppet to say) the words from a page of text that you want the children to count. Repeat them again as you (or a puppet) move out one item at a time to correspond to your stated word. Then you (or a puppet) count out loud the number of blocks moved to get the word count. Gradually allow the children to do the counting by themselves. Use words directly from a page of the text in hierarchical order to the desired word length. Some words from the text to count include

Waves lap	Sheep can't sail	It rains and hails
Sails flap	Make a raft	They chop a mast
Sheep slide	The storm lifts	Not far to go
Sheep trip	The raft drifts	
Sheep collide	Sheep jump off	
Sheep paddle		

PLAY **Rearrange-It.**

Children rearrange, in correct word order, a scrambled phrase or sentence from a portion of the text.

For example, say

(continues on next page)

PLAY **Rearrange-It.** *Continued*

Ship on a sheep
Is that right? Can you help me say the words in the right order?
That's right. *Ship on a sheep* should really be *Sheep on a ship.*

More words to rearrange include

Nap sheep	Sheep off jump
Sheep sail can't	Sheep up wake
	Sheep map a read

PLAY **The Same-Sound game.**

Children identify whether word pairs begin with the same sound. For example, say

sheep, ship
Do they start with the same sound? (Yes)

Intersperse nonmatched pairs into the following list of matched pairs. To make an unmatched pair, exchange one of the following words with another word from the text.

sail, sea	map, mast	ship, shark
sag, sail	land, lap	wave, wake
read, rain	deep, day	deck, dark

PLAY **Word-Search.**

Children search the picture for the word you are thinking of that begins with the sound of a given word. For example, say

I see something in this picture that starts with the same sound as *ship.*
What other word starts with *Sh?* (Give phoneme/sound only.)
Search for the word. (sheep)
That's right. *Sheep* is a word that starts with *Sh.*

Use the alliterative words provided in the Same-Sound game as well as other words found on the pages of the text.

PLAY **Say-the-Sound.**

Children identify beginning sounds in a series of words (and related words) from the text. For example, ask

What sound do you hear at the beginning of *short, sheep,* and *shark?*
Hear it, then say it.
That's right. *Sh* is the sound at the beginning of *short, sheep,* and *shark.*

In addition to the following three-word strings, use two-word strings provided in the Same-Sound game.

sheep, ship, shake	sail, set, sag, sea
lap, lift, land, leap	map, make, mast, mop
deep, dark, deck, day	port, paddle, porpoise, pan

PLAY **Which-One-Rhymes?**

Children select a rhyming word out of a word string that matches the target word you present. For example, say

> Which word rhymes with *sheep*?
> trip, shark, deep
> That's right. *Deep* rhymes with *sheep*.

More word strings include

ship (flap, slide, trip)	sail (wave, hail, collide)
wash (slosh, port, raft)	wave (form, save, cloud)
nap (sheep, lap, port)	sea (no, she, sail)
lift (wave, storm, drift)	chop (lift, seaweed, shop)
drip (climb, treasure, trip)	

PLAY **Rhyming-Ings.**

Children rhyme root words with added *-ing* suffixes using words of the text (root + added suffix, if necessary). Give initial phoneme or cluster cues and picture prompts if needed. Accept any nonsense word that rhymes. For example, say

> The sheep are sleeping on the ship. (Stress *sleeping* and show the picture.)
> What word rhymes with *sleeping*? (*beeping, weeping, keeping, sweeping, creeping,* etc.)

Other words include

> napping (flapping, slapping, tapping, trapping)
> sailing (mailing, jailing, bailing, wailing, nailing)
> raining (gaining, staining)
> sliding (hiding, riding, siding)
> crashing (slashing, dashing, mashing)
> drifting (sifting, shifting)

PLAY **Clap-and-Count.**

Children clap to, and then count, the number of syllables heard in selected words from the illustrations and text. Demonstrate by clapping to a word and then asking children how many parts they heard. For example, clap and say

> crash
> How many parts in the word? Clap it out. (one)
> Crash. One.

Clap and say

> crashing
> How many parts in that word? Clap it out. (two)
> Crash-ing. One, two.

(continues on next page)

Clap-and-Count. *Continued*

Stress and elongate syllables when presenting words such as

anchor	sailing
dolphin	disaster
lightning	telescope
sailboat	attention
collide	suddenly
napping	

PLAY **Find-the-Little-Words.**

Children listen for "little" words within compound and two-syllable words of the text. Stress and elongate syllables when presenting the word. For example, say

> sailboat
> Can you hear any little words in *sailboat*? (sail, boat)
> That's right. *Sail* is a little word in *sailboat*.
> *Boat* is another little word in *sailboat*.

Continue with two-syllable words, changing the stress as necessary so the children can hear all the "little" words. Some two-syllable words are as follows:

> dol-phin (doll, fin)
> crash-ing (crash)
> napp-ing (nap)
> sail-ing (sail)
> sleep-ing (sleep)
> slipp-ing (slip)
> rain-ing (rain)

PLAY **Leave-It-Out.**

Children say a compound or two-syllable word, then leave out the beginning or final part to create a smaller word. For example, say

> Say *sailboat*.

Then say

> Now, say *sailboat*, but leave out *boat*.
> What little word is left? (sail)

Then say

> Now, say *sailboat*, but leave out *sail*.
> What little word is left? (boat)

Continue with the list of two-syllable words provided in Find-the-Little-Words.

> **PLAY** **Add-It-On.**
>
> Children put two syllables together to make two-syllable words. For example, say
>
> > Say *sail*.
>
> Then say
>
> > Now, say *sail*, and add *boat*.
> > What new word can you make? (sailboat)
>
> Then, reverse the order in which the words are presented. For example, say
>
> > Put *boat* at the end of *sail*. What word do you have? (sailboat)
>
> Continue with the two-syllable words provided in Find-the-Little-Words.

> **PLAY** **Turn-It-Around.**
>
> Children reverse the parts of words they previously analyzed and synthesized, for example,
>
> > Put the word *fin* at the beginning of *doll*.
> > What silly word do you have? (findoll)
> > What was it before we turned it around? (dolphin)

☛ See the catalog for Grades 1 through 5 for continuing activities in the hierarchy of phonological awareness.

Note: Read also *Sheep in a Jeep, Sheep in a Shop,* and *Sheep Out to Eat* by the same author. Use the words of the text and adapt them to the PA games in the same manner they are listed here.

Silly Sally

by Audrey Wood
San Diego, CA: Harcourt Brace, 1992

Suggested Grade and Interest Level: Pre-K

Skill Builders:

Vocabulary	Grammar and syntax
Adjectives	Tenses, present and past
Prepositions	
Antonyms	

Synopsis: "Silly Sally went to town, walking backwards, upside down" goes the opening lines of the text. From there, it only gets zanier, and the repetition builds as a pig dances a jig, a dog plays leapfrog, a loon sings a silly tune, and more friends join the silly girl on her fun-loving journey. The rhyming, cumulative text is ideal for repetition.

Method: Before the read-aloud, have children describe Sally, pictured on the cover of the book doing a somersault. What is she doing? What kind of a girl might she be?

During the read-aloud, pause to have children repeat the text and use the prepositions in their own phrases and sentences. Prepositions include *backwards, upside down, forwards,* and *right side up.*

Also, encourage use of past-tense verbs in the text, including *met, sang, tickled,* and *woke.*

After the reading, have children say in their own words how Sally got to town, who she encountered, and what they did. What words describe Sally? How did she get to town?

For antonyms, ask children to give the opposite word for the following:

> upside down (rightside up)
> backwards (forwards)
> silly (serious, normal, regular, etc.)

For practice using prepositions at the sentence level, begin with the lines of text, having children finish the sentence. For example, say

> Sally Sally went to town, dancing . . .
> Silly Sally went to town, leaping . . .
> Silly Sally went to town, singing . . .

Add other verbs to the ones already used from the text, having children finish the sentence. Examples include

> Silly Sally went to town, skipping . . .
> Silly Sally went to town, hopping . . .

Make alliterative sentences with children's names and include different locations in the sentence starters. Encourage children to repeat the entire sentence, such as

> Artistic Arthur went to school, singing . . .
> Happy Jose went to the park, skipping . . .
> Curteous Katie went to her grandmothers, jumping . . .

Sing, Sophie!

by Dayle Ann Dodds
Cambridge, MA: Candlewick Press, 1997, 1999

Suggested Grade and Interest Level: Pre-K

Topic Explorations: Cowboys and cowgirls; Family relationships; Music, musicians, and musical instruments; Sounds; Weather, Storms

Skill Builders:

Vocabulary	Grammar and syntax	Phonological awareness
Attributes	Two- and three-word utterances	
Synonyms	Noun–verb agreement	
	Present tense	

Synopsis: Sophie is a hoot. She loves her guitar and at any moment she may break into song—one of her own, unique songs, like, "My dog ran off/My cat has fleas/My fish won't swim/and I hate peas." However, no one in her family likes to listen to them—nor to her loud voice. Then, during a fierce thunderstorm, Sophie's singing calms her baby brother, and her family puts a new spin on their little shining star. This is a great book to help show children how to create songs or poems from their own experience and to express their thoughts and language! Yippie-ki-yo!

Method: Before the read-aloud, ask children what they know about cowboys and cowgirls. Elicit background knowledge about the term *caterwauling*. Draw children's attention to the syllables in the word as they practice saying it. Give a definition, such as "long, loud, shrieking, wailing sounds that cats and other animals sometimes make." Then ask the children to listen to the story. As soon they hear the word, they can all say it after you.

During the read-aloud, limit interaction so that the words and rhythm of Sophie's songs can be thoroughly enjoyed. Pause at the word *caterwauling,* and after the children all repeat it, ask what they think Sophie's brother means when he says that her "caterwauling will scare all the fish away."

After the read-aloud, describe Sophie, including her 20-gallon hat, cowboy boots, and trusty guitar. Include a list of her attributes. Is she

quiet or loud?	lively or boring?
shy or bold?	happy or sad?
a bother or a hoot?	

Shape children's descriptions into target syntactical forms, building grammar and syntax skills. Some examples include

Sophie sings.
Loud Sophie sings.
Sophie sings loudly.
Sophie sings her songs.
Sophie sings in the cornfield.
Sophie plays.
Happy Sophie plays.
Sophie plays happily.
Sophie plays her guitar.
Sophie wails.
Sophie caterwauls.
Sophie wails when she is singing.
Sophie scares the fish.

For synonyms, brainstorm other words for noise, such as

sound
racket
caterwauling
clatter (as in the poem, *The Night Before Christmas,* ". . . there arose such a clatter . . .")
clamor
commotion
din (as in ". . . they made such a din" in *Who Sank the Boat*)
hubbub
hullabaloo

Reread some of Sophie's songs and use portions of them in games for phonological awareness training. For example,

"I'm a cowgirl	"But I'm a cowgirl
Through and through	Don't you know!
Yippie-ky-yee!	Yippie-ky-yee
Yippie ky-yuu!"	Yippee-ky-yo!"

PLAY **Word-Count.**

Children count the number of words in a short verse. Demonstrate by assigning one word to one finger as you say the words. For example, say

> Sophie

as you hold up one finger. Ask

> How many words did I say? (one)

Then say

> Sing, Sophie

for a two-finger count. Gradually allow the children to do the counting by themselves.

If children don't have one-to-one correspondence, give each child a collection of manipulables (i.e., blocks, felt squares, buttons, etc.) to use for representing each of the stated words. Demonstrate by saying (or use a puppet to say) the words from a page of text that you want the children to count. Repeat them again as you (or a puppet) move out one item at a time to correspond to your stated word. Then you (or a puppet) count out loud the number of blocks moved to get the word count. Gradually allow the children to do the counting by themselves. Use words directly from a page of the text in hierarchical order to the desired word length. Use the short text for word sources.

PLAY **Rearrange-It.**

Children rearrange, in correct word order, a scrambled phrase or sentence from a portion of the text.

For example, say

> Cowgirl I am
> Is that right? Can you help me say the words in the right order?
> That's right. *Cowgirl I am* should really be *I am a cowgirl.*

Then say

> I'm going to say the words to part of Sophie's song, but I might get it a little mixed up. If I do, help me rearrange it so I can get it right.
> "But I'm a cowgirl
> Don't you know
> Yippie-ky-yee
> Yippie-*yo-ky.*" (Yippie-ky-yo)

Continue mixing up part of the text for the children to rearrange.

PLAY **The Same-Sound game.**

Children identify whether word pairs begin with the same sound. For example, say

> cow, coat
> Do they start with the same sound? (Yes)

(continues on next page)

PLAY **The Same-Sound game.** *Continued*

To make unmatched pairs, replace one of the following words with another word from the text.

cow, coat
bump, bug
know, not
peas, pass
socks, cider
cow, kite

lost, liver
nose, knee
ran, rug
scared, skinny
crow, cry

PLAY **Finish-the-Rhyme.**

Children supply the rhyming word you leave out at the end of a verse. Provide the initial phoneme cue and picture prompt if needed. For example, say

Help me say the words of Sophie's poem:
"My kite got stuck
I ate a bug
I spilled red cider
On the (r)_____." (rug)

PLAY **Rhyme-It-Again.**

Children identify the rhyming word you read after each set. For example, say

Bug rhymes with _____. (rug)

PLAY **Make-a-Rhyme.**

Children supply another rhyming word after a set of two is presented. Give initial phoneme cues if needed. Accept any nonsense word. For example, ask

What word rhymes with *bug*? *Bug, rug,* (m) _____

Then ask

What are some other words that rhyme with *bug*? (*tug, dug, hug, jug, lug, mug, pug,* and any nonsense word)

PLAY **Clap-and-Count.**

Children clap to, and then count, the number of syllables heard in words from the text and illustrations. For example, clap and say

cow
How many parts in the word? Clap it out. (one)
Cow. One.

(continues on next page)

PLAY Clap-and-Count. *Continued*

Clap and say

> cowgirl
> How many parts in that word? Clap it out. (two)
> Cow–girl. One, two.

Stress and elongate syllables when presenting words, such as

corn-field	li-ver	bro-ther
thun-der	roo-ster	ca-ter-waul
spi-nach	ski-nny	ca-ter-waul-ing

And part of Sophie's song:

yippie	yee	Yippie-ky-yee
ky	yippie-ky	

PLAY Find-the-Little-Words.

Children listen for "little" words within compound and two-syllable words of the text. Stress and elongate syllables when presenting the word. For example, say

> cowgirl
> Can you hear any little words in *cowgirl*? (cow, girl)
> That's right. *Cow* is a little word in *cowgirl*.
> *Girl* is another word in *cowgirl*.

Continue with the following compound and two-syllable words, changing the stress as necessary so the children can hear all the "little" words.

cowboy (cow, boy)	cornfield (corn, field)
spinach (spin)	skinny (skin, knee)
yippie (yip)	caterwaul (cat, wall)

PLAY Leave-It-Out.

Children say a compound or two-syllable word, then leave out the beginning or final part to create a smaller word. For example, say

> Say *cowgirl*.

Then say

> Now, say *cowgirl*, but leave out *girl*.
> What little word is left? (cow)

Then say

> Now, say *cowgirl*, but leave out *cow*.
> What little word is left? (girl)

Continue with the compound and two-syllable words provided in Find-the-Little Words.

(PLAY) Add-It-On.

Children put two syllables together to make two-syllable words. For example, say

> Say *cow*.

Then say

> Now, say *cow*, and add *girl*.
> What bigger word can you make? (cowgirl)

Then, reverse the order in which the words are presented. For example, say

> Put *girl* at the end of *cow*. What word do you have? (cowgirl)

Continue with the two-syllable words provided in Find-the-Little-Words.

(PLAY) Turn-It-Around.

Children reverse the parts of the compound words they have previously analyzed and synthesized, for example,

> Put the word *girl* at the beginning of *cow*.
> What word do you have? (girlcow)
> What was it before we turned it around? (cowgirl)

Continue with the compound and two-syllable words in Find-the-Little-Words.

(PLAY) Switch-It.

Children delete part of a compound or two-syllable word and exchange it with a new part to make another compound word. Prompt with cues as necessary. For example, say

> Say *cowgirl*.
> Now, say *cowgirl*, only take out *girl* and put in *boy*.
> What new word can you make? (cowboy)

Some word exchanges include

> Say *cornfield*, only take out *field* and put in *cob*. (corncob)
> Say *cornfield*, only take out *field* and put in *flakes*. (cornflakes)
> Say *cornfield*, only take out *corn* and put in *wheat*. (wheatfield)
> Say *yippie*, only take out *yip* and put in *skip*. (skippie)

☛ See the catalog for Grades 1 through 5 for continuing activities in the hierarchy of phonological awareness.

Extended Activity: Have children make up their own cowgirl (or cowboy) songs. You may even want to accompany them with a guitar. First establish a pattern for children to simply fill in the ending words to starter lines. The words don't necessarily have to rhyme, or make sense! Some suggestions include

My dog _____ (went meow)	But I'm a cowgirl (cowboy)
My cat _____ (wears jeans)	Don't you know
My fish _____ (ran off)	Yippie-ky-yee
I hate _____ (beans)	Yippie-ky-yo.

The Snopp on the Sidewalk and Other Poems

by Jack Prelutsky
New York: Greenwillow Books, 1976, 1977

Suggested Grade and Interest Level: Pre-K

Topic Exploration: Humor

Skill Builders:
    Phonological awareness   **Articulation,** *G* and *F*

Synopsis: Vignettes in rhyming verse are illustrated with imaginary creatures that are always a hit.

Method: After you have read the rhyme a few times, play a few phonological awareness games.

The rhyming words of the verses come close together, making them more memorable. Some rhyming games include the following:

> (PLAY) **Finish-the-Rhyme.**
>
> Children supply the rhyming word left out at the end of a familiar verse.

> (PLAY) **Rhyme-It-Again.**
>
> Children identify the rhyming word you read after each set.

> (PLAY) **The Same-Sound game.**
>
> Children identify whether two words (or three-word strings) selected from the text begin with the same sound. For example, say
>
> > gibble, gobble
> > Do they start with the same sound? (Yes)

For articulation of *F*, read "Flonster Poem" and "The Frummick and the Frelly" to practice *F*. Play a game of repeating the silly target words two and three times.

For articulation of *G*, read "The Gibble" and "The Gobbles." Use the alliteration for repeated sound identification and production.

The Snowy Day

by Ezra Jack Keats
New York: Viking Press, 1962, 1976

Suggested Grade and Interest Level: Pre-K

Topic Explorations: Seasons, Winter; Weather

Skill Builders:

Grammar and syntax	Language literacy
Noun–verb agreement	Relating personal experiences
Tenses, present and past	Sequencing

Synopsis: A child's delight at winter's first snowfall is richly depicted by this award-winning author and illustrator.

Method: For noun–verb agreement and present and past tenses, structure phrases and sentences from the short text for repetition.

For sequencing, ask children what they think the boy will tell his mother about his adventures in the snow when he returns home. What are some of the things the boy did? For example,

> He saw snow outside when he woke up.
> He put on his snowsuit.
> He walked through the snow.
> He made tracks.
> He found a stick.

Ask children to tell how this boy's adventure is like their own experiences in the snow. What's the first thing they do when they want to go outside and play in the snow? Then what do they do? Continue to elicit a complete series of events. Encourage children to share stories about playing in the snow.

Note: This book is also published in Spanish, titled *Un dia de nieve* (Picture Puffins, 1991).

Snowy Flowy Blowy: A Twelve Months Rhyme

Illustrated by Nancy Tafuri
New York: Scholastic Press, 1999

Suggested Grade and Interest Level: Pre-K

Topic Explorations: Birds; Months of the year; Seasons; Weather

Skill Builders:

Vocabulary	Grammar and syntax	Language literacy
Adjectives	Two- and three-word utterances	Relating personal experiences
Morphological units	Noun–verb agreement	Sequencing

Synopsis: The simple, flowing words of an old rhyme by Gregory Gander (1745–1815) are accompanied by Nancy Tafuri's size-enhanced, trademark watercolors. Enlarged, strikingly visual birds are featured in the foreground of each double-page spread that features both the name of the month and a one-word phrase of the poem, which is the sole text. Characters in the background provide the action. In March, for example, a red-breasted robin sits in the foreground on a sap bucket of a maple tree. In the background, the snow is partially melted, revealing the grassy ground where children fly kites in their jackets and mittens. *Blowy* is the single featured word. In September, black crows are featured among the bright red apples of a tree. Behind their large shapes are two children leaving their rural home as a yellow school bus waits behind the fence. This is an ideal book for a variety of language activities.

Method: Before the read-aloud, talk about the seasons of the year and their corresponding months. Ask children what they know about the seasons. Demonstrate the months of the year with a large picture calendar, showing the present month. Refer to the weather outside and the season you are presently experiencing.

During the read-aloud, pause at each page to structure two- and three-word utterances and phrases for noun–verb agreement, such as

Ducks quack   Birds chirp
Children play   The girl swings
The boy reads   Children fly kites
People get married Kids go fishing

Use the text's adjectives in short phrases (using your own discretion, as the poet definitely used poetic license here)

Flowy river
Blowy wind
Showery day
Flowery backyard in May
Bowery branch (leafy branch)

After the read-aloud, do a picture walk-through and talk about each month and events that happen during the months. Ask children to relate their own experiences of things that happen during the months and seasons. Assist in their constructions by starting them off and using scaffolding with words such as *once, then,* and *and finally.*

Review the pages once again, reciting the months in sequential order. Use the events previously discussed while talking about the sequence. For example,

At the beginning of the year it is snowy
In spring the snow melts and
After spring come the summer months
After the summer months it becomes fall
Then leaves fall from the trees and people harvest pumpkins
Next comes freezy winter

Teach awareness of the morphological unit –*y* with the use of the text and illustrations. Use the month of October and the illustrations, for example. Focus on the word and ask

How many parts do you hear in the word *breezy*?
What little word do you hear in *breezy*? (breeze)
What part of the word do you hear after *breeze*? (y, sounds like *ee*)

Explain one meaning of the little sound –*y* (*ee*) when used at the end of a word as a way to describe something (e.g., January has snow. It's snow<u>y</u>.). Give examples of other –*y*-ending words. For example,

sun, sunny   wind, windy
ice, icy   breeze, breezy
flower, flowery   mess, messy
scratch, scratchy

Encourage children to use the words in sentences within the immediate context of their lives.

PLAY The Suffix game.

Put –*y* after *wind*. What word is it now? (windy)
Put –*y* after *sun*. What word is it now? (sunny)
Use the previous word list and some words of your own.

Spot's Birthday Party

by Eric Hill
New York: Putnam, 1982

Suggested Grade and Interest Level: Pre-K

Skill Builders:

Vocabulary	**Grammar and syntax**
Prepositions	Possessive nouns

Synopsis: Join Spot as he meets all his friends in unexpected places on his romp through the house in search of his birthday party.

Method: Children can't wait to lift the peek-a-boo flaps to find

> An alligator under the carpet.
> The bear behind the curtain.
> The snake in the cupboard.

Structure phrases for repetition, using prepositions and possessive nouns in the context of the story.

Note: Read also *Spot's Alphabet, Spot's Busy Year, Spot's Toys, Spot's Toy Box, Spot's Friends, Spot's Big Book of Words,* and other Spot stories to work on the same target objectives.

Swimmy

by Leo Lionni
New York: Pantheon, 1963; Knopf, 1987

Suggested Grade and Interest Level: Pre-K

Topic Explorations: Friendship; Sea and the seashore

Skill Builders:

Vocabulary	**Language literacy**
Attributes	Storytelling
Morphological units	Problem solving

Synopsis: Swimmy, who looks different from all the other fish in the sea, loses his family to a big tuna fish. Alone, he sets out to explore the underwater world until he finds a school of fish just like his old family. But they're afraid to play with Swimmy until he solves the big old scary fish problem. Using his uniqueness and a clever ploy, he persuades them all to swim away together in one big fish formation, while he poses as the giant fish's eye.

Method: Before the read-aloud, ask children to make story predictions. Elicit background information about oceans.

During the read-aloud, pause to clarify meaning. Discuss the vocabulary of the text, including the following:

Medusa	jellyfish
lobster	invisible
seaweed	eel
sea anemones	school (of fish)

After the read-aloud, teach morphological word endings and comparatives by discussing the concepts of *big, little, bigger than,* and *smaller than.* Encourage children to use the words in sentences about Swimmy, such as

Swimmy was *smaller* than the big tuna fish.
The tuna fish was bigger than all the other fish.

Also, ask children to name something in the ocean that is bigger than they are. What is in the ocean that is smaller than they are?

For storytelling and problem solving, discuss the story elements.

Who is the story about?
Where did it take place?
What happened to start the story?
How did Swimmy feel about that? What did he do?
What happened next?
How did Swimmy "think things through" to solve the problem?
How did the fish change?

Extended Activity: Gather an assortment of sea objects (sand, starfish, sand dollars, etc.), some of which Swimmy may have seen on his underwater journey. Put them in a paper bag. Have children take turns feeling the items (without looking at them) and think of attributes to describe them, such as *rough, smooth, big,* and *prickly.* Then, reveal the items, naming them along with their attributes.

Ten, Nine, Eight

by Molly Bang
New York: Greenwillow Books, 1983, 1991

Suggested Grade and Interest Level: Pre-K

Topic Explorations: Colors; Number concepts; Shapes and visual images

Skill Builders:

Vocabulary	**Phonological awareness**
Adjectives	**Fluency**
Prepositions	**Voice**
Grammar and syntax	
Two- and three-word utterances	
Singular and plural nouns	

Synopsis: A father prepares his little girl for bed with a countdown of rhyming text. This Caldecott Honor and ALA Notable book is ideal for language structuring.

Method: Use the illustrations and the rhythmic, rhyming verse to encourage repetition of the text as you read, for example,

> "9 soft friends in a quiet room."
> "8 square windowpanes with falling snow."
> "7 empty shoes in a short, straight row."
> "6 pale seashells hanging down."
> "5 round buttons on a yellow gown."
> "4 sleepy eyes which open and close."

For adjectives and early utterances, encourage children to repeat the part of the text on each page. Prompt with the following:

> What kind of room?
> What kind of window?

What other words can you use to describe the friends? For example,

> stuffed (animals)
> fuzzy
> cuddly

For phonological awareness training, play the following:

PLAY **Word-Count.**

Children count the number of words in a short line from the text. Demonstrate by assigning one word to one finger as you say the words. For example, say

> soft

as you hold up one finger for the word. Ask,

> How many words did I say?

Then say

> soft friends

for a two-finger count. Gradually allow the children to do the counting by themselves.

If children don't have one-to-one correspondence, give each child a collection of manipulables (i.e., blocks, felt squares, buttons, etc.) to use for representing each of the stated words. Demonstrate by saying (or use a puppet to say) the words from a page of text that you want the children to count. Repeat them again as you (or a puppet) move out one item at a time to correspond to your stated word. Then you (or a puppet) count out loud the number of blocks moved to get the word count. Gradually allow the children to do the counting by themselves. Use words directly from a page of the text in hierarchical order to the desired word length. Some words from the text to count include

soft friends	short, straight row
empty shoes	seven empty shoes
seven shoes	buttons on a gown
quiet room	buttons on a yellow gown

PLAY **Rearrange-It.**

Children rearrange, in correct word order, a scrambled phrase or sentence from a portion of the text. For example, say

> Nine friends soft.
> Is that right? Can you help me put the words in the right order?
> That's right. *Nine friends soft* should really be *Nine soft friends*.

Ask children to rearrange other words you scramble from the short lines of text.

PLAY **The Same-Sound game.**

Children identify whether word pairs begin with the same sound. For example, say

> toes, ten
> Do they start with the same sound? (Yes)

Intersperse nonmatched pairs into the following list of matched pairs:

> bear, big
> cat, kiss
> bear, button
> book, bear
> shoes, shells
> short, shoes
> four, five
> six, seven
> soft, six
> nine, night

PLAY **Odd-One-Out.**

Children select from a string of alliterative words the one that does not belong. For example, say

> six, seven, gown
> Which word has a different beginning sound? (gown)
> That's right. *Gown* is the odd one out.

Use the word pairs provided for two-word strings, inserting a word with a different initial sound for the children to identify. Use the following words to make three-word strings, inserting an odd one for the children to identify:

> six, seven, sew
> ten, two, time
> bear, button, book
> round, row, room
> shoes, shells, short

PLAY Which-One-Rhymes?

Children select a rhyming word out of a word string that matches the target word you present. For example, say

> Which word rhymes with *jar*? (soft, car, gown)

More word strings include

eyes (shoes, ties, empty)	close (shoes, yellow, nose)
shoes (use, two, row)	box (nine, blue, sox)
round (snow, found, bear)	row (snow, pale, shell)
room (sea, boom, blue)	down (frown, gown, close)
short (shoes, sport, straight)	

PLAY Clap-and-Count.

Children clap to, and then count, the number of syllables heard in selected words from the illustrations and text. Demonstrate by clapping to a word and then asking children how many parts they heard. For example, clap and say

> two
> How many parts in the word? Clap it out. (one)

Clap and say

> seven
> How many parts in that word? Clap it out. (two)
> Se–ven. One, two.

Stress and elongate syllables when presenting words, such as

> yellow
> hanging
> buttons
> window
> seashells

PLAY What's-the-Word?

Children synthesize two syllables into a word. Use the words and pictures of the book as cues. Present the syllables, inserting a clear pause between them, and have children say them quickly and repeatedly until they can guess the word. Demonstrate by saying

> yell–ow
> What's the word?
> Say it until you hear it. *Yelllll–ow. Yell-ow. Yellow.*
> *Yellow* is the word.

Continue with the two-syllable words in Clap-and-Count.

PLAY **Find-the-Little-Words.**

Children listen for "little" words within two-syllable words of the text. Stress and elongate syllables when presenting the word. Change stress if necessary so children can hear all the "little" words. For example, say

> yellow
> Can you find any little words in *yellow.* (yell, oh)
> That's right. *Yell* is a little word in *yellow.*
> *Oh* is another little word in *yellow.*

Continue with the following words:

> window (win, dough)
> windowpane (win, dough, window, pain)
> seashell (sea, shell)
> hanging (hang)

PLAY **Leave-It-Out.**

Children say a compound or two-syllable word, then leave out the beginning or final part to create a smaller word. For example, say

> Say *yellow.*
> Now, say *yellow,* but leave out *oh.*
> What little word is left? (yell)

Then say

> Now, say *yellow,* but leave out *yell.*
> What little word is left? (oh)

Continue with the words provided in Clap-and-Count and Find-the-Little-Words.

PLAY **Add-It-On.**

Children put two syllables together to make two-syllable words. For example, say

> Say *win.*
> Now, say *win,* and add *dough.*
> What word can you make? (window)

Then, reverse the order in which the words are presented. For example, say

> Put *dough* at the end of *win.*
> What word do you have? (window)

Continue with the words provided in Clap-and-Count and Find-the-Little-Words.

PLAY **Turn-It-Around.**

Children reverse the parts of the words they have analyzed and synthesized, such as

> Put the word *oh* at the beginning of *yell*.
> What word do you have then? (ohyell)
> What was it before we turned it around? (yellow)

Continue with the compound and two-syllable words provided.

Extended Activity: Go around the room and find or arrange groups of objects. Make up phrases about the groups for repetition. For example,

> 6 wet paintbrushes in a glass jar.
> 5 nice books on a big chair.
> 4 red balls in a cardboard box.
> 3 quiet children on a blue rug.
> 2 little peeps in a cage by the door.
> 1 yellow sun on a happy day.

Note: This book is also available in a Spanish-language translation, titled *Diez, nueve, ocho.*

The Tenth Good Thing About Barney

by Judith Viorst
New York: Atheneum, 1971, 1987

Suggested Grade and Interest Level: K

Topic Explorations: Death and dying; Family relationships; Pets

Skill Builders:

Vocabulary	Language literary
Attributes	Relating personal experiences
Grammar and syntax	Storytelling
Past tense	Drawing inferences

Synopsis: The cycle of life and death is explored in this story of a boy who grieves for his cat, Barney. After a funeral, where he tells of nine good things about Barney, he thinks of a tenth thing, after pondering and questioning the concept of death.

Note: This book is particularly helpful for encouraging discussion with children dealing with the issue of loss in any form.

Method: Before the read-aloud, ask whether any of the children have had a pet that died. What happened? How did they feel about it? Explain that this story is about a boy who is sad and misses his cat, Barney.

Read the entire story aloud, without pausing for interaction. Then, have children recall the words the boy used to describe his cat, such as *brave, smart, cuddly,* and *clean.* Ask children whether they can think of 10 good things about their pet, a class pet, a friend, or other people. Brainstorm as a group and record the adjectives on the board.

For past tense, recount the events of the story, structuring target sentences as necessary. For example,

> The cat died.
> The boy cried.
> The boy went to bed.
> The boy did not watch TV.
> Mother wrapped Barney in a scarf.
> Father buried Barney.

For storytelling, encourage children to recount the story while you provide scaffolding as needed. Ask what the problem was. Draw inferences about the boy's behavior. For example, ask

> How did the boy resolve the problem?
> Was it enough just to bury Barney?
> What helped the boy feel better about his missing cat?

That's Good! That's Bad!

by Margery Cuyler
New York: Henry Holt, 1991, 1993

Suggested Grade and Interest Level: Pre-K

Topic Explorations: Animals, Jungle; Zoos

Skill Builders:

Vocabulary	Language literacy	Fluency
Antonyms	Relating personal experiences	
	Predicting	
	Sequencing	
	Cause-and-effect relationships	
	Verbal expression	

Synopsis: A little boy goes to the zoo, where his parents buy him a balloon. Suddenly, the balloon lifts him into the sky. It carries him into a jungle and bursts on a prickly tree, leading the boy to some good and bad adventures. The funny pictures and the "Oh, that's good! No, that's bad" theme offer lots of opportunities for participation, as do the "noisy" words in the text, such as *slurp, snore, purr,* and *sob.*

Method: Before the read-aloud, talk about antonyms and brainstorm a few (e.g., *up* and *down, backward* and *forward, good* and *bad*). Present the book and its cover, and encourage children to predict what the story might be about.

Read aloud and interact by asking,

> What's the bad thing about _____? (e.g., sliding down the neck of a giraffe and falling into quicksand)
> What's the good thing about _____? (e.g., falling into quicksand next to an elephant)

Point out and name other animals in the background, including the macaw, ladybug, aphid, kudu, and sable antelope.

For cause-and-effect relationships, build a predictable pattern of adventure and misadventure. Ask

What happened when the giraffe bent down to take a drink? (or, Oh dear, the boy fell into the quicksand. What caused this to happen?)
What do you think will happen next? What makes you think so?

If necessary, point out the clues presented in the pictures.

After the read-aloud, recall the events, again emphasizing the cause-and-effect relationships that create the story sequence.

For fluency, have the child participate in the predictable, repetitive verse. Use the "that's good, that's bad" theme to shape progressively longer responses produced on a sustained breath stream.

There's an Alligator Under My Bed

by Mercer Mayer
New York: Dial Books for Young Readers, 1987

Suggested Grade and Interest Level: Pre-K

Skill Builders:

Vocabulary	**Language literacy**
Prepositions	Predicting
Grammar and syntax	Sequencing
Tenses, present and past	Cause-and-effect relationships
	Problem solving

Synopsis: A little boy insists there's an alligator living under his bed. He conquers his bedtime fears by coaxing the alligator from under his bed, down the stairs, and into the garage, using some pretty clever thinking.

Method: Before the read-aloud, ask children to make predictions about the story based on the book's title and cover illustration. Could an alligator really be under the boy's bed? Why might he think so?

During the read-aloud, pause briefly to teach verb tenses as you model or shape sentences from the illustrations.

After the read-aloud, review the pages and locate the alligator and the boy, modeling and shaping phrases based on the text and illustrations, such as

> under the bed
> beside the bed
> across the hall
> in the refrigerator
> on top of the board

For problem solving, ask the children to explain how the boy solved the problem of having an alligator under his bed. For sequencing and cause-and-effect relationships, ask children to recall the events that took place in order for him to get rid of the alligator. Help them to connect the events with words, such as *because* and *so,* to express the causal relationships.

Read also *There's a Nightmare in My Closet* and *There's Something in the Attic* by the same author.

The Thing That Bothered Farmer Brown

by Teri Sloat
New York: Orchard Books, 1995; First Orchard Paperbacks, 2001

Suggested Grade and Interest Level: Pre-K

Topic Explorations: Animals, Farm; Farms; Sounds and listening

Skill Builders:

Vocabulary	**Language literacy**
Synonyms	Relating personal experiences
Grammar and syntax	Predicting
Two- and three-word utterances	Sequencing
Noun–verb agreement	Cause-and-effect relationships
Past tense	Drawing inferences
	Phonological awareness

Synopsis: What makes that "tiny, whiny, humming sound" and prevents Farmer Brown from getting his sleep? Follow the pages of the amusing, rhyming, repetitive, and cumulative verse until the answer is revealed—or guessed! A fun book you will want to read again and again. It's easy to see why it is an American Bookseller Kids' Pick of the Lists book.

Method: Before the read-aloud, explore the book's cover. What can be said about Farmer Brown from his appearance? Talk about the dog and cat asleep in the bed behind the frazzled-looking farmer. Read the title and predict what might happen in the story. Infer from the picture and title what the book is about.

During the read-aloud (and once the pattern of Farmer Brown hitting the wall to stop the "tiny, whiny, humming sound" becomes established), have children predict what he will do next. For example, after reading

> "But the thing exhausting Farmer Brown
> Was something flying round and round
> With a tiny, whiny, humming sound."

Pause before turning the page and ask, What do you think he will do next? or Why do you think he's hitting the wall with a swat and a whack? What will happen next?

After the read-aloud, teach synonyms by talking about how the author used several words in the story to tell how Farmer Brown felt about the tiny, whiny, humming mosquito. Read the title and start with *bothering*. What's another word for *bothered*? Use it in another sentence. Review the text to discuss synonyms *annoying* and *disturbing*. Brainstorm other synonyms, including *irritating* and *bugging*.

To build sequencing skills, do a picture walk-through, rereading portions of the text. The words on several successive pages detail the actions the farmer took that evening. For instance, he ate his soup and bread, put his nightshirt on, climbed into bed, pulled up the sheet, and so on. Ask a child to tell part of the story, sequencing the actions from the illustrations and shaping two- and three-word utterances, noun–verb agreement, and past-tense structures.

> Horse neighed
> Donkey brayed
> Old goat bucked
> Chickens clucked
> Doves cooed
> Cows mooed

The horse neighed.
The donkey brayed.
The farmer snapped his sheet.
It startled the grumpy goat.
It made the hens flutter.
The farmer whacked the wall.

Have a discussion about the sounds of insects. Use descriptive words to identify different insect sounds. Recall the sounds of crickets, bees, flies, cicadas, and mosquitoes, to name a few. Have children relate personal experiences about a tiny (or not so tiny) insect sound. Was it bothersome? Where were they? What were they doing? Why did it bother them? What did they (or an adult) do about it?

For phonological awareness training, use the words of the text to play the following games:

PLAY **Word-Count.**

Children count the number of words from the verse. Demonstrate by assigning one word to one finger as you say the words. For example, say

old horse

as you hold up one finger for each word until two fingers are showing. Ask

How many words did I say?

Then say

The old horse neighed

for a four-finger count. Gradually allow the children to do the counting by themselves.

If children don't have one-to-one correspondence, give each child a collection of manipulables (i.e., blocks, felt squares, buttons, etc.) to use for representing each of the stated words. Demonstrate by saying (or use a puppet to say) the words from a page of text that you want the children to count. Repeat them again as you (or a puppet) move out one item at a time to correspond to your stated word. Then you (or a puppet) count out loud the number of blocks moved to get the word count. Gradually allow the children to do the counting by themselves. Use words directly from a page of the text in hierarchical order to the desired word length. Use words of the text of varying lengths for the children to count.

PLAY **The Same-Sound game.**

Children identify whether word pairs begin with the same sound. For example, say

cows, cat
Do they start with the same sound? (Yes)

Intersperse nonmatched pairs into the following list of matched pairs:

cows, cat	hens, head
neigh, night	whack, whiny

(continues on next page)

PLAY The Same-Sound game. *Continued*

horse, hum	hand, horse
snap, snore	sleep, slow
dairy, dog	doves, donkey
brown, brayed	chickens, chores
farmer, feathers	wall, weary

PLAY Finish-the-Rhyme.

Children supply the rhyming word left out at the end of a verse. Teach children to use the meaningful clues in the pictures as well as the meter of the verse to rhyme the word. If necessary, prompt with picture cues and with the initial phoneme, then gradually remove the scaffolding. For example, say

The cat yowled,	The doves cooed,
The dog _____, (howled)	The cows _____, (mooed)
The old goat bucked,	The old horse neighed,
The chickens _____, (clucked)	The donkeys _____. (brayed)

PLAY Rhyme-It-Again.

Children identify the rhyming word heard after a rhyming set is given. For example, after reading "The doves cooed, the cows mooed, the old horse neighed, the donkey brayed. . ." say,

Cooed rhymes with (m)_____. (mooed)
Neigh rhymes with (br)_____. (brayed)

PLAY Make-a-Rhyme.

Children supply another rhyming word after a set of two is presented. Give initial phoneme cues, if needed. Accept any nonsense word. For example, ask

What word rhymes with *neigh*? Neigh, bray, (m) _____.

Have children supply more rhyming words. For example, "What else rhymes with *neigh*?" (*hay, jay, Kay, lay, gay, pay, ray, say, way, sleigh, stay, stray,* and *clay*).

PLAY Rhyming-Ings.

Children rhyme root words with added *–ing* suffixes using words of the text (root + added suffix, if necessary). Give initial phoneme or cluster cues and picture prompts if needed. For example, say

What word rhymes with *humming*? (*coming, drumming, bumming, numbing, summing, strumming,* and other nonsense words that rhyme)

(continues on next page)

PLAY **Rhyming-Ings.** *Continued*

Other –*ing* words include

> closing (nosing, posing, dozing)
> flying (buying, tying, sighing, lying, frying, drying, prying, trying, dying)
> eating (meeting, seating, beating, cheating)
> sleeping (beeping, keeping, weeping, seeping, leaping)
> snoring (boring, pouring, roaring, soaring, storing, warring)
> cooing (mooing, doing, suing, booing)

PLAY **Clap-and-Count.**

Children clap to, and then count, the number of syllables heard in selected words from the illustrations and text. Demonstrate by clapping to a word and then asking children how many parts they heard. For example, clap and say

> farm
> How many parts in the word? Clap it out. (one)

Clap and say

> farmer
> How many parts in that word? Clap it out. (two)
> Farm-er. One, two.

Stress and elongate syllables when presenting words, such as

brown	sound	cow
coo	swat	whack
feathers	tiny	whiny
bucket	humming	pillow
donkey	bothered	chicken
pitchfork	sunflower	disturbing
exhausting	mosquito	

PLAY **What's-the-Word?**

Children synthesize two syllables into a word. Use the words and pictures of the book as cues. Present the syllables, inserting a clear pause between them, and have children say them quickly and repeatedly until they can guess the word. Demonstrate by saying

> pill-ow
> What's the word?
> Say it until you hear it. *Pilllll-ow. Pill-ow. Pillow.*
> *Pillow* is the word.

Continue with any clearly illustrated word on a page, such as *chicken, farmer, window, pitchfork,* and *mosquito.*

PLAY **Find-the-Little-Words.**

Children listen for "little" words in the compound words of the text. Stress and elongate syllables when presenting the word. For example, say

> nightshirt
> Can you find any little words in *nightshirt*? (night, shirt)
> That's right. *Night* is a little word in *nightshirt*.
> *Shirt* is another little word in *nightshirt*.

Continue with compound words of the text and illustrations, including

something	pitchfork	Butterball (the donkey)
newspaper	overhear	sunflower

Then present two-syllable words, changing the stress as necessary so children can hear all the "little" words, including

pillow (pill, low)	farmer (farm)	tiny (knee)
whiny (whine)	humming (hum)	

PLAY **Leave-It-Out.**

Children say a compound or two-syllable word, then leave out the beginning or final part to create a smaller word. For example, say

> Say *nightshirt*.
> Now, say *nightshirt*, but leave out *shirt*.
> What little word is left? (night)

Then say

> Now, say *nightshirt*, but leave out *night*.
> What little word is left? (shirt)

Continue with the compound and two-syllable words provided.

PLAY **Add-It-On.**

Children put two syllables together to make two-syllable words. For example, say

> Say *night*.
> Now, say *night*, and add *shirt*.
> What bigger word can you make? (nightshirt)

Then, reverse the order in which the words are presented. For example, say

> Put *shirt* at the end of *night*.
> What word do you have? (nightshirt)

Continue with the compound and two-syllable words provided.

PLAY **Leave-It-Out.**

Play this game with words that have morphological endings. Children delete the marker and identify the root word. Refer to the previous game, Leave-It-Out. Some words from the text include

farm-er	fly-ing
humm-ing	whin-y
slow-ly	sleep-ing

☛ See the catalog for Grades 1 through 5 for continuing activities in the hierarchy of phonological awareness activities.

Things That Are Most in the World

by Judi Barrett
New York: Atheneum Books for Young Readers, Simon & Schuster, 1998; First Aladdin Paperbacks, 2001

Suggested Grade and Interest Level: Pre-K

Skill Builders:
 Vocabulary
 Morphological units

Synopsis: "The wriggliest thing in the world is a snake ice-skating." "The silliest thing is a chicken in a frog costume." The quietest thing, the prickliest thing, the hottest thing, and more are all depicted on the pages of this wonderful book of superlatives. From the author of *Cloudy with a Chance of Meatballs*.

Method: Present the book by asking the children to explain what *most* means, soliciting any number of assorted re-sponses. Then, read the text aloud, pausing to comment on each of the illustrations, including things that are the

oddest	teensie-weensiest
longest	jumpiest
smelliest	nearest

Encourage children to make up their own examples for each superlative. Encourage a complete sentence to elicit the morphological ending. Use classroom articles for ideas and themes such as food or toys. For example, say

 I think the silliest thing in the world is pizza with pickles.
 I think the oddest thing in the world is a bullfrog on a bicycle.

After the read-aloud, revisit the pages. Structure new sentences for repetition that include suffixes, with all of the comparative forms of the word, as well as the root word. For example, say

 A quiet thing is a library.
 A quieter thing is a boy sleeping in a library.
 The quietest thing is a boy sleeping in a library when a worm is chewing on his peanut butter sandwich.

As the last page of the book suggests, have children fill in what the ____est thing in the world is about them-selves. Prompt with some beginning sentences, such as

 The happiest thing about me is ____.
 The cutest thing about me is ____.
 The smartest thing about me is ____.

The chewiest thing about me is my _____ .
The loudest thing about me is my _____ .
The softest thing about me is my _____ .
The silliest thing about me is _____ .

Then have them repeat the following: The very best thing in the world about me is me!

This Is the House That Jack Built

by Pam Adams
Swindon, England: Child's Play, 1977

Suggested Grade and Interest Level: Pre-K

Topic Explorations: Fairy tales and nursery rhymes

Skill Builders:
    Articulation, *K*   **Fluency**

Synopsis: A version of the ever-popular nursery rhyme with progressively longer verses. Children love to repeat the rhythmic verse, such as

> "This is the dog,
> That worried the cat,
> That killed the rat,
> That ate the malt,
> That lay in the house
> That Jack built."

Method: Read the text and view the illustrations. Then go back and have the child retell from memory as much of the tale as possible while you provide scaffolding, as necessary.

For articulation of *K*, first select words from the rhyme for auditory bombardment of the target phoneme. Practice words at the one-word level before reading the story, then have children repeat more and more of the verse as it becomes increasingly familiar, using their target sounds.

The rhyme naturally builds fluency because one phrase is added to the repetitive, rhythmic verse on each page. Each page gives the child an opportunity to practice maintaining airflow during progressively longer utterances containing familiar words.

Note: There are many versions of this tale written by various authors. Versions can also be found in many books of nursery rhymes. You may wish to review them all and select a personal favorite.

The Three Billy Goats Gruff

by Peter Asbjornsen
New York: Harcourt Brace & World, 1957, 1991

Suggested Grade and Interest Level: Pre-K

Skill Builders:
    Vocabulary   **Articulation, *G***
    Morphological units   **Voice**
    Language literacy
    Predicting
    Sequencing
    Storytelling

Synopsis: This is the familiar tale of the three billy goats—with successive sizes and successively louder voices—who outsmart the troll under the bridge.

Method: Before the read-aloud, elicit background knowledge about the story to determine how much the children already know about the familiar tale. Talk about the cover and make story predictions, especially pointing out the sizes of the three billy goats. Discuss vocabulary words, such as *hooves, butted,* and selected words from your version of the text, by using them to talk about the cover.

During the read-aloud, pause to make predictions, point out information, and briefly discuss words that help children understand the meaning of the story.

After the read-aloud, bring awareness to morphological units *-er, -ier,* and *-iest* in root words such as *gruff* and *heavy* by reviewing the billy goats' voices, sizes, and weights. Have children use the words in their own sentences, including some of the following:

> The smallest, tiniest, quietest billy goat.
> The bigger, larger, heavier, louder, "gruffer" billy goat.
> The biggest, largest, loudest, heaviest, "gruffest" billy goat.

Have children sequence the episode of each goat's encounter with the troll, including some of the dialog. Provide scaffolding as necessary, progressively withdrawing support as children are able to supply their own words. For example, say

> The first billy goat walked across the bridge.
> Trip, trap, trip, trap!
> "Who's that crossing over my bridge?" roared the Troll.
> "It is I," said the tiniest billy goat.
> The Troll said he was going to gobble him up.
> The tiniest billy goat told him to wait for the second billy goat because he was much bigger.

Help children develop story schema by asking questions that enable their storytelling skills. If necessary, revisit the text and illustrations. Some sample questions include

> Who is the story about? (three billy goats named *Gruff*)
> Where does the story take place? (in a valley, meadow, on a hillside, etc.)
> What happened to start off the story? (They wanted to go up to the hillside where there was grass to eat.)
> What was the problem? (They had to cross a bridge to get there and a troll lived under the bridge.)
> What did the billy goats do about it? (repeat the sequenced episodes)
> What happened when the biggest billy goat came across the bridge?
> How did the story end?

For articulation of *G,* begin with auditory bombardment of words with the *G* phoneme, including *goat, gruff, grass, ugly* (some additions), *big, bigger, biggest,* and other target words found in your version. Reread the text and pause to allow the children to fill in the *G* words, either with a prompt or without, as they anticipate the target words. Use carrier phrases such as

> The smallest billy goat ____.
> The bigger billy goat ____.
> They biggest billy goat ____.

For voice training, portray the billy goats' and troll's voices to demonstrate different vocal qualities. Demonstrate a "small" (very soft) voice for the first billy goat, a "not-so-small" voice for the second billy goat, and "an ugly hoarse voice" for the big billy goat, as described in the text. Compare and contrast the roaring troll's voice with those of all three billy goats and discuss how the child feels about the characters or people who have these different vocal qualities. Use the smallest or "not-so-small" billy goat's voice to target easy onset of voice in progressively larger linguistic units.

Note: There are several versions of this tale, written by authors such as Paul Galdone and illustrated by artists such as Janet Stevens and Stephen Carpenter (the latter version is edited by Bruse Asbjornsen). Although Peter Asbjornsen's version is ideal to use for vocal awareness, it may not be available in your library. If you use another version, change the text by reading "hoarse" for the third billy goat's voice, as well as for the troll's.

Extended Activities: This is an excellent story for children to retell on a felt board. Cut out felt pieces for the troll and the three billy goats. Use an illustration from the book and a photocopier to outline and create templates for three successively larger goats and the troll. Attach bright-orange frayed yarn to the felt troll's head. Cut out a mountain, some green grass, and a bridge, and you are all set. During the storytelling, one child can move a goat over the bridge and say the goat's lines while another child can move the troll out from under the bridge and say its lines. You might even take small green felt pieces to put in the billy goats' mouths as they come back from the hillside, having found their grass to eat!

To Market, To Market

by Anne Miranda
San Diego, CA: Harcourt Brace, 1997; Voyager Picture Books, 2001

Suggested Grade and Interest Level:	Pre-K

Topic Explorations:	Fairy tales and nursery rhymes; Food; Vegetables

Skill Builders:

Vocabulary	**Language literacy**
Prepositions	Sequencing
Grammar and syntax	**Phonological awareness**
Tenses, present and past	**Articulation—*K*, *G*, and *P***

Synopsis: Here's a new twist on a classic nursery rhyme. A woman makes a simple trip to the market that turns into utter chaos after she buys the "fat pig" and returns for other animal ingredients to make her meal. The fat pig, red hen, plump goose, and so on all run amuck in her home until she does the smart thing and fetches the vegetables instead—and she finally gets her lunch!

Method: Before the read-aloud, ensure that children are familiar with the nursery rhyme for background knowledge. Read it a few times if necessary, then discuss what it might have been like long ago when people had no supermarkets and had to raise animals and grow vegetables for their food. Introduce the book and make predictions about what will happen in the story based on the cover illustration.

During the read-aloud, keep interaction to a minimum so that the flow of the verse and the rhyming pattern are easily identified. Point out features or clarify as necessary.

After the read-aloud, do a picture walk-through. Describe the funny scenes in the book to work on structures such as present and past tense. Structure responses to elicit prepositional phrases, such as "to the market, toward the market, inside, around, back home," and so on.

Play the following games for phonological awareness training.

PLAY The Same-Sound game.

Children identify whether word pairs begin with the same sound. For example, say

cow, coat
Do they start with the same sound? (Yes)

Intersperse nonmatched words into the following list of matched pairs:

duck, do   fat, find
hen, hat   goose, goat
peas, pass   pea, pods
luck, lamp

PLAY Finish-the-Rhyme.

Children supply the rhyming word left out at the end of a verse. Teach children to use the meaningful clues in the pictures as well as the meter of the verse to rhyme the word. If necessary, prompt with picture cues and with the initial phoneme, then gradually remove the scaffolding. For example, say

To market, to market, to buy a fat pig
Home again, home again, jiggity, _____. (jig)

PLAY Rhyme-It-Again.

After each rhyming set, ask students to identify a rhyming word. For example,

Pig rhymes with _____. (jig)

Rhyming words include

pig, jig   trout, out
hen, pen   goose, loose
lamb, swam   cow, now
duck, luck   goat, coat
shoe, zoo

PLAY Make-a-Rhyme.

Children supply another rhyming word after a set of two is presented. Give initial phoneme cues, if needed. Accept any nonsense word. For example, ask

What rhymes with *hen*? (pen)
What are some other words that rhyme with *hen*? (*Ben, den, men, ten*, etc.)

Continue with the rhyming words presented in Rhyme-It-Again.

PLAY **Clap-and-Count.**

Children clap to, and then count, the number of syllables heard in selected words from the illustrations and text. Demonstrate by clapping to a word and then asking children how many parts they heard. For example, clap and say

> mark
> How many parts in the word? Clap it out. (one)

Clap and say

> market
> How many parts in that word? Clap it out. (two)
> That's right. Mar–ket. One, two.

Stress and elongate the two syllables when presenting words from the text, such as *pepper* and *garlic*.

☛ See the catalog for Grades 1 through 5 for continuing activities in the hierarchy of phonological awareness.

Truck

by Donald Crews
New York: Puffin, 1980, 1985 (paperback)

Suggested Grade and Interest Level: Pre-K

Topic Explorations: Journeys; Transportation

Skill Builders:
   Vocabulary   **Language literacy**
   Categories   Verbal expression
   Grammar and syntax
   Two- and three-word utterances
   Noun–verb agreement

Synopsis: A wordless book follows the journey of a red trailer-truck, from loading to unloading, in action-packed illustrations that lead to plenty of conversation.

Method: This book is appropriate for very young children. For early utterances, structure short phrases as you show the story. Talk about how the truck stops at the stop sign, drives past a city, past neon signs, drives in the rain, past rural areas, and on a freeway. Here are some examples:

Big truck	Red truck	Truck stops
Truck goes	Truck gets gas	Rains on truck
Truck doors open	Truck has tricycles	Truck delivers

For prepositions, describe how the red truck

goes through a tunnel	goes over the bridge	stops next to the stop sign
stops beside the gas pump	has boxes of tricycles inside it	stops at the stop sign

For categories, talk about vehicles and name the other types of vehicles on the road. See how many different cars and trucks the children can name and categorize.

For verbal expression, journey along with the truck driver to find out what he delivers. Discuss each page of the story, then talk about how we get toys from the store and how the store gets them from a factory or a warehouse. Discuss how important trucks are in delivering goods.

The Very Busy Spider

by Eric Carle
New York: Philomel Books, 1984

Suggested Grade and Interest Level: Pre-K

Topic Explorations: Animals, Farm; Insects and spiders

Skill Builders:

Vocabulary	**Language literacy**
Associations	Sequencing
Adjectives	Cause-and-effect relationships
Grammar and syntax	Compare and contrast
Two- and three-word utterances	**Articulation, *V***
Negative structures	
Question structures	

Synopsis: When a spider begins to "spin a web with her silky thread," the nearby farm animals test her resolve by inviting her to join them in play. But the spider is so intent on her web that she doesn't even answer. Her patience pays off when she shows them the fruits of her labor. Not only does she create a beautiful web, which the children can feel by touching the pages, but she also catches a delicious fly for her dinner. The repetitive text, the animal noises that you can encourage children to make, and the silky-to-the-touch web make this an exceptional book to encourage interaction.

Method: Before the read-aloud, ask children, "What can you think of that goes with a spider?" Elicit children's background knowledge about spiders and spider webs. Why do spiders make webs? What do they look like? How are they made?

During the read-aloud, pause to shape two- and three-word utterances, structuring interaction around portions of the text, such as "take a nap," "chase a cat," "go for a swim," and "very busy."

Also use the text to encourage repetition of negative and question structures.

For associations, ask children to associate the animals with their sounds.

For vocabulary and adjectives, encourage repetition of portions of the text, such as "busy spider," "pesky fly," and "silky thread." Other combinations to structure include "brown horse," "wooly sheep," and "beautiful web."

For articulation of *V*, have children join in on the phrase "very busy spinning her web," which is repeated on every double-page spread, or structure responses to include the target word *very* while talking about how busy the spider is.

After the reading, ask children to recall the story and tell why the spider didn't answer the farm animals. What happened to the pesky fly at the beginning of the story? Why did she fall asleep after she caught the fly? Have you ever seen a spider web? Where have you seen spider webs?

Have children sequence some of the events in the story. What happened first? Then what happened? What happened at the end of the story? Encourage children to express cause-and-effect relationships with words such as *so* and *because.* Some examples include

She didn't talk to the horse because she was busy making her web.
She made the web so she could catch the fly.
She fell asleep because she was tired.

Extended Activity: Make spiders! All you'll need are head and body shapes precut from construction paper (traced from the cover of the book). Next, cut eight strips of black yarn for the legs of each spider. Include a six-inch piece of white silky thread for the spider web.

Have the children glue the head to the body and glue four legs to each side of the spider's body. Tape one end of the silky thread to each spider so that they can be hung from the ceiling, or glue the spiders to a white piece of paper with the threads dangling from their bodies. As the children make their spiders, ask them to explain what a spider does with its silky thread and the purpose of a web. Compare spiders to insects by looking at their legs and body shapes. How are they alike? How are they different?

The Very Hungry Caterpillar

by Eric Carle
New York: Philomel Books, 1969, 1981

Suggested Grade and Interest Level: Pre-K

Topic Explorations: Days of the week; Fruit; Insects and spiders

Skill Builders:

Vocabulary	**Grammar and syntax**	**Language literacy**
Beginning concepts (spatial size and quantity)	Two- and three-word utterances	Sequencing
	Singular and plural nouns	Cause-and-effect relationships
Adjectives	Present tense	**Articulation, *K* and *V***
Categories		
Prepositions		
Morphological units		

Synopsis: A very hungry caterpillar eats its way through everything, including the pages of the book, until it makes its amazing transformation.

Method: Before the read-aloud, choose one of the following concepts in the story to discuss on the first reading: eating and growing, the days of the week, caterpillars, foods and food groups, quantities of things, and sizes of things. Introduce the book by leading into one of the chosen themes.

During the read-aloud, concentrate on one or two concepts at a time. For example, while teaching eating and growing and discussing beginning concepts of size, pause to teach morphological endings with words such as *big and bigger* and *hungry and hungrier.*

After the read-aloud, teach prepositions by talking about how the caterpillar ate *through* the food, going in one end (or side) and out the other. Show both sides of the pages that the caterpillar has eaten through. Talk about trains going through tunnels and people walking through one room to get to another. Have children demonstrate crawling "through" a hoop or cut-out box.

Teach adjectives by talking about other words that describe the caterpillar. Ask children how they feel when they're hungry. Have they ever eaten something and still been hungry? Perhaps that will give them an idea of why the caterpillar needed to eat so much.

Categorize different kinds of food. Show the small pages of fruit and ask children to name each type. Elicit the category name *fruit* by asking, What are all these things together called? What are ice-cream sundaes and cakes and pies all called? Repeat for other categories of food.

Have children sequence parts of the story by telling what the caterpillar did first. Then what did it do? What happened at the end of the story? Encourage children to express cause-and-effect relationships with words such as *so* and *because*. Some examples include

> The caterpillar ate up all the food because it was hungry.
> The caterpillar was hungry so it ate more food.
> The caterpillar ate through all the food so it could grow (and turn into a butterfly).

On another occasion, do a picture walk-through to review the story, then continue the teaching of morphological word endings by playing phonological awareness games, such as the following:

PLAY **The Suffix game.**

Count the number of parts using the concepts of *big* and *hungry*. For example, ask

> How many parts in the word *big*?
> How many parts in the word *bigger*?
> How many parts in the word *biggest*?

Continue with these words:

> large, larger, largest
> heavy, heavier, heaviest
> hungry, hungrier, hungriest
> full, fuller (he became fuller and fuller)

PLAY **Find-the-Little-Word.**

For example, ask

> Do you hear any little words in *bigger*? (big)
> Do you hear any little words in *biggest*? (big)

PLAY **Sentence-It.**

Have children generate sentences using the words *big, bigger,* and *biggest*. Some examples include

> The caterpillar became *big* (when he ate the pear).
> The caterpillar became *bigger* (when he ate the strawberry).
> The caterpillar was *biggest* right before it became a butterfly.

For articulation, elicit responses using the *k* phonemes in *caterpillar* and the *v* phoneme in *very* during reading and in structured conversations.

Extended Activity: After the read-aloud, pass out old magazines. Ask children to find pictures of food and either cut or tear them out of the magazines. Assist children in punching a hole through each picture with a hole punch, then have the children collect all the pictures in a basket.

Return to the story circle and choose a child to come to up and hold the basket of pictures. Choose another child to pick the pictures out of the basket one by one and show them to the class. Start the story by telling of the very hungry caterpillar. As each picture is taken out of the basket, assist the children to include that food item in the things the hungry caterpillar ate. For instance, say, "On Sunday, the very hungry caterpillar ate through a bunch of bananas and a plate of macaroni and cheese." Ask whether the caterpillar was full. When the children respond "No," ask, "And then what happened?" as the child pulls out the next item of food.

Note: This book is available in many translations, including Arabic, Bengali, Chinese, French, Italian, Japanese, and Spanish (*La oruga muy hambrienta*).

The Very Lazy Ladybug

by Isabel Finn and Jack Tickle (Illustrator)
London: Little Tiger Press, 1999; Wilton, CT: Tiger Tales, ME Media LLC, 2001

Suggested Grade and Interest Level: Pre-K

Topic Exploration: Insects and spiders

Skill Builders:

Vocabulary	**Language literacy**
Synonyms	Predicting
Grammar and syntax	Sequencing
Two- and three-word utterances	Cause-and-effect relationships
Tenses, present and past	**Articulation, *V* and *L***
Negative structures	

Synopsis: A lazy ladybug has spent all of her time sleeping and not learning how to fly, so when she decides to sleep somewhere else, the only way she can get there is to hop. She hops first into a kangaroo's pouch, but because the kangaroo likes to jump, it is too bumpy to sleep. She continues to hop from one animal to the next, unable to find the perfect napping place, until an unexpected event prompts her to fly.

Method: Before the read-aloud, elicit children's background knowledge of the word *lazy*. What does it mean? What are some examples of laziness? Show the book cover and introduce children to a ladybug that is very lazy. Be sure to point out the names of the authors when introducing the book (e.g., the author's last name is Finn. Is there another meaning for the word *fin*? The illustrator's name is Jack Tickle. Is there another meaning for the word *tickle*?).

During the read-aloud, structure questions to elicit desired responses to increase grammar and syntax skills and encourage predictions easily allowed by the repetitive text (e.g., when the ladybug finds that her spot is not to her liking, prompt with a question such as, "What do you think she said?" to elicit the answer, "I can't sleep here." When another animal comes along, seeming to offer a better place, prompt with the question, "What do you think she did?" for the prediction, "She hopped onto his . . .").

After the read-aloud, to further increase vocabulary, grammar, and syntax skills (including noun–verb agreement, present or past tense), do a picture walk-through and describe what each animal is doing when it passes by. Children can describe the actions and movements of the animals in the pictures—even act them out. Model and shape target structures. Phrases with verbs describing movement include

Kangaroo bounded by	Tiger padded by	Tortoise plodded by
Monkey swung by	Bear ambled by	
Elephant walked by	Crocodile swam by	

Shape responses, if necessary, by repeating the text (e.g., say "a crocodile swam by" and then ask, "How did he pass by?" to elicit desired response, "He swam by.").

For synonyms, once the words of the story have been discussed and used, ask the children to say another word for the following:

sleep (nap)	snooze (nap, sleep)
Walk by slowly (amble, plod)	bound (hop)
swish (swing)	pouch (pocket)

Revisit the text to sequence events and to explore and express cause-and-effect relationships. While reading, pause to talk about the conditions that caused the ladybug to move on (e.g., What caused the ladybug to hop out of the kangaroo's pouch and onto the tiger's back? What caused her to leave the monkey's head and hop onto the crocodile's tail? [Because the monkey was swinging too much.] What happened to the ladybug because the monkey was swinging so much? [She got dizzy.]).

For generalization and story comprehension, ask children if that would be a good place to nap. Why not?

For articulation of V and L phonemes, capitalize on the sounds of the words, *very lazy ladybug*, in eliciting responses containing the target sounds.

Extended Activities: Cut out felt pieces for the ladybug and different animals to use on a felt-board story. Have children participate in telling the story with the felt animals.

The Very Worst Monster

by Pat Hutchins
New York: Greenwillow Books, 1985, 1988

Suggested Grade and Interest Level: Pre-K

Topic Explorations: Family relationships

Skill Builders:

Vocabulary	**Pragmatic language**
Adjectives	**Articulation, V**
Morphological units	
Grammar and syntax	
Present tense	

Synopsis: Hazel's sibling rivalry leads her to prove to her family that she is the worst monster. Her *bad, worse,* and *worst* behavior doesn't seem to get her any attention at all.

Method: Before the read-aloud, talk about appropriate ways that children can get attention from adults. Lead into the story by introducing Hazel on the cover and asking children to listen so that they can decide for themselves whether she was the very worst monster.

During the read-aloud, elicit present-tense structures by talking about the actions taking place in the illustrations. Emphasize the words *bad, worse,* and *worst* as they are used in the story. Encourage children to use the words in their own sentences.

After the read-aloud, use Hazel's behavior in the story for a lesson in language pragmatics. Talk about what Hazel could have said and how she could have said it to get her the good kind of attention from her family members. Even though she may not have been the very worst monster if she used good manners, ask children whether it is a good idea to know what to say and how to say it when in other places with other people.

Continue developing morphological endings by using the story to structure other sentences. For example, ask

> Would Hazel get more attention with a loud voice?
> What if she used a louder voice?
> What if she used her loudest voice?
> Would Hazel get her family to notice her if she made a big mess?
> What if she made a bigger mess?
> What if she made the biggest mess you ever saw?
> Would Hazel's family pay more attention to her if she made a big frown?
> What if she made a bigger frown?
> What if she made the biggest frown she could possibly make?

Other comparatives with which to structure sentences include

good, better, best	lots, more, most
long, longer, longest	short, shorter, shortest
small, smaller, smallest	warm, warmer, warmest
cold, colder, coldest	

For articulation of *V*, elicit utterances containing the words *very worst, very loud, very messy,* and so on, in increasingly longer linguistic units.

What the Moon Saw

by Brian Wildsmith
New York: Oxford University Press, 1978, 1986

Suggested Grade and Interest Level: K

Topic Exploration: Nighttime

Skill Builders:
Vocabulary
Antonyms

Synopsis: Pairs of opposite concepts are presented with one-sentence text and illustrated in Brian Wildsmith's vivid and unique style.

Method: Use the illustrations to teach opposite concepts, which include

many, few	heavy, light
patterned, plain	outside, inside

Extend the activity to name other opposites, such as

empty, full	near, far	happy, sad
tall, short	narrow, wide	wet, dry
hot, cold	hard, soft	
soft, rough	fat, thin	

Where Once There Was a Wood

by Denise Fleming
New York: Henry Holt, 1996

Suggested Grade and Interest Level:	Pre-K
Topic Explorations:	Animals; Conservation; Woods

Skill Builders:

Vocabulary	**Grammar and syntax**	**Phonological awareness**
	Two- and three-word utterances	
	Noun–verb agreement	
	Past tense	

Synopsis: Once there was a wood, a meadow, and a creek, with wildlife creatures engaged in their usual activities. Exquisite illustrations, made of handmade paper art, depict the scenes, and the brief, lyrical verse eventually reveals what has displaced them—a new housing development. Encourages children to protect nature.

Method: Before the read-aloud, read the title and discuss the illustration on the cover. Talk about the meaning of the word *wood* and elicit children's background knowledge about and experience with woods and meadows. Have children name creatures that live in the woods, then discuss what the word *habitat* means (i.e., a home for creatures in the natural environment). Other vocabulary words include

wood	meadow	creek
habitat	unfurl	speared
glittering	slithered	slipped
rambled	rummaged	

During the read-aloud, pause briefly, if necessary, to supply definitions of vocabulary words, to comment on a page of illustrations, or to discuss a word in the text. Pause to build grammar and syntax skills by structuring utterances for children to repeat. For noun–verb agreement, model phrases for children to repeat, such as "the fox rests," "the owl hunts," "the heron fishes," "the raccoon rummages," and so on.

For two- and three-word utterances and past-tense formations, prompt with a question at the end of the text before turning the next page. For example, read

> "Where once the red fox rested and closed his eyes to sleep," and then ask,
> "What did the brown fox do?"

Read another page of text, such as

> "Where once the brown snake slithered and slipped out of sight,"
> and then ask, "What did the snake do?" to elicit responses from the words of the text.

After the read-aloud, discuss the meaning of the story. Talk about displacement, and provide examples to assist children in understanding the concept of something being replaced by something else.

> What does the title, *Where Once There Was a Wood?* mean?
> Where might the creatures go if they lost their homes?
> What might happen if there were already too many creatures at the spot where they moved?
> Would there be enough food?

Reread the story, pausing to interact and use the words of the verse in creative ways, continuing to generate oral language.

Use the alliterative words of the text for phonological awareness training.

PLAY The Word-Count game.

Children count words from a short line of text. Demonstrate by assigning one word to one finger as you say the words. For example, say

>   red fox

as you hold up one finger for each word until two fingers are showing. Ask

>   How many words did I say? (two)

Then say

>   red fox rested

for a three-finger count. Gradually allow the children to do the counting by themselves.

If children don't have one-to-one correspondence, give each child a collection of manipulables (i.e., blocks, felt squares, buttons, etc.) to use for representing each of the stated words. Demonstrate by saying (or use a puppet to say) the words from a page of text that you want the children to count. Repeat them again as you (or a puppet) move out one item at a time to correspond to your stated word. Then you (or a puppet) count out loud the number of blocks moved to get the word count. Gradually allow the children to do the counting by themselves. Use words directly from a page of the text in hierarchical order to the desired word length. Word sources are easy to select from on each page.

PLAY The Same-Sound game.

Children identify whether word pairs begin with the same sound. For example, say

>   was, wood
>   Do they start with the same sound? (Yes)

Intersperse nonmatched pairs into the following list of matched pairs:

red, rest	fox, fern	horn, hunt
pheasant, feed	slither, slip	once, was, wood
horn, hunt, hungry	red, rest, raccoon	fox, fern, fish
raccoon, ramble, rummage	where, once, was, wood	

PLAY Word-Search.

Children search the picture for the word you are thinking of that begins with the sound of a given word. For example, say

>   I see something in this picture that starts with the same sound as *fern*.
>   Search for the word that starts with *f*. (Give phoneme/sound only.)

(continues on next page)

PLAY Word-Search. *Continued*

Provide names of other things that start with the same sound for cues, such as

> It's not a *pheasant*, it's not a *fish*, and so on.
> That's right. *Fox* is the word.

PLAY Clap-and-Count.

Children clap to, and then count, the syllables heard in selected words from the story. Demonstrate by clapping to a word and then asking children how many parts they heard. For example, clap and say

> wood
> How many parts in the word? Clap it out. (one)

Clap and say

> woodchuck
> How many parts in that word? Clap it out. (two)
> Wood-chuck. One, two.

Stress and elongate syllables when presenting words, such as

once	ramble	slithered
wood	woodchuck	woodpecker
wing	meadow	grasshopper
waxwing	hungry	glittering
raccoon	rummaged	

PLAY What's-the-Word?

Children synthesize two syllables into a word. Use the words and pictures of the book as cues. Present the syllables, inserting a clear pause between them, and have children say them quickly and repeatedly until they can guess the word. Demonstrate by saying

> sli–ther
> What's the word?
> Say it until you hear it. *Sllliiiiii–ther. Slliii–ther. Slither.*
> *Slither* is the word.

Continue with any clearly illustrated word, such as *pheasant, woodpecker,* and *raccoon.*

PLAY Find-the-Little-Words.

Children listen for "little" words in compound words of the text. Stress and elongate syllables when presenting the word. For example, say

> *Waxwing* is the name of a bird.
> Can you find any little words in *waxwing*? (wax, wing)

(continues on next page)

PLAY Find-the-Little-Words. *Continued*

That's right. *Wax* is a little word in *waxwing*.
Wing is another word in *waxwing*.

Continue with the following compound and two-syllable words:

woodchuck (wood, chuck)
outside (out, side)
sunshine (sun, shine)
afternoon (after, noon)
grasshopper (grass, hop, hopper)
woodpecker (wood, peck)
raccoon (rack)
purple (purr)
berries (bear)
slithering (slither)

PLAY Leave-It-Out.

Children say a compound or two-syllable word, then leave out the beginning or final part to create a smaller word. For example, say

Say *woodchuck*.
Now, say *woodchuck*, but leave out *chuck*.
What little word is left? (wood)

Then say

Now, say *woodchuck*, but leave out *wood*.
What little word is left? (chuck)

Continue with the words provided in Find-the-Little-Words, beginning with the compound words and continuing with two-syllable words, if indicated.

PLAY Add-It-On.

Children put two little words or two syllables together to make a bigger word. For example, say

Say *wood*.
Now, say *wood*, and add *chuck*.
What bigger word can you make? (woodchuck)

Then, reverse the order in which the words are presented. For example, say

Put *chuck* at the end of *wood*.
What word do you have? (woodchuck)

Continue with the words provided in Find-the-Little-Words.

> **PLAY** Turn-It-Around.
>
> Children reverse the parts of the word they have analyzed and synthesized, as in
>
> > Put the word *chuck* at the beginning of *wood.*
> > What word do you have? (chuckwood)
> > What was it before we turned it around? (woodchuck)

> **PLAY** Switch-It.
>
> Children delete one part of a word and substitute a new part to make another word. Prompt with cues as necessary. For example, say
>
> > Say *woodchuck.*
> > Now say *woodchuck,* only take out *chuck* and put in *pile.*
> > What new word can you make? (woodpile)
>
> Some word exchanges include
>
> > Say *woodchuck,* only take out *chuck* and put in *work.* (woodwork)
> > Say *woodchuck,* only take out *chuck* and put in *pecker.* (woodpecker)
> > Say *outside,* only take out *out* and put in *in.* (inside)
> > Say *grasshopper,* only take out *hopper* and put in *land.* (grassland)

☛ See the catalog for Grades 1 through 5 for continuing activities in the hierarchy of phonological awareness.

Extended Activities: On the last pages of the book, there are suggestions for communities and schools to create backyard habitats. The pages also list plants and trees that will provide shade and flowers that will attract hummingbirds and butterflies. Classrooms can contact wildlife habitat programs for further suggestions. Engage in activities that will foster a natural habitat and keep a classroom journal of the events and types of birds and butterflies observed.

Where's My Teddy?

by Jez Alborough
London: Walker Books, 1992; Cambridge, MA: Candlewick Press, 1994

Suggested Grade and Interest Level: Pre-K

Topic Explorations: Bears; Woods

Skill Builders:

Vocabulary	Grammar and syntax	Phonological awareness
Morphological units	Two- and three-word utterances	
	Noun–verb agreement	
	Possessive pronouns	
	Present tense	

Synopsis: Little Eddie goes into the woods searching for his lost teddy bear. He finds a huge teddy, sitting right in the middle of the forest and much too large to bring home and cuddle. When a real, gigantic bear, also searching for *his* teddy, comes along, each discovers that the other has his teddy. All ends well when they leave the forest with their rightful, cuddly teddy bear and go home to their beds.

Method: Before the read-aloud, lead into the story with a discussion about losing something that is important. Perhaps children have lost a stuffed animal and know how it feels to want it back.

Then, read the short, rhyming text without interruption. Children will connect with the illustrations and the story without a break in the rhythm and flow of the verse.

After the read-aloud, discuss what happened in the story. Who had whose bear? How did the boy get his teddy back? How did the bear get his teddy back? Do a picture walk-through and model and shape target grammar and syntax structures appropriate to each page of the story. Some two- and three-word utterances include

Eddie's teddy	Huge bear	Where's my teddy?
He tiptoed	What's that?	Giant teddy bear
Look out	"A boy!"	Lost his teddy
Giant teddy	"My teddy!"	Found his teddy

Examples for noun–verb agreement include

Eddie walks	They look at each other
He tiptoes	Eddie looks at the bear
He finds a teddy	They run back home
They sit in the forest	The boy runs back home
He sits on the bear	They sleep in their own beds
He hears a sound	The boy sleeps in his own bed

For teaching the morphological structures of comparatives and superlatives, point out the sizes of the boy, the bear, and the two teddies. Sentences with target structures include

Eddie's teddy is small.
Eddie's teddy is the small*est*.
The bear's teddy is big.
The bear's teddy is the big*gest*.
The bear's teddy is big*ger* than Eddie's teddy.
Eddie's teddy is small*er* than the bear's teddy.
The bear is big*ger* than the boy.
The boy is small*er* than the bear.

For possessive pronouns, elicit target structures, such as the following:

Eddie has his teddy.
The bear has his teddy.
They both have their teddies.

For phonological awareness training, first reread the text. Then play the series of games, depending on the level of phonological sensitivity of the students.

PLAY Word-Count.

Children count the number of words in a short line from the text. Demonstrate by assigning one word to one finger as you say the words. For example, say

teddy

(continues on next page)

PLAY **Word-Count.** *Continued*

as you hold up one finger for the word. Ask

How many words did I say?

Gradually work up to four words, adding the word *is* (instead of using the contraction *'s*) to the title, such as

Where is my teddy?

for a four-finger count. Then, transfer the counting to the children to do by themselves.

If children don't have one-to-one correspondence, give each child a collection of manipulables (i.e., blocks, felt squares, buttons, etc.) to use for representing each of the stated words. Demonstrate by saying (or a puppet can say) the words from a page of text that you want the children to count. Repeat them again as you (or a puppet) move out one item at a time to correspond to the stated word. Then you (or a puppet) count out loud the number of blocks moved to get the word count. Gradually allow the children to count by themselves. Use words directly from a page of the text in hierarchical order to the desired word length. Some examples of words to count include

"MY TED!"
gasped the bear
"A BEAR!"
screamed Eddie

PLAY **Stand-Up-to-the-Word.**

Children demonstrate awareness of a word by standing up when the word to which they are assigned is spoken. Choose four children and assign each child to one of the words in the altered title, *Where is my Teddy?* Begin by stating the first word of the title, *where*. The child assigned to *where* stands and repeats *where*. Then, state the word *is* and have the child assigned to that word stand up and repeat *is*. Continue until all the designated children are standing, then have each standing child repeat his or her word again, repeating until the altered four-word title, *Where is my Teddy?* is readily understood by the children.

PLAY **Which-Word-Is-Missing?**

Children identify the word in a word string that has been omitted from a previously given string. Choose two to four words from the illustration and text to make up a string. Repeat the words, leaving one out for the children to identify, such as

Eddie, Freddie, bed, woods
Eddie, bed, woods
Which one is missing? (Freddie)

Some word lists from the text include

teddy, stop, dark, lost
woods, forest, path, trunk
path, huddle, stop, lost
small, voice, yell, cry
bear, path, until, tiptoe
yell, home, fast, dark

PLAY **Rearrange-It.**

Children rearrange, in correct word order, a scrambled phrase or sentence from a portion of the text. For example, say

Teddy my
Can you help me say it in the right order?
That's right. *Teddy my* should really be *My teddy.*

More words to rearrange:

Surprise what a	Bed I my want	He woods through the ran
Teddy where is my	He's too cuddle to big	

PLAY **Odd-One-Out.**

Children select from a string of alliterative words the one that does not belong. For example, say

big, bed, ran
Which word has a different beginning sound? (ran)
That's right. *Ran* is the odd one out.

Use the words provided in the Same-Sound game. Insert an additional word from the story with a different initial sound for the children to identify, such as

woods, want, big	dark, bear, boy	want, was, yell
what, where, bed	yell, lost, left	dark, big, dear
big, dark, bear	ran, woods, run	lost, path, pat
gasp, go, path		

PLAY **Word-Search.**

Children search the picture for the word you are thinking of that begins with a given sound. For example, say

I see something in this picture that starts with a *b*. (Give phoneme/sound only.)
Can you find it?

Provide names of other things that start with the same sound for cues, if needed, such as

It's not a boy, it's not a basket, it's not a bat, and so on.

PLAY **Finish-the-Rhyme.**

Children supply the rhyming word left out at the end of a verse. Teach children to use the meaningful clues in the pictures as well as the meter of the verse to rhyme the word. If necessary, prompt with picture cues and with the initial phoneme, then gradually remove the scaffolding. For example, say

Eddie's off to find his teddy.
Eddie's teddy's name is (Fr)_____ . (Freddie)

"Help!" said Eddie. "I'm scared already!
I want my bed! I want my (t)_____." (teddy)

PLAY **Rhyme-It-Again.**

Children identify the rhyming word heard after a rhyming set is given. For example, say

> *Teddy* rhymes with _____. (Freddie)
> *Already* rhymes with _____. (teddy)

PLAY **Do-They-Rhyme?**

Children identify whether word pairs rhyme. Intersperse the following rhyming words from the text with unmatched sets:

Eddie, teddy	Teddy, Freddie
huddle, cuddle	would, could
until, still	

PLAY **Make-a-Rhyme.**

Children supply another rhyming word after a set of two is presented. Give initial phoneme cues if needed. For example, ask

> What word rhymes with *teddy*?
> *Teddy, Freddie,* (r)_____ (ready)

Encourage children to make other rhyming words, such as *steady*, and nonsense words, such as *meddie, feddie,* and *weddie*. Continue using the rhyming words from the text, some of which are provided above.

PLAY **Clap-and-Count.**

Children clap to, and then count, the syllables heard in selected words from the story. Demonstrate by clapping to a word and then asking children how many parts they heard. For example, clap and say

> some
> How many parts in the word? Clap it out. (one)

Clap and say

> somewhere
> How many parts in that word? Clap it out. (two)
> Some–where. One, two.

Stress and elongate syllables when presenting words, such as

tiptoe	teddy
Freddie	huddle
darkness	sobbing
cuddle	already
stomping	

PLAY **Find-the-Little-Words.**

Children listen for "little" words within compound words of the text. Stress and elongate syllables when presenting the word. For example, say

> somewhere
> Can you find any little words in *somewhere*? (some, where)
> That's right. *Some* is a little word in *somewhere*.
> *Where* is another little word in *somewhere*.

More compound words include

> tiptoe
> already

Also, use two-syllable words, changing the stress as necessary so the children can hear all the "little" words, including

> darkness (dark)   Teddy (Ted)
> sobbing (sob)   stomping (stomp)
> Eddie (Ed)

PLAY **Leave-It-Out.**

Children say a compound or two-syllable word, then leave out the beginning or final part to create a smaller word. For example, say

> Say *somewhere*.
> Now, say *somewhere*, but leave out *where*.
> What little word is left? (some)

Then say

> Now, say *somewhere*, but leave out *some*.
> What little word is left? (where)

Continue with the compound and two-syllable words provided in Find-the-Little-Words.

PLAY **Add-It-On.**

Children put two little words or syllables together to make a word. For example, say

> Say *some*.

Then say

> Now, say *some*, and add *where*.
> What word can you make? (somewhere)

(continues on next page)

(PLAY) Add-It-On. *Continued*

Then, reverse the order in which the words are presented. For example, say

> Put *where* at the end of *some.*
> What word do you have? (somewhere)

Continue with the compound and two-syllable words provided in Find-the-Little-Words.

(PLAY) Turn-It-Around.

Children reverse the parts of compound words they previously analyzed and synthesized. For example, say

> Put the word *where* at the beginning of *some.*
> What funny word do you have? (wheresome)
> What was it before we turned it around? (somewhere)

Continue with the compound words provided in Find-the-Little Words.

➤ See the catalog for Grades 1 through 5 for continuing activities in the hierarchy of phonological awareness.

Read also the sequel to this story, *It's the Bear,* that is featured in this catalog. *Note:* This book is also available in a Spanish version, titled, *¿Donde esta mi osito?*

Who Is the Beast?

by Keith Baker
New York: Harcourt Brace Jovanovich, 1990, 1991 (big book)

Suggested Grade and Interest Level: Pre-K

Topic Explorations: Animals, Jungle; Conservation

Skill Builders:

Vocabulary	Language literacy	
Categories	Cause-and-effect relationships	Compare and contrast
Attributes	Problem solving	Discussion

Synopsis: In richly illustrated scenes, a tiger lumbers through the dense and colorful vegetation of the jungle. One by one, the animals flee from the tiger who begins to suspect that he is feared. So he returns to the animals to point out the things he has in common with each of them.

Method: Before the read-aloud, introduce the book by showing its cover and talking about the jungle and how it is similar to a rain forest. In the rain forests, there are many lush plants and trees, so many that the forest becomes thick and dense. Because of this, the animals that live there are mostly hidden, just like the tiger on the cover of the book. Discuss how rain forests are disappearing because people are cutting them down and how the animals are losing their homes, or *habitat.* Teach other applicable vocabulary words such as *equator* and *conservation.*

During the read-aloud, interact with the children, clarifying meaning where needed. When the text suggests similarities among the animals (e.g., "I see eyes, green and round. We both have eyes to look around"), ask in what other ways the animals (i.e., a tiger and a snake) are similar. What are some ways that they are different? Include vocabulary words, such as *habitat, equator,* and *conservation.*

After the read-aloud, talk about the parts of the tiger that were shown and discussed in the book (e.g., whiskers, eyes, tail, paws, stripes, legs, fur, etc.) and help children describe the tiger's attributes.

For problem solving, discuss what's happening to rain forests today and what their destruction is doing to the animals that live there. Talk about ways to solve this problem so that no more of the rain forests are destroyed. Some examples are recycling, planting trees, making room for animals, and educating people.

Extended Activities: Cut out pictures of jungle animals from magazines, either beforehand or as part of the class activity. Gather the pictures and have the class form a circle, choosing one child to be the jungle animal in the center. Attach an animal picture to the back of the child. The child must guess the animal as the other children give attributes and descriptions without giving away the name.

Play the Imagine game. Ask the children to close their eyes and to imagine their bathrooms as home. Draw analogies to the shrinking rain forest, for example, say

Pretend that 80 different plants are in your bathroom. Put in 10 monkeys, 15 beautiful butterflies, 3 tigers, 7 frogs, 40 spiders, 2 snakes, and 3 bats. Turn on the shower in your bathroom and let it fill up with steam. Now, open your eyes. What is your habitat like? Elicit descriptive words, such as *warm, sticky, crowded,* and *uncomfortable.* Ask how it would feel to be one of these animals in this habitat.

Who Sank the Boat?

by Pamela Allen
New York: Coward McCann, 1982; Putnam & Sons, 1990; Paper Star, 1996

Suggested Grade and Interest Level: Pre-K

Topic Explorations: Animals, Farm; Boats

Skill Builders:

Vocabulary	Grammar and syntax	Language literacy
Homonyms	Question structures	Predicting
(multiple-meaning words)		Cause-and-effect relationships
Antonyms		

Synopsis: As a cow, a donkey, a sheep, a pig, and a little mouse get into a rowboat one by one, the author asks, "Do you know who sank the boat?" The text is overflowing with speculation and opportunities for language stimulation as questions prepare the children for each successive event.

Method: For prediction and question structures, simply present the book and read the text, "Do you know who sank the boat?"

Introduce vocabulary words: *din* (noise), *balance, sink,* and *float.*

For antonyms, discuss the opposite concepts of *sink* and *float.*

When does a boat sink in water? (When the boat is too heavy in front or in back, or when it tips.)

When does a boat float in water? (When it is light.)
Why did the boat in the story sink?
What would happen if all the animals got into the back of the boat? Would it be balanced?
What would happen if all the animals got into the front of the boat? Where would it be too heavy?
What would happen?
What would have happened if the sheep had gotten into the boat without balancing her weight?
What would have happened if the mouse had gotten into the boat and balanced its weight like the sheep did?
Would the boat have sunk?

For homonyms and multiple-meaning words, discuss the word *sink* and ask children to tell another meaning for the word. More multiple-meaning words to associate with the story include *rock, float, weight* (wait), and *yarn.*

Section 2

Books Are for Talking with Children in Grades 1 Through 5

* Using Picture Books To Build Oral Communication Skills and Literacy Achievement

* Looking for Books That Help Build Communication Skills and Literacy Achievement

* Suggestions for Book Talk with Children in Grades 1 Through 5

* A Catalog of Picture Books for Children in Grades 1 Through 5

Using Picture Books

To Build Oral Communication Skills and Literacy Achievement

*The talk is the site of learning; the book reading
is important because it is the site of the talk.*

—Snow (1994, p. 270)

Numerous studies conducted during the past few decades conclude that joint picture book reading—whether conducted by parents at home, day-care providers, interventionists, or teachers in the classroom—contributes to strong language growth and literacy achievement in elementary school-aged children (Fey, Windsor, & Warren, 1995).

Spoken Language

With careful selection, planning, and facilitation, the use of picture books can address any of the components of spoken language, including the following:

To Develop the Components of Spoken Language

- Vocabulary: To acquire words, especially different kinds of words, such as nouns, verbs, prepositions, pronouns, and so on.
- Phonetics: To produce speech sounds.
- Phonology: To learn how to change the structure of sounds in words and to learn how sounds are distributed and changed when making one word into another (as discussed under phonological awareness).
- Morphology and syntax: To learn the rules for arranging words in sentences and to learn the meaningful parts that make up words.
- Semantics: To learn the meanings of words, including concepts, words with multiple meanings, synonyms, antonyms, and figurative language.
- Pragmatics: To learn how to engage in an interchange of language for social purposes.

Literacy Achievement

To Develop a Literate Discourse Style

A literate language style is essential for comprehending text. Literate language differs from oral language in that it contains more specific and descriptive vocabulary (such as multiple words to express various shades of meaning) and more complex syntactic structures (such as conjunctive sentences and relative clauses) (Westby, 1999). Westby writes,

> In order to develop a literate language style, children must hear literate language and have the opportunity to use it in meaningful communicative contexts. Children may be exposed to a literate style in the language spoken by adults around them and in stories that are read to them. (p. 189)

To Develop an Understanding of Narrative Schema

A literate language style also encompasses the ability to comprehend and produce schematic structures, such as narratives. The conceptual knowledge underlying narrative text involves being able to understand and produce a hierarchy of discourse skills. The picture book genre of children's literature can provide children with opportunities to hear and use literate language through the following discourse skills:

- Relating personal experiences: To tell of past personal experiences that children are reminded of when learning about of the characters' experiences in storybooks.
- Verbal expression: To explain meanings, express thoughts, and relate events that the children encounter in a picture book.
- Predicting outcomes: To state what might happen next in the story based on evidence or familiarity of experience.
- Sequencing: To organize and report the events of the story in logical, temporal relationships. Many stories entail a string of sequenced events that children can retell, such as *The Carrot Seed*, by Ruth Krauss, and *Good Night, Gorilla*, by Peggy Rathmann.
- Cause-and-effect relationships: To understand and express causal links between the actions and reactions of characters in stories. *Martha Speaks*, by Susan Meddaugh, is an example of a book that can be used to draw the connection (although fanciful) between a dog eating alphabet soup and then being able to speak as a result of it.
- Storytelling: To produce narratives containing all the essential story grammar elements of a complete episode (Applebee, 1978). To understand and express the characters' motivations toward their goals and how their feelings motivate their behavior.
- Problem solving: To state facts about a problem, think of ways to solve the problem, and provide evidence to defend potential solutions to the problem. To comprehend and retell a goal-based story, children must be able to identify the problem and the attempts the character or characters make in responding to it. *Miss Fannie's Hat*, by Jan Karon (whose character cannot decide which hat to donate to charity), and *The Gardener*, by Sarah Stewart (whose character must figure out a way to bring her country garden to a city apartment during the Great Depression), are books that require an understanding of the problem and the characters' attempts at solving it.
- Drawing inferences: To comprehend intended meaning from the literal meaning by filling in information from one's background knowledge. *Home Run*, by Robert Burleigh—a book that uses poetic verse to describe the great baseball player Babe Ruth—is an example of a text that makes use of inferences from which the reader must draw meaning.

To Develop a Sufficient Lexicon Base

Building a strong vocabulary is crucial for eventual reading success. More than simply relying on context when reading, skilled readers are able to decode *"when the meaning of the word is adequately established in memory"* (Stanovich, 1993, p. 283). Other research substantiates that vocabulary size contributes more to early reading ability than age or general developmental level does and that an insufficient vocabulary base can impede the development of phonological awareness (Snow et al., 1998). Vocabulary size includes not only the *quantity* of words but also the *kinds* of words, such as nouns, verbs, articles, and prepositions.

Achieving literacy entails understanding text, not simply decoding words on a printed page. A reader must understand the meaning of the words in relation to the real world and in relation to other words. In describing ways to teach vocabulary and the meaningful relationships among words, Moats (2000) states that "verbal knowledge is organized in networks of associations that have definable structures. Words and concepts are known in relation to one another, not as isolated units" (p. 112).

Landauer and Dumais (1997) have found that the acquisition of vocabulary knowledge from text not only adds new words to one's vocabulary but alters and refines the semantic representations of words already acquired. Their experiment showed that "three fourths of children's vocabulary gain from reading a passage was in words not found in the paragraph at all" (p. 234).

Using words in context, discussing their meanings, and using the words in association with other words can be facilitated through reading aloud, and talking, too! Areas to include in building vocabulary skills are as follows:

- Synonyms: Words that have the same meaning, or are near-perfect substitutes.
- Antonyms: Words that have opposite meanings.
- Homonyms and multiple-meaning words: Words that have more than one meaning.
- Categories of words: Words that share the same semantic class or network. For example, words that have to do with temperament include *tense, relaxed, explosive, laconic, hostile,* and *cautious.*
- Associations: Words that share the same thematic associations.
- Compare and contrast: Words can be expressed and defined on the basis of their shared attributes and contrasted on the basis of their contrasting features.
- Figures of speech: Figures of speech include idioms (words used as a unit that convey a specific meaning, although not literally), similes (words used as a unit that make use of the words *like* or *as* to show an implied connection or comparison between an idea and an unusual referent), and metaphors (words that have an implied connection or comparison between an idea and unusual referent that don't use *like* or *as*).

To Develop the Metalinguistic Aspects of Language

Linguistic knowledge, or the ability to speak a language, is an unconscious process and does not require a speaker to define what he or she knows about the act of speaking. Metalinguistic knowledge, on the other hand, is conscious knowledge about, and insights into, language. Children's metalinguistic skills begin to develop in all of the spoken language components during the elementary school years as they begin to think about, analyze, and manipulate language. "Indeed, literacy growth, at every level, depends on learning to treat language as an object of thought, in and of itself" (Snow et al., 1998, p. 45). Awareness of each of the following components unfolds over time at varying rates and can be facilitated through the use of selected works of children's literature:

- Metasemantic awareness: To develop an understanding of what a word is and that words are distinct from their referents. Ways to think about words include the introduction of synonyms, antonyms, multiple meanings, thematic associations, idioms, and other forms of figurative language. "Deep, rich knowledge of words and varied experiences with their uses are necessary for proficient reading" (Moats, 2000). For example, *A Cache of Jewels and Other Collective Nouns,* by Ruth Heller, explains how one word can be used for a collection or group of things and helps children think about the aspects of language.
- Phonological awareness: To develop an appreciation and sensitivity to the sounds of speech as distinct from their meaning. It is further used to define a whole spectrum of skills that culminate in phonemic awareness, meaning "the understanding that words are

made up of individual sounds and the ability to manipulate these phonemes, either by segmenting, blending or changing individual phonemes within words to create new words." (Chard & Dickson, 1999)

Scientific research substantiates that achievement in phonological awareness levels is the best predictor of early reading success, including that of IQ (Stanovich, 1993). Children's picture books can be ideal material with which to develop carefully planned, systematic instruction in the following hierarchy of phonological awareness:

- Appreciating rhymes and alliteration
- Reciting rhyme and making rhyming words
- Sentence segmentation (using the portions of the text to count words)
- Syllable segmentation and blending (using words of the text to segment and blend syllables into words)
- Onset-rime, blending, and segmentation
- Blending and segmenting individual phonemes
- Manipulating phonemes as in adding, deleting, and substituting to generate a word from the remainder

Recently published picture books abound with the elements of sounds in their text and titles. Examples include *Click, Clack, Moo: Cows That Type; Sing, Sophie!; Zin! Zin! Zin! A Violin; Gabriella's Song; Ten Go Tango;* alliterative titles such as *Mouse Mess; Counting Crocodiles; Piggie Pie;* and a host of books with rhyming texts, such as *The Adventures of Taxi Dog* and *The Thing That Bothered Farmer Brown.*

- Morphological awareness. Phonological awareness facilitates morphological awareness in young children, and both are closely linked in intervention (Carlisle & Normanbhoy, 1993; Moats & Smith, 1992). Teaching derivational morphologies to sharpen connections between meaning and written material in order to enhance comprehension abilities is both supported and encouraged in the literature (Adams, 1990). Snow et al. (1998) state that sensitivity to morphology may be an important aspect for early readers in identifying words when reading and, more important, in learning the meanings of words. Young children begin to be sensitive to word derivations and to think about how words are built from other words. For example, the word *swim*, and Swimmy, the name of the fish in Leo Lionni's picture book by the same name, can be seen as related. *Things That Are Most in the World,* by Judi Barrett, is another instance of a picture book designed to help children focus on the morphological (*-est*) aspects of language.

- Syntactical awareness. To develop an awareness of word order in sentences and that variations in syntax affect the meaning of a message. Five-year-old children begin to develop the rudimentary ability to correct syntactic errors (Ely, 2001). Young children also become aware of syntactic structure in their ability to identify the subject of a sentence (Ferreira & Morrison, 1994). Adams (1990) states that sensitivity to the syntactic system helps children to link word order and meaning in a systematic way and may be especially critical in mastering spelling. Books like *Jabberwocky,* by Lewis Carrol, can be used to develop children's awareness of sentence subjects and predicates, even when nonsense words are used. Other picture books that enhance parts of speech include those in Ruth Heller's language series, such as *Many Luscious Lollipops: A Book About Adjectives* and *Up, Up and Away: A Book About Adverbs.*

- Metapragmatic awareness: To develop an awareness of the relationship between language and the social context in which it is used—including the ability to explain with specificity the rules of social language—whether or not behavior demonstrates adherence to those rules (Ely, 2001). For example, *It's a Spoon, Not a Shovel,* by Caralyn Buehner, offers children the opportunity to select an appropriate verbal response to a social situation. *Martha Speaks,* by Susan Meddaugh, can be used in giving children the opportunity to express why Martha's family becomes frustrated with her lack of turn-taking in conversation.

Speech Production

With a bit of planning and preparation, a carefully chosen picture book can also help to achieve almost any objective in the area of speech–sound production, including the following:

To Improve Articulation

- To discriminate the target sound. Before reading, the text and illustrations can be used for auditory bombardment to stimulate target sounds. Throughout the reading, attention can be drawn to target sounds in the text by stressing their production.
- To produce the target sound in words and structured phrases and sentences. After stressing target sounds within the text and before turning each page, the reader can pause to have the child
  - repeat words in the story that contain the target sound,
  - say a carrier phrase appropriate to the story, or
  - answer a question that elicits a word or words from the text.
- To produce the target sound in conversation. After reading, the story's events can be discussed in language that contains the target sound.

To Speak Fluently

Metrical verses help children learn the natural rhythm of speech. Books that call for a rhythmic, melodic, or singsong type of response are beneficial.

Many alphabet and counting books are also excellent for this purpose (e.g., *Ten, Nine, Eight,* by Molly Bang). They can be used creatively to help a child maintain airflow in responses that increase in length from a single word, to a short phrase, to a full sentence.

Keep in mind that, while using a picture book to systematically increase the length of fluent responses, joint book talk can incorporate other objectives, such as improving eye contact and communication appearance.

To Improve Vocal Quality and Minimize Vocal Abuse

Adults can use books for shaping vocal quality as well as for fluency by having the child use the optimal voice in progressively longer responses. Some stories make reference to the characters' voices. *Cuckoo: A Mexican Folktale,* by Lois Ehlert, and *The Three Billy Goats Gruff,* by Peter Asbjornsen, are examples of stories with characters whose voices are described as "golden" and "raspy" or "hoarse" and "loud."

They can be used to draw a young child's awareness to vocal quality and intensity and to model various manners of vocal production to add further meaning and to generalize knowledge about the uses of voice in other contexts.

Regardless of the objectives in attaining the desired communication skills and early literacy achievement, they undoubtedly can be facilitated through thoughtful planning and careful selection of a picture book from within the immense domain of children's literature.

Looking for Books

That Help Build Communication Skills and Literacy Achievement

---

Searching for the right picture books—those that hold potential for interaction and facilitate a variety of specific communication and literacy skills during a limited time frame—takes time. The Catalog of Picture Books in this section and the Skills index were created to save you time in your search. You will undoubtedly add your own favorites, and when making additional selections for elementary school-aged children, keep in mind the following.

Find the books that you love. The value of sharing your love and enthusiasm for literature is perhaps the foremost prescription for helping children to build language and literacy skills.

Choosing a limited text has advantages. Although lengthier texts can create outstanding stories, picture books with shorter texts and creative language afford greater opportunities for interaction, dialogic reading, and intervention that occur within certain time constraints. Many high-quality picture books have excellent but relatively brief texts and are well suited for elementary school-aged children.

For younger school-aged children, look for books with words and actions that appear over and over again. These books have

- repetition, rhyme, and verse;
- sequenced events; and
- allow for both spoken and imitated speech.

Examples of books that meet these criteria are *Suddenly!* by Colin McNaughton; *Sing, Sophie!* by Dayle Ann Dodds; and *The Thing That Bothered Farmer Brown,* by Teri Sloat.

For older school-aged children, look for books with excellent stories that children can relate to and interact with the reader by

- responding to modeled or shaped sentences at appropriate intervals,
- discussing story grammar elements (e.g., who did what, who felt what, how the story began and ended, etc.), and
- using critical thinking skills to identify the problem and the cause of the problem, suggest solutions, predict outcomes, and draw inferences.

A few examples that meet this criteria include *Piggie Pie,* by Margie Palatini; *The Gardener,* by Sarah Stewart; *Imogene's Antlers,* by David Small; *Miss Fannie's Hat,* by Jan Karon; and *One Grain of Rice: A Mathematical Folktale,* by Demi.

Many picture books suitable for this age group combine both the features of rhyming verse and story elements, such as *George Washington's Cows,* by David Small; *Barn Dance!* by Bill Martin Jr. and John Archambault; and *Home Run,* by Robert Burleigh.

Search for picture opportunities. Be sure the book's text is supported by good illustrations. The best illustrations are representational, easily interpreted, and appealing. To assist children in focusing on the oral language of the text, look for books in which

- each line of text has pictures to illustrate its meaning, and
- the pictures provide more language opportunities than the text alone.

Examples of such books are *Tough Boris,* by Mem Fox; *Officer Buckle and Gloria,* by Peggy Rathmann; and *The Thing That Bothered Farmer Brown,* by Teri Sloat. These wordless picture books can facilitate picture descriptions, cause-and-effect relationships, problem identification, and storytelling skills.

Examples of outstanding wordless books (or near-wordless books) include *You Can't Take a Balloon Into the Metropolitan Museum,* by Jacquiline Preiss Weitzman; *Tuesday* and *Sector 7,* by David Wiesner; and *Time Flies,* by Eric Rohmann.

Be sure the story is relevant. The text and illustrations are most effective when they

- reflect the child's surrounding culture,
- make sense to the child, and
- relate to the child's personal experiences.

Cull through many genres. Picture books can be found in many sections of a library or bookstore. Don't forget to check the

- junior section (e.g., *Seven Brave Women,* by Betsy Gould Hearne, and *Home Run,* by Robert Burleigh),
- folklore section (e.g., *The Paper Crane,* by Molly Bang, and *Arrow to the Sun,* by Gerald McDermott),
- science section (e.g., *Cloud Dance,* by Thomas Locker),
- history section (e.g., *If a Bus Could Talk: The Story of Rosa Parks,* by Faith Ringgold),
- language section (e.g., *Hairy, Scary, Ordinary: What Is an Adjective?* by Brian P. Cleary, and *Behind the Mask: A Book About Prepositions,* by Ruth Heller),
- sports section (e.g., *Casey at the Bat,* by Ernest Lawrence Thayer), and the
- poetry section (e.g., *Noisy Poems,* by Jill Bennett).

Look for award winners. Not all of the books that are ideal for promoting communication and literacy skills win awards, but lists of award-winning books can help you begin your search. Lists of Caldecott Medal winners, Children's Notables, and other award-winning books are available online, including the following Web sights:

- Association for Library Service to Children (ALSC): www.ala.org
- MacKin Library Media: www.mackin.com
- Booksellers such as Amazon.com (www.amazon.com) and Barnes & Noble (www.bn.com).

Make books a topic of conversation. Adults love to talk about good children's books. Ask friends, colleagues, librarians, and parents to share titles of books they have enjoyed reading aloud.

Suggestions for Book Talk
with Children in Grades 1 Through 5

Talking about storybook reading helps children to link stories to their everyday lives. Actively engaging children in read-aloud sessions enhances meaning and language learning, and it can also promote many dimensions of literacy achievement. Snow et al. (1998) reported studies in which read-aloud sessions included discussion activities before the reading, during the reading, and after the reading. Each picture book in the catalog for Grades 1 through 5 has a methods section that lists ways for promoting a wide variety of language and literacy skills before, during, and after the read-aloud. Here are some suggestions to keep in mind when reading picture books:

Introduce the book. Before the reading,

- ask children what they know about the topic of the book,
- find out what questions they may have before you begin,
- give background information if necessary,
- talk about other books that relate to the same topic, and
- read the title and names of the author and illustrator and give further details about them.

Pause to ask questions. Modify story reading to encourage children's active participation in the following ways:

- Ask prediction questions about the story
- Ask open-ended questions about the story
- Elicit picture descriptions and action sequences

Give feedback. In addition to the question-and-answer format, Fey (2001) suggests the following ways to give feedback to children:

- Request clarification of a child's utterances
- Recast the child's sentences
- Recast and recap the story content

Elaborate on the language. Elaborating on both the text and the children's utterances facilitates meaning. Ways to elaborate on the language during and after the reading include the following:

- Facilitate connections of new words and concepts to children's background knowledge
- Facilitate the use of the new word or concept by assisting children in paraphrasing and giving examples
- Relate the story to the children's experiences and interests
- Assist children in expressing their ideas with the use of scaffolding
- Follow a child's lead without being sidetracked (Arnold & Whitehurst, 1994)

Help structure and scaffold narratives. Questions based on story grammar elements (Applebee, 1978) can help develop story schema. Sample questions to elicit storytelling include

- Setting: Where does the story take place?
- Characters: Who is the story about?
- External Attempts: What happened to start the story?
- Internal Attempts: How did the character(s) feel about this? What did the character(s) do?
- Consequences: What happened at the end?
- Outcome: How did the character(s) feel at the end and how did they change?

Reread the story. Rereading enables younger children to become familiar with predictable language, thereby allowing them to better acquire the concepts and gain an understanding of the story (Neuman et al., 2000). When children can anticipate what is coming next in a story or line of verse, they begin to have a sense of mastery over books (Cullinan & Bagert, 1996). Several ways to allow children to participate are suggested by Fey (2001) and include having them

- fill in the blanks during "cloze" activities ("I know an old lady who swallowed a _____"),
- recite the words in unison (choral reading), and
- retell the story (with *and* without the aid of pictures).

For older children, rereading the story often better enables them to

- discuss features of the story,
- retell the story sequence,
- explain cause-and-effect sequences,
- formulate the problem and ways the character(s) overcome the problem or attempt to achieve the goal,
- answer comprehension questions, and
- participate in storytelling activities.

Stay with the book-related activities. Depending on the type or genre, continue to use the book for more than one day or one session throughout various language and literacy activities. Suggestions for multiple sessions include the following:

- Introduce the book, discuss its topic, and read it aloud in the first session.
- Reread the book, pausing to ask comprehension questions, and engage in discussions in another session.
- Do a picture walk-through and retell the story in another session.
- Engage in phonological awareness activities with the words of the story in successive sessions.
- Do an extended activities project, such as making class murals of the story's setting or dramatizing the story over successive sessions.
- The American Speech-Language-Hearing Association (ASHA, 2001) guidelines advocate role-playing during which children have opportunities to act out parts of characters in order to give them a sense of story. In an interesting study, Rose, Parks, Androes, and McMahon (2000) found that role-playing and the dramatic techniques of imagery-based learning significantly improved reading comprehension levels in elementary students compared with students who did not participate in the activities.

Collaborate with others. Special educators can coordinate books and topics with those of classroom teachers to facilitate language and literacy skills while aiding in academic success. ASHA (2001) has guidelines on collaborating with teachers, speech-language pathologists, and special educators so that language and literacy-based activities are relevant to the classroom curriculum and to Individualized Education programs.

A Catalog of Picture Books for Children in Grades 1 Through 5

Abuela

by Arthur Dorros
New York: Puffin Books, 1991

Suggested Grade and Interest Level: 1 through 3

Topic Explorations: Cities, New York; Culture and history, Hispanic

Skill Builders:

Vocabulary	**Grammar and syntax**	**Language literacy**
Semantics	Present tense	Relating personal experiences
Categories		Sequencing
Morphological units		

Synopsis: While riding on a bus, a little girl sits next to her *abuela* (Spanish for *grandmother*), who speaks mostly Spanish. Soon she is imagining that they are carried up into the sky, looking down on the sights of New York City. The text is interspersed with Spanish vocabulary and sentences such as *"El parque es lindo"* (The park is beautiful) and *"Sí, quiero volar"* (Yes, I can fly). The charming, colorful pictures of the city, as seen through the child's eyes, are an intricate patchwork of color. There is a lot of action, leaving much to describe in the detailed illustrations. A list of Spanish words and their pronunciations are provided on the back page.

Method: Introduce the book by talking about different languages. Many children have parents or grandparents that came from places where they spoke a language besides English. Elicit children's background knowledge about different languages and ask them to share the word for *grandmother* in another language. Some include *la nonna* and *grandmere.*

During the read-aloud, develop vocabulary by pointing out the features of the city illustrated in the book. Have children identify them, or give them the word to use as they describe what's happening in the illustrations. Include

downtown	building	parks
airport	factories	trains
the sea	Statue of Liberty	loading dock

Point out the activity in the pictures and pause briefly to structure sentences of present tense within the context of the story. Use the verbs of the text and illustrations, including

swooping	flying	gliding
pointing	soaring	circling
sailing	loading	
visiting	flapping	

After the read-aloud, have a discussion. The narrator explained that her grandmother liked adventure. Talk with children about the word *adventure* and what it means. Give examples of an exciting experience. Have children relate their personal experiences. Perhaps they have also been to a city, or they live in a city and have traveled to another part on a bus. Perhaps their grandmother or grandfather came from a different country and told them about life there. Perhaps the class has gone on an adventure together.

Do a picture walk-through while children sequence the events of the story, telling what Rosalba and her grandmother saw over New York City. Encourage the use of words *first, then,* and *next* so that children can connect the visual sequence in words.

Teach morphological units with the use of the word *higher,* as portrayed in the illustrations of Rosalba and her grandmother flying "higher than tall buildings downtown." Use the opportunity of the text to talk about how the characters ascend over the city. Focus on the word and ask,

> How many parts do you hear in the word *higher?*
> What little word do you hear in *higher?*
> What part of the word do you hear after *high?*

Explain one meaning of the word *–er* when it is used at the end of a word (a way to make a comparison to something else). Rosalba and her grandmother went high in the sky. Then they went higher. Give examples and demonstrate visually with objects:

> small, smaller
> big, bigger
> low, lower
> bright, brighter

Encourage children to use the words in sentences within the immediate context or their lives.

Play the Suffix game. For example, say

> Put *–er* after *loud.* What word is it now?
> Put *–er* after *tall.* What word is it now?
> And so on.

For increasing the ability to categorize, have children name the fruit, such as bananas, mangos, and papayas (all Spanish words), and have them supply the name for what they are all called. Look for other things to categorize in the illustrations of the city, such as vehicles and buildings. Have the children label them and ask, "What are they all called?"

The Adventures of Taxi Dog

by Debra Barracca and Sal Barracca
New York: Dial Books for Young Readers, 1990

Suggested Grade and Interest Level: 1 through 3

Topic Explorations: Animals, Dogs; Cities, New York City; Careers; Community; Transportation

Skill Builders:

Vocabulary	**Language Literacy**	**Phonological awareness**
Semantics	Relating personal experiences	
Idioms	Sequencing	
Similes and metaphors	Point of view	
Grammar and syntax	Discussion	
Tenses, present and past		

Synopsis: In delightful, rhyming verse, Maxi tells his story of how he came to belong to Jim, the taxi driver. No longer a stray "avoiding the pound," he now rides around New York City all day long. The story is based on the authors' experience of a New York City taxi ride with a driver and his dog that sat next to him in the front seat. Maxi, like the real taxi dog, travels with Jim to any number of different places. Follow them around, from airport to theater to hospital, and meet the characters Maxi meets from all walks of life and in all sorts of circumstances and predicaments.

Method: Before the read-aloud, elicit the children's background knowledge of taxicabs and big cities such as New York. If children have been in a big city before, encourage them to relate their experiences. Explain what a taxicab is and how it works.

During the read-aloud, allow children to experience the story so that the flow of the text, the rhythm and rhyme, is not interrupted.

After the read-aloud, reread the story, pausing after each page to discuss vocabulary, including

> roam
> avoid
> fare

Discuss idioms such as

> Cleaned the plate
> Start life anew
> Broke into a song
> Put on a show

Talk about similes and what each might mean, as in

> Like lightning we flew
> It's just like a dream

Describe the colorful characters that get into the taxi. Recall their occupations. Point out all the activity in the city and have children describe the action depicted in the illustrations. Model and shape grammatical structures. Then see if children can find the black cat that is hiding on every page.

Talk about a story's point of view and ask children to decide who told this story. From whose eyes was it seen?

Hold a discussion about the importance of being kind to animals. What might have happened to Maxi had Jim never found him? Do you think that dogs respond differently when people are nice to them than when they are mean and angry toward them?

Use the words of the text to play phonological awareness games. See the entry in the Pre-K catalog for activities that address earlier phonological awareness levels.

PLAY Odd-One-Out.

Children select from a string of words ending in the same sound the one that does not belong. For example, say

> plate, eat, right, dog
> Which word has a different ending sound? (dog)
> That's right. *Dog* is the odd one out.

Some four-word strings follow. Reduce to three-word strings if needed.

quick, back, look, roa*m*	name, hea*d*, Jim, home	dream, bar*k*, come, home
dar*k*, pat, spot, put	sing, sang, ring, tri*p*	hurr*y*, quick, back, look
Murray, taxi, city, do*g*	lady, Maxi, hotdo*g*, taxi	
stopped, roa*m*, barked, ate	ki*ss*, head, found, cleaned	

PLAY **Say-It-Until-You-Hear-It.**

Children synthesize one-syllable words divided into onset-rime. Present the word with a clear pause between the onset and rime. Demonstrate how to elongate the parts to blend them together, saying them a little quicker each time until they are readily identified. Provide scaffolding until children are ready to do it on their own. For example, say

> Put these two parts together: *s–it.*
> Say it until you hear it. *Sssss . . . iiit. Sss . . . it. Sit.*

Continue with these one-syllable words beginning with a single consonant sound:

r-ide	w-ay	l-and
r-oam	s-ick	s-ide
w-ide	s-ing	
b-oss	l-ook	

Then demonstrate how to synthesize one-syllable words divided into onset-rime beginning with a two-consonant cluster until children are ready to do it on their own. Words include

fl-ight (flight)	gl-ad (glad)	cl-ean (clean)
pl-ate (plate)	tr-eat (treat)	dr-eam (dream)
dr-ive (drive)	sp-ot (spot)	

PLAY **Roll-It-Out.**

Children synthesize a C–V–C word by blending each of its phonemes. Demonstrate by elongating the phonemes and blending them together in shorter and shorter sequences until children can identify the word. For example, say

> r-ī-d
> What's the word? Roll it out.
> *Rrrrr . . . īīīī . . . d. R-ī-d. Ride.*

Once children are able to blend the sounds, present the word by saying each phoneme separately so the children can "roll it out" on their own and identify the word. In addition to the C–V–C words provided above, words from the story include

r-oa-m	s-i-t	s-i-de
l-oo-k	f-ood	s-i-ck
t-i-p	d-o-g	h-o-me

PLAY **Break-It-Up.**

Children analyze one-syllable C–V–C words in order to identify the beginning, middle, and ending sounds. Begin activities with initial sounds, and then proceed to middle and ending sounds. For an example on how to demonstrate finding the middle sound in the word *ride*, ask

> What's the sound in the middle of *ride*?
> Break it up: *Rrrrrr–iiiiii–d. R-ī-d.*
> *ī* is the middle sound in *ride.*

(continues on next page)

PLAY **Break-It-Up.** *Continued*

Continue to present one-syllable C-V-C words provided above so children can "break them up" and identify the sounds in each position.

In the last stage of the game, children identify all the sounds in the word. Demonstrate how to elongate the sounds and then break them up in order to identify each one. For example, ask

> What are all the sounds in the word *ride*?
> Roll it out and break it up: *Rrrrr–iiiiii–d. R-ī-d.*
> *R-ī-d* are the sounds in *ride.*

PLAY **Delete-It.**

Children omit the first sound in one-syllable words from the text. Demonstrate by saying the word slowly, then leaving off the initial sound. To demonstrate using the word *ride,* for example, say

> Listen to how I can make *ride* become *I'd.*
> I delete the first sound. *Ride. –ide.* (as in *I'd*)
> Now you delete it. *Ride.*

Use the lists of one-syllable words provided above. Then practice with two-syllable words *Maxi* and *taxi* for the following game, both of which become *–axi.*

PLAY **Switch-It.**

Children delete the initial sound of the word and exchange it with a new sound to make another word. Demonstrate first, then prompt with cues as necessary. For example

> Say *dog.*
> Now say *dog,* only take out *d* and switch it with *f.*
> What new word can you make? (fog)

Play the game with words *Maxi* and *taxi.* Using *f,* their part will sound like this:

> Faxi and Faxi Fog.

Remember to go slowly! Other possibilities include

> Naxi. Naxi Nog   Waxi. Waxi Wog   Laxi. Laxi Log
> Saxi. Saxi Sog   Haxi. Haxi Hog

Have fun!

Read also *Maxi, the Hero; Maxi, the Star;* and *A Taxi Dog Christmas.* This book is also available in a Spanish version, titled *Las aventuras de Maxi: El perro taxista.*

Ah-Choo

by Mercer Mayer
New York: Dial Books for Young Readers, 1976, 1977

Suggested Grade and Interest Level: 1 through 3

Skill Builders:
    Language literacy   **Articulation, *Ch***
    Predicting
    Sequencing
    Cause-and-effect relationships
    Storytelling

Synopsis: An elephant's disastrous sneezes cause havoc in the town until he saves the day by winning the heart of a lady hippo. Pictures tell the story in this wordless book, which is excellent for stimulating language.

Method: Before the read-aloud, elicit background knowledge about allergies and things that make people sneeze. Lead into the story by having children make predictions based on the title.

Read aloud, pausing to interpret the story from what is implied in the pictures. Allow the children to supply the sneezing sounds. Ask what might happen next. Ask what caused the sneezes and what caused the police officer and judge to get mad.

For storytelling, use story grammar questions as scaffolding. For example,

> Who is the story about?
> Where does it take place?
> What happened to start the story off?
> How did the characters feel about this?
> What did the police officer want to do with the elephant?
> Was the police officer successful?
> How did the story end?
> Now how do the characters feel? How did they change?

For articulation of *Ch*, allow the child to supply the *Ah-choo* word where indicated in the story.

Alexander and the Terrible, Horrible, No Good, Very Bad Day

by Judith Viorst
New York: Atheneum, 1972, 1987

Suggested Grade and Interest Level: 1 through 5

Topic Explorations: Daily activities; Family relationships; Feelings

Skill Builders:
    Grammar and syntax   **Language literacy**   **Articulation—*R, S,* and *Z***
    Tenses, present and future   Sequencing
                                Storytelling
                                Problem solving
                                Drawing inferences

Synopsis: It's no wonder this book is a classic. Who can't relate to having a terrible, no good, very bad day? The story tells of the trials of Alexander and his repeated solution: "I think I'll move to Australia."

Method: Before the read-aloud, introduce the idea that every now and then, we all have days when everything seems to go wrong. This is the story of such a day for a boy named Alexander.

For verb tenses, pause to describe the events portrayed in the illustrations. Model and shape target structures.

For problem solving, pause at each episode to have children state the problem and Alexander's solution. Are there other ways to handle the problem? Name a few. Could the problem have been avoided? How? For drawing inference, pause to infer meaning from the text. For example, what does it mean when Alexander says he drew a picture of an invisible castle? What about when he describes his lunch and says, "Guess whose mother forgot to put in dessert?"

For sequencing, help children recall the events in Alexander's day. For example, first he wakes up, then he has breakfast, then he gets a ride to school, and so on. Have them say what horrible things happened in each episode.

For discussion, after reading aloud, ask children whether they have ever had a day like Alexander's. Encourage them to talk about their experiences. How did they solve their problems?

For articulation, practice words (such as *terrible, horrible, Australia,* and *Alexander*) before the read-aloud. While reading, interject questions to elicit these and other target words that appear in the text.

Extended Activities: Using the story's pictures for scaffolding, have children tell how Alexander's day might be better tomorrow. For example, when he gets out of bed, he won't have gum in his hair or trip over the skateboard. Maybe this time the tooth fairy will give him two-dollar bills. And maybe at breakfast he will get the prize in the cereal box while his brothers get only cereal. Review each episode and create a sequel to it. Ask the children to collaborate in creating a new title, perhaps "Alexander's Wonderful, Fantastic, Incredibly Good Day."

Have each child fold a piece of paper into four sections. Label the first two sections "Alexander's Very Bad Day." In these two sections, the child draws an episode from the book and Alexander's response. Label the next two sections "Tomorrow Is a Better Day." Under this title, each child draws a picture of an improved episode in the first section and next to it draws a picture of Alexander's new response. Encourage the children to color the pictures creatively and write dialog beneath each picture.

Anansi the Spider: A Tale from the Ashanti

Retold by Gerald McDermott
New York: Henry Holt, 1972

Suggested Grade and Interest Level: 1 through 4

Topic Explorations: Folklore, African and African American; Insects and spiders

Skill Builders:

Vocabulary	**Language literacy**
Semantics	Storytelling
Attributes	Verbal expression
Grammar and syntax	Drawing inferences
Tenses, present and past	**Articulation—*R, S* and *Z, Sh***

Synopsis: The folk hero Anansi overcomes seemingly insurmountable obstacles with the help of his six sons. Then he must decide which one to reward. The brief, poetic verse is ideal for shaping language and discussing meaning.

Method: Before the read-aloud, introduce the book by talking about folktales and the ways different cultures long ago explained the nature of life through the telling of stories.

During the reading, pause to build grammar and syntax skills by asking children to describe the actions in the pictures. Recast portions of the text as necessary to elicit and shape structures such as present or past tense.

For attributes, have students think of words that describe the characters.

> What kind of spider was Anansi?
> Fair or unfair? Timid or brave?
> What words can you use to describe his sons?

For storytelling, encourage retelling of the folktale by relating that a long time ago, people made up a story about how the moon got in the sky. Ask the students to retell the folktale of Anansi as if they were making it up long ago. Have them take turns sequencing parts of the story. Use scaffolding where necessary.

For drawing inferences, ask questions that draw meaning from the story's pictures and text. For example, "Why were the sons named Road Builder and River Drinker?" "What do we call the beautiful white light in the story?"

For articulation, pause to ask questions that elicit responses containing the target sounds. Before reading the story, use the following words from the text for auditory bombardment of *S* and *Z*.

Anansi	sea
spider	sky
six	forest
sons	rescue
See Trouble	swallow
Game Skinner	prize
Stone Thrower	always
soft	

These words are useful for auditory bombardment of *R*:

spider	trouble
See Trouble	water
Road Builder	brother
River Drinker	road
Game Skinner	prize
Stone Thrower	rescue

For auditory bombardment of *Sh*, use the following words:

Ashanti	fish
cushion	splash
ocean	shining

Animalia

by Graeme Base
New York: Abrams, 1986, 1987

Suggested Grade and Interest Level: 1 through 3

Topic Explorations: Alphabet; Animals, Zoo

Skill Builders:

Vocabulary	**Articulation**
Semantics	General articulation
Phonological awareness	**Fluency**
	Voice

Synopsis: An extraordinary alphabet book presents an amazing array of animals and objects beginning with particular letters along with alliterative sentences.

Method: Before the read-aloud, talk about the boy in the striped shirt hidden within the pages illustrating words beginning with an alphabet letter. Encourage the children to search for him among the objects and animals depicted.

During the read-aloud, have children seek out and name as many objects and animals as possible whose names begin with the alphabet letter named. Use the book to teach new vocabulary words and put them in sentences, using the alliterative verse as much as possible.

Use the words of the text to play phonological awareness games. See the entry in the Pre-K catalog for activities that address earlier phonological awareness levels.

> **PLAY** Say-It-Until-You-Hear-It.
>
> Children synthesize one-syllable words divided into onset-rime. Start with words that begin with a continuous single consonant sound. An example using the "R" page:
>
> First, identify as many of the *r* words as you and the children can find. Talk about their meanings and use them in sentences. Then take the one-syllable words beginning with a single sound from illustrations and the text (shortening two-syllable words where needed) and divide them into onset-rime. Demonstrate by producing each part and showing children how to blend the parts until they can identify the word. Elongate the parts, inserting a clear break between them. For example, say
>
> > Put these two parts together: *r-ed.*
> > Say it until you hear it. *Rrrr . . . eeeed. Rr-ed. Red.*
>
> Continue with words
>
> > r-ide (ride)
> > r-ose (rose)
>
> More words can be readily found on each page.
>
> Children can blend one-syllable words divided into onset-rime beginning with a two-consonant cluster. An example using the "P" page:
>
> *(continues on next page)*

PLAY Say-It-Until-You-Hear-It. *Continued*

> Put these two parts together: *pr–oud.*
> Say it until you hear it. *Prrrr . . . oud. Prr-oud. Proud.*

Continue with words such as

> pr-een (preen)
> pl-ume (plume)

More words can be readily found on each page.

PLAY Roll-It-Out.

Children synthesize a previously given consonant–vowel–consonant word by blending its individual phonemes. Demonstrate by elongating the phonemes and blending them together in shorter and shorter sequences until children can identify the word. For example, say

> r– ō–z
> What's the word? Roll it out.
> *Rrrr . . . oooo . . . zzzz . . . R . . . o . . . z. Rose.*

Once children are successful, present each of the phonemes separately so they can "roll them out" on their own, in shorter and shorter sequences, to find the word. Word sources are plentiful on each page. Some words from the *R* page include

r-a-m	r-i-ch	r-o-d
r-ou-te	r-oa-d	
r-u-g	r-e-d	

PLAY Break-It-Up.

Children analyze one-syllable consonant–vowel–consonant words in order to identify the beginning, middle, and ending sounds. Begin with initial sounds, then proceed to middle and then ending sounds. For an example on how to demonstrate finding the middle sound in *red,* ask

> What's the sound in the middle of *red*?
> Break it up: *Rrrrrr . . . eeeeee . . . d. R . . . e . . . d.*
> *ĕ* is the sound in the middle of *red.*

In the last stage of the game, children identify all the sounds in the word. Demonstrate how to elongate the sounds and break them up in order to identify each one. For example, ask

> What are all the sounds in the word *red*?
> Roll it out and break it up: *R . . . e . . .d. R-e-d.*
> *R-ĕ-d* are the sounds in the word *red.*

PLAY **Delete-It.**

Children omit the first sound in one-syllable words from the text. Demonstrate by saying the word slowly, then leaving off the initial sound. For an example using *two* from the short text of the "T" page, show how to leave off the beginning sound, saying

> Listen to how I can make *two* become *oo*.
> I delete the first sound. *Two. oo.*
> Now you delete it. *Two . . .*

Use part of the alliterative words of the text on each page to play the game, slowly working up to the whole line. First have children say only part of the verse—slowing—leaving off the initial sounds. For example, "Two Tigers Taking the Train (to Timbuktu)" would sound like this:

> Oo Igers
> Oo Igers Aking (sounds like *aching*)
> Oo Igers Aking the Ain
> Oo Igers Aking the Ain oo Imbuk-oo

PLAY **Switch-It.**

Using the same words found on the "T" page, have children replace the initial *t* with another designated sound. For example, switch *t* with *m*. Their part will sound like this:

> Moo Migers Making the Main
> Moo Migers Making the Main moo Mimbuk-moo

Antarctica

by Helen Cowcher
New York: Farrar, Straus & Giroux, 1990

Suggested Grade and Interest Level: 1 through 3

Topic Explorations: Animals, Endangered; Conservation; Sea and the seashore

Skill Builders:

Vocabulary	**Language literacy**
Semantics	Compare and contrast
	Discussion

Synopsis: Dazzling illustrations and lines of beautiful text tell of life in the antarctic, including seals and penguins, and how their environment is being threatened by an unaccustomed visitor—humans.

Method: Begin by talking about the environment of the south pole. Explain that the climate is so cold that people cannot live there permanently. Point out Antarctica on a globe. Brainstorm words that give a picture of life in the antarctic. Ask students to imagine the kinds of animals that might live there.

Read aloud, pausing to model and shape target structures. Interact with children about the vocabulary words in the text, including

emperor penguins	leopard seals
Adelie penguins	Weddell seals

After the read-aloud, ask children what they now know about the place called Antarctica. List descriptive words. Ask questions such as these:

> How is Antarctica like a cold day at the lake or ocean? How is it different?
> How are the animals that live in the antarctic like the animals that live in forests, in the mountains, in jungles, and in the desert?
> What common dangers do many of these animals share?

Extended Activity: Break into learning groups. Tell the students to imagine that they are going on an expedition to the south pole. Have each child in the group take on a particular responsibility on his or her trip. Discuss what students would like to see most on the trip. What would they like to discover about the environment in the antarctic? What would they like to do there? What do they imagine they would find? Then have each group present to the class what their responsibilities were and what they saw and did on their expedition.

Arrow to the Sun

by Gerald McDermott
New York: Puffin Books, 1984

Suggested Grade and Interest Level: 3 through 5

Topic Exploration: Folklore, Native American

Skill Builders:

Language literacy	**Articulation— *R, S,* and *Th* (voiced and voiceless)**
Sequencing	
Cause-and-effect relationships	
Problem solving	
Critical thinking	

Synopsis: The universal hero myth is embodied in this story of a boy who is rejected because he has no father and leaves on a quest to find him. When he is sent to the Lord of the Sun, his true father, he is not acknowledged until he undergoes a series of trials to prove his identity. Having accomplished them, he returns to earth with his father's spirit, and everyone rejoices with the Dance of Life.

Method: Pause to identify the problem in the story, asking

> What events caused the problem to happen?
> What facts can you state about the problem?
> How does the boy solve his problem?
> Recall in order the series of trials the boy underwent to prove he was his father's son.
> How did the boy change?
> What brought this change about?
> What caused the people to celebrate the boy's return with the Dance of Life?

For articulation, pause to elicit target words found in the text. Have students use them in sentences reflecting the story. *Th* words include

father	mother
earth	through
nothing	this

Extended Activities: Bring in materials to familiarize the children with Pueblo art and then compare the illustrations to Pueblo art. What qualities do they have in common?

Discuss elements that are common to the hero motif in folktales. What ingredients does the story have that fit with the hero motif? How is it like other hero myths?

Arthur's Nose

by Marc Brown
Boston: Little, Brown, 1976, 1986

Suggested Grade and Interest Level: 1 through 4

Topic Explorations: Careers; Friendship; Self-esteem

Skill Builders:

Grammar and syntax	Language literacy	Articulation—*R, S,* and *Th* (voiced and
Possessive nouns	Problem solving	voiceless)
Pronouns—personal, possessive, and reflexive	Critical thinking	

Synopsis: Arthur is an aardvark whose family loves him. That includes his nose, which Arthur happens to detest. Even his schoolmates laugh at it. So Arthur visits the rhinologist to find a new nose, while his friends wait anxiously outside. When he comes out, everyone is surprised. Arthur's nose hasn't changed a bit. "I'm just not me without my nose!" he exclaims.

Method: For possessive nouns and pronouns, model structures directly from the text, such as "Arthur's house," "Arthur's family," "Arthur's friends," and so on. Shape responses such as the following:

> He didn't like his nose.
> She thought his nose was funny.
> She wanted to change her seat.
> He wasn't himself without his nose.
> Arthur liked himself now.

For problem solving and critical thinking, ask questions about the meaning of the story.

> What was Arthur's problem?
> How did Arthur feel about himself?
> What did Arthur decide to do about his problem?
> Arthur's friends express concern that he may change if he gets a new nose. Why were Arthur's friends worried?
> What caused Arthur to change his mind and keep his own nose?
> How did Arthur feel about himself after he decided to keep his nose?
> What did Arthur learn from this experience?

Note: Read also *Arthur's Eyes, Arthur's First Sleepover, Arthur's New Puppy, Arthur's Tooth, Arthur's Pet Business,* and other books in this series.

Aunt Harriet's Underground Railroad in the Sky

by Faith Ringgold
New York: Crown Books, 1993

Suggested Grade and Interest Level: 1 through 5

Topic Explorations: Culture and history, African and African American;
Family relationships; Journeys

Skill Builders:

Vocabulary	**Language literacy**
Similes and metaphors	Cause-and-effect relationships
	Drawing inferences

Synopsis: Cassie, wanting to reunite with her brother, BeBe, retraces the steps that scores of slaves walked in their escape to freedom on the Underground Railroad. Her journey is guided by a dreamlike Harriet Tubman, who relates the history of slavery and Cassie's cultural background with interesting facts about the escape route and the Civil War era.

Method: Before the read-aloud, talk about similes as a tool an author can use in creating powerful images. Discuss the cover, making predictions about the story based on it.

> What do we already know about the story?
> What do you think the story will be about?
> What makes you think so?

For identifying cause and effect, ask students what caused slaves to follow the Underground Railroad to Canada.

> What effect did the Underground Railroad have on the lives of the people who escaped and on our history?
> What caused the Underground Railroad to be so successful?
> What would the effects have been if the slaves had not escaped?

For drawing inferences, ask why the author portrayed Cassie as being able to fly at the beginning and ending of the story. What does flying bring to mind? How would it feel to be able to fly?

Extended Activity: Discuss similes. Ask students to close their eyes and recall what was most interesting about the story. What are the images they remember most? What words did the author use to convey those images? Go back and review the similes in that part of the story. Then have the students think of and write their own. Develop associations for some key words to get them started. For example,

> Slavery reminds me of _____.
> When I think of slavery I think of _____.
> Slavery is like _____.

> Flying reminds me of _____.
> When I think of flying, I think of _____.
> Flying is like _____.

> The Underground Railroad reminds me of _____.
> When I think of the Underground Railroad, I think of _____.
> The Underground Railroad is like _____.

Harriet Tubman reminds me of _____.
When I think of Harriet Tubman, I think of _____.
Harriet Tubman is like _____.

Note: Read also *Harriet and the Promised Land,* by Jacob Lawrence. See that catalog entry for another extended activity. Compare and contrast the two books. What do they have in common in terms of characters, setting, plot, mood, theme, and literary style?

The Baby Uggs Are Hatching!

by Jack Prelutsky
New York: Greenwillow Books, 1982, 1989

Suggested Grade and Interest Level: 1 through 4

Topic Exploration: Humor

Skill Builders:

| Vocabulary | Grammar and syntax | Articulation—*S, Sh,* and *Ch* |
| Attributes | Present tense | |

Synopsis: A collection of silly rhymes about imaginary creatures, such as sneepies, snatch-its, and sneezy snoozers.

Method: For articulation, read aloud verses loaded with a student's target sounds. For example,

> The sneezy snoozer sneezes
> as the sneezy snoozer chooses
> it snoozes as it pleases
> and it sneezes as it snoozes.

For adjectives and attributes, have the children make up their own crazy critter. Then brainstorm a list of adjectives for the critter and some actions it performs. (*Note:* You may want to establish rules that limit the type of language used.) For example,

> Is it affectionate? Does it give hugs?
> Does it wink and smile?
> Is it noisy?
> Does it buzz or sing? Clink or slurp?
> How many feet does it have?
> Does it have fur or scales?
> Does it share or hoard?
> Does it shrink or expand?

Construct short sentences expressing the attributes and actions the children suggest. Vote on a class mascot after class members contribute whimsical names.

Extended Activity: Have children draw pictures of how they envision the critter. Then make a list of the attributes and sentences the students brainstormed earlier and have them write poems about their critters. Have the students present their poems. Gather the works and make a class book, or have all the students contribute to one class poem. Display the poem on a large poster board.

Barn Dance!

by Bill Martin Jr. and John Archambault
New York: Henry Holt, 1986

Suggested Grade and Interest Level: 1 through 3

Topic Explorations: Animals, Farm; Country life; Music, musicians, and musical instruments; Nighttime; Owls; Seasons, Autumn

Skill Builders:

Vocabulary	Language literacy	Articulation, general, especially
Semantics	Verbal expression	*Sh*, *Ch*, and *J*
Categories	**Phonological awareness**	
Attributes		

Synopsis: Late at night, with the moon shining bright, everything seems quiet out by the old barn. Or is it? As a boy listens to the sounds of the night from his bedroom window, an owl comes to lead him out across the fields and into the barn. There he sees a scarecrow hosting some mighty fine, western-style dancin'. This book is great for tapping out rhythms and is perfect for autumnal reading.

Method: Before the read-aloud, ask children what they know about barn dances. Discuss harvest festivals and how farmers celebrated finishing their work of harvesting corn and picking pumpkins off the vines with music and dancing in the barn. Show the cover of the scarecrow with his fiddle and a boy crawling through the rails of a fence in the moonlight. Have children predict what the story will be about.

During the read-aloud, demonstrate the rhythm of the text by tapping it out with your foot or playing it on a small instrument as you read the lines. Encourage children to join in. For vocabulary, talk about what a fiddle is and the type of music the scarecrow is playing on it. Discuss how barn dancing differs from other kinds of dancing. Other words include

kin	hound dog	wonderment
partner	curtsey	

For verbal expression, pause in the reading to discuss the story. When the boy arrives at the barn, let the children find where he is hiding. Ask what the boy sees from his perspective. Point out the autumnal details, including scarecrows, apples in a barrel, pumpkins, and dried corn.

After the read-aloud, ask children to describe a barn dance with attributes such as *lively*, *active*, and *happy*.

For categories, recall the items mentioned or shown in the story that can be found on a farm. Then divide these items into categories, such as farm animals (cows, chickens, pigs), produce (corn, pumpkins, apples, wheat), and structures (barn, fence, house, loft, silo).

Use the text to play phonological awareness games. See the entry in the Pre-K catalog for activities that address earlier phonological awareness levels.

> **PLAY**   Say-It-Until-You-Hear-It.
>
> Children synthesize one-syllable words divided into onset-rime. Present the word with a clear pause between the onset and rime. Demonstrate how to elongate the parts to blend them together, saying them a little quicker each time until they are readily identified. Provide scaffolding until children are ready to do it on their own. For example, say

(continues on next page)

PLAY **Say-It-Until-You-Hear-It.** *Continued*

Put these two parts together: *m-oon.*
Say it until you hear it. *Mmmmm . . . oooon. Mm . . . oon. Moon.*

Continue with these three- and four-sound words from the text beginning with a single sound:

s . . .-ing	f . . .-arm	k . . .-id
n . . .-ight	r . . .-ound	b . . .-arn
ch . . .-in		d . . .-ance

Then demonstrate how to synthesize one-syllable words divided into onset-rime beginning with a two-consonant cluster, as in

tr-ee (tree)	sl-eep (sleep)	bl-ink (blink)
cl-ose (close)	gr-ab (grab)	sp-in (spin)
cr-ow (crow)	pl-ink (plink)	st-yle (style)
br-ight (bright)		

PLAY **Roll-It-Out.**

Children synthesize a consonant–vowel–consonant (C–V–C) word by blending each of its phonemes. Demonstrate by elongating the phonemes and blending them together in shorter and shorter sequences until children can identify the word. For example, say

m-oo-n
What's the word? Roll it out. *Mmmmm . . . ooooo . . . nnnn. . . . Moon.*

Continue with the following words from the text.

night	right	dog
hide	pig	bed
light	kid	

PLAY **Break-It-Up.**

Children analyze a one-syllable C–V–C word in order to identify the beginning, middle, and ending sounds. Begin activities with initial sounds, and then proceed to middle and ending sounds. For an example on how to demonstrate finding the middle sound in *moon*, ask

What's the sound in the middle of *moon*?
Break it up: *Mmmmm-oooo-nnnnn. M-oo-n.*
oo is the sound in the middle of *moon*.

Use words provided in Roll-It-Out.

In the last stage of the game, children identify all the sounds in the word. Demonstrate how to elongate the sounds and then break them up in order to identify each one. For example, ask

What are all the sounds in the word *moon*?
Roll it out and break it up: *Mmmm . . . oooo . . . nnn. . . . m-oo-n.*

> PLAY   **Delete-It.**

Children omit the first sound in one-syllable words from the text. Demonstrate by saying the word slowly, then leaving off the initial sound. To demonstrate using the four-sound word *dance*, for example, say

> Listen to how I can make *dance* become *–ants*.
> I delete the first sound. *Dance. –ance.* (as in *ants*)
> Now you delete it. *Dance* . . .

Continue with the words provided in Roll-It-Out. Then practice with the words *barn* and *dance* together to make the following title:

> _arn _ants (sounds like *Arn Ants*)

Once children become proficient in playing the game, play it again with the owl's short verse as it coaxes the boy out of his room. Their part will sound like this:

> _ome a _ittle _oser (sounds like *um-a-ittle-oser*)
> _ome a _ittle _oser
> _isten _o the _ight

Go very slowly!

> PLAY   **Switch-It.**

Children delete the initial sound of the word and switch it with a new sound to make another word. Demonstrate first, then prompt with cues as necessary. For example,

> Say *dance.*
> Now say *dance*, only delete the *d* and switch it with *m*.
> What funny word can you make? (mance)

Then play Switch-It with the owl's verse. Their part will sound like this:

> Mum a middle moser

Other possibilities include

Fum a fiddle foser	Num a nittle noser
Gum a giddle goser	Dum a diddle doser

For *Sh* articulation therapy, use the words and illustrations to elicit the target sound. Phoneme *Sh* words and pictures include *shinin', pushin' shadows*, and *sheep.*

For articulation of *Ch*, include *chin, chicken, chit 'n chatter, much, branch, questions, stretched, kitchen, patchwork* (quilt).

For articulation of *J*, include *magic* and *jump.*

Bear Noel

by Olivier Dunrea
New York: Farrar, Straus & Giroux, 2000

Suggested Grade and Interest Level: 1 through 3

Topic Explorations: Animals, Bears; Holidays, Christmas; Seasons, Winter; Sounds and listening

Skill Builders:

Vocabulary	Grammar and syntax
Semantics	Tenses, present and past
Similes and metaphors	Question structures

Synopsis: A lovely book for the holiday season and ideal for encouraging children's participation at story time. The quiet story, with its breathtaking, snowy scenes, is set in the north woods on Christmas Eve. Wolf, Hare, Fox, Boar, Hedgehog, Possum, Owl, and Mole listen in anticipation for Bear Noel (a clever pun on Pere Noel, the French Father Christmas). "This is the night when all creatures may come together without fear," declares the big jovial bear. The repetitive text is an accumulation of what each animal hears Bear Noel doing as he comes closer and closer. When Bear Noel appears, he brings a feast for them to share as they put away their quarrels and find joy in celebrating the season together.

Method: Before the read-aloud, set the stage and prepare children to listen to the sounds of Bear Noel, just like the animals in the forest. Talk about the quietness of snow falling and little sounds that can be heard in the silent forest. When all is quiet, what could the animals hear? Then show the first few pages and invite children to describe the snowy scenes with their own words.

During the read-aloud, encourage children to chime in on the repetitive, cumulative verse. Pause occasionally to briefly define a word or point out a detail. For children working on question structures, have them repeat the predictable lines of the text after the words, "He is coming." Children ask, "Who is coming?"

After the read-aloud, go back through the pages and shape past-tense structures (regular and irregular) by having children recast the lines of the story, such as

> He laughed
> He sang
> He tramped through the snow
> He jingled his bells
> He got nearer
> He brought something wonderful

Review the vocabulary in context. Some phrases to discuss include the metaphor, "Snow blankets the forest." Tell how metaphors use words in a comparison but don't say *like* or *as*. In this example, the author uses a metaphor for what the snow in the forest is like without using many words. Another way of saying the sentence is using a simile that the "snow looks *like* a white blanket across the ground in the forest."

"Wolf lopes toward him" (toward Hare). Have children guess at what the word *lopes* means. Moving fast or slow? What other animal in the story might lope? Have children construct sentences with the word or demonstrate the wolf's stride.

"Into the clearing strides Bear Noel." Talk about the forest behind Bear Noel and go back to the first pages of the book to give the children a sense of where he has just been in the thick trees. Then ask children to describe what a clearing is (land that contains no trees or bushes). Have children construct simple sentences about Bear Noel using the word in relation to where he is standing in the picture.

"His furry feet sweep a broad path through the snow." Ask children if they can hear what Bear Noel sounds like when he comes into the clearing. Is it a quiet sound? A whooshing sound? What other words do the children have for it? Ask what the snowy ground looked like after Bear Noel walked on it to enable children to use all or part of the words, "a broad path in the snow."

" . . . his bells faintly ringing in the quiet night." Have children guess at what the word *faintly* means. Do the bells sound loud or soft? Far away or near? Have children construct sentences with the word.

Extended Activity: Hold a reader's theater with several children taking the parts of the animals and saying their lines. When Owl asks, "Who is coming?" the other children in the audience can say, "Bear Noel!" adding whatever embellishments they want to create and add to the text.

Berlioz the Bear

by Jan Brett
New York: Putnam, 1991; Scholastic, 1992

Suggested Grade and Interest Level: 1 through 3

Topic Explorations: Animals, Bears; Careers; Community; Music, musicians and musical instruments

Skill Builders:

Vocabulary	**Language literacy**
Categories	Cause-and-effect relationships
Grammar and syntax	Problem solving
Present tense	Verbal expression
Pronouns, personal and possessive	**Articulation, Z and –er**

Synopsis: Berlioz has been practicing his double bass for weeks. When the day comes for the orchestra to play at the village ball, the musicians load into the bandwagon. Meanwhile, border pictures show the townspeople busy with their preparations. But the wagon is held up when the mule decides to stall. Will the musicians get there in time?

Various animals try to help. At last a strange phenomenon coming from Berlioz's bass causes them to get to the ball on time.

Method: Before the read-aloud, discuss the cover and have children make predictions about the story. Elicit any prior knowledge about the instruments on the cover. What other instruments do the children know about? Perhaps they will recognize some in the story as you turn the pages.

For verbal expression and present progressive tense, pause to interact about the story and its characters. Talk about what a border is and point out the story within the border. Ask the children to describe the preparations for the ball that are depicted in the border. Shape and model target structures within the context of the story.

For problem solving and identifying cause-and-effect relationships, pause during the story and ask the children to define each problem. The first problem arises when Berlioz can't get the bee out of his bass. The second problem arises when the mule will not budge. For each problem, brainstorm possible solutions. See whether the children can explain how the problems are related.

After the story, discuss what might have happened if the bee had not stung the mule (which then brought the musicians to the party in time) and solved both problems. What effect would arriving late for the ball have on the story? Have the children recount the different ways they thought of to get the musicians to the party. How else might the musicians have gotten to the party? Could they have done something else to solve the problem? Which solution do the children think is best?

For articulation of *Z* and *–er*, encourage responses that include the name of the head musician, Berlioz, in progressively longer utterances as children interact with the story.

Extended Activity: Play a recording of Rimsky-Korsakov's *The Flight of the Bumblebee.* Talk about how the members of the symphony orchestra who play on the recording are like the musicians in *Berlioz the Bear.* Turn to one of the last pages in the book to identify and categorize the musical instruments, including the bass, violin, french horn, oboe, drum, and trombone. Talk about how *The Flight of the Bumblebee* tells a story—not with words but with musical notes. See whether the children can identify one or more of the musical instruments in the recording. Ask children to describe the music. What words can they think of to describe the sounds of the bumblebee? Where might the bumblebee be? What might the bumblebee want to do? How might the bumblebee feel?

The Big Orange Splot

by Daniel Manus Pinkwater
New York: Scholastic, 1977, 1993; Hastings, 1992

Suggested Grade and Interest Level: 1 through 5

Topic Exploration: Community

Skill Builders:

Vocabulary	**Language literacy**
Idioms	Cause-and-effect relationships
Grammar and syntax	Storytelling
Past tense	Problem solving
	Drawing inferences

Synopsis: Mr. Plumbean unsettles the neighbors on his street when he paints his house to "make it look like all his dreams." A highly colorful and imaginative story with a message.

Method: Before the read-aloud, talk about the word *neighborhood* and elicit background knowledge about different communities and their characteristics.

For past tense, pause during the reading to model or shape some of the following sentences from the text and illustrations:

> The seagull flew over the house.
> The seagull dropped the paint.
> He looked outside.
> He flipped his lid.
> He planted palm trees.
> He bought a hammock.
> He made lemonade.
> He drank lemonade.
> He talked to the neighbor.

After the reading, talk about the expression "flipped his lid," encouraging children to explain what a literal meaning of the expression might be and contrasting that to the figurative meaning. How might the expression accurately describe someone "under pressure"?

For critical thinking skills, talk about the events that led to the problem and how Mr. Plumbean solved it.

What facts can you state about Mr. Plumbean's problem?
What other ways could he have solved his problem?
Was Mr. Plumbean's solution the best one for him?
Why do you think so?
What can you tell about how he feels?
What would you have done if you were Mr. Plumbean?

For storytelling, encourage children to retell the story. Provide scaffolding by asking questions relating to Mr. Plumbean's actions and feelings.

The Boy Who Held Back the Sea

Retold by Lenny Hort
Paintings by Thomas Locker
New York: Dial Books, 1987

Suggested Grade and Interest Level: 2 through 5

Topic Explorations: Community; Long ago and far away

Skill Builders:
   Language literacy
   Problem solving
   Drawing inferences
   Critical thinking

Synopsis: This is the popular tale of a boy in 17th-century Holland who discovers water trickling through a hole in the dike. Lenny Hort has created a story within a story as he weaves together the circumstances surrounding the boy's single-handed efforts to save his town. Thomas Locker's oil paintings are reminiscent of the Dutch masters.

Method: Before the read-aloud, ask students what they know of the story about the Dutch boy who stuck his finger in the dike. Have them make predictions about the story based on the book's title. Talk about the cover illustration, especially the windmill in the background, as you discuss the setting for the story.

During the read-aloud, pause to clarify inferences and identify the problem in the story. Is there more than one problem? What facts can the students state about each?

After the read-aloud, ask students to think about the significance of Jan sneaking off to read to Mr. Schuyler while the town honored him in a festival.

> How did Jan change?
> Why could Pieter hardly wait for dinner to be over so he could keep watch over the dike?
> How are Jan and Pieter alike in this story?
> How might Pieter's life have changed after his grandmother's story about the brave boy, Jan?

Caps for Sale

by Esphyr Slobodkina
New York: Harper & Row, 1940, 1947, 1968; Scholastic, 1987

Suggested Grade and Interest Level: 1 through 2

Topic Explorations: Clothing; Colors

Skill Builders:

Vocabulary	**Language literacy**	**Phonological awareness**
Prepositions	Predicting	**Fluency**
	Sequencing	

Synopsis: An unusual peddler carries his wares on his head, calling, "Caps! Caps for sale! Fifty cents a cap!" When he falls asleep under a tree, monkeys in the tree do what monkeys do—monkey business, of course! Kids love to imitate the peddler as he tries to retrieve his caps in this all-time favorite.

Method: Before the read-aloud, talk about the types of caps people wear, including baseball caps, and encourage children to describe a cap they may own and wear. What does it look like? What color is it? Where did the cap come from?

During the read-aloud, pause to briefly discuss vocabulary words or words with multiple meanings, including

peddler	wares	upset
refreshed	checked	

Model prepositions from the text, such as "He looked *in back* of him," "He looked *behind* the tree," and "He pulled *off* his cap." Also pause to structure phrases based on the illustrations, such as "on his head," "in the tree," "under the tree," "up in the sky," and "beside the pond."

For predicting, ask children what the monkeys will do when the peddler shakes his fist, throws his cap on the ground, and does other predictable events.

After the read-aloud, children can practice sequencing skills by describing how the peddler puts the caps on his head—first his own checked cap, then the gray caps, then the blue caps, and so on, as shown in the text and pictures.

Use the words of the text to play phonological awareness games. See the entry in the Pre-K catalog for activities that address earlier phonological awareness levels.

> **PLAY**   **Say-It-Until-You-Hear-It.**
>
> Children synthesize one-syllable words divided into onset-rime. Present the word with a clear pause between the onset and rime. Demonstrate how to elongate the parts to blend them together, saying them a little quicker each time until they are readily identified. Provide scaffolding until children are ready to do it on their own. For example, say
>
> > Put these two parts together: *s-ale.*
> > Say it until you hear it. *Sssss. . . . aaale. Sss. . . . ale. Sale.*
>
> Continue with these (C–V–C) words from the text beginning with a single continuous sound:
>
> *(continues on next page)*

PLAY **Say-It-Until-You-Hear-It.** *Continued*

w-ares (sounds like *airs*)	f-eel	w-alk
s-un	w-oke	r-ight
l-eft	l-ook	th-ink
sh-ook		

Then demonstrate how to synthesize one-syllable words divided into onset-rime beginning with a two-consonant cluster. Begin with three-sound words with continuant sound clusters, then stop sound clusters, then four-sound words, then four-sound words with stop clusters. Words include

sl-ow (slow)	gr-ay (gray)	sp-oke (spoke)
sl-eep (sleep)	br-own (brown)	st-and (stand)
sl-ept (slept)	br-anch (branch)	
gr-ound (ground)	bl-ue (blue)	

PLAY **Roll-It-Out.**

Children synthesize a consonant–vowel–consonant word by blending each of its phonemes. Demonstrate by elongating the phonemes and blending them together in shorter and shorter sequences until children can identify the word. For example, say

s–ā–l
What's the word? Roll it out. *Sssss. . . . āāāāā. . . . lllll. Ss. . . . āā . . . ll. Sale.*

Once children are successful, present each of the phonemes separately so they can "roll them out" on their own, in shorter and shorter sequences, to find the word. Continue with the following words:

sun	woke	cap
walk	give	
back	right	

PLAY **Break-It-Up.**

Children analyze one-syllable C-V-C words in order to identify the beginning, middle, and ending sounds. Begin activities with initial sounds, and then proceed to middle and ending sounds. For an example on how to demonstrate finding the middle sound in *sale*, ask

What's the sound in the middle of *sale*?
Break it up: *Sssss. . . . āāāāā. . . . lll. S–ā–l.*
ā is the sound in the middle of *sale*.

Continue with the words listed in Roll-It-Out.

Then have children identify all the sounds in the word. Demonstrate by showing them how to elongate the sounds in words and break them up to identify them. For example, ask

What are all the sounds in the word *sale*?
Roll it out and break it up: *Ssss. . . . āāāā. . . . llll. S–ā–l.*
S–ā–l are the sounds in *sale*.

(continues on next page)

PLAY **Break-It-Up.** *Continued*

Continue to present one-syllable C–V–C words provided in Roll-It-Out so children can break them up and identify the sounds in each of the positions.

In the last stage of the game, children identify all the sounds in the word. Demonstrate how to elongate the sounds and then break them up in order to identify each one.

PLAY **Delete-It.**

Children omit the first sound in one-syllable words from the text. Demonstrate by saying the word slowly, then leaving off the initial sound. To demonstrate using *sale*, for example, say

> Listen to how I can make sale become *-ale.* (as in *ginger ale*)
> I delete the first sound. *Sale. -ale.*
> Now you delete it. *Sale . . .*

Use the list of one-syllable words provided in Roll-It-Out. Also practice with the two-syllable word *fifty*, slowly building up to the entire phrase, "Fifty cents a cap." The children's part will sound like this:

> _ifty _ents a _ap

PLAY **Switch-It.**

Children delete the initial sound of the word and switch it with a new sound to make another word. Demonstrate first, then prompt with cues as necessary. For example,

> Say *sale.*
> Now say *sale,* only delete the *s* and switch it with an *m.*
> What new word can you make? (male)

Play the game with words "fifty cents a cap," slowly building up to the phrase. Their part will sound like this:

> Mifty ments a map

Other possibilities:

> Wifty wents a wap
> Nifty nents a nap
> Tifty tents a tap

Go slowly!

Note: A Spanish version of this book is available, titled *Sevenden gorras: La historia de un vendedor ambulante, unos monos y sus travesuras.*

A Chair for My Mother

by Vera B. Williams
New York: Greenwillow Books, 1982, 1988, 1993

Suggested Grade and Interest Level: 1 through 3

Topic Explorations: Careers; Community; Family relationships; Money

Skill Builders:

Vocabulary	Language literacy	Articulation
Similes and metaphors	Drawing inferences	Carryover for any target sound

Synopsis: The goodness of people during hard times is a rare theme in picture books. This story centers on how family, friends, and neighbors pull together as a child and her mother save coins to buy a chair after a fire destroyed their home.

Method: Before the read-aloud, discuss the word *community* and the people and places a community is made up of. Have students share characterizations of their own communities.

Read the story aloud. For drawing inferences, pause to ask questions that can only be answered by applying background knowledge and putting it into meaningful relationships. Encourage the use of *when* and *because*. For example,

> Q: Why does Mother look worried when she counts her tip money, and it is not as much as on other days?
> A: Maybe she's afraid she won't have enough to buy a chair.

Other possible questions: The story says there were fire engines in front of their house and that later the whole house was spoiled. What does that mean? What happened? How do we know this? The story says the apartment they lived in after the fire was empty. How do we know this?

For similes, discuss the description of feeling like Goldilocks when trying all the chairs in the furniture store. How might the girl and her mother feel once the chair is home? Brainstorm adjectives such as *happy, content,* and *warm.* Then have students create their own similes. Some possibilities are

> They felt as happy as Cinderella in new clothes. They were as content as two cats by the fire or a couple of bugs on a rug.

For articulation carryover, pause to interject conversation-eliciting target phonemes.

Note: This story is also useful for discussing the concepts of "more" and "less." For example, how does Grandmother have money to put in the savings jar after she finds a bargain on tomatoes or bananas?

Charlie Needs a Cloak

by Tomie de Paola
Englewood Cliffs, NJ: Prentice Hall, 1973

Suggested Grade and Interest Level: 1 through 5

Topic Explorations: Clothing; Sheep

Skill Builders:

Vocabulary	Language literacy	Articulation, *Sh* and *Ch*
Semantics	Sequencing	
	Storytelling	

Synopsis: Charlie the shepherd shears his sheep, cards and spins the wool, weaves and dyes the cloth, and sews a beautiful new cloak for himself. Meanwhile, the antics of his sheep keep the reader and listeners continually amused. Vocabulary words are presented and defined on the last page.

Method: Before the read-aloud, activate children's prior knowledge by asking what they know about wool.

> Where does it come from?
> How is it made?
> What do we do with it?
> In what kind of climate is it worn?

Before the read-aloud, create the semantic web described in the Extended Activities section. Then present the book's cover, suggesting that more questions may be answered after the book is read.

Read aloud and pause to talk about the steps of turning wool into yarn, yarn into cloth, and cloth into clothes. (Don't forget to talk about what the little mouse is up to on each page!)

Have students use new vocabulary in sentences based on the context of the story. Vocabulary includes

> shear
> weave
> card
> sew
> spin
> cloak

After the read-aloud, have children tell the story of how Charlie made his new cloak, using story grammar questions to scaffold the narration. For articulation of *Ch,* interact with children about the story parts, using the pages to elicit speech containing the target sounds, especially from the words *sheep, sheer, sheers, shorn,* and *Charlie.*

Extended Activities: Make a semantic web by diagramming children's questions related to sheep. One way is to start with the word *sheep* circled on the board. Then associate ideas as you talk about sheep. What do the children want to know? For example, do they want to know what sheep give us? How wool is made? Where the yarn comes from? Write each question around the word *sheep,* and draw a line from the circle to each of the questions.

Another way is to group ideas and questions under several subheadings. For instance, perhaps they want to know all the different places one can find sheep. If so, draw a line in the direction of another circle labeled *environment.* Then have children brainstorm such places as farms, ranches, fields, and zoos. Perhaps the children want to know what sheep eat. If so, draw a line in the direction of another circle labeled *habits* and write questions concerning what sheep eat under this subheading. List answers that children already know, such as grass and oats. Help the children generate questions in order to model the self-learning strategy of posing questions before reading, then looking for the answers in the text.

Then read the story and ask students to listen and see if they can find the answers to their questions. After reading, go back to the map and answer some of the questions by generating statements about sheep from the information in the text. For example,

> Sheep are animals that live _____.
> Sheep like to eat _____.
> Sheep are used for _____.
> Wool cloth is made by _____.

Encourage use of varied and complex sentence structures. For example,

> Shearing is like giving the sheep a very short haircut.
> Wool, which we need for clothing, comes from sheep.
> After a sheep's wool is shorn, it is carded.

For teaching sequencing, ask children to identify some of the key parts of the story and the key steps in the process of making the cloak. Either collaboratively or individually, have children create their own illustrations for each part of the process (shearing, carding, dyeing, etc.). Have the children put their completed illustrations in order to tell the story of Charlie's new cloak. They can then take turns retelling the story using these sequenced illustrations. Children can write or dictate a text for the story beneath the illustrations.

Chato's Kitchen

by Gary Soto
New York: Putnam, 1995

Suggested Grade and Interest Level: 1 through 5

Topic Explorations: Animals, Cats; Culture and history, Hispanic; Food; Literacy

Skill Builders:

Vocabulary	**Language literacy**
Idioms	Compare and contrast
Similes and metaphors	Drawing inferences
Grammar and syntax	Retelling events
Past tense	**Articulation—*S, Z, R,* and *Ch***

Synopsis: When a family of mice move in next to Chato, a cool, "low-riding cat with six stripes," they appear to fall for his nicely worded invitation to dinner. They accept, asking if they can bring along a guest. Chato graciously obliges, and he and his friend, Navio Boy, prepare an elaborate Mexican feast to go along with their *ratoncitos* supper. But it turns out the mice were more thoughtful than they at first let on. When the mice arrive on the back of a "low, road-scraping dog," Chato and Navio leap onto the curtains in fear. Chorizo's presence at the dinner table changes their dinner plans. Unable to dine on their guests, the cool (but wary) cats settle on enjoying the meal—the one they'd prepared in Chato's kitchen.

Method: Before the read-aloud, talk about some of the food items from the Mexican culture that the children are familiar with. Introduce more of the items in Spanish from the glossary in the front of the book.

During the read-aloud, pause to clarify meaning of the words. Vocabulary includes words such as

spied (he spied five mice)	slinking	grooming
cowered	threshold	scrape (of tiny feet)
mambo	gems (in Navio Boy's collar)	suppressed (a meow)

Pause to clarify the meaning of the idiom "shot off" as the story tells that the sparrow was frightened and "shot off into the tree." Ask the children to tell another way of saying something happened very quickly. Encourage the use of the expression in other sentences.

There are many similes in the text. Pause to point out the author's use of words in describing such events as how the mice left their house for the *fiesta*. ("As if in a limousine they cruised out of their jungly yard. . . . ") Ask children what a limousine is and to use the word *like* in the description when retelling the story. Other similes include

They began to shiver like leaves in the wind.
The mice dropped like gray fruit.

Much of the text is not explicitly stated, so there are opportunities to help children draw inferences by associating situations they have experienced and their general knowledge to the story's meaning. Some examples include

In Chato's invitation, he first referred to his mice guests as "tasty." Why did he change it to "lovely"?

When Chato saw the mice family move in next door, "His whiskers vibrated with pleasure. . . . " Direct children's attention to the illustration of Chato's whiskers. Ask what *vibrate* means and why his whiskers shook.

The text reads:

"When they [Chato and Navio Boy] heard a rap on the door they grinned at each other. It was like a delivery service with mice instead of pizza."

Ask students why the cats grinned at each other. To enable children to use language to compare and contrast, ask them how the rap on the door was like a pizza delivery.

After the reading, be sure to look over Chato's menu at the front of the book where the glossary of Spanish words in the story is listed. Then ask children to retell some of the events of the story.

For articulation of *S, Z, R,* and *Ch,* read the story and interact with the children, encouraging them to use the target words at their own levels.

Chicken Soup with Rice

by Maurice Sendak
New York: Harper & Row, 1962; Scholastic, 1986, 1991

Suggested Grade and Interest Level: 1 through 3

Topic Explorations: Months of the year; Seasons

Skill Builders:

Grammar and syntax	**Articulation—*S, R,* and *Ch***
Present tense	**Fluency**
Phonological awareness	

Synopsis: The repetition and rhyming in this whimsical collection of verses lend themselves nicely to speaking in unison. Each picture depicts a different action, scene, and verse about a month of the year. Ideal for modeling sentence structures or sound production. This book will become a favorite you'll use again and again.

Method: Before the read-aloud, talk about the different kinds of soups the children like to eat and ask children to tell about when they like to eat soup.

During the read-aloud, pause to model or structure present tense, such as

> He is riding an elephant (and dreaming about soup)
> He is pouring soup (on the roses)
> He is sprinkling the roses (with the soup)
> He is pepping up the roses (with the soup)
> The whale is spouting (hot soup)
> The wind is blowing (down the door)
> He is paddling ("down the chicken soupy Nile")

After the read-aloud, children can practice sequencing the months of the year and the seasons as you show the illustrations.

Use the words of the text to play phonological awareness games. See the entry in the Pre-K catalog for activities that address earlier levels.

PLAY **Say-It-Until-You-Hear-It.**

Children synthesize one-syllable words divided into onset-rime. Present the word with a clear pause between the onset and rime. Demonstrate how to elongate the parts to blend them together, saying them a little quicker each time until they are readily identified. Provide scaffolding until children are ready to do it on their own. For example, say

> Put these two parts together: *r–ice.*
> Say it until you hear it. *Rrrrrr . . . ice. Rrr . . . ice. Rice.*

Continue with these consonant–vowel–consonant (C–V–C) words beginning with a single sound.

n-ice	s-ip	s-oup
r-ide	wh-ale	s-ell
h-ot	ch-eap	c-ook

Then demonstrate how to synthesize one-syllable words divided into onset-rime beginning with a two-consonant cluster, as in

sl-ide (slide)	dr-eam (dream)	dr-ess (dress)
bl-ow (blow)	tw-ice (twice)	fl-op (flop)
dr-oop (droop)	sl-ip (slip)	sp-ill (spill)
fl-ip (flip)		

PLAY Roll-It-Out.

Children synthesize a C–V–C word by blending each of its phonemes. Demonstrate by elongating the phonemes and blending them together in shorter and shorter sequences until children can identify the word. For example, say

> r-ī-s
> What's the word? Roll it out. *Rrrrr . . . īīīī . . . sss. Rice.*

Once children are successful, present each of the phonemes separately so they can "roll them out" on their own, in shorter and shorter sequences, to find the word. Use the one-syllable C–V–C word list provided in Say-It-Until-You-Hear-It.

PLAY Break-It-Up.

Children analyze one-syllable C–V–C words in order to identify the beginning, middle, and ending sounds. Begin activities with initial sounds, and then proceed to middle and ending sounds. For an example on how to demonstrate finding the middle sound in *rice,* ask

> What's the sound in the middle of *rice*?
> Break it up: *Rrrr . . .-īīīī . . .- ssss . . . R -ī-s.*
> *ī* is the sound in the middle of *rice.*

Continue to present the one-syllable C–V–C words provided in Say-It-Before-You-Hear-It so children can break them up and identify the sounds in each position.

In the last stage of the game, children identify all the sounds in the word. Demonstrate how to elongate the sounds and then break them up in order to identify each one. For example, ask

> What are all the sounds in the word *soup*?
> Roll it out and break it up: *Ssss . . .-oooo . . .-p. . . . S-oo-p.*
> *S-oo-p* are the sounds in *soup.*

PLAY Delete-It.

Children omit the first sound in one-syllable words from the text. Demonstrate by saying the word slowly, then leaving off the initial sound. To demonstrate using *rice,* for example, say

> Listen to how I can make *rice* become *-ice.*
> I delete the first sound. *Rice. _ice.*
> Now you delete it. *Rice. . . .*

Use the list of one-syllable words provided. Then practice with the two-syllable word *chicken,* and slowly build on the words to the phrase "chicken soup with rice." The children's part will sound like this:

> Icken Oop with Ice

Also practice the repetitive refrain, as in "Sipping once, sipping twice. . . ." The children's part will sound like this:

> -ipping unce, ipping ice, ipping icken oop with ice.

Practice with the other, similar refrains.

PLAY Switch-It.

Children delete the initial sound of the word and replace it with a new sound to make another word. Demonstrate first, then prompt with cues as necessary. For example,

> Say *soup*.
> Now say *soup*, only delete the *s* and switch it with *m*.
> What funny word can you make? (moop)

Play the game with the words of the title. Continuing to switch the initial sounds of the word with the *m* sound, their part will sound like this:

> Micken moop with mice

Other possibilities:

> Nicken noup with nice
> Bicken boop with bice
> Dicken doop with dice

Continue with the refrain, building on each word, until the children's part sounds like this:

> Bipping bunce, bipping bice, bipping bicken boop with bice!
> Dappy dunce, dappy dice, dappy dicken doop with dice!
> Rowing runce, rowing rice, rowing ricken roup with rice!

Chimps Don't Wear Glasses

by Laura Numeroff
New York: Scholastic, 1995

Suggested Grade and Interest Level: 1 through 2

Topic Explorations: Animals; Imagination

Skill Builders:
Grammar and syntax   **Phonological awareness**
Present tense
Negative structures
Question structures

Synopsis: A series of animals are depicted in outrageously silly acts while the text, in short rhyming verse, proclaims differently.

Method: Before the read-aloud, read the title, *Chimps Don't Wear Glasses*, and ask children to describe what's happening in the book's cover. (Children will describe animals driving cars on the freeway, two of which are chimps wearing crazy sunglasses.) You might reply, "Hmmm, let's discover what this book is all about."

During the read-aloud, pause at natural intervals for interaction about the text and pictures. Rhyming verses often are completed on a two-page spread and, together with the pictures depicting the text, make for a natural pause in the reading. This allows children an opportunity to observe and talk about what's going on in the illustrations.

For teaching negative structures, read the text, "Chimps don't wear glasses," and have the children repeat the line of text (i.e., "Chimps don't wear glasses."). After the line is repeated, ask, "They don't? But what's happening here?" to elicit picture descriptions of cool chimps performing in a rock band with wild and crazy glasses.

For present tense, state the negative phrase of the text, such as, "Chimps don't wear glasses," and have children respond to the contrary, as illustrated in the book. For example,

> But the chimps *are* wearing glasses
> But the kangaroo is reading a book
> But the horses *are* hang gliding
> But the llama *is* shopping
> And so on

After the read-aloud, play a fun game in the spirit of the book by using the illustrations to teach question structures. Go back over the pages and demonstrate how to change the text into a question. You or the other children must answer the children's (or child's) question. For example, on a two-page spread, the text reads

> And zebras don't cook
> And you won't see a kangaroo reading a book.

Prompt children to look at the illustration of a zebra cooking and ask, "Do zebras cook?" to which the class responds, "Yes, zebras cook!" Another child can play the game on the facing page and ask, "Does a kangaroo read a book?" to which the class answers, "Yes, a kangaroo reads a book!"

Turn the page and read, "Horses don't hang glide." Prompt a child to ask, "Do horses hang glide?" to which the class responds, "Yes, horses hang glide!" Once children get the hang of it, they can expand on their answers.

Use the words of the text to play phonological awareness games. See the entry in the Pre-K catalog for activities that address earlier phonological awareness levels.

(PLAY) Odd-One-Out.

From a string of words ending in the same sound, children select the one that does not belong. Exaggerate ending sounds. For example, say

> boat, kite, don't, book
> Which word has a different ending sound? (book)
> That's right. *Book* is the odd one out.

Some three-word strings include

cook, book, pig	dine, boat, sign	horse, dance, king
mop, mug, pug	hat, shop, boat	hang, sing, pole

PLAY **Word-Search.**

Children search the picture for a word that ends with a designated sound. Provide clues if needed. For example, say

> I'm searching for something in this picture that ends with the sound *t*.
> Can you help me find it?
> That's right. *Hat* is a word that ends with *t*. (Possibilities include *hat, cat, scout.*)

Children can search for other words with different end sounds on each page.

PLAY **Say-It-Until-You-Hear-It.**

Children synthesize one-syllable words divided into onset-rime. Present the word with a clear pause between the onset and rime. Demonstrate how to elongate the parts to blend them together, saying them a little quicker each time until they are readily identified. Provide scaffolding until children are ready to do it on their own. For example, say

> Put these two parts together: *w–air.*
> Say it until you hear it. *Wwww . . . . air. Ww . . . . air. Wear.*

Continue with the following consonant-vowel–consonant (C-V-C) words from the text beginning with a single sound:

sh-ow (a C-V word)	m-op	m-ug
m-ice	s-ing	s-ale
s-ave	r-ide	f-ull

Then demonstrate how to synthesize one-syllable words divided into onset-rime beginning with a two-consonant cluster, as in

fl-y (fly)	fl-oat (float)	squ-are (square)
gl-ide (glide)	cl-ean (clean)	st-ilts (stilts)
dr-eam (dream)		sk-ate (skate)
dr-ive (drive)		sc-out (scout)

PLAY **Roll-It-Out.**

Children synthesize a C-V-C word by blending each of its phonemes. Demonstrate by elongating the phonemes and blending them together in shorter and shorter sequences until children can identify the word. For example, say

> m-o-p
> What's the word? Roll it out. *Mmmm . . . ooo . . . p. Mop.*

Once children are successful, present each of the phonemes separately so they can "roll them out" on their own, in shorter and shorter sequences, to find the word. In addition to the C-V-C words provided above, more include

shop	sight	mug
made	kite	pug
book	ham	boat

PLAY **Break-It-Up.**

Children analyze one-syllable C–V–C words in order to identify the beginning, middle, and ending sounds. Begin activities with initial sounds, and then proceed to middle and ending sounds. For an example on how to demonstrate finding the middle sound in *ride,* ask

> What's the sound in the middle of *ride?*
> Break it up: *Rrrrrr-ī ī ī ī ī ī –d. R–ī–d.*
> *ī* is the sound in the middle of *ride.*

Continue to present one-syllable C–V–C words provided in Say-It-Until-You-Hear-It so children can break them up and identify the sounds in each position.

In the last stage of the game, children identify all the sounds in the word. Demonstrate how to elongate the sounds and then break them up in order to identify each one. For example, ask

> What are all the sounds in the word *ride?*
> Roll it out and break it up: *Rrrrr-ī ī ī ī ī ī –d. R –ī–d.*
> *R–ī–d* are the sounds in *ride.*

PLAY **Delete-It.**

Children omit the first sound in one-syllable words from the text. Demonstrate by saying the word slowly, then leaving off the initial sound. To demonstrate using *wear,* for example, say

> Listen to how I can make wear become *air.*
> I delete the first sound. *Wear. Air.*
> Now you delete it. *Wear . . .*

In addition to the one-syllable words provided in Say-It-Until-You-Hear-It, practice with the word *chimps* to create *imps.* Put it into the title, and the name of the book will sound like this:

> Imps don't wear glasses

PLAY **Switch-It.**

Children delete the initial phoneme of the word and exchange it with a new phoneme to make a different word. Demonstrate like this:

> Say *wear.*
> Now say *wear,* only delete the *w* and switch it with *t.*
> What new word can you make? *Wear, tear* (as in *rip*)

Continue with the one-syllable words in Roll-It-Out until children experience success. Then play the game with the words of the title. Begin with *chimps,* switching the initial phoneme. For example, when using a *g,* their part will sound like this:

> Gimps don't wear glasses

(continues on next page)

> **PLAY** **Switch-It.** *Continued*
>
> Other possibilities include
>
> > Blimps don't wear glasses
> > Simps don't wear glasses
> > Frimps don't wear glasses
>
> Then play the game with the main words of the title. Using the *t*, the children's part will sound like this:
>
> > Timps don't tear tasses

A Chocolate Moose for Dinner

by Fred Gwynne
Englewood Cliffs, NJ: Prentice Hall, 1976

Suggested Grade and Interest Level: 2 through 5

Skill Builders:
> **Vocabulary**
> Semantics
> Idioms
> Homonyms (multiple meanings)

Synopsis: Here's a witty collection of homonyms shown from a child's bewildered perspective. How else would a child conceptualize "Mommy toasting Daddy" than as her squeezing him into a toaster?

Method: Read the book and pause to discuss each homonym. Also discuss the idioms presented and their meanings.

Extended Activities: Have students make up some ambiguous phrases of their own and illustrate them the way the author did. Start off by brainstorming other homonyms and mixing up their meanings. Here are a few.

pear, pare: Pear an apple
beau, bow: Bring your bow to the party
sole, soul: Do you feel it in your sole?

Then think of some idioms and decide how they could be interpreted literally. Examples are

> Catch your breath   The cat's got your tongue
> Stick your neck out   Afraid of your shadow
> The apple of your eye

Have students draw pictures illustrating the literal interpretations of these idioms. Have them write the idiom on the back of the picture illustrating it. Display the completed pictures around the room. Have the class view the pictures and try to guess what idiom each one illustrates. Afterward, allow each student to present his or her picture, then turn it over to reveal the idiom written on the back.

Note: Also read *The King Who Rained, The Sixteen Hand Horse,* and *A Little Pigeon Toad,* by the same author.

Click, Clack, Moo: Cows That Type

by Doreen Cronin
New York: Simon & Schuster Books for Young Readers, 2000

Suggested Grade and Interest Level: 1 through 2

Topic Explorations: Farms, Animals; Literacy

Skill Builders:

Vocabulary	Language literacy	Phonological awareness
Semantics	Relating personal experiences	
	Problem solving	
	Verbal expression	

Synopsis: Typing cows turn life on Farmer Brown's farm upside down when their demand note is tacked up in the barn. What they want is better working conditions in the form of electric blankets. When the farmer doesn't budge, they go on strike and refuse to give milk. Duck, the neutral party, waddles over to deliver the farmer's ultimatum to the cows. A mutually agreeable solution is achieved, but wait—all does not end there. Word spreads, and soon "click, clack, moo" turns to "click, clack, quack." Look what the cows have started! What a great way to show the rewards of literacy—and compromise! A Caldecott award winner.

Method: Before the read-aloud, ask children to predict what they think the story will be about based on the title. Talk about what a typewriter is and have children share their experiences, if applicable.

Read and enjoy the book, pausing to let the children chime in with the "click, clack, moo" refrain. Clarify meaning where necessary.

After the read-aloud, build vocabulary skills by talking more about words children may not have heard, like *demand, ultimatum,* and *neutral.* Use the words in the context of the story and in real-life contexts. Add the word *compromise.*

Ask the children to identify the problem. Discuss whether the animals and the farmer did the right thing by compromising. Encourage verbal expression and problem-solving skills by asking children to decide whether it was a fair agreement. Do the children have other ideas about how Farmer Brown could have solved the problem? What would have happened if the farmer and the cows had not compromised?

Children can relate personal experiences of having resolved issues by compromising. When might they have had to agree on doing something differently than the way they expected? Talk about classroom events that have happened in the past to give examples.

For phonemic awareness training, ask children to describe what cows typing on a typewriter might sound like (computer keyboards make a similar click-clack sound), then use the text to play phonological awareness games. See the entry in the Pre-K catalog for activities that address earlier phonological awareness levels.

PLAY   **Say-It-Until-You-Hear-It.**

Children synthesize one-syllable words divided into onset-rime. Present the word with a clear pause between the onset and rime. Demonstrate how to elongate the parts to blend them together, saying them a little quicker each time until they are readily identified. Provide scaffolding until children are ready to do it on their own. For example, say

(continues on next page)

(**PLAY**) **Say-It-Until-You-Hear-It.** *Continued*

Put these two parts together: *n–ote.*
Say it until you hear it. *Nnnnnnn–oooote. Nnn-ote. Note.*

Continue with these one-syllable words beginning with a single continuant sound:

m . . . -oo (C-V word)	(k)n . . . -ock	w . . . -ait
h . . . -en	n . . . -ight	f . . . -un
m . . . -ilk	f . . . -arm	t . . . -ype

Then demonstrate how to synthesize one-syllable words divided into onset-rime beginning with a two-consonant cluster, as in

sn-oop	cl-ick	cl-ack
gr-ow	cl-ose	str-ike

(**PLAY**) **Roll-It-Out.**

Children synthesize a consonant–vowel–consonant (C–V–C) word by blending each of its phonemes. Demonstrate by elongating the phonemes and blending them together in shorter and shorter sequences until children can identify the word. For example, say

n–ō–t
What's the word? Roll it out.
Nnnnnnn . . . ōōōōō . . . t. Nnnn . . . ōō . . . t. N-ote. Note.

Once children are successful, present each of the phonemes separately so they can "roll them out" on their own, in shorter and shorter sequences, to find the word. Use the one-syllable C-V-C word list provided in Say-It-Until-You-Hear-It.

(**PLAY**) **Break-It-Up.**

Children analyze one-syllable C-V-C words in order to identify the beginning, middle, and ending sounds. Begin activities with initial sounds, and then proceed to middle and ending sounds. For an example on how to demonstrate finding the middle sound in *note*, ask

What's the sound in the middle of *note*?
Break it up: *Nnnnn . . .-ōōō . . .-t. Nnnn-ōō-t. Note.*
ō is the sound in the middle of *note.*

Continue to present one-syllable C-V-C words provided above so children can break them up and identify the sounds in each position.

In the last stage of the game, children identify all the sounds in the word. Demonstrate how to elongate the sounds and then break them up in order to identify each one. For example, ask

What are all the sounds in the word *note*?
Roll it out and break it up: *Nnnn . . . ōōō . . . t. N–ō–t.*
N–ō–t are the sounds in the word *note.*

PLAY **Delete-It.**

Children omit the first sound in one-syllable words from the text. Demonstrate by saying the word slowly, then leaving off the initial sound. To demonstrate using *cow*, for example, say

> Listen to how I can make *note* become *oat*. (as in *oatmeal*)
> I delete the first sound: *Note. Oat.*
> Now you delete it. *Note . . .*

Continue with words that make smaller words first, such as *cow* (*ow*), *wait* (*ate*), and *farm* (*arm*).

Continue with the one-syllable C–V–C words in Say-It-Until-You-Hear-It, then play the game with the alliterative words of the title. Repeat the demonstration, leaving out the initial sounds in the words

> click, clack, moo

to make

> ick, ack, oo

And finish with the rest of the title.

PLAY **Switch-It.**

Children delete the phoneme blend in the initial part of the word and exchange it with a new phoneme to make a different word. Demonstrate with words of the title, for example,

> Say *click*.
> Now say *click*, only delete the *cl* and switch it with *t*.
> What new word can you make? *Click, tick.*

Continue with the remaining title, switching the essential words, which will sound like this:

> Tick, Tack, Too: Tows That Type

Demonstrate with other sounds until children experience success. Other possiblities include

> Nick, Nack, New: Nows That Nype
> Sick, Sack, Sue: Sows That Sype
> Mick, Mack Moo: Mows That Mype
> Wick, Whack, Woo: Wows That Wipe
> Bick, Back, Boo: Bows That Bike

Come Away from the Water, Shirley

by John Burningham
New York: Crowell, 1977; Trophy, 1983

Suggested Grade and Interest Level: 1 through 5

Topic Explorations: Boats; Pirates; Sea and the seashore

Skill Builders:

Grammar and syntax	**Language literacy**	**Articulation,** *Sh*
Present tense	Sequencing	
	Storytelling	
	Drawing inferences	

Synopsis: As Mother and Father sit in their beach chairs, continually reminding Shirley not to go in the water, Shirley has a harrowing adventure at sea. The text consists of Mom's nagging dialog, printed on the left. Action-packed scenes on board a pirate ship are pictured on the right. As the reader reads the dialog, the children who are listening can tell of Shirley's adventures using the striking illustrations.

Method: While reading, encourage children to tell the other half of the story from the illustrations. Shape or model appropriate target structures. After the read-aloud, ask children what was really happening throughout the story.

> Was Shirley's story real, or was she fantasizing?
> What makes you think she was fantasizing?
> What do you think Shirley really wanted to do?

Encourage storytelling by asking scaffolding questions that elicit story grammar elements.

For articulation, stress words in the text that contain the target sound. Include others from the pictures, such as

ocean	ship
push (the pirate over)	shovel
sharp (sword)	wishes (she were at sea)
shells	

Extended Activity: This is a good book for story mapping. Help children recall the story parts, telling what happened first and then sequencing the events. On a large sheet of drawing paper, have the children chart Shirley's adventure with pictures, starting with her walking onto the beach, then staring at the boat on the shore, rowing out to sea, and so on. Connect the story sequences with a colored line, then caption the work and share it with the class.

Note: Read also *Time to Get Out of the Bath, Shirley,* by the same author.

Corduroy

by Don Freeman
New York: Viking, 1968, 1993

Suggested Grade and Interest Level: 1 through 2

Topic Explorations: Animals, Bears; Careers; Family relationships; Money

Skill Builders:

Vocabulary	**Grammar and syntax**	**Language literacy**
Semantics	Pronouns, personal and possessive	Relating personal experiences
Categories	Tenses, present and past	Storytelling
Prepositions		

Synopsis: Corduroy the teddy bear wants someone to take him home from the department store. When a little girl shows interest, her mother points out that the bear is missing a button on his overalls. That night, Corduroy goes to the furniture section to look for a button. The night watchman finds him and returns him to the shelf. All ends well when the little girl returns. Corduroy finds a home with a friend who loves him—with or without a button.

Method: Before the read-aloud, ask children to bring in and share their favorite stuffed animals. Compare features of the different stuffed animals and encourage children to relate their histories.

During the read-aloud, pause to clarify meaning and teach prepositions by talking about where Corduroy is (on the shelf, beside the bunny), where he goes (up and down the escalator), where the girl and mother go, where the night watchman flashes his flashlight (under the beds), and so on.

After the read-aloud, do a picture walk-through so children can tell the story. Ask questions to provide scaffolding and elicit responses containing target structures. Children can also relate their personal experiences about wanting something and paying for it with their own money.

Teach categories by naming sections commonly found in a department store. Name various items for children to place in the section where they are most likely to be found.

Note: For an extended activity, see the entry in the Pre-K catalog.

Counting Crocodiles

by Judy Sierra
New York: Scholastic, 1997

Suggested Grade and Interest Level: 1 through 2

Topic Explorations: Folklore, Pan-Asian; Number concepts; Trickster tales

Skill Builders:

Vocabulary	**Language literacy**
Semantics	Storytelling
Grammar and syntax	Drawing inferences
Tenses, present and past	**Phonological awareness**

Synopsis: A monkey on an island in the Sillabobble Sea spies another island close by. Seeing a sweet stack of bananas on a tree, he wants to take a trip across the sea. But how will he get there? Cleverly. The monkey tricks the crocodiles into forming a bridge across the water under the pretext of counting them. Written in rhyming verse, the whimsical illustrations show every crocodile (or group of crocodiles) engaged in an activity or sporting an unusual style of dress. Plenty to describe and lots of possibilities from which to spin off language activities.

Method: Before the read-aloud, ask children to predict where the story takes place. Talk about islands and their special features.

Read the story aloud, pausing briefly to define vocabulary words, state what the monkey's goal is, and describe how he tricked the crocodiles.

After the read-aloud, go back over the illustrations, allowing the children to describe what is happening in the illustrations. Slightly reshape the text to match the illustration, recasting the text to elicit target syntactic structures. Examples include

> Two crocs are resting on rocks.
> Three crocs are rocking in a box.
> Four crocs are building with blocks.
> Five crocs are tickling a fox.

Use the activity taking place in the pictures to further describe the characters' actions. This example is from "nine crocks with chicken pox":

> A nurse is looking in one croc's ear.
> Crocs are using back scratchers to itch themselves.
> The monkey is pouring calamine lotion over one croc's head.
> One croc is reading a story to another croc eating soup in bed.

There's a fox living on the island with the monkey, who assists the clever character in his attempt to get across the sea. Go back over the pages to describe what the fox was doing all along to help. Use past tense for these structures, as in

> He brought the monkey lemonade.
> He tossed a lemon into the air.
> He caught the crocodiles' attention.
> He dove in the water.
> He wrote on the crocodile's tummy.
> He carried the bananas back home.
> He put a stake in the ground that labeled the lemon tree a "banana" tree.

For drawing inferences, ask the students to infer what the monkey really meant when he asked aloud, "I wonder, are there more crocodiles in the sea, or monkeys on the shore?" Infer what the crocodiles really meant when they asked, "Will you count us, please?"

> What does the monkey really want?
> What do the crocodiles want?
> After the monkey got to the island, what did it really mean when it said, "Line up now, crocodiles! I need to count you *one more time*."

For storytelling, ask children to retell the folktale as if it might have been told long ago. Have them take turns telling parts of the story. Provide scaffolding where necessary.

> Where did the story take place? Who was the story about?
> What started the story off? What did the characters do about it?
> What was the result? What happened next?
> How did the story end? How did they feel?

Once the text has been read several times, use the familiar words for phonological awareness training, beginning at the child's development skill level. See the entry in the Pre-K catalog for activities that address earlier phonological awareness levels.

> **PLAY** Say-It-Until-You-Hear-It.

Children synthesize one-syllable words divided into onset-rime. Present the word with a clear pause between the onset and rime. Demonstrate how to elongate the parts to blend them together, saying them a little quicker each time until they are readily identified. Provide scaffolding until children are ready to do it on their own. For example, say

> Put these two parts together: *w–ide.*
> Say it until you hear it. *Wwwwww . . . ide. Wide.*

Continue with these consonant-vowel-consonant (C–V–C) words from the text beginning with a single sound (shortening two-syllable words where needed):

l-ove	s-ide	r-ock
l-ine	f-ive	n-ine
h-ome	sh-ore	t-op

Then demonstrate how to synthesize one-syllable words divided into onset-rime beginning with a two-consonant cluster until children are ready to do it on their own. Words include

cr-oc (croc)	tr-ee (tree)	sc-owl (scowl)
tr-ip (trip)	sl-ime (slime)	st-ack (stack)
sm-ile (smile)	sw-eet (sweet)	
cr-oss (cross)		

> **PLAY** Roll-It-Out.

Children synthesize a C–V–C word by blending each of its phonemes. Demonstrate by elongating the phonemes and blending them together in shorter and shorter sequences until children can identify the word. For example, say

> w-ī-d
> What's the word? Roll it out. *Wwwww . . . īīīī . . . d. Wide.*

Once children are successful, present each of the phonemes separately so they can "roll them out" on their own, in shorter and shorter sequences, to find the word. Use the one-syllable C–V–C word list provided above.

> **PLAY** Break-It-Up.

Children analyze one-syllable C–V–C words in order to identify the beginning, middle, and ending sounds. Begin activities with initial sounds, and then proceed to middle and ending sounds. For an example on how to demonstrate finding the middle sound in *wide*, ask

> What's the sound in the middle of *wide?*
> Break it up: *Wwwww . . .-īīīī . . .-d . . . W-ī-d.*
> *ī* is the sound in the middle of *wide.*

Continue to present one-syllable C–V–C words provided in Say-It-Until-You-Hear-It so children can break them up and identify the sounds in each of the positions.

(continues on next page)

PLAY Break-It-Up. *Continued*

In the last stage of the game, children identify all the sounds in the word. Demonstrate how to elongate the sounds and then break them up in order to identify each one. For example,

> What are all the sounds in the word *wide*?
> Roll it out and break it up: *Wwwww . . . -īīīī . . . d. W-ī-d.*
> *W-ī-d* are the sounds in *wide*.

PLAY Delete-It.

Children omit the first sound in one-syllable words from the text. Demonstrate by saying the word slowly, then leaving off the initial sound. To demonstrate using *wide*, for example, say

> Listen to how I can make *wide* become *I'd*.
> I delete the first sound. *Wide. _ide.*
> Now you delete it. *Wide . . .*

Use the list of one-syllable words provided. Also practice deleting the *m* in the words *mind* and *manners* for the game that follows.

PLAY Switch-It—or in this case—"Make Monkey Talk."

Children delete the initial sound of the word and exchange it with a new sound to make another word. Demonstrate first, then prompt with cues as necessary. For example,

> Say *wide*.
> Now say *wide*, but delete the *w* and switch it with *s*.
> What new word can we make from *wide*? (side)
> *Wide, side.*

Once children experience success, use the words of the monkey as he scolds the crocodiles ("Mind your manners!"). Have the children replace the initial *m* in *mind* and *manners* with another designated sound. For example, say

> Repeat what the monkey told the crocodiles, only this time, when the monkey says "mind your manners," you will switch the beginning *m* sound in the words with a *f*, as in

> Find your fanners!

Other possibilities to "Make Monkey Talk" include

> Nine your nanners!
> Wined your wanners!
> Dined your danners!
> Pined your panners!

A Country Far Away

by Nigel Gray
New York: Orchard, 1989

Suggested Grade and Interest Level: 1 through 5

Topic Explorations: Community; Culture and history, African and African American; Daily activities

Skill Builders:

Vocabulary	Language literacy	Articulation
Higher-level concepts	Verbal expression	Carryover for any target sound
Grammar and syntax	Compare and contrast	
Present tense	Discussion	
Advanced syntactic structures		

Synopsis: A wordless book of side-by-side contemporary scenes that portray the lives of two boys—one in the United States, the other in an African village. Ideal for promoting conversation and promoting the concept that people all over the globe, no matter how different their lives are, have much in common.

Method: Before the read-aloud, tap children's knowledge of other customs and ways of life they may have experienced. Ask children to think of how children's lives in other countries are similar to the lives and experiences they have in this country. How are they dissimilar?

During the read-aloud, encourage the children to describe the action in each scene. Then demonstrate how to compare the two scenes using words such as *same, different, similar, yet, in common,* and *compared to.* Ask

> How are the children's lives different?
> How are they the same?

For higher-level concepts, talk about the simultaneousness of time depicted in the pictures. Discuss the word *simultaneous* and its meaning (i.e., occurring at the same time). Use the word and others, such as *meanwhile,* to construct sentences about events taking place at the same time, but in different places of the world.

Also talk about the concepts of the *commonality* and *universality* of all human beings and the characters, feelings, interests, and desires that apply to all people. Help students imagine what the students in the book might be interested in at school, what they might be interested in doing during free time, and what they may hope for in the future. Encourage students to draw parallels from their own lives to people living in other countries.

Facilitate the use of complex syntactic structures with conjunctions such as *and, but,* and *because* and dependant clauses and adverbial phrases beginning with *while, after,* and *although.*

After the read-aloud, encourage discussion of different customs in other countries besides the one depicted in the book.

Deep in the Forest

by Brinton Turkle
New York: Dutton, 1976

Suggested Grade and Interest Level: 1 through 3

Topic Explorations: Animals, Bears; Fairy tales and nursery rhymes

Skill Builders:
Language literacy

Predicting	Storytelling
Sequencing	Compare and contrast

Synopsis: This wordless book tells the story of a little bear that discovers a log cabin in the forest. The inhabitants, a family of three, have gone out for a walk. Follow the little bear as it explores Mama's, Papa's, and Baby's bowls of porridge, chairs, and beds in a reversal of the *Goldilocks* tale.

Method: Introduce the book by recalling the story of *Goldilocks and the Three Bears*. Explain that this book tells another story about a baby bear and that the children will get to tell this bear story because there are no words to read.

During the read-aloud, encourage predictions by recalling the story of Goldilocks.

After the read-aloud, have the children recall the sequence of events or have the children tell the story as you provide scaffolding when needed. Compare and contrast this story with *Goldilocks*. How are the stories alike? (Both took place in a house, with the character trying porridge, chairs, etc.) How are they different? (In our story, the main character is the little bear. In *Goldilocks*, it is the little girl.) What is different about a bear wandering into a strange house versus a girl entering a strange house?

Extended Activity: Younger children can dramatize the tale using the following props: three bowls on a table, three chairs, and three beds (mats). Have three children act the parts of the family members who decide to go for a walk after tasting their porridge. Have one child act the part of the little bear. The actors can pantomime while the audience tells the story (prompted by you).

Older children can illustrate several events from the story in sequential order. Have them write an internal monologue of what the little bear is thinking as it goes from place to place.

Dog Breath: The Horrible Trouble with Hally Tosis

by Dav Pilkey
New York: Scholastic, 1994

Suggested Grade and Interest Level: 1 through 5

Topic Explorations: Animals, Dogs; Family relationships

Skill Builders:
Vocabulary

Semantics	Homonyms
Idioms	Morphological units

Synopsis: The Tosis family is in a terrible predicament. Their dog, Hally, has the worst breath imaginable. Hally causes all kinds of trouble: She breathes on the fish and it dies, breathes on Gradma Tosis and makes her spill her tea, and causes the neighborhood children to walk on the other side of the street so they don't come near the Tosis's smelly house. The children try to solve the problem by taking her to a mountaintop with a breathtaking view, showing her a movie that would leave her breathless, and bringing her to a carnival where they hoped the roller coaster would make her lose her breath. But these things just don't work, and it looks as if they would have to get rid of her. Finally, Hally solves her own problem when she annihilates the bad guys who came to rob the house and makes front-page news. The puns in this book will keep children entertained and generate lots of laughs.

Method: Before the read-aloud, read the title and have a discussion about the word *halitosis* and define what it means. Read the subtitle and ask children to explain the meaning of the dog's name. Why is Hally a good name for a stinky dog of the Tosis family?

Many children have difficulty understanding puns because of the nature of their use and also because of misunderstanding or not knowing about the word itself. After the read-aloud, first build vocabulary skills by reviewing the meaning of the words used as puns, like *breathtaking*. After defining the word (*thrilling, beautiful, astonishing, remarkable*), use it in a sentence and see if children can explain why it is funny when used in connection with Hally. What is Hally's problem? What would the children in the story like to do about Hally's breath? Would showing Hally a breathtaking view really take her breath away?

Talk about how homonyms sometimes can be used in funny ways and the meaning of the last page of text: "Because life without Hally Tosis just wouldn't make scents." Ask children what the funny thing about that sentence is. Discuss the two meaning of *scents* and *sense*. Brainstorm other homonyms.

Talk about idioms used in the story, such as "take my breath away." Explain that they most often cannot be explained literally. Does a movie really leave one breathless? Can you really "catch your breath"? Other idioms to talk about are "save your breath," "barking up the wrong tree," and "by the skin of your teeth."

For building morphological skills, use the words of the story to talk about root words and their endings, or suffixes, which alter the meaning. Give other examples of words like *breathless* that have the same suffix, like *speechless, careless,* and *weightless*.

Extended Activity: Have children make up their own puns; to help them, brainstorm a list of homonyms. Then use the word in a sentence, but switch the meaning of the words so that the sentence is silly. For example, talk about the words *hall* and *haul* and the meaning of each. Use each word in a sentence. Then associate the first word with an expression and apply it to the second word. For instance, "Why did the dump truck need to go to the office?" (Answer: "It needed a haul pass.") Also, read the books by Fred Gwynne listed in these catalogs, such as *A Chocolate Moose for Dinner* and *The King Who Rained*. Have students draw pictures illustrating the literal interpretations of the idioms in *Dog Breath*, such as Hally watching a movie and having her breath leave her. Have them label the picture with the pun and present it to the class with an explanation.

Dogteam

by Gary Paulsen and Ruth Paulsen
New York: Delacorte Press, 1993

Suggested Grade and Interest Level: 1 through 5

Topic Explorations: Animals, Dogs; Careers

Skill Builders:

Vocabulary
Attributes
Similes and metaphors

Language literacy
Verbal expression

Articulation— L, R, and S

Synopsis: Three-time Newbery winner Gary Paulsen, who twice has run the Iditarod across Alaska, portrays the excitement and danger of dogsled racing at night. The repetition and rhythm in this prose poem give the reader a sense of what these dogs love to do.

Method: Before the read-aloud, set the stage by asking students what they know about dog racing in Alaska. Explain that dogs are prepared and trained for the Iditarod all year long.

After the read-aloud, brainstorm words that describe dogsled racing at night. How do you think the dogs experience the event? How would you experience it?

For articulation, students can repeat the words of the text and respond to questions that elicit target phonemes.

Discuss the author's use of similes and metaphors, such as

> . . . small songs of excitement when the harnesses are put on . . .
> Straining to join the snow and the moon and the night . . .
> Frozen and flat and white as the moonlight we slip out of the woods.

Extended Activity: From the list of words that describe dogsled racing, have students write prose poems. Encourage them to use repetition and rhythm and to use a phrase for a topic heading as the authors did. Have them include a metaphor and a simile in the poem.

Dreams

by Peter Spier
New York: Doubleday, 1986

Suggested Grade and Interest Level: 1 through 5

Topic Explorations: Clouds; Shapes and visual images; Weather

Skill Builders:

Grammar and syntax
Tenses, present and past

Language literacy
Verbal expression

Fluency

Synopsis: A list of children's picture books wouldn't be complete without the work of Peter Spier. This wordless masterpiece illustrates a cloud formation on each two-page spread. It generates lots of possibilities for creative sentences and makes a perfect sequel to *It Looked Like Spilt Milk*.

Method: Model or shape appropriate structures based on the illustrations. Make up a separate story about each illustration. For verbal expression, have children describe the cloud formations and make up stories about what's happening in the sky.

For fluency, elicit sentence repetitions or responses to questions based on the illustrations, and systematically increase the length of phrases to sentences, having the children maintain airflow.

Extended Activity: On a day when there are many cumulus clouds in the sky, let the class take a walk outside and sit down to watch cloud formations. While they stare at the clouds for several minutes, encourage the children to use their imaginations to see shapes in the clouds. Encourage them to make up stories about what they see.

The Eyes of the Dragon

by Margaret Leaf
New York: Lothrop, Lee & Shepard, 1987

Suggested Grade and Interest Level: 3 through 5

Topic Explorations: Community; Culture and history, Chinese; Folklore, Chinese

Skill Builders:
Language literacy
Cause-and-effect relationships
Predicting
Problem solving
Discussion

Synopsis: The village magistrate's grandson is caught writing on the town wall. In order to save face, the magistrate commissions an artist to embellish the wall with a dragon that will bring prosperity to the villagers. The artist agrees to paint the wall on the condition that the magistrate accept his finished work. The magistrate agrees. When the magnificent dragon is done, however, the magistrate insists that eyes be painted on the creature. The consequence of this action creates a dramatic ending.

Method: Before the read-aloud, discuss the significance of the dragon and the positive influence it connotes in the Chinese culture. Talk about the huge paper dragons that are part of Chinese New Year celebrations.

During the read-aloud, pause to ask comprehension questions. For problem solving, after the magistrate lets his grandson go, ask students what facts they can state about the problem. What events led to the problem? When the artist finishes painting the dragon, target cause-and-effect relationships by pausing to ask what happened because of the problem. When the magistrate insists that eyes be painted on the dragon, pause to ask about the possible consequences. What do the children think the effect will be if the artist puts them in? What do they think the effect will be if he doesn't? What caused the dragon to come to life and the wall to crumble? What was the effect of the broken promise?

After the read-aloud, review the problem of the story and the facts that led to the problem. Ask children what ways the characters came up with to solve the problem. Are there other possibilities not mentioned in the book?

Discuss the outcome.

What is the author saying about life?
What would have happened if the magistrate had accepted the painting as the artist had asked?
If you were the magistrate, what would you have done? Why?
What do you think the results would have been?

Extended Activity: Have a Chinese celebration with paper lanterns and Chinese food. Demonstrate how to stir-fry vegetables in a wok and eat them with chopsticks. Invite children from Chinese families to share some of their belongings showing the dragon motif, such as kites and chopsticks.

The Fall of Freddie the Leaf

by Leo Buscaglia
Thorofare, NJ: Slack, 1982; New York: Henry Holt, 1982

Suggested Grade and Interest Level: 2 through 5

Topic Explorations: Death and dying; Seasons

Skill Builders:
    Language literacy
    Relating personal experiences   Drawing inferences
    Sequencing   Discussion

Synopsis: Warm and wise, *The Fall of Freddie the Leaf* is the story of the cycle of life and death, with death being portrayed as a regenerative process. The photographs of trees capture the magnificence of nature.

Method: Before the read-aloud, talk about loss and ask students to share their experiences. Sample questions include

> Have you ever lost something special to you?
> Have you ever lost a special person?
> What was that like?

Read aloud without initiating interaction. Then discuss how listeners felt about the story and what images came to them. Talk about loss and what happens when you lose something or someone special.

> What did you gain from the experience of knowing the person?
> If you lost a special thing, what did that special thing give you?
> What transpired because of this?

Reread the story, pausing to reflect on how the author draws parallels between leaves on a tree and life. What is the author saying about life?

Farmer Duck

by Martin Waddell
Cambridge, MA: Candlewick Press, 1992

Suggested Grade and Interest Level: 1 through 3

Topic Explorations: Animals, Farm; Feelings; Humor; Speaking and communicating

Skill Builders:

Vocabulary	**Language literacy**	**Articulation,** *H*
Prepositions	Storytelling	**Voice**
Grammar and syntax	Problem solving	
Tenses, present and past	Verbal expression	
	Drawing inferences	

Synopsis: A humorous tale of a lazy farmer who makes his duck do all the work so he can stay in bed. The other animals, feeling sorry for the poor duck, decide to take matters into their own hands and do something about the injustice. A jewel in your repertoire of read-alouds, you'll pull this book out again and again.

Method: Read the story, having the children describe the duck's chores and make the quacking response. Shape responses to elicit target structures and sounds.

After reading the book through, discuss the problem in the story. Talk about how the other animals felt about the duck having to do all the work. Discuss what the "quack" of the duck might mean and what the rest of the animals might be saying. What did they do to solve the problem? Discuss the story elements and let children take turns retelling the story.

Reread the book with greater class participation. Have one side of the class repeat the text and the other side repeat the duck's quack. Let the children decide what the duck might say about the work if he could speak. Use the dialog to elaborate the duck's response. For example, "Quack. There sure is a lot of work." "Quack. I'm getting awfully tired." "Quack. Can't keep up with it." "Quack. Can't talk now."

For articulation, initiate auditory bombardment of speech sounds before reading aloud. Then read and pause to ask questions that elicit answers containing the target sound. Words beginning with *H* include *hen, house, hard* (work), *hall, whole* (story), and *hill.*

For voice, have children initiate the sentence, "How goes the work?" with an easy onset each time it is introduced in the story.

A Fish in His Pocket

by Denys Cazet
New York: Orchard Books, 1987, 1991

Suggested Grade and Interest Level: 1 through 4

Topic Explorations: Death and dying; Feelings; School activities; Seasons, Autumn

Skill Builders:

Grammar and syntax	Language literacy	Articulation, *Sh*
Pronouns, personal and possessive	Relating personal experiences	
Tenses, present and past	Cause-and-effect relationships	
	Problem solving	
	Drawing inferences	

Synopsis: What is Russell to do with the little orange fish he inadvertently took to school with him from the pond? Plagued by this dilemma, his distraction keeps him from schoolwork until he figures out a way to return it to the pond. With so much left unsaid in this touching story, you'll want to allow plenty of time to discuss its meaning and implications.

Method: Read and interact, shaping responses that contain target structures. Pause to infer what is causing Russell to lose his place in reading and leave his lunch uneaten. Why is he bothered? What do you think he wants to do? Have children brainstorm ideas Russell could have about what to do with the fish and predict what he will do. Also ask the children whether they believe the fish is still alive. Why or why not?

After the story, discuss how Russell handled his problem. Did his solution resemble the children's predictions? What did the teacher say when Russell told her about his accident? How did he show that he would "take care"?

Talk about accidents, caring for others, and how Russell showed that he cared for the fish. Talk about what effect finding the fish had on Russell. How was this shown?

For relating personal experiences, ask volunteers to share experiences similar to Russell's. Perhaps a pet died. How did they show that they cared for the pet after it died? Why was it important to do this?

For articulation of *Sh,* use the repetition of the word *fish* and the illustrations of the book to practice *Sh* in the final position of the word at word, phrase, sentence, and discourse levels.

For Laughing Outloud: Poems To Tickle Your Funnybone

Compiled by Jack Prelutsky
New York: Knopf, 1991

Suggested Grade and Interest Level: 1 through 5

Topic Exploration: Humor

Skill Builders:
  Phonological awareness   **Articulation—*H, L, R, S, Z, Ch, Sh,* and *Th***   **Fluency**

Synopsis: Jack Prelutsky's selection of crazy poems, many from authors you will recognize, are sure to delight both reader and listener.

Method: For phonological awareness training, use the poems to play the sound game activities. The following picks up from where the activities left off in the Pre-K catalog, using the poem "The Pancake Collector."

> **PLAY** **Say-It-Until-You-Hear-It.**
>
> Children synthesize one-syllable words divided into onset-rime. Present the word with a clear pause between the onset and rime. Demonstrate how to elongate the parts to blend them together, saying them a little quicker each time until they are readily identified. Provide scaffolding until children are ready to do it on their own. For example, say
>
>> Put these two parts together: *l–ight.*
>> Say it until you hear it. *Lllllll . . . ight. Ll . . . ight. Light.*
>
> Continue with these consonant–vowel–consonant (C–V–C) words from the text beginning with a single sound:
>
>| l-et | b-ake | b-ook |
>|------|-------|-------|
>| n-ice | p-ack | p-an |
>| m-ore | b-ag | c-ake |
>
> Then demonstrate how to synthesize one-syllable words divided into onset-rime, beginning with a two-consonant cluster until children are ready to do it on their own. Words include
>
>| fl-uff (fluff) | fl-ake (flake) | pr-ess (press) |
>|----------------|----------------|----------------|
>| cr-epe (crepe) | dr-ape (drape) | st-uff (stuff) |

PLAY **Roll-It-Out.**

Children synthesize a C–V–C word by blending each of its phonemes. Demonstrate by elongating the phonemes and blending them together in shorter and shorter sequences until children can identify the word. For example, say

> l-ī-t
> What's the word? Roll it out. Lllll . . . $\overline{iiii}$ . . . t. Light.

Once children are successful, present each of the phonemes separately so they can "roll them out" on their own, in shorter and shorter sequences, to find the word. Use the one-syllable C–V–C word list provided in Say-It-Until-You-Hear-It.

PLAY **Break-It-Up.**

Children analyze one-syllable C–V–C words in order to identify the beginning, middle, and ending sounds. Begin activities with initial sounds, and then proceed to middle and ending sounds. For an example on how to demonstrate finding the middle sound in *light,* ask

> What's the sound in the middle of *light*?
> Break it up: Lllll . . .-$\overline{iiii}$ . . .-t. L–i –t.
> $\overline{i}$ is the sound in the middle of *light.*

Continue to present one-syllable C–V–C words provided in Say-It-Until-You-Hear-It so children can break them up and identify the sounds in each of the positions.

In the last stage of the game, children identify all the sounds in the word. Demonstrate how to elongate the sounds and then break them up in order to identify each one. For example, ask

> What are all the sounds in the word *light*?
> Roll it out and break it up: Llll . . . -$\overline{iiii}$ . . . -t. L–i–t.
> L–ī-t are all the sounds in *light.*

PLAY **Delete-It.**

Children omit the first sound in one-syllable words from the text. Demonstrate by saying the word slowly, then leaving off the initial sound. To demonstrate using *nice,* for example, say

> Listen to how I can make *nice* become *ice.*
> I delete the first sound. *Nice. Ice.*
> Now you delete it. *Nice . . .*

Use the list of one-syllable words provided above. Once children experience success, practice with the words in the titles of the poems, especially the alliterative ones. Children will say the title slowly, leaving off the initial sound from the main words. For example, "How to Tell a Tiger" will sound like this:

> Ow to Ell a Iger

> **PLAY** **Switch-It.**
>
> Children delete the initial sound of the word and replace it with a new sound to make another word. Demonstrate first, then prompt with cues as necessary. For example,
>
> > Say *light*.
> > Now say *light*, only delete the *l* and switch it with *n*.
> > What new word can you make? *Light, night*.
>
> Continue with the one-syllable words provided until children experience success. Then play the game with titles of poems. For example, switch the *t* in "How to Tell a Tiger" with an *m* sound to get
>
> > How to Mell a Miger
>
> Ask children to tell you what the words were before you changed them. Other possibilities include
>
> > How to Bell a Biger
>
> Then switch initial phonemes in the words of the title with consonant blends. For example, using *fr*, the children's part will sound like this:
>
> > How to Frell a Friger
>
> Remember to go slowly!

For articulation, look in the title index in the back for a list of poems heavily loaded with any sound you wish to target. Here are a few selections:

> "Habits of the Hippopotamus"   "Raising Frogs for Profit"
> "Chimney Squirrels"   "Thunder and Lightning"

For example, use the poem "When Ice Cream Grows on Spaghetti Trees" for articulation of *S* and *Z*.

> When ice cream grows on spaghetti trees,
> And the Sahara Desert grows muddy,
> When cats and dogs wear B.V.D.'s
> That's the time to study. (anonymous)

For *L*: "Eels"

> > Eileen Carroll
> > Had a barrel
> > Filled with writhing eels
> > And just for fun
> > She swallowed one:
> > Now she knows how it feels. (Spike Mulligan)

Use *H* illustrations to practice onset of phonation. Ask questions to elicit responses containing target words. Have children maintain the easy voice while building alliterative sentences or telling stories heavily loaded with the target sounds.

For fluency, use the target words on a page of illustrations to practice sustaining airflow during production of words, phrases, and sentences.

Extended Activity: Have students make up alliterative phrases about a favorite animal. Include in the phrases something about what the animal does, then set them to rhyme. Begin by brainstorming a few examples with the class. Then have each student create a graphic that illustrates the rhyme, write the words, and add a fancy border. Let students read their poems to the class and display them.

Fortunately

by Remy Charlip
New York: Parents Magazine Press, 1964; Aladdin, 1993

Suggested Grade and Interest Level: 1 through 3

Topic Exploration: Journeys

Skill Builders:

Vocabulary	**Language literacy**	**Articulation,** *Ch*
Adverbs	Relating personal experiences	
Antonyms	Predicting	
Morphological units	Verbal expression	
Grammar and syntax	**Phonological awareness**	
Past tense		

Synopsis: Through a series of fortunes and misfortunes, Ned somehow gets to a surprise party, which turns out to be for him!

> Fortunately a friend loaned him an airplane
> Unfortunately the motor exploded
> Fortunately there was a parachute in the airplane
> Unfortunately there was a hole in the parachute . . .

Method: Before the read-aloud, explain the meaning of the word *fortunately* and use it in a sentence. Discuss how sometimes our experiences can at first seem unfortunate but later turn out to be fortunate.

For verbal expression, ask what is good about Ned's parachute breaking. (He can land on the haystack.) Then ask what will be the bad thing about Ned falling into the haystack. (He will fall on the pitchfork.) Build grammar and syntax skills by modeling appropriate structures from the text.

For adverbs and antonyms, ask children to make up sentences based on experiences similar to Ned's. (For example, "Unfortunately I missed the bus. Fortunately my dad could bring my to school.")

Note: The following activities can be enhanced by first engaging in the Extended Activity found at the end of this book entry.

First talk about the meaning of the root word *fortune* and encourage children to generate sentences using the word. Some examples include

> Did Ned have good fortune? Why do you think so?
> Did Ned have bad fortune? Why do you think so?
> What kind of fortune did Ned have in the end of the story?
> Have you ever had good fortune? What happened?

Then use the "fortunate" words to play phonological and morphological awareness games. See the entry in the Pre-K catalog for activities that address earlier levels.

PLAY **Sentence-It.**

Generate a sentence using the words *fortunate, fortunately,* and *unfortunately.* Some examples include

> Ned was *fortunate* that the party was for him.
> *Fortunately,* the party was for Ned.
> *Unfortunately,* Ned's party was far away.

PLAY **Leave-It-Out.**

Say the two-syllable word *fortune* and have the child delete the beginning or final part. For example,

> Say *fortune* without saying *tune.* (pronounced *chun*)
> What little word is left? (for)
> Now say *fortune* without saying *for.*
> What sound is left? (pronounced *chun*)

PLAY **Leave-It-Out.**

Use the three-syllable word *fortunate.*

> Say *fortunate* without saying *ate.* (pronounced *et*)
> What word is left? (fortune)
> Say *fortunately* without saying *–ly.*
> What little word is left? (fortunate)

PLAY **Add-It-On.**

Say part of the word and have the child supply the rest. For example,

> Say *for* and add *tune.* (sounds like *chun*)
> What word do you have? (fortune)
> Say *fortune* and add *ate.* (pronounced *et*)
> What word do you have? (fortunate)
> Say *fortunate* and add *–ly.*
> What word do you have? (fortunately)
> Say *un* and add the word *fortunate.*
> What word do you have? (unfortunate)
> Say *un* and add the word *fortunately.*
> What word do you have? (unfortunately)

This activity is a good introduction to antonyms and adverbs that contain the prefix *un–.* Here are a few.

cover, uncover	dress, undress	tie, untie
known, unknown	real, unreal	willing, unwilling

For articulation of *Ch,* use repetition of the word *fortunately* and the many derivational forms of the word *fortunate* to practice *Ch* in the medial positions of words.

318

Extended Activity: Discuss shared unfortunate/fortunate experiences. An example from one second-grade class follows:

> Unfortunately I got in trouble with my teacher at school. Fortunately it was 3:00 and time to go home.

Then demonstrate with an example about how to draw a picture of these experiences. Fold a large sheet of paper in half. Draw a picture of the unfortunate experience on one half of the paper (simple marking pen drawings turn out best). Show the experience turning out to be fortunate on the other side of the paper. Have children dictate a brief story underneath. Title the project "My Story." Have each child present his or her story to the class as you provide scaffolding and elaboration as needed.

Note: The methods for teaching morphological units correspond nicely to that of *Suddenly!* by Colin McNaughton, listed in this catalog.

Frederick

by Leo Lionni
New York: Knopf, 1967; Dragonfly Books, 1995

Suggested Grade and Interest Level: 1 through 2

Topic Explorations: Creativity; Seasons; Self-esteem

Skill Builders:
    Vocabulary   **Phonological awareness**
    Semantics

Synopsis: Just because Frederick sits quietly collecting words and colors into his thoughts while his family works hard gathering food doesn't mean Frederick is lazy. He is simply artistic and imaginative, qualities that also are important in life. When winter comes, the food the family has gathered sustains them at first but eventually runs out. Frederick's memories of the colors and sights of spring, shaped into poems and stories, take the others' minds off their troubles and get them through winter. The story of Frederick reminds us of the importance of nurturing the creative spirit. It is just as powerful and popular today as it was in 1967, when this classic was first published.

Method: Before the read-aloud, play the Imagine game. Talk about what happens when you imagine. Have children close their eyes and imagine *warm*. What pictures do they see in their minds? What are some words to describe the pictures? (A toasty fire? A cat in your lap?) Now imagine *cold*. What do they see in their mind's eye? What words can they use to describe *cold*? (Snow? Running water from a hose?)

Then show the book's cover and tell children they are going to hear a story about a family gathering supplies for the winter. Talk about the meaning of the word *supplies*. Give examples, such as paints, paintbrushes and paper for making a picture, and bread, tuna, potato chips, plastic wrap, and paper sacks for packing a lunch. Make predictions about what supplies a family of mice might need during the winter.

During the read-aloud, increase vocabulary and story comprehension by briefly pausing to talk about the words of the text. In addition to words already noted, discuss the meanings of the following in context:

stones (stone wall)	graze (cows grazed)	chatty (a chatty family)
abandoned (an abandoned barn)	granary	hideout
except	reproachfully	memory

After the read-aloud, reinforce the learning of new vocabulary. Explain expressions of speech and the meaning of the phrases "stood empty," "take their hideout in the stones," and "the corn was only a memory."

For generalization and story comprehension, ask the students questions such as the following:

> What happened when winter came?
> Why didn't anyone feel like chattering?
> How did Frederick's family feel when he entertained them with his poem?
> Why did gathering words and colors of spring turn out to have been a good thing?
> How does one "gather" words?
> How does one "gather" colors?
> Where did Frederick put the words and colors he gathered?

Recall your earlier discussion about supplies. If you were Frederick, what would you say if your family asked you, "What about your supplies, Frederick?"

What words would you gather about spring or summer?

Use the words of the text to play phonological awareness games. See the entry in the Pre-K catalog for activities that address earlier phonological awareness levels.

⬭PLAY⬭ Word-Search.

Children identify a word from the story that begins with a designated sound. For example, say

> I'm thinking of a word in the story that starts with *m*. (Give phoneme/sound only.)
> What word starts with *m . . . mmmmm . . .*?
> That's right. *Mouse. Mouse* starts with *mmmmm. . . .*

Give clues and prompts as necessary. For example,

> I see a word on this page that starts with *k*.

Show the page of the mice carrying the corn. Say

> I see see something that starts with *k*.

Or show the page of the mice thinking about colors.

Some suggestions for *m* include

> mouse
> mice

For *w:*

> wall
> white

(continues on next page)

PLAY Word-Search. *Continued*

For *b*:

berry
butterfly

For *s*:

sun
snow

PLAY The Same-Sound game.

Children identify whether word pairs end with the same sound. For example, say

sun, gone
Do they end with the same sound?

To make an unmatched pair, exchange one of the following words with another word from the text.

nut, cat	warm, home	dark, work
paint, throat	bush, blush	mice, voice
fell, wall	mind, field	corn, ran

PLAY Odd-One-Out.

From a string of words ending in the same sound, children select the one that does not belong. For example, say

stone, barn, corn, nut
Which word has a different ending sound? (nut)
That's right. *Nut* is the odd one out.

Some four-word strings follow. Reduce to three-word strings as necessary.

night, sun, gone, ran	wall, bush, fell, we'll	mice, voice, once, five
home, warm, bush, came	wheat, took, nut, eat	cat, throat, off, paint
dark, sleep, work, Frederick	word, mind, field, corn	

PLAY Say-It-Until-You-Hear-It.

Children synthesize one-syllable words divided into onset-rime. Start with words that begin with a single consonant sound. Demonstrate by presenting each part of the word separately. Show children how to elongate the onset part to blend the two parts together, saying them a little quicker each time until they are readily identified. For example, say

Listen to how I can put these two parts together:
M-$\bar{\imath}$ce. Mmmmmmmm . . . . $\overline{\imath\imath\imath\imath\imath}$ . . . . s. Mmm . . . $\overline{\imath\imath\imath}$ . . . sss. Mice.
Now you do it. *M-ice.*
Say it until you hear it. *Mmmmm . . . . ice. Mice.*

(continues on next page)

PLAY **Say-It-Until-You-Hear-It.** *Continued*

Continue with these C-V-C words from the text beginning with a single sound:

m-oon	m-ouse	n-ice
f-eet	l-ight	s-un
f-all	sh-ake	

Then demonstrate how to synthesize one-syllable words divided into onset-rime, beginning with a two-consonant cluster, as in

dr-eam (dream)	sn-ack (snack)	gr-aze (graze)
fl-ake (flake)	sn-ap (snap)	st-one (stone)

PLAY **Roll-It-Out.**

Children synthesize a C-V-C word by blending each of its phonemes. Demonstrate by elongating the phonemes and blending them together in shorter and shorter sequences until children can identify the word. For example, say

m-i-s
What's the word? Roll it out. *Mmmm . . . iiii . . . s. Mice.*

Once children are successful, present each of the phonemes separately so they can roll them out on their own, in shorter and shorter sequences, to find the word. Use the one-syllable C-V-C word list provided in the game above.

PLAY **Break-It-Up.**

Children analyze one-syllable C-V-C words in order to identify the beginning, middle, and ending sounds. Begin activities with initial sounds, and proceed to middle and ending sounds. For an example on how to demonstrate finding the middle sound in *mice,* ask

What's the sound in the middle of *mice?*
Break it up: *Mmmmm . . . -iiii . . .-ssss . . . M-ī-s.*
ī is the sound in the middle of *mice.*

Continue to present one-syllable C-V-C words provided above so children can break them up and identify the sounds in each position.

In the last stage of the game, children identify all the sounds in the word. Demonstrate how to elongate the sounds and then break them up in order to identify each one. For example, ask

What are all the sounds in the word *mice?*
Roll it out and break it up: *Mmmmm . . . -iiii . . . -sss. . . . M-ī-s.*
M-ī-s are all the sounds in *mice.*

PLAY **Delete-It.**

Children omit the first sound in one-syllable words from the text. Demonstrate by saying the word slowly, then leaving off the initial sound. To demonstrate using *feet,* for example, say

(continues on next page)

Delete-It. *Continued*

> Listen to how I can make *feet* become *eat*.
> I delete the first sound. *Feet.* _*eat.*
> Now you delete it. *Feet* . . .

Practice with Frederick's name. Demonstrate how to delete the two-consonant cluster *fr* in "Frederick" to get "Ed-erick." Once children are successful, use the list of one-syllable words provided.

 Switch-It.

Children delete the initial sound of the word and replace it with a new sound to make another word. Demonstrate first, then prompt with cues as necessary. For example,

> Say *feet*.
> Now say *feet*, only delete the *f* to get *eet*.
> Switch it with *m* to get *meet*.
> What new word did I make from *feet*? (meet)
> That's right. *Feet, meet.*

Continue with the one-syllable words until children experience success. Then demonstrate how to play the game with the words "Frederick the Mouse," switching the initial phonemes. For example, when using a *d* and then the consonant cluster *dr*, the new names will like look this:

> Dederick the Douse. Drederick the Drouse.

Other possibilities include

Brederick the Brouse	Trederick the Trouse
Prederick the Prouse	Shrederick the Shrouse

Note: Be sure to check the inside of the cover of the paperback edition by Dragonfly Books for some more activities and interesting facts. Here's one: Do you know where the word *mouse* came from? A Sanskrit word meaning *thief*!

Also note: This book is available in a Spanish version under the same title.

Frog on His Own

by Mercer Mayer
New York: Dial Books for Young Readers, 1973, 1980

Suggested Grade and Interest Level: 1 through 4

Topic Exploration: Pets

Skill Builders:

Grammar and syntax	Language literacy	Fluency
Tenses, present and past	Predicting	
	Sequencing	
	Cause-and-effect relationships	
	Storytelling	

GRADES 1–5

Synopsis: This small wordless book shows how a pet frog escapes from his owner and makes mischief in the park—to his own disadvantage.

Method: Model or shape target structures as the children tell the story from the illustrations. Have them make predictions based on the preceding events.

For storytelling, present the book and ask the children to tell the story. Provide organizational structure to their stories by asking questions to elicit story grammar elements.

> Who is the story about?
> Where does it take place?
> What happens to start the story off?
> How do the characters respond?
> How is the problem solved?
> How do the characters feel?

After the read-aloud, assist children in recalling the events of the story in sequential order. Provide scaffolding as necessary.

For fluency, elicit responses to questions or repetitions of words, phrases, and sentences that increase in length and complexity based on the pictures in the story. Practice maintaining airflow during production of increasingly longer responses.

Note: Read also the following wordless books by the same author: *A Boy, a Dog, a Frog, and a Friend; Frog Goes to Dinner; Frog, Where Are You?* and *One Frog Too Many.*

Gabriella's Song

by Candace Fleming
New York: Simon & Schuster, 1997; Aladdin Paperbacks, 2001

Suggested Grade and Interest Level: 1 through 3

Topic Explorations: Boats; Careers; Community; Music, musicians, and musical instruments; Sounds and listening

Skill Builders:

Vocabulary	Grammar and syntax	Language literacy
Semantics	Tenses, present and past	Compare and contrast
Categories		
Idioms		
Homonyms		

Synopsis: A young girl finds delight in all the sounds around her as she walks through her hometown of Venice, Italy. With sounds in her head and joy in her heart, she mingles them together and turns them into a song. Singing her song as she walks through the city, she delights her neighbors, one of whom is a composer who is so inspired that he writes a symphony. A heartwarming story that teaches children not only to listen to the beauty of sounds around them but also how songs are "born."

Method: Before the read-aloud, introduce the book by talking about far-away places in other countries, some of which are very unique and beautiful. Introduce the city of Venice and explain that it was once called "the city of music," because opera was first performed there. Explain how it was built on small islands that are close together, and people today use the waterways or canals to get from one island (part of the city) to another. Show the cover of the book and describe the boats called *gondolas* that the people travel in.

During the read-aloud, pause to briefly talk about words that give the meaning of the story. The beginning page will set the stage.

"Ah, Venice. The Piazza San Marco. The Grand Canal. St. Mark's Cathedral."

Vocabulary words include

gondolas	gondoliers	composer
marketplace	tethered	
symphony	canals	

After the read-aloud, go back for a picture walk through the book. Describe what is happening on the pages, shaping present and past tense.

Talk about idioms, or expressions of speech, to gain greater meaning from the story. What did the baker mean when he said, "It makes my heart light and my feet feel like dancing"? Can feet really feel like dancing? Elicit children's interpretations on the meaning. Give explanations such as

It is the author's way of saying the baker felt his troubles go away. He felt so good that he wanted to dance when he heard Gabriella's song.

For homonyms, talk about what the baker meant when he said, "It makes my heart light. . . ." Explain that the word *light* can mean cheerful or happy, as in lighthearted. Talk about other homonyms, ones that can be used with examples from the story. For example,

road, rowed—"A road is something you travel on. In our story, the roads in Venice are really water roads. *Rowed* sounds just like it and means that someone rowed a boat, much like what the gondoliers did in the story when they paddled or rowed the gondolas."

flour, flower—"Flour is what the baker needed for bread, and another word that sounds just like it is *flower.* Flowers are often sold at stands in Venice."

bow, bow—"A bow is the front part of the boat. Another word that sounds just like it is *bow,* which is what an actor, conductor, or composer, like Giuseppi in our story, does when they acknowledge applause from the audience."

story, story—"A story is what we just heard that is told or written down, like it was in this book. A word that sounds just like it is another kind of story, like the level or floor of the building on which Gabriella lived."

hear, here—"*Hear* is what you do when you listen to someone, or listen to the sounds of the city, as Gabriella did. *Here* can also mean come here, or come home, like where Gabriella's mother wanted her to come to."

For developing categories, categorize types of music, such as rock, rap, country-western, and classical, like the music of the composer in the story. Categorize places to hear music, including on the car radio, and musical instruments. Make use of all of the people in the story to categorize jobs that people hold in their communities. Also categorize different types of stores in a mall and compare that to a marketplace, where everything is sold in one place.

Have children compare and contrast Gabriella's community with the one in which the children live. How is it the same? How is it different?

Extended Activity: Play a favorite classroom song, a child's favorite CD, or one of your favorites (perhaps even classical) that you want to share with the children. Ask the children how it makes them feel. Is it a happy song? Recall how Gabriella's song made the baker feel like dancing.

The Gardener

by Sarah Stewart
New York: Farrar, Straus & Giroux, 1997; Sunburst, 2000

Suggested Grade and Interest Level: 2 through 5

Topic Explorations: Careers; Cities; Growing cycles and planting; History, American; Hobbies; Literacy

Skill Builders:

Vocabulary	**Language literacy**
Semantics	Storytelling
Higher-level concepts	Problem solving
Adjectives	Drawing inferences
Idioms	Retelling events
Proverbs	

Synopsis: In just 20 double pages, this multiple award winner, a richly conceived story set in the backdrop of the Great Depression, brings inspiration to all who read it. The book's text consists of a series of letters from Lydia Grace Finch to her family. Together with David Small's illustrations of dramatic and unusual perspective, it "speaks volumes about the vast impact one small individual can make," states *Publisher's Weekly.* Because her family has been hit by hard times, Lydia is sent to live in the city with Uncle Jim. She takes her love of gardening with her, and in trying to please her dour uncle and bring a smile to his face, she secretly creates a magnificent rooftop garden. In the end, her efforts are doubly rewarded. (Readers are also comforted to know that she eventually returns home, having touched the lives of her hardworking uncle and all those around her.)

Method: Use in conjunction with a classroom history lesson on the Great Depression. Before the reading, elicit background knowledge about the Great Depression in the 1930s. Talk about the era and help children understand that it was a sad time in history because so many people had no jobs.

After the reading, use the illustrations that further underscore the poignancy of this story and help lend understanding to the era. Teach inferencing skills for improving reading and language comprehension with the use of the illustrations. Encourage children to make the leap in understanding what is meant but not directly stated. Assist them in linking what is said in the text to what is highlighted in the illustrations to what they already know based on similar experiences.

For example, show the picture of Lydia on the train in one of the first pages of the book. A small child, alone on a train bound for her uncle's apartment in the city, she looks dwarfed by her surroundings. The people around her and the activities in which they are engaged further highlight her situation. A mother tends to her child on one side, and on the other side a young couple sit close together, visibly intent on one another. And there is Lydia, with the seat beside her empty.

> Why did the artist portray the scene this way?
> What did the artist want to tell the reader?

Have the students been in a similar situation before, perhaps not on a train but by themselves with people they didn't know? (If they cannot recall, can they pause for a moment to think about how Lydia might have experienced that?)

Ask students to describe how Lydia might feel in such a situation.

> What is her expression?
> What is remarkable about Lydia? (brave, positive attitude)

Also observe how the artist draws Lydia throughout the entire book. While she is drawn small and assumed to be young, observe her actions, clothing, and attitude. What else does this tell the reader/viewer about how she faced her situation and the era and the times in which she lived?

To teach storytelling skills, an important skill for language literacy, discuss the story grammars. For example,

> Who was the story about? (Lydia Grace Finch)
> Where did it take place? (It began at Lydia's house on a farm.)
> When? (During the Great Depression)
> What happened to start the story off? (Lydia had to leave her home to live with her Uncle Jim because her father lost his job.)
> How did the character(s) feel about it? (Lydia's mother looks sad. Lydia seems to be trying to make the best of it.)
> What was the character's goal in the story? (Lydia wanted to continue her hobby of growing her garden, but it seemed there was nowhere to grow one in a city apartment. Also, she wanted to please her Uncle Jim and make him smile.)
> What were her attempts to reach her goal? (She found a spot on the roof and she asked her family to send seeds.)
> What was the next thing the character did? (She performed her chores and grew beautiful plants on the rooftop in pots and tubs and planter boxes.)
> What was the result? (She transformed the rooftop into a splendid place.)
> How did the story end? (She made not only Uncle Jim happy, but she transformed the lives of those around her. Uncle Jim smiled in his own way, and she received a beautiful birthday cake decorated with a multitude of flowers.)
> How did the characters feel then? (Happiness in an otherwise sad time due to the spirit and positive attitude of a remarkable young girl.)

Students can take turns retelling the story as they are prompted with features in the illustrations and scaffolding questions as needed. Encourage use of words *and, then, so,* and *because.* After the story has been retold, ask students what made them feel good about it.

Each child in a small group can also retell the main events of the story. One can begin by explaining the events that led to Lydia's move to the city. Another can retell the events of her journey to the city. And another can retell the events of her life in the city.

Discuss what Lydia's problem was, what she wanted to achieve, and how she achieved it in the story. What was Lydia's goal? How did she achieve it?

Teach vocabulary words from pictures showing the city in all its variety. Students can learn words such as *push-cart, pigeons, packing crates, fire escapes, awnings, nuns, bums, bakery, rooftop,* and higher-level concepts such as *transformation.*

In teaching the concept of transformation, begin at a concrete level with an example such as a caterpillar transforming into a cocoon and then into a beautiful, splendid butterfly. Then apply the concept to that of the story, the process of turning the litter-strewn rooftop into the glorious garden that it became. Have children use variations of the word in sentences. Some examples include

> The empty, dirty rooftop was transformed into a beautiful garden.
> Lydia wanted to transform the rooftop into a gorgeous garden and make her uncle smile.
> Transforming the rooftop into a beautiful garden, Lydia made her uncle smile.

Then apply the concept of transformation to the characters. How did Lydia transform the people around her?

Start with her uncle's frown at the beginning of the story and point to his expression at the end of the story. How did he transform?

Lydia brought smiles to the faces of the customers in the bakery. What sentences can the children construct using the word *transformation* in connection with these characters?

The moral of the story can be explained in several idioms, proverbs, or expressions of speech. Some examples include

> Brighten the corner where you are
> Make the best of it
> Actions speak louder than words

Use the words in sentences to further underscore the meaning of the story and use the expressions in situations involving the children's own lives.

George and Martha: Back in Town

by James Marshall
Boston: Houghton Mifflin, 1984

Suggested Grade and Interest Level: 1 through 4

Topic Explorations: Friendship; Humor; Speaking and communicating

Skill Builders:

Grammar and syntax	**Language literacy**
Possessive nouns	Storytelling
Pronouns—personal, possessive, and reflexive	Drawing inferences
	Articulation—*R, J,* and *Th*
Tenses, present and past	

Synopsis: More short stories about the two hippos, the famous friendship couple, and how they sensitively resolve their problems with a sense of humor.

Method: Use the male and female characters and their belongings to model and shape possessive nouns, pronouns, and present and past tenses.

This series is excellent for teaching beginning storytelling skills because of the simple story lines and brevity of the stories. To teach story grammar components, first ask children to describe the characters. Then have them give the setting information and the problem one or both of the characters have. Ask how the characters respond to the situation, how they attempt to solve the problem, and what the final outcome is.

Many of the stories leave much to infer because of the relationship between the two hippos. For example, in one story, Martha sees a little box on the kitchen table with a note from George saying, "Do not open." She can't resist the temptation, so she opens it to find Mexican jumping beans, which she must scramble to retrieve when they all spill out all over the floor. When George gets home and asks why Martha is out of breath, she responds, "You don't think I opened that little box, do you?" to which George says, "Of course not." Martha tells George that she is not the nosey type, and the story ends with the words, "George didn't say a word."

Ask students why George might have asked Martha why she was out of breath, what her response meant, and whether George believed Martha. Also ask students why they think George left the little package on the table in the first place.

For articulation, use the couple's names to reinforce *R, Th,* and *J.* Capitalize on the short stories by having each child in a group either read aloud or retell one story, producing the target sound in connected speech.

Note: Also read other books in the series, including *George and Martha, George and Martha One Fine Day, George and Martha Rise and Shine, George and Martha Round and Round,* and *George and Martha Tons of Fun.*

George Washington's Cows

by David Small
New York: Farrar, Straus & Giroux, 1994; Sunburst, 1997

Suggested Grade and Interest Level: 3 through 5

Topic Explorations: History, American; Holidays, Presidents' Day; Famous people

Skill Builders:

Vocabulary	Grammar and syntax	Language literary
Adjectives	Past tense	Compare and contrast
Adverbs	Advanced syntactic structures	
Morphological units		

Synopsis: At George Washington's home of Mt. Vernon, the farm animals take the upper hand. Dressed in historical garb, the anthropomorphic cows, hogs, and sheep provide the hilarity. The pampered cows won't give milk until they've been moved into the finest quarters of the house, outfitted in lavender gowns, sprayed with expensive cologne, and bedded on cushions of silk! The hogs, "on the other hand/Were a genteel and amiable group/Delighted to help with the household chores/If a servant had fever or croup." But the sheep, the scholars, top it off with their academic lesson to the ladies and gentlemen of the day. The zany text, marvelous watercolors depicting expressions and gestures of the characters and the impeccable details of the site, and George's response to it all make this book one of the most entertaining read-alouds on anyone's library shelf.

Method: The book is an ideal February read-aloud to incorporate into the theme of Presidents' Day. It offers historical accuracy of Mt. Vernon and the culture and dress of the day. The text presents the following vocabulary words:

scones	obsequious (tones)	genteel
amiable	croup	impeccably (dressed)
scholar	impressive	degrees
ferried	muttered	despair

Before the reading, gather students' background knowledge as you talk about the times, the style of living, dress, manners, and occupations.

Read the book, pausing to point out a feature or two where appropriate. After the reading, build a fun lesson around the vocabulary. For example, using the word *obsequious*, first define the word, explaining that if some- one acts obsequious, the person is acting as if he or she were inferior to another. Have students act out the word, saying "Yes, whatever you say," fawning over the person, and saying "Oh, you are so _____ (a word students will relate to). If only I were as good as you!" (be sure to reverse the roles). Use the word in a sentence. Talk about what it means within the context of the story. Ask questions such as

Why is it funny that the servants at Mt. Vernon had to speak in "obsequious" tones to the cows?
How might one speak to a cow in an obsequious tone?
What might the servants of Mt. Vernon say in an obsequious way?

Increase grammar and syntax skills by developing a lesson around the words of the story. Learning to use long words is often viewed by children as a fun activity. For example, use the word *obsequious* as an adjective to describe the servants and create the beginning of a past-tense sentence for the students to fill in. For example, say

"The obsequious servants _____" and ask the students to finish the thought by referring to the illustrations. Suggestions include

_____ begged the cows (to give milk).
_____ sprayed the cows (with perfume).
_____ made the cows clothes (such as lavender gowns).
_____ dressed the cows (in lavender gowns).
_____ made the cows' beds (and fluffed up their pillows).

Then have the students begin and end a few sentences on their own.

To teach adverbs, change the adjective *obsequious* by adding the *–ly* suffix. This time, the *obsequious* word will describe *how* the servants attended to the cows.

The servants _____

Suggestions include

_____ obsequiously attended the cows.
_____ obseqiously begged the cows to give their milk.
_____ obsequiously made the cows' beds.

Note: Use the vocabulary word *impeccably* to illustrate an adverb here as well. *How* were the pigs dressed? Impeccably!

Show students how to create sentences with more complex syntactical form. First create a verb phrase or adverbial phrase. For example, ask *when* the servants attended the cows.

Suggestions include

when working at Mt. Vernon
every morning

Turn these words into phrases with which students can begin a sentence. For example, state the adverbial phrase

When working at Mr. Vernon, _____

Students can complete the thought using the previous sentences.

When working at Mt. Vernon, the servants obsequiously attended the cows.
Every morning, the servants obsequiously begged the cows to give their milk.

Improve students' language literacy skills by assisting them as they compare and contrast George Washington's cows to his hogs. How were his cows and hogs alike?

Suggestions include

They both dressed up in fine clothes.
They both acted like people.
They both took control of his house.

What was different in the behavior of the cows and hogs?

> The cows had an attitude, but the hogs were pleasant.
> The cows didn't work, but the hogs worked hard and enjoyed it.
> The cows didn't socialize or communicate with anyone, but the pigs like hosting parties.

Extended Activity: Bring in materials and pictures of Mt. Vernon to familiarize the children with colonial times. Compare the material and photographs to the illustrations in the book. What qualities do they have in common? What details were captured by the artist? Have students illustrate one of the sentences they created. Use the sentence as a graphic on the illustration. Highlight the adverb, adverbial clause, or adjective so that it stands out from the rest. Complete the picture with a border that looks like a frame. Ask students to share their drawings and point out one detail of colonial times in their artwork.

Good Dog, Carl

by Alexandra Day
La Jolla, CA: Green Tiger Press, 1985

Suggested Grade and Interest Level: 1 through 5

Topic Explorations: Humor; Loyalty; Pets

Skill Builders:

Vocabulary	**Language literacy**
Prepositions	Sequencing
Grammar and syntax	Storytelling
Possessive nouns	Verbal expression
Tenses, present and past	Point of view
Advanced syntactic structures	**Articulation**
	Carryover for any sound

Synopsis: A trustworthy dog in the role of a baby-sitter understands a child's desire to make mischief. So the good dog Carl takes the baby for a romp. The reader gets to supply most of the words to a nearly wordless book.

Method: Before the read-aloud, encourage children to make story predictions. Then present the book, inviting a different child to be the narrator for each page of this nearly wordless story. Encourage children to use lots of dialog in their narratives. (Have them make up dialog about what Carl and the baby are feeling, thinking, and using when involved in one activity and planning the next.) Field questions pertaining to story grammar elements so children learn to cue themselves when structuring narratives.

Pause to model and shape target structures. As the children describe each picture (as in "Carl is running down the stairs"), pause to praise their story construction. Then invite them to restructure the sentence or elaborate on it to offer more information. (As in "Carl, who is a good baby-sitter, races down the stairs to meet the baby.") Invite other children to vary the words within the same format. (As in "Carl, the trustworthy dog who takes good care of the baby, races down the stairs.")

After the read-aloud, have children sequence the events of the story. What are some of the events that took place while Carl looked after the baby? Encourage the use of connective words such as *first, then, next,* and *finally.*

Also encourage the use of connective words such as *however, while,* and *because* to describe the temporal and causal relationships between the events. For example,

The baby is listening to the music while Carl is listening to make sure Mom isn't coming back.

Carl cleans up the mess in the kitchen because he doesn't want Mom to come home and see it.

Extended Activity: Once students are familiar with the "Carl" books, present a lesson on point of view. Have students create their own sequel called "Carl Talks to His Canine Friends" or "Carl Raps with His Buddies." Have them create an amusing story that tells how Carl feels about Mother leaving him with the baby and his reasons (point of view) for wanting to take part in the mischief while she is away.

Have children break into cooperative groups to create the story. Students must come up with the following ingredients:

Carl's point of view	time sequence	external response
the other characters in the story	initiating event	consequences
story location	internal response	reaction

The children might decide, for example, to start off the story with Mother dropping Carl off at the kennel saying, "Have a good time with your friends, Carl. I'll be back for you tomorrow." The other characters can be the kennel owner who receives Carl and the other dogs in the kennel. The focus must remain on the interaction between Carl and the other dog or dogs so that Carl's side of the story can be told. The students can act out their sequel or illustrate it on butcher paper, with dialog and story line beneath each illustration.

Be sure children understand that this story is make-believe and that in real life, dogs, even rottweilers, don't baby-sit children.

Also by the same author: *Carl Goes Shopping, Carl's Afternoon in the Park, Carl's Christmas, Carl's Masquerade, Carl Goes to Day Care,* and *Carl's Scrapbook.*

Good-Night, Owl!

by Pat Hutchins
New York: Macmillan, 1972; Aladdin, 1990

Suggested Grade and Interest Level: 1 through 3

Topic Explorations: Nighttime; Owls

Skill Builders:

Vocabulary	**Language literacy**	**Articulation, *L* and *S***
Categories	Storytelling	
Grammar and syntax	Drawing inferences	
Past tense	Discussion	

Synopsis: With bees buzzing, squirrels cracking nuts, and crows croaking, how can a night owl ever get any sleep? The repetition of "Owl tried to sleep" on each page provides consistency for structuring language. When all the animals have finished their noisemaking, the complete text—every sentence—is repeated on the last page. Then, when night falls and all is silent, guess what? SCREECH!

Method: The text is all you'll need to model sentences in past tense. Ask children to tell a simple story about how the owl was kept up all day by noisy animals. Be sure children can infer what kept the owl awake. Discuss owls and their sleeping habits. Brainstorm names of other animals that sleep during the day, such as bats, leopards, opossums, and raccoons.

Extended Activity: Have each child create a puppet representing one of the noisy animals that kept the owl awake. Draw the outline of each animal on a paper bag or paper plate for the children to color in. Affix a craft stick to the paper plate. Reread the story in a circle as children participate with their puppets. Each child can repeat the lines of the text that relate to his or her puppet and make the appropriate animal noises while holding up the puppet. For example, read, "The bees buzzed. Buzz buzz." Then the child or children holding bee puppets repeat the lines and make the noises. Encourage the whole class to echo the repeated line, "And Owl tried to sleep."

Gorilla

by Anthony Browne
New York: Knopf, 1985, 1989

Suggested Grade and Interest Level: 1 through 5

Topic Explorations: Careers; Family relationships; Gorillas; Zoos

Skill Builders:

Grammar and syntax	**Language literacy**
Tenses, present and past	Drawing inferences
	Critical thinking

Synopsis: Hannah is so fascinated with gorillas that reading about them isn't enough. She wants to see the real ones at the zoo with her father. When the answer is no, the neglected and lonely girl turns her wishes into a dream in which her toy gorilla comes to life. What better way for the story to end than for her dream to come true and her real wish to be fulfilled?

Method: Before the read-aloud, ask children whether they ever imagined doing something or going somewhere and later found that Mom or Dad was thinking the same thing—and their wish came true. What are some reasons both they and their parents were thinking this? Share an experience with the class, then encourage children to relate their experiences. Lead into the story by showing the book cover and having students read the title and make predictions about the story.

Read aloud and pause to interact about how the girl feels and why. Ask questions such as these:

> What's happening to Hannah?
> What kind of girl is she?
> How do we know this?
> What is the problem in the story?
> What happened because of the problem?
> What are some ways Hannah might solve her problem?
> What does Hannah's dream tell us about her?
> What can we infer about Hannah's father before he takes her to the zoo?
> What can we infer about him when he takes her to the zoo?
> How does she feel at the end of the story? Why?

Encourage the use of conjunctions such as *when* and *because* to express temporal and causal relationships.

Grandfather's Journey

by Allen Say
Boston: Houghton Mifflin, 1993

Suggested Grade and Interest Level: 1 through 5

Topic Explorations: Culture and history, Japanese; Family relationships; Journeys; Memory and remembering

Skill Builders:

Vocabulary	Language literacy	Compare and contrast
Attributes	Relating personal experiences	Drawing inferences
	Cause-and-effect relationships	Point of view
	Problem solving	Discussion

Synopsis: A Japanese American recounts his grandfather's journey to America, which he later undertakes as well. The 1994 Caldecott medal–winning illustrations are highly evocative of the America and Japan of the past—from the railways, to the riverboats, to the storefronts of American towns, to the rubble of war-torn Japan. The scenic landscapes splendidly contrast the two cultures and underscore the men's dual heritage as well their love of two cultures.

Method: Before the read-aloud, ask children what they know about the word *journey.* What ways do people travel and why do people like to travel? Discuss ways two countries can be different and how both may have many good and beautiful things about them. Look at the cover and discuss the title of the story, asking questions such as

> What does the young man's dress imply?
> Where is he?
> What does the title mean?
> What do you think the story will be about?

For likenesses and differences, pause during the read-aloud to compare and contrast the two cultures. For example, on one page the young man is shown in Japanese dress, whereas on the opposite page he is shown in European dress. Discuss how both men were torn between their love of two countries.

> What did the grandfather like about America when he was in Japan and missed America?
> What did the grandfather like about Japan when he was in America and missed Japan?
> What would you do if you were the grandfather in the story?
> How are Japan and America alike?
> How are Japan and America different?

For drawing inferences, pause to elucidate meaning implied in the words of the story. When he was in America, why did the grandfather surround himself with songbirds? What was their importance? When the grandfather was in Japan, why did he raise warblers and silvereyes? When he grew older, why didn't the grandfather keep songbirds anymore?

For relating personal experiences, ask whether students have ever been anywhere where they felt homesick.

> What did they miss?
> How did they feel?
> What did they do?
> How was the experience like the grandfather's in the story?
> How was it like the grandson's?

For problem solving, ask what facts the children can state about the problem in the story. How did the grandfather attempt to solve the problem? Can they think of other solutions that might have helped the grandfather overcome the feeling of being torn between two countries?

For identifying cause and effect, ask what happened because of the grandfather's internal conflict. What effect did it have on his daughter? What effect did it have on her son?

For attributes, elicit words that describe the grandfather. What words describe the grandson?

For point of view, ask from whose point of view the story is being told. How do the students think the grandson knew so much about his grandfather's journey? How do you suppose he came to learn about it?

Extended Activity: Send home a short letter to parents explaining that students are learning about different heritages. Encourage parents to share their ancestries with their children. Did their grandparents come from another state? Another city? Another country? Have each student put together a journal of his or her family history. Encourage students to share their journals and their backgrounds in oral presentations to the class.

Hairy, Scary, Ordinary: What Is an Adjective?

by Brian P. Cleary
Minneapolis, MN: Carolrhoda Books, 2000

Suggested Grade and Interest Level: 1 through 5

Skill Builders:

Vocabulary	**Phonological awareness**
Categories	
Adjectives	
Morphological units	

Synopsis: The "nifty" rhyming text explains what an adjective is with loads of examples. It's accompanied by whimsical illustrations to enhance the meaning of each one. Here's an example from the text:

> "Adjectives help tell us more,
> Like narrow street or favorite store,
> Hilly, chilly, fast and fun,
> Undercooked and overdone."

Illustrations show humorous characters and creatures, settings, and actions that exemplify such things as the narrow street, the favorite "Kool Kitty Toys" store, a sled ride down a snowy mountain, a bowl of charred rolls, and a bowl of a runny, undercooked who-knows-what substance.

Method: Before the read-aloud, elicit background knowledge of adjectives to see if children can define what an adjective is. Briefly discuss the concept of words that describe. Brainstorm examples from around the room. Introduce the book by telling children they will hear and see many more examples for using them in the book.

During the read-aloud, pause briefly to point out an adjective or detail in the illustration, make comments, or ask questions with adjectives. Also pause at new vocabulary words such as *modify*.

After the read-aloud, continue to talk about adjectives, brainstorm a few from the book, and see if children can come up with more. Continue to discuss the concept of words that describe. Then go back through the book and reread part of the text. Spend several days discussing the adjectives and talking about how they are illustrated on several pages. After each double page of rhyming verse, pause to discuss the examples. Have children use them in phrases or sentences to describe the creatures or situations in the pictures. Then have them use the word in phrases or sentences to describe something in their own lives or from their own experience. For example,

> From the picture: The frisky puppy is jumping up to eat the dog bone.
> From experience: My frisky puppy jumps up on me when I come home from school.

For increasing the ability to categorize, have children name all the adjectives they can think of, and then have them supply the name for what they are all called. Look for other things to categorize in the illustrations. For example, read the text

> "Herringbone, pinstriped or plaid."
> What else can they all be called? (designs)

Another example is,

> "Crabby, excited or glad."
> What are they all called? (emotions, feelings)

Teach morphological units by examining root words that can be added to by using –y (long *ee* sound), such as

> airy, scary, leaky, squeaky
> easy, breezy, hilly, chilly
> silly, fizzy, busy, yummy
> baggy, saggy, stretchy, flashy
> trashy, spunky, clunky, junky
> speedy, thrifty, nifty, crabby
> stuffy, funny, puny, tiny

Say each word and ask,

> What part of the word do you hear after the first part?
> What little word do you hear in *crabby*?

Explain that sometimes adding a long *ee* sound to a word (spelled with the letter *y*) enables us to use it in another way—the adjective way.

For example,

> Our door has a *squeak*.
> It is a *squeaky* door.

Create basic sentences for children to fill in with an adjective, such as the following:

It is a ＿＿ book.	It is a ＿＿ day.
It is a ＿＿ piece of cake.	It is a ＿＿ room.
It is a ＿＿ shirt.	It is a ＿＿ drink.
It is a ＿＿ person.	

PLAY **Leave-It-Out.**

Children say a two-syllable word ending in –y, then leave out the suffix –y to reveal the root word. For example, say

> Say *leaky* without saying –y.
> What little word is left? (leak)

Continue using the previously provided list of two-syllable words ending in –y. Begin with C–V–C words.

PLAY **Add-It-On.**

Children put root word plus suffix together to make a two-syllable word. For example, say

> Put –y (sounds like *ee*) after *leak*.
> What word is it now? (leaky)

For phonological awareness training, use the words in the text that the children have become familiar with and understand the meanings for in activities. Begin at the developmental level of the child.

The following games begin at the syllable level using these compound words found in the text and illustrations:

kickball	bathtub	ballgame
pinstripe	milkshake	downright
undercooked	overdone	tablecloth
herringbone		

PLAY **Clap-and-Count.**

Children clap to and then count the syllables heard in the compound words. Demonstrate by clapping to a word and asking children how many parts they heard. Stress and elongate the syllables. For example, say and clap

> kick
> How many parts in the word? Clap it out. (one)

Clap and say

> kickball
> How many parts in that word? Clap it out. (two)
> Kick–ball. One, two.

Stress and elongate the syllables when presenting the compound words provided in Add-It-On.

PLAY **Find-the-Little-Words.**

Children listen for little words within compound words of the text. Stress and elongate syllables when presenting the word. For example,

> kickball
> Can you hear any little words in *kickball*? (kick, ball)
> That's right. *Kick* is a little word in *kickball*.
> *Ball* is another word in *kickball*.

Continue with compound words provided in Add-It-On.

PLAY **Leave-It-Out.**

Children say a compound word, then leave out the beginning or final part to create a smaller word. For example, demonstrate this way:

> Say *ballgame*.
> Now say *ballgame* but leave out *game*.
> What little word is left? (ball)

Then say

> Now say *ballgame* but leave out *ball*.
> What little word is left? (game)

Continue with the compound words provided in Add-It-On.

PLAY **Add-It-On.**

Children put two syllables together to make a two-syllable word. For example,

> Say *ball*.
> Now say *ball* and add *game*.
> What bigger word can you make? (ballgame)

Then reverse the order in which the words are presented. For example,

> Put *game* at the end of *ball*. What word do you have? (ballgame)

Continue with the compound words provided.

PLAY **Turn-It-Around.**

Children reverse the parts of the compound word *ballgame*, which they previously analyzed and synthesized.

> Put the word *game* at the beginning of *ball*.
> What word do you have then? (gameball)
> What was it before we turned it around? (ballgame)

PLAY **Switch-It.**

Children delete part of a compound word and exchange it with another part to make a new word. Prompt with cues as necessary. For example,

> Say *pinstripe.*
> Now say *pinstripe,* only take out *stripe* and put in *ball.*
> What new word can you make? (pinball)

Some word exchanges include

> Kickball: Switch *kick* with *base* (baseball).
> Bathtub: Switch *tub* with *room* (bathroom).
> Ballgame: Switch *game* with *room* (ballroom).
> Milkshake: Switch *milk* with *hand* (handshake).
> Downright: Switch *down* with *all* (alright).
> Undercooked: Switch *under* with *over* (overcooked).
> Overdone: Switch *over* with *under* (underdone).
> Tablecloth: Switch *cloth* with *spoon* (tablespoon).
> Herringbone: Switch *herring* with *dog* (dogbone).

The following games continue to advance through the spectrum of phonological awareness levels to the phoneme level.

PLAY **Say-It-Until-You-Hear-It.**

Children synthesize one-syllable words divided into onset-rime. Present the word with a clear pause between the onset and rime. Demonstrate how to elongate the parts to blend them together, saying them a little quicker each time until they are readily identified. Provide scaffolding until children are ready to do it on their own. For example, say

> Put these two parts together: *f–un.*
> Say it until you hear it. *Fffff . . . un. Fff . . . un. Fun.*

Continue with these words from the text beginning with a continuous single sound:

l-oose	w-ink	c-up
h-ot	c-ow	t-all
l-ean	t-an	

Then demonstrate how to synthesize one-syllable words divided into onset-rime, beginning with a two-consonant cluster, as in

dr-ink (drink)	sm-all (small)	bl-ue (blue)
gr-ay (gray)	gr-een (green)	cl-ean (clean)
bl-ack (black)	fl-at (flat)	
br-ight (bright)	sm-ooth (smooth)	

Once this level is achieved, children can continue segmenting, blending, and changing individual phonemes in the words to create new words.

PLAY **Roll-It-Out.**

Children synthesize a C-V-C word by blending each of its phonemes. Demonstrate by elongating the phonemes and blending them in shorter and shorter sequences until children can identify the word. For example, say

> f-u-n
> What's the word? Roll it out. *Fffff . . . uuu . . . nnn. Fun.*

Once children are successful, present each of the phonemes separately so they can "roll them out" on their own, in shorter and shorter sequences, to find the word. Use the one-syllable C-V-C word list provided.

PLAY **Break-It-Up.**

Children analyze one-syllable C-V-C words in order to identify the beginning, middle, and ending sounds. Begin activities with initial sounds, and then proceed to middle, and ending sounds. For an example on how to demonstrate finding the middle sound in *fun,* ask

> What's the sound in the middle of *fun?*
> Break it up: *Fff . . . -uuu . . . - nnn . . . f-u-n.*
> *ŭ* is the sound in the middle of *fun.*

Continue to present one-syllable C-V-C words provided above so children can break them up and identify the sounds in each of the positions.

In the last stage of the game, children identify all the sounds in the word. Demonstrate how to elongate the sounds and then break them up in order to identify each one. For example, ask

> What are all the sounds in the word *fun?*
> Roll it out and break it up: *Ffff . . . -uuu . . . -nn . . . F-u-n.*
> *F-ŭ-n* are all the sounds in *fun.*

Note: For an additional list of words, shorten the adjectives with *-y* endings to form one-syllable words, such as *hair, leak,* and *yum.*

Note: Read also *A Mink, a Fink, A Skating Rink: What Is a Noun?* and *To Root, to Toot, to Parachute: What Is a Verb?* by the same author. Also by the same author, books on puns: *It Looks a Lot Like Reindeer* and *Jamaica Sandwich?*

The Hallo-wiener

by Dav Pilkey
New York: Scholastic, 1995

Suggested Grade and Interest Level: 1 through 4

Topic Explorations: Animals, Dogs; Holidays, Halloween

Skill Builders:

Vocabulary	Grammar and syntax
Semantics	Pronouns, personal and possessive
Prepositions	Tenses, present and past
Homonyms	

Synopsis: Oscar the Wiener Dog, "half-a-dog tall and one-and-a-half dogs long," doesn't like it when the other dogs make fun of him. Even his mother calls him her little Vienna sausage. When Halloween comes, Oscar is looking forward to all the fun, especially dressing up for trick-or-treating. Excitedly he opens the box in which his mother has put his costume and discovers a giant hotdog bun with a big yellow ribbon of mustard down the center. Not wishing to hurt his mother's feelings, he wears the silly costume and is made fun of most of the night until he rescues the other dogs from some masquerading cats. That's when the other dogs change his nickname to Hero Sandwich. This is a delightful Halloween book that children will thoroughly enjoy.

Method: Before the read-aloud, lead into the story with discussions of Halloween activities. Then present the book's cover with the illustration of the dachshund inside the giant hotdog looking glum while other dogs are laughing. Have children infer what the story is about.

During the read-aloud, pause briefly, if appropriate, to point out details in the illustrations, like the trick-or-treat bag dangling from Oscar's tail when he shows up on Halloween night. Use humor to elicit and shape grammar and syntax structures from the children's responses. For example, at doggy school, one pupil writes on the board, "I will not sniff my neighbor." Ask the children to explain why he is writing on the chalkboard (i.e., "He was sniffing dogs."). Talk about the picture of Oscar on the wall at his house and ask why it was framed in three parts, with the longest part in the middle (Oscar is too long to get into one picture). Talk about what gave the monster away ("Oscar saw the cat paws.").

For prepositions, point out the locator words (such as *inside, beside, along, within, by,* etc.) in the text and illustrations and encourage children to use them in their constructions.

After the read-aloud, reread the pages that use the puns in the text to develop vocabulary and comprehension of homonyms. For instance, when Oscar shows up in his Halloween costume, the text reads, "Then Oscar showed up, looking quite frank." Ask children to explain why the words are funny. Discuss the meaning of the word *frankfurter.* Also discuss why Oscar's name was changed to Hero Sandwich. What is a hero? What is a hero sandwich? Why is it funny to change his name?

Harriet and the Promised Land

by Jacob Lawrence
New York: Simon & Schuster, 1968, 1993

Suggested Grade and Interest Level: 3 through 5

Topic Explorations: Art, artists, and architecture; Creativity; Culture and history, African and African American; History, American; Journeys

Skill Builders:

Vocabulary	Grammar and syntax	Language literacy
Semantics	Past tense	Drawing inferences
Attributes	Advanced syntactic structures	Answering *why* questions
		Discussion

Synopsis: The masterful paintings in this book are done by a celebrated American artist whose work is exhibited in museums around the world. Accompanying them are short verses that tell the story of Harriet Tubman, the slave who led people to freedom.

Method: This is an excellent book to use in conjunction with a classroom history lesson on the Civil War. On each page, pause to reflect on the symbolism the artist uses to convey his message. For example, look at Harriet scrubbing the floor. Why did the artist exaggerate the floor and her hand over the rag? Why is her head down, with her face hidden from view?

Point out the extraordinary nature of the book in that the illustrations are a series of paintings by a great American artist known for painting in a series of works. Talk about an artist's perspective and the qualities that distinguish great art. Talk about how artists can often "tell" a story with pictures rather than words and create feelings in people that can help them understand the complexities of a situation.

To teach advanced syntactic structures, have students create sentences based on the phrases of the verse. For instance, when young Harriet holds the infant in her arms, use the verse and painting to form sentences such as

> Harriet had to sweep.
> Harriet had to rock her master's baby to sleep.
> Harriet had to sweep and rock her master's baby to sleep.
> Although Harriet was a child, she had to sweep and rock her master's baby to sleep.
> When Harriet was a child, she had to sweep and take care of her master's baby.

Extended Activities: Brainstorm attributes to describe Harriet Tubman. A few suggestions include *brave, inspired, intelligent, focused,* and *determined.* Have students give examples to justify why they selected each word. Ask students what else they want to know about Tubman's experiences as a child or as an adult.

Break into learning groups. Have students put together a list of questions they would ask if they could interview Harriet Tubman. (Read also *Aunt Harriet's Underground Railroad in the Sky.*) You may choose to allow students time to research their questions in the library.

Each group can select a student to play the role of Harriet Tubman. Then pretend to go back in time in a time machine. Have Ms. Tubman answer the students' questions based on knowledge gained in other readings and awareness of the conditions at that time. Ask groups to present their interviews to the class.

Harry and the Terrible Whatzit

by Dick Gackenbach
New York: Clarion, 1977, 1979, 1984

Suggested Grade and Interest Level: 1 through 3

Skill Builders:

Vocabulary	Grammar and syntax	Language literacy
Prepositions	Past tense	Problem solving
		Drawing inferences

Synopsis: Harry confronts his fears of a monster and finds a "double-headed, three-clawed, six-toed, long-horned Whatzit." This story is nice for all types of language structuring as well as stimulating conversation about children's fears.

Method: Some past-tense sentences to model and shape include

He waited by the door.	He saw the Whatzit.	He smacked the Whatzit.
The Whatzit shrank.	It climbed on the washer.	He hit it.
He pulled its tail.	He chased it away.	He found her glasses.
He looked outside.		

Some prepositions to model and elicit are

in	inside	behind
on	outside	beside

Adjectives to model and elicit include

> dark and damp
> bright (sunlight)
> awful (yell)

For drawing inferences, direct children's attention to the story told in the illustrations. Ask what Harry might be thinking and track the change in his feelings and behavior. Why is the Whatzit hiding behind the furnace? What do you think the monster is afraid of? What do you think the Whatzit will do after it leaves Harry's house? For problem solving, ask children to state the problem in the story. What did Harry do to solve his problem?

Harry the Dirty Dog

by Gene Zion
New York: Harper & Row, 1956, 1976

Suggested Grade and Interest Level: 1 through 3

Topic Explorations: Community; Pets

Skill Builders:

Language literacy	**Articulation, *H* and *R***
Relating personal experiences	**Voice**
Storytelling	
Discussion	

Synopsis: Harry the dog gets so dirty in his adventures that even his own family doesn't recognize him.

Method: Before the read-aloud, encourage children to relate some of their own stories about giving their dogs a bath. Do their dogs like being given a bath? When working on articulation, use the words listed below in activities that focus on auditory bombardment of the *R* sound.

During the read-aloud, pause to have the children imitate target words and phrases in the story for the following words:

bury	run away	crawled through the fence
dirty	dirtier	dirtiest
tired and hungry	wonder	really
ran away tricks	clever	strange
rolled over	corner of the garden	wonderful
scrubbing brush	under pillow	girl and her father

After the read-aloud, encourage children to relate the story to their own experiences. Ask questions such as

> What kind of dog is Harry? What makes you think so?
> Why do you think he likes to get dirty?
> What are some ways you like to get dirty?
> What happens when you get dirty?
> What other animals do you know that like to get dirty?
> What does Harry do that shows he's a smart dog?
> What does your pet do that shows it's smart?

For voice and articulation of *H,* have students practice initiating airflow prior to phonation on the word *Harry.* Use a carrier phrase to have children practice gradually increasing the length of utterance while maintaining vocal quality. Pause during the read-aloud to allow a child to fill in the dog's name.

Extended Activity: Encourage students to make up a similar story about "Harriet the Messy Mouse" or "Rita the Klutzy Cat." What would that story be about? Would she have adventures similar to Harry's? Make a game out of imagining what some of them might be. Then take the information and construct a story with all the essential story grammar elements.

Note: Read also *No Roses for Harry* and *Harry by the Sea* by the same author.

Here Come the Aliens!

by Colin McNaughton
Cambridge, MA: Candlewick Press, 1995

Suggested Grade and Interest Level: 1 through 4

Topic Explorations: Humor; Outer space

Skill Builders:

Vocabulary	Grammar and syntax	Articulation, *L* and *S*
Attributes	Past tense	

Synopsis: A group of colorful, warty-looking aliens are on their way to Earth, out to conquer the human race. In rhyming text, the story is told about these unique looking characters whose trip is cut short before they land. Finding something floating in space, they pick it up and are frightened to see a group of Earth children making goofy faces at them. The order is issued—"Fleet Retreat!!!"—and the aliens are gone. A good book to motivate the young sci-fi set.

Method: Before the read-aloud, discuss the various aliens on the cover and elicit picture descriptions, including colors, sizes, shapes, and distinguishing features. Also elicit descriptions of the outer space scene on the cover.

During the read-aloud, pause to have children fill in the predictable, repetitive text, "The aliens are coming."

After the read-aloud, go back over the pages, read the verse beneath the illustrations, and encourage children to describe the aliens using their own words. For example,

> The green-warted alien is an admiral with a jacket full of medals and a nose like a big pickle.
> The first mate is a yellow alien with puffs of gasses coming out of his head and sides wearing a red belt and star buckle.

When pages tell what the aliens do, structure sentences with tenses found in the text. For example,

> The aliens slobbered during their lunch.
> The aliens gobbled their disgusting food at lunch.
> The aliens had no table manners at lunch.

For articulation of *L,* allow children to repeat the repetitive text, "The aliens are coming," on each double-page spread. Also pause for repetition of the text, heavily loaded with *L* words. For articulation of *S,* simply read and discuss the text, which is heavily loaded with the target sound.

Hester

by Byron Barton
New York: Greenwillow Books, 1975

Suggested Grade and Interest Level: 1 through 4

Topic Exploration: Holidays, Halloween

Skill Builders:
Grammar and syntax	**Fluency**
Possessive pronouns	**Voice**
Articulation—*H, –er,* and *R*	

Synopsis: Here's a perfect Halloween tale. Follow Hester the alligator on her visit to a very spooky place to see some very spooky creatures and take a very spooky ride.

Method: To elicit pronouns, when the text reads, "This is my favorite room," ask

> Whose room is it?
> Whose clothes are they?
> Whose hat is it?
> Whose broom is it?

For articulation of *R*, read the text, stressing the *R* sounds. Ask questions to elicit target words such as

arrived	monsters
crash	party
favorite	ride
friends	room
Hester	trick or treat
hurried	wonderful

For voice and articulation of *H,* have children practice initiating the airstream prior to phonation on the words *Hester, her,* and *Halloween.* Pause in the reading of the text to elicit answers to the questions listed above.

For fluency, practice initiating and maintaining airflow during production of the same three words. Gradually increase the length of utterance the child can produce with uninterrupted airflow.

Hey, Al

by Arthur Yorinks
New York: Farrar, Straus & Giroux, 1986

Suggested Grade and Interest Level: 3 through 5

Topic Explorations: Careers; Journeys; Pets

Skill Builders:
Vocabulary	**Language literacy**	Drawing inferences
Semantics	Predicting	Answering *why* questions
Idioms	Sequencing	Discussion

Synopsis: Al and his dog, Eddie, live in a little one-room apartment on New York's West Side. Discontented with their life and its struggles, they complain bitterly. Out of the blue, a huge, colorful bird presents itself at their window, ready to change their fortunes. Ferried to a gorgeous island in the sky, they soon discover that the grass is just a little too green in paradise.

Method: Interact by posing questions about what might happen next and why the two become disenchanted on the island. When asking *why* questions, encourage students to express the information in meaningful relationships. For example,

> Q: Why was Al sulking in his room?
> A: Al was sulking in his room because he didn't think his life was exciting, and he felt like he was
> in a rut.

After the read-aloud, have students retell the story. Use the illustrations to help sequence events, if necessary. Discuss situations in the children's own lives that are similar to Al's.

> How is Al like someone you know?
> What would you do if you were Al?
> How many ways could Al look positively upon his life and his situation?

Discuss the meaning of these idioms in the text: "Ripe fruit soon spoils" and "Paradise lost is sometimes heaven found." Also discuss the meaning of the cliché, "The grass is always greener on the other side of the fence." Discuss how the cliché applies to the story of Al and Eddie.

Hey! Get Off Our Train

by John Burningham
New York: Crown, 1989, 1990

Suggested Grade and Interest Level: 1 through 3

Topic Explorations: Animals, Endangered; Conservation; Journeys; Trains; Transportation

Skill Builders:

Vocabulary	Grammar and syntax	Articulation, *H*
Semantics	Tenses, present and future	Voice
Categories	Language literacy	
	Predicting	

Synopsis: At bedtime, a young boy takes a trip on board his train and rescues many endangered animals. The repetitive pattern of animals wanting to come on board enables frequent use of prediction skills.

Method: Before the read-aloud, ask children to say what they know about endangered animals. What does *endangered* mean? Ask whether they can name any animals they know are endangered. Present the book's cover and suggest they will soon discover more.

For tenses, pause to model or shape target structures. Many of the wordless illustrations depict actions. Interact by asking questions that require responses in the present and future tenses. Also ask students to rephrase each animal's explanation of why it wants to board the train (e.g., a hunter will shoot the polar bear for its fur. People will pollute the water, so the seal will have nothing left to eat.).

Elicit predictions about the next animal that will want to come aboard. After the characters yell, "Hey! Get off our train," elicit predictions about why the animal wants to get on. After the animal explains its endangered status, make predictions about what will happen next. Will the other characters let it on board? Why do you think so?

Categorize these and other animals by their endangered status, habitat, and species.

For voice and articulation of *H*, practice onset of air prior to phonation with the word *hey*. Pause in the reading to allow the child to gradually increase repetition of the repetitive words, "Hey, get off our train."

Hiccup

by Mercer Mayer
New York: Dial Books for Young Readers, 1976

Suggested Grade and Interest Level: 1 through 3

Skill Builders:

Grammar and syntax	**Language literacy**	**Articulation, *H***
Personal pronouns	Relating personal experiences	**Voice**
	Predicting	
	Storytelling	
	Drawing inferences	

Synopsis: In this wordless book, a gentleman hippo invites a lady friend for a row in his boat. His not-so-gentlemanly attempts to stop her hiccups teach that turnabout is fair play and that it's a good idea to remember the golden rule.

Method: Use the lady and gentleman hippo characters to elicit "he" and "she" and the sequence of events to predict further mishaps. Relate personal experiences of having the hiccups and what measures were or might have been taken to overcome them. Ask the children to draw inferences about the characters and their feelings from their actions. Also discuss how people may not always be aware of how their actions affect others. Ask how we can make others aware of the effects of their actions.

For voice and articulation of *H*, practice onset of air prior to phonation with the word *hiccup*. Pause in the telling of the story to allow the child to fill in the lady hippo's dialog—which is "hiccup." Have the child gradually increase the length of utterance while maintaining vocal quality.

Home Run

by Robert Burleigh
San Diego, CA: Silver Whistle, Harcourt Brace, 1998

Suggested Grade and Interest Level: 3 through 5

Topic Explorations: Baseball; Famous people, Heroes

Skill Builders:

Vocabulary	**Grammar and syntax**	**Language literacy**
Semantics	Advanced syntactic structures	Drawing inferences
Similes and metaphors		Retelling events
Morphological units		Discussion

Synopsis: This is a poetic account of one of the world's greatest sports figures, the legendary Babe Ruth. The verses use imagery and figurative language to describe how the mighty player prepares to hit a home run. On each page is superimposed a vintage-style baseball card with another short story included on it. Interesting and little-known facts are presented, not only about his hitting but also about his excellent pitching record and his legendary breakfasts, which "might include a dozen eggs and half a loaf of toast."

Method: Before the reading, elicit background information on the game of baseball and Babe Ruth. Provide meaning and establish connections to the story through personal experiences and knowledge of such players as Barry Bonds and Mark McGwire.

During the reading, pause briefly to define a word, leaving interaction to a minimum so listeners gain a sense of the language used in the poetic text. Point out the use of metaphors, such as in the first line of the following verses:

> The ball cracks off the bat.
> It soars far up in the air
> As it passes first base.
> Going, going.

Point out the "sound" reference in the use of the word *cracks*. Help children hear and visualize the scene. Establish the emotional connection of the game and with the player himself.

Next, do a picture walk-through and pause to read the information on the baseball cards. Ask comprehension questions and hold discussions on facts such as how the baseball great came to be called "Babe." After a discussion, use the facts to encourage children to rephrase and retell the events.

For drawing inferences, reread the text to discuss the following:

> The fans crane their necks to follow
> But Babe already knows.
> The perfectness.
> The feeling.
> The boy-fire inside the body of a man.

Ask children to think about what the author is saying and how he chooses his words to express what Babe feels as he hits the ball. Draw inferences about what it is that Babe "already knows." How does Babe know he will hit a home run? Provide meaning through personal connections. Talk about what the author is referring to when he uses the word *perfectness*.

To work on morphological units and metalinguistic awareness, talk about the syllables in the word *perfectness*. Identify the root word and the suffix. Ask or demonstrate how many words can be generated from the word *perfect* (e.g., *perfectly, perfected, perfectedly, perfecter, imperfect, imperfectable,* and *imperfection*). Talk about the word's relationship with other words such as *complete* and *unique*. Generate lists of words that can be combined with the suffix *-ness* (e.g., *like, sad, happy, quiet, loud, neat, crooked, tart,* etc.). Use the word in combination with a unit on U.S. government while discussing the U.S. Constitution's words, "In order to form a more perfect union."

Discuss the similes used and draw inferences in other lines of text, such as

> Then it is as it should be.
> Smooth as silk,
> Easy as air on the face,
> Right as falling water.

Encourage students to use the similes as they generate advanced syntactic structures. Assist students by starting sentences with an adverbial phrase. Have them finish the sentence with a simile, such as

When Babe Ruth hit the ball with the bat *it was as smooth as silk.*
When Babe Ruth hit a home run *it felt as right as falling water.*
When Babe Ruth felt the ball hit the bat *it was as easy as air on the face.*

Support sentence constructions with scaffolding and gradually withdraw as children's mastery increases.

I Read Signs

by Tana Hoban
New York: Greenwillow Books, 1983

Suggested Grade and Interest Level: 1 through 5

Topic Exploration: Community

Skill Builders:

Vocabulary	Language literacy
Semantics	Relating personal experiences

Synopsis: A series of photographs shows how traffic signs and signals, street signs, and signboards convey meaning in our culture. This is also a good book to use with students who are developmentally delayed.

Method: This book is excellent for young children and students with developmental disabilities. Present the book and talk about what the signs mean and children's experiences seeing these signs. Also talk about hypothetical situations and contexts in which children might observe each sign and why understanding it would be important.

Extended Activity: Take a walk around the community with the class. Observe what signs are present and what they tell about the community. Observe the traffic signs. Are any of them similar to the ones in the book? Look at the street signs. What do they tell us and why are they necessary? Observe store signs. Why are they important? Observe signs on people's houses, such as "For Sale" signs and the numbers on the house or sidewalk that tell the address. Upon your return, have children recall all the various signs and have a discussion about why it's important to look at signs in the community.

I Wish I Were a Butterfly

by James Howe
San Diego, CA: Harcourt Brace Jovanovich, 1987

Suggested Grade and Interest Level: 1 through 3

Topic Explorations: Feelings; Friendship; Insects and spiders; Self-esteem

Skill Builders:

Vocabulary	Grammar and syntax	Language literacy
Attributes	Advanced syntactic structures	Cause-and-effect relationships
Antonyms		Problem solving
		Drawing inferences

GRADES 1-5

Synopsis: The author acknowledges a group of Ohio schoolchildren for giving him the idea for this tale. A cricket who believes he is ugly wants to be a beautiful butterfly. With the help of a wise spider, he learns where beauty comes from. Only then does he begin to love himself and others and come to know how special he is.

Method: Before the read-aloud, ask the children what they know about crickets. Elicit many descriptions and stories about different experiences. Tell the children that the story you will read is the story of a cricket and introduce the book's cover. Based on what they know of crickets, ask children to predict what the story will be about.

For problem solving, pause during the read-aloud to identify the problem. What facts can be stated about it? (E.g., The cricket doesn't want to come outside. He doesn't want to make music. He doesn't want to be a cricket.) Identify how the cricket is trying to solve his problem. Ask students whether they have better ideas for how the cricket might come to feel good about himself.

For cause-and-effect relationships, pause to ask what happened to the cricket because of how he felt about himself. What happened that finally caused him to feel good? How did that happen? What effect did the spider's friendship have on the cricket?

After the read-aloud, assist children in drawing inferences about the story by talking about the cricket's feelings based on his actions and thoughts. Talk about the frog who told the cricket he was an ugly creature. What might have caused the frog to say that? When the spider told him he was beautiful and the cricket looked at his reflection, "his ugliness began to fade away." What does this mean? Was he really ugly? To whom? Who is most important in the way we feel about ourselves?

For advanced syntactic structures, assist children in creating the beginnings of sentences with subordinate clauses, such as

> If I were a cricket, I'd be happy _____. (with my musical voice)
> If I were a spider, I'd be happy _____. (with my delicate webs)
> If I were a butterfly, I'd be happy _____. (with my beautiful wings)

For attributes and antonyms, have children describe the different insects presented in the pictures. What words can they use to describe the dragonfly? The glowworm? The ladybug? Can they think of antonyms for these words? For example, *beautiful/ugly, colorful/dull, quiet/loud,* and *melodic/monotonous.*

If a Bus Could Talk: The Story of Rosa Parks

by Faith Ringgold
New York: Simon & Schuster Books for Young Readers, 1999

Suggested Grade and Interest Level: 1 through 5

Topic Explorations: Culture and history, African and African American; Famous people, Heroes; History, American; Holidays, Martin Luther King Jr. Day

Skill Builders:

Vocabulary	Grammar and syntax	Language literacy
Semantics	Advanced syntactic structures	Cause-and-effect relationships
Beginning concepts		
Attributes		

Synopsis: The biography of the famous African American woman is set into a story about a girl named Marcie who steps onto a bus that can talk. The bus tells her she is riding on the Rosa Parks Bus, named for the woman who changed the course of American history when she wouldn't give up her bus seat to a White man in 1955. The voice explains how Rosa Park's actions led to a 381-day boycott in Montgomery, Alabama; the Montgomery Bus Boycott; and ultimately the beginning of Martin Luther King Jr.'s leadership in the civil rights movement. At the end of Marcie's ride, she meets Rosa Parks herself at a birthday party with several distinguished guests. This is a wonderful book to present in January for Martin Luther King Jr. Day. Ringgold delivers Parks's story as a life lived with pride, conviction, and dignity.

Note: Although the book has been criticized by some reviewers as being too gimmicky and thereby not doing justice to the incredible life of Rosa Parks, most agree that Ringgold's vividly colored, richly textured acrylic paintings are noteworthy. For children with language-learning disabilities, there is value in these bold illustrations and the story-within-a-story concept, as it better enables them to understand the concept of time and past events, the fictional story of Marcie, and the reality of Mrs. Rosa Parks. Older children will relate to interesting information about her life, including her work as a community activist in Detroit with a congressman helping the homeless find housing, jobs, and services and her bronze statue at the Smithsonian Institute.

Method: Before the read-aloud, access children's background knowledge about Rosa Parks. Talk about what the children already know of this hero in American history. Talk about the concept of freedom for all Americans and help enable children to grasp a sense of history and what went on before this day and time.

During the read-aloud, pause to clarify words, relate them to the children's own lives, and expand on the text where necessary. Shape or model morphosyntactic structures as children talk about the story and illustrations.

After the read-aloud, discuss the concepts of *dignity, freedom, prejudice, courage,* and *consequences.* The book tells about the prejudice of the South and makes clear what consequences were in store for Mrs. Parks when she refused to give up her seat. Illustrate her bravery by talking of something equivalent, such as facing an enemy and knowing the consequences, so that children can relate and fully understand what this American hero did. Ask children to tell what this shows about Rosa Parks's character.

Ask children to give Mrs. Parks qualities or attributes. Make sentences with the words. Older students can use linking words such as *because* and *when* in order to link attributes with information about her life. Some examples include

> Mrs. Parks was brave (courageous) *because* she did not give up her seat on the bus.
> Rosa Parks was dignified *when* she refused to give up her seat.
> Rosa Parks was caring (compassionate) *because* she helped people find houses and jobs.

Then vary the syntactic structure, as in

> *Because* she believed in herself, Rosa Parks had dignity.
> *When* she didn't give up her seat on the bus, Rosa Parks showed courage.
> *When* she didn't give up her seat, Rosa Parks knew the consequences of her refusal.

If You Give a Mouse a Cookie

by Laura Numeroff
New York: Harper & Row, 1985

Suggested Grade and Interest Level: 1 through 3

Skill Builders:

Vocabulary	Grammar and syntax	Language literacy
Associations	Tenses, present and future	Predicting
	Advanced syntactic structures	Sequencing
		Storytelling

Synopsis: Children love this story about a demanding little mouse that makes a series of requests after a boy gives him a cookie. In fact, Californians voted it one of their favorites, for which it won the Young Reader's Medal.

Method: Interact with the children, using present progressive tense to discuss what the mouse is doing. Then go back over the story and model or shape future-tense sentences. For example,

> Q: What will he do when you give him the milk?
> A: He'll ask for a straw.
> Q: What will he do when he looks in the mirror?
> A: He'll ask for some scissors.

For advanced syntactic structures, model and shape sentences with connective phrases using the words *if* and *then*, such as

> *If* you give a mouse a glass of milk, *then* he's going to ask for a straw.
> *If* you give a dog a biscuit, *then* it's going to want another one to go with it.
> *If* you want to go outside, *then* you're going to need a jacket.

For sequencing, close the book and see whether the children can remember the series of events that resulted from giving the mouse a cookie.

Extended Activity: Help children make up their own stories using the same format. For example, have children brainstorm things that go with a flower (such as *bees, water, scent,* and *vase*). Write the ideas on the board. Then have children incorporate this list of ideas into a story that begins, "If you give an opossum a flower, she'll . . ." or "If you give a hippo a suitcase he'll . . ." or any other creative starters you or the children may offer.

Note: Read also *If You Give a Moose a Muffin, If You Give a Pig a Pancake,* and *If You Take a Mouse to the Movies,* all by the same author.

This book is also available in a Spanish version, titled *Si le das una galletita a un raton,* along with *Si llevas un raton al cine.*

Iktomi and the Boulder

Retold by Paul Goble
New York: Orchard Books, 1988

Suggested Grade and Interest Level:	2 through 5	

Topic Explorations: Folklore, Native American; Humor; Trickster tales

Skill Builders:

Language literacy		
Storytelling	Drawing inferences	**Articulation, *R* and *-er***
Verbal expression	Point of view	

Synopsis: The Indian trickster Iktomi incurs the wrath of a huge boulder when he takes away the gift he gave to it. The boulder pins him by rolling onto his legs, and all the animals that try to help cannot push it off. When the bats appear, Iktomi enrages them by telling them that the boulder "has been saying rude things" about them. The bats attack the boulder and break it into little chips of rock. The legend says that's why bats have flattened faces and why there are rocks scattered all over the Great Plains.

Method: Iktomi stories are excellent for interaction as they are strongly rooted in the oral tradition from which the stories came. Where the text changes to italics, students are invited to comment on Iktomi's words, thoughts, and deeds. The small text that represents Iktomi's thoughts can be read by a student, especially one who is practicing carryover of articulation skills.

Ask students to draw inferences about what kind of man Iktomi is based on his thoughts (such as, "I'm looking my very best today" and "I'll look great at the dance tonight"). Also have them draw inferences about what Iktomi really means when he tells the bats that the boulder has been saying rude things about them.

Discuss from whose point of view the story is told. Does the point of view change? What makes the students think so?

For articulation, use the text heavily loaded with *R* and *–er* sounds to elicit target structures.

Extended Activity: Create a reader's theater by having several participants re-create the roles of Iktomi and the animals, using the book as a guide. Drape a blanket over a beanbag chair to represent the rock. Have the audience tell the story and the Iktomi character perform the actions and repeat the dialog, both internal and external. Prompt the actors to enhance their performances with facial gestures and body language, especially Iktomi, the mischiefmaker who is so full of himself.

For a small group, do a dramatic retelling of the story with one member being the storyteller and the others creating the dialog of Iktomi and the animals.

Note: Be sure to read and enjoy *Iktomi and the Berries* and *Iktomi and the Buffalo Skull* by the same author.

Imogene's Antlers

by David Small
New York: Dragonfly Books, 1985

Suggested Grade and Interest Level:　1 through 4

Topic Explorations:　Daily activities; Family relationships; Humor; Self-esteem

Skill Builders:

Vocabulary	Grammar and syntax	Language literacy
Semantics	Tenses—present, past, and future	Storytelling
Prepositions	Question structures	
Homonyms (multiple meanings)		

Synopsis: One day Imogene wakes up and finds she had grown antlers—very, very big antlers. And life with antlers is not exactly easy. First she has to get out of her bedroom door and down the stairs. Then she has to deal with her mother fainting all the time. She must also listen to her brother announce that she has turned into a rare form of miniature elk. But then, her antlers do come in handy when she needs a clothesline to dry the clothes and holders for all of the cook's doughnuts. Antlers don't seem to phase the delightful, self-accepting Imogene, although not so with her mother. She has the answer, though: Call the milliner to make a hat to disguise them. What a hat it is! With a kiss goodnight she goes to bed, and the next morning the antlers are surprisingly gone. But that's not the end. Imogene only trades her antlers in for another problem!

Method: Before the read-aloud, present the cover and after the laughter subsides, ask the children to explain what is funny about Imogene having antlers. How did she get her head out the window, and what might life be like with a big set of antlers on your head?

During the read-aloud, because the text is brief and allows for plenty of embellishing from the pictures, pause occasionally to allow the children to explain in more detail what is happening to Imogene. For instance, in getting dressed, her slip gets hung up on one of the extensions. In getting down the stairs, she decides to go by the way of the banister (while the cat takes to walking), only to get hung up (literally) in the chandelier. For increasing grammar and syntax skills, use the opportunity for interaction to shape target grammatical structures.

After the read-aloud, do a picture walk-through and increase vocabulary comprehension and expression by talking about the words of the text. Use the words in context. What is a milliner? What did her brother do when he "consulted the encyclopedia"? What does it mean when the principal has no advice to give? What is *advice*? Do the children have advice to give Imogene? Ask the children to use the word in a sentence. Start the sentence with, "The advice I would give Imogene would be to _____."

To teach question formations, have students ask each other, "What advice would you give to Imogene?"

Discuss the multiple meanings of the word *deck,* such as an open platform, "on deck" (meaning "next to bat" in baseball), and "decked out." Mrs. Perkins, the cook, "decked her out" (Imogene) with more doughnuts. What does it mean to be "decked out" (to make something fancy)? What else can be decked out? A person in their dress-up clothes and jewelry? A house at Christmas time? Start a sentence with, "Imogene was all decked out in her _____" and have the children finish the sentence (fancy antlers, antlers full of doughnuts).

To teach storytelling skills, a necessary skill for literacy, discuss the story grammars. For example,

> Who was the story about? (Imogene and her family)
> Where did it take place? (Imogene's house)
> When? (On Thursday)
> What happened to start the story off? (Imogene woke up with antlers.)
> How did the character(s) feel about it? (She feels OK about it. She has fun with them, but her mother is so upset she faints.)
> What did the character do to solve her problem? (Because her mother was the one who had the problem with the antlers [she continually fainted], her mother tried to solve it by calling a milliner to make her a hat.)
> What was the result? (The antlers didn't go away.)
> What was the next thing the character did? (She went to bed.)
> What was the result? (She woke up in the morning and her antlers were gone.)
> How did the story end? (She went downstairs without her antlers—only she had grown a tail of peacock feathers this time.)
> How did the characters feel then? (Everyone was shocked, including the milliner, but Imogene didn't seem to mind.)

Have students take turns retelling the story, prompting them with features in the illustrations and providing scaffolding as necessary. Encourage use of words *and, then, so,* and *because.*

After the story has been retold, ask a question to provide feedback to the child, such as, "What might you do if you had antlers?" Any response is acceptable, because the story is lighthearted.

The Important Book

by Margaret Wise Brown
New York: Harper & Row, 1949

Suggested Grade and Interest Level: 1 through 2

Topic Exploration: Self-esteem

Skill Builders:

Vocabulary	**Language literacy**
Semantics	Relating personal experiences
Categories	Verbal expression
Associations	

Synopsis: Here's a classic that teaches children how to describe a familiar word from the world of the senses. For example,

The important thing about a shoe is that you put your foot in it. You walk in it, and you take it off at night, and it's warm when you take it off. But the important thing about a shoe is that you put your foot in it.

Method: Read and interact about each definition presented. Talk about the children's own experiences. Ask the children to make up their own definitions. For example, "Is there anything else that's important about a shoe?" Then use the same format to define additional words. What's the important thing about a hamburger? A book? Roller skates? A leprechaun?

Introduce categories by naming types of shoes or things that go on your feet (sandals, slippers, boots, etc.). Do the same for the other words that are defined (e.g., "An apple is a fruit. What other kinds of fruit are there?").

For associations, ask children to think of things that go with each pictured item. For example, what goes with an apple? (tree, teacher, worm, etc.)

Extended Activity: Make books entitled "The Important Thing About Me." Have each child fold a piece of paper lengthwise and write the title on the cover. Children can color the covers if they choose. Inside, have each one draw a self-portrait and write a sentence or more about what they value in themselves. This activity also makes a nice gift for Mother's Day or Father's Day. Have children make books entitled "The Important Thing About My Mom (or Dad)."

In the Haunted House

by Eve Bunting
New York: Clarion Books, 1990

Suggested Grade and Interest Level: 1 through 3

Topic Exploration: Holidays, Halloween

Skill Builders:

Vocabulary	**Language literacy**
Prepositions	Sequencing
Grammar and syntax	**Phonological awareness**
Past tense	

Synopsis: A walk inside a haunted house reveals all sorts of scary features and creatures. At the end of the story, a girl and her father come out of what is now recognized as a Halloween House. The text is in a fun, quick-paced rhyming verse.

Method: Before the read-aloud, have children relate personal stories about Halloween houses.

During the read-aloud, allow children to experience the story so that the flow of the text, the rhythm and rhyme, is not interrupted.

After the read-aloud, go back over the text and ask children to tell the story by walking through the Halloween house just as the girl and her father did. Use their feet shown in each illustration to sequence the sights that they saw. Include connecting words such as *then they . . . next they . . .* and *so they. . . .*

For grammar and syntax, especially past tense, shape responses to form target structures. Make use of the opportunities the illustrations provide to construct prepositional phrases. Some examples include

> Inside the house
> Up the stairs
> Behind the door
> Inside the box
> On top of the box
> Behind the box (the telltale sign of the can of paint)
> Through the door
> Under the floor boards

For phonological awareness training, review the earlier levels of activities in the Pre-K catalog, if necessary. Then begin at the child's developmental level with the following.

PLAY **Say-It-Until-You-Hear-It.**

Children synthesize one-syllable words divided into onset-rime. Present the word with a clear pause between the onset and rime. Demonstrate how to elongate the parts to blend them together, saying them a little quicker each time until they are readily identified. Provide scaffolding until children are ready to do it on their own. For example, say

> Put these two parts together: *f-eet.*
> Say it until you hear it. *Ffff . . . eet. Fff-eet. Feet.*

Continue with these C–V–C words from the text beginning with a single sound:

f-un	f-ound	h-ouse
w-itch	l-ift	l-ook
w-ings	s-ound	w-ink

Then demonstrate how to synthesize one-syllable words divided into onset-rime beginning with a two-consonant cluster, as in

cr-eep (creep)	cr-ack (crack)	fr-ight (fright)
pl-ay (play)	cl-aw (claw)	sc-are (scare)
cr-awl (crawl)	br-ave (brave)	st-airs (stairs)

PLAY **Roll-It-Out.**

Children synthesize a C–V–C word by blending each of its phonemes. Demonstrate by elongating the phonemes and blending them together in shorter and shorter sequences until children can identify the word. For example, say

> f-ee-t
> What's the word? Roll it out. *Ffff . . . eee . . . t. Feet.*

(continues on next page)

PLAY Roll-It-Out. *Continued*

Once children are successful, present each of the phonemes separately so they can "roll them out" on their own, in shorter and shorter sequences, to find the word. Use these one-syllable C–V–C words provided above as well as these additional words from the text.

web	sun	bat
look	wall	tomb
wink	roof	

PLAY Break-It-Up.

Children analyze one-syllable C–V–C words in order to identify the beginning, middle, and ending sounds. Begin activities with initial sounds, and then proceed to middle and ending sounds. For an example on how to demonstrate finding the middle sound in *web*, ask

What's the sound in the middle of *web*?
Break it up: *Wwwwww . . . -eeeeee . . . -b. . . . W-e-b.*
ĕ is the sound in the middle of *web*.

Continue to present one-syllable C–V–C words so that children can break them up and identify the sounds in each of the positions.

In the last stage of the game, children identify all the sounds in the word. Demonstrate how to elongate the sounds and then break them up in order to identify each one. For example, ask

What are all the sounds in the word *web*?
Roll it out and break it up: *Wwww . . . -eee . . . -b. . . . W-e-b.*
W-ĕ-b are all the sounds in the word *web*.

PLAY Delete-It.

Children omit the first sound in one-syllable words from the text. Demonstrate by saying the word slowly, then leaving off the initial sound. To demonstrate using *feet*, for example, say

Listen to how I can make *feet* become *eat*.
I delete the first sound. *Feet. Eat.*
Now you delete it. *Feet . . .*

Use the list of one-syllable words provided. Also practice with the individual words in the title of the book. Once children are successful, present all the words in the title, "In a Haunted House." Demonstrate how to remove the first consonant sound in *haunted* and *house* to get

In a Aunted Ouse

Ask the children what the title was before you removed the first sounds. Encourage them to stress the *h* sound in responding, "In a *H*aunted *H*ouse."

(**PLAY**) **Switch-It.**

Children delete the initial sound of the word and replace it with a new sound to make another word. Demonstrate first, then prompt with cues as necessary. For example,

> Say *house*.
> Now say *house*, only delete the *h* sound and switch it with *m*.
> What new word can you make? (mouse)

Continue with the words provided until children experience success. Then play the game with the words of the title. For example, when switching the *h* to *m*, their part will sound like this:

> In a Maunted Mouse

For other possibilities, switch the *h* to a

w: wanted wouse	*d:* daunted douse	*p:* paunted pouse
fr: fraunted frouse	*bl:* blaunted blouse	

Is It Rough, Is It Smooth, Is It Shiny?

by Tana Hoban
New York: Greenwillow Books, 1984

Suggested Grade and Interest Level: 1 through 2

Skill Builders:
> **Vocabulary**
> Semantics
> Adjectives
> Antonyms

Synopsis: Here is a beautiful collection of photographs for stimulating language and teaching the meaning of opposites and adjectives, including those in the title.

Method: Present the photographs to teach words and concepts in meaningful contexts. Capitalize on the realism in the photographs when teaching new vocabulary words. For adjectives, use the words in sentences depicting the illustrated objects for the children to repeat. Encourage the children to create other sentences using the featured adjective with other familiar objects.

Extended Activity: Play the game of opposites with things around the room, asking such questions as

> What do you see that is rough?
> What do you see that is shiny?
> What do you see that is soft?
> What do you see that is hard?

Then go outside and observe. Ask similar questions, such as, "What do you see that is shiny?" "What do you see that is dull?"

Is Your Mama a Llama?

by Deborah Guarino
New York: Scholastic, 1989, 1991, 1992

Suggested Grade and Interest Level: 1 through 3

Topic Explorations: Animals, Zoo; Family relationships

Skill Builders:

Vocabulary	Grammar and syntax	Articulation, *L*
Attributes	Negative structures	
	Question structures	

Synopsis: A baby llama learns about life as it questions its friends about whether their mamas are llamas. In rhyming verse, the friends describe what their mothers do, and the baby llama learns that all mothers are different.

Method: Pause at appropriate places in the text to model and shape target structures.

To teach attributes, play an animal guessing game. Recall which animals the baby llama encountered in the book. Then describe each animal. What does it look like? What does it do? Describe other animals, too.

For articulation, reinforce target phonemes by using the text for auditory bombardment and by encouraging children to recite the repetitive text, as well as other target words.

Note: In Spanish, *ll* is pronounced like the letter *y*. Therefore, the book may not be appropriate for *L* remediation with certain students.

It's a Spoon, Not a Shovel

by Caralyn Buehner
New York: Dial Books for Young Readers, 1995

Suggested Grade and Interest Level: 1 through 3

Topic Exploration: Manners and etiquette

Skill Builders:

Pragmatic language	Phonological awareness

Synopsis: This manners book, in quiz format, is a great way to have fun. The text escorts children through a series of social situations, humorously depicted by the vivid illustrations. Children select from the appropriate and not-so-appropriate (in some cases, downright rude) behavior by selecting the correct letter. The answers are obvious, but after all, shouldn't manners be, too? To double-check the answer, children will find the correct letter selection hidden within each page—and other little creatures, too.

Method: This is an ideal book to use for language pragmatics (making use of the lighthearted vein is effective). Before the read-aloud, ask children to recall some rules about behaving in appropriate ways. Then let go and prepare for laughs.

During the read-aloud, read the text and present the quiz without interruption, as in "Marty Mouse has been saving crumbs for weeks to give to Elmer Elephant for his birthday. Elmer exclaims: a. 'Your whiskers are twitching.'

b. 'Rats! That's not what I wanted!' c. 'Thank you, Marty!'" The location of the correct answer, *c,* is found inside the elephant's eye. For a list of locations of all answers, see the back of the book.

After the read-aloud, continue to address language pragmatics. Go back to a few preselected pictures and ask children to express in their own words what good manners should be used by the characters in the situation. For example, ask, "When Karla Kangaroo played hide-and-seek in the bushes and didn't see Harold Hyena, what should she have said when she accidentally hopped right on top of him?" Ask the children what the consequences might have been if she'd said one of the other—incorrect—selections.

Use the words of the text to play phonological awareness games. See the entry in the Pre-K catalog for activities that address earlier phonological awareness levels.

PLAY **Say-It-Until-You-Hear-It.**

Children synthesize one-syllable words divided into onset-rime. Present the word with a clear pause between the onset and rime. Demonstrate how to elongate the parts to blend them together, saying them a little quicker each time until they are readily identified. Provide scaffolding until children are ready to do it on their own. For example, say

> Put these two parts together: *n–ot.*
> Say it until you hear it. *Nnnnn . . . oot. Nnn-ot. Not.*

Other words from the text beginning with a single sound include the following:

s-am	w-eeks	h-ide
r-ats	s-eek	t-ooth
sh-ove		

Then demonstrate how to synthesize one-syllable words divided into onset-rime beginning with a two-consonant cluster, as in

sm-all (small)	sm-ooth (smooth)	sn-ap (snap)
br-eath (breath)	tw-itch (twitch)	pl-ay (play)
Sm-ith (Smith)	cr-umbs (crumbs)	sp-oon (spoon)

PLAY **Roll-It-Out.**

Children synthesize a consonant–vowel–consonant (C-V-C) word by blending each of its phonemes. Demonstrate by elongating the phonemes and blending them together in shorter and shorter sequences until children can identify the word. For example, say

> n-o-t
> What's the word? Roll it out. *Nnn . . . ooo . . . t. Not.*

Once children are successful, present each of the phonemes separately so they can "roll them out" on their own, in shorter and shorter sequences, to find the word. Use the one-syllable C-V-C word list provided in Say-It-Until-You-Hear-It.

PLAY **Break-It-Up.**

Children analyze one-syllable C–V–C words in order to identify the beginning, middle, and ending sounds. Begin activities with initial sounds, and then proceed to middle and ending sounds. For an example on how to demonstrate finding the middle sound in *not,* ask

> What's the sound in the middle of *not?*
> Break it up: *Nnnn . . . -ŏŏŏŏ . . . -t. N–ŏ–t.*
> *ŏ* is the sound in the middle of *not.*

Continue to present one-syllable C–V–C words so children can break them up and identify the sounds in each position.

In the last stage of the game, children identify all the sounds in the word. Demonstrate how to elongate the sounds and then break them up in order to identify each one. For example, ask

> What are all the sounds in the word *not?*
> Roll it out and break it up: *Nnnn . . . -ŏŏŏŏ . . . -t. . . . N–ŏ–t.*
> *N–ŏ–t* are all the sounds in *not.*

PLAY **Delete-It.**

Children omit the first sound in one-syllable words from the text. Demonstrate by saying the word slowly, then leaving off the initial sound. To demonstrate using the name "Sam," for example, show children how to leave off the beginning sound. Say

> Listen to how I can make *Sam* become *am.*
> I delete the first sound. *Sam. Am.*
> Now you delete it. *Sam . . .*

Continue with the list of C–V–C words provided. Once children are successful, demonstrate with two-syllable names in the text, such as Larry and Tina and Victor, creating words and nonsense words such as *airy, eena,* and *ictor.* Then use the full names of characters to delete initial phonemes. For example,

> *Marty Mouse* becomes *Arty Ouse*
> *Tina Tarantula* becomes *Ina Arantula*
> *Melissa Mandrill* becomes *Elissa Andrill*
> *Buster Bunny* becomes *Uster Unny*
> *Karla Kangaroo* becomes *Arla Angaroo*
> *Cory Cobra* becomes *Ory Obra*
> *Walter Warthog* becomes *Alter Orthog*
> *Larry Lion* becomes *Airy Ion*

PLAY **Add-It-On.**

Children insert a new sound into a word to make a new word. For example, say

> Listen to how I can make *Sam* become *slam.*
> I start with *s,* and then roll out *llll–am.*
> Then I have *sssssssslllaaammm. Slam.*
> Now you try it.

(continues on next page)

PLAY **Add-It-On.** *Continued*

Continuing with the word *Sam:*

>>> Add a *w* to make *swam*
>>> Add a *c* to make *scam*
>>> Add a *p* to make *Spam*

For the work *seek,*

>>> Add *n* to make *sneak*
>>> Add *l* to make *sleek*

PLAY **Switch-It.**

Children delete the initial sound of the word and replace it with a new sound to make another word. Demonstrate first, then prompt with cues as necessary. For example,

>>> Say *Sam.*
>>> Now say *Sam*, only delete the *s* and switch it with *p.*
>>> What new name did I make from *Sam? Pam.*
>>> *Sam, Pam*

Continue with one-syllable words until children experience success. Some ideas include

>>> sh-ove—Switch *sh* with *l.* (love)
>>> s-eek—Switch *s* with *w.* (week)
>>> r-ats—Switch *r* with *h.* (hats)
>>> w-eeks—Switch *w* with *ch.* (cheeks)
>>> h-ide—Switch *h* with *r.* (ride)
>>> t-ooth—Switch *t* with *r.* (Ruth)

Then play the game with two-syllable names. Begin with the names used in the Delete-It activities, switching the initial phoneme. For example,

>>> Marty: Switch *m* with *p.* (party)
>>> Tina: Switch *t* with *n.* (Gina [or Nina])
>>> Cory: Switch *k* with *l.* (Laurie)
>>> Larry: Switch *l* with *h.* (Harry)
>>> And so on

Once children are successful, use the alliterative, two-word names of the characters to switch initial phonemes in words. For example, switch the intial phoneme with an *m:*

>>> *Victor Vulture* becomes *Micter Mulcher*

More suggestions include

>>> Switch *m* in Marty Mouse to *p.* (Party Pouse)
>>> Switch *t* in Tina Tarantula to *b.* (Bina Barantula)
>>> Switch *m* in Melissa Mandrill to *t.* (Telissa Tandrill)

(continues on next page)

PLAY **Switch-It.** *Continued*

Switch *b* in Buster Bunny to *d.* (Duster Dunny)
Switch *k* in Karla Kangaroo to *t.* (Tarla Tangaroo)
Switch *c* (*k* sound) in Cory Cobra to *sh.* (Shory Shobra)
Switch *w* in Walter Warthog to *p.* (Palter Porthog)
Switch *l* in Larry Lion to *b.* (Barry Bion)

The Itsy Bitsy Spider

by Iza Trapani
Boston: Whispering Coyote Press, 1993

Suggested Grade and Interest Level: 1 through 2

Topic Exploration: Insects and spiders

Skill Builders:

Vocabulary	Grammar and syntax	Language literacy
Prepositions	Past tense	Cause-and-effect relationships

Synopsis: The famous little spider who struggles up the waterspout is back for further adventures. Follow her up a kitchen wall, a yellow pail, a green rocker, and finally a maple tree, where she decides to give it one more try. At last, her web is spun, and, oh, how sweet it is! Play the game of finding the spider in each beautiful picture, rendered from the perspective of an itsy-bitsy being.

Method: When each mishap happens, pause to talk about what caused the spider to fall down the wall, off the pail, and so on. Encourage the use of words such as *because* and *since* to place information in meaningful temporal relationships.

Encourage the use of prepositions to describe the spider's direction or position in the pictures.

For past tense, pause to have children repeat the verbs in the text, which include

wove	spun	climbed
slipped	plopped	knocked
fell	flicked	

Jambo Means Hello: Swahili Alphabet Book

by Muriel Feelings
New York: Dial Books for Young Readers, 1974, 1985; Pied Piper, 1981, 1985

Suggested Grade and Interest Level: 1 through 5

Topic Exploration: Culture and history, African and African Americans

Skill Builders:

Vocabulary	Language literacy
Semantics	Verbal expression
	Compare and contrast

Synopsis: Twenty-four Swahili words are presented, one for each letter of the alphabet. They include words for *school, beauty, friendship,* and *respect.* Don't worry—an easy pronunciation key accompanies each entry. Beautiful black-and-white illustrations capture the essence of African culture.

Method: Introduce children to the countries of Africa where Swahili is spoken. Read the Swahili word along with the interpretation, and pause to discuss its meaning. Compare and contrast U.S. culture with African cultures. What are the similarities and differences?

Also discuss cultures of other countries and how two cultures may have the same item, but their manners and customs of use differ. A broom is a broom in the United States and in Africa as well. But look at the picture. How are the African brooms different? Include a discussion of greetings in your culture lesson. Begin by listing greetings in English—such as "hi," "hello," and "welcome." Then elicit students' knowledge of greetings in other countries, such as China, Japan, France, and Italy.

Extended Activity: Brainstorm important classroom words. Some suggestions are *respect, feelings, self-esteem, inform, learn, fact, opinion, justice,* and *equality.* (You may want to choose a theme related to the students' dominant culture.) Have students go to the dictionary to look up the words. Using a separate sheet of paper for each word, have students create individual classroom dictionaries, then copy the definition, include a pronunciation key, and illustrate the word using a format similar to the book. Ask students to present their work to the class, either individually or in groups.

Joyful Noise: Poems for Two Voices

by Paul Fleischman
New York: Harper & Row, 1988

Suggested Grade and Interest Level: 4 through 5

Topic Exploration: Insects and spiders

Skill Builders:

Vocabulary	Grammar and syntax	Articulation
Semantics	Advanced syntactic structures	Carryover for any sound
Similes and metaphors	**Language literacy**	**Fluency**
Synonyms	Drawing inferences	**Voice**

Synopsis: Members of the insect world, their characteristics and activities, are set to verse for two voices to read aloud (different words are spoken by each speaker simultaneously). The resulting harmony of sounds is a remarkable vocal celebration. This book is highly deserving of its Newbery Award.

Method: Present the book by explaining how the poems are meant to be read by two voices at the same time but that the words will often differ, or the timing of the words spoken will be different for both speakers. Before beginning each poem, review the vocabulary. Then allow for plenty of practice reading aloud in this unique way.

Read the text, practicing target skills. After the reading, assist children in developing more syntactical variety and complexity in sentence structures. Have them create their own sentences with adverbial phrases and embedded phrases based on the short poetic text. For example, the poem "Whirligig Beetles" reads

> We're whirligig beetles
> we're swimming in circles,
> black backs by the hundred.

We're spinning and swerving
as if we were on a
mad merry-go-round.

Start sentences for students to finish with a phrase like the one in the poem that contains a simile. For example,

They're (whirligig beetles) swimming in circles like _____ (crazy wind-up toys).

Use the words of the text to construct embedded sentences, as in

Whirligig beetles, since they swim in circles, look like they're on a mad merry-go-round.
Whirligig beetles, spinning and swerving, never get dizzy.

The poem also presents a variety of words that pertain to a circling motion. List all the vocabulary words that are used to define the beetles and use them creatively in sentences about the water beetles. Words include

spinning	swirling
swerving	whirling
weaving	wheeling
turning	revolving
curving	twirling
gyrating	

For fluency, have a student read one column of text while you read the other. The duetlike verse provides excellent practice for speaking in rhythm, as each speaker must maintain a separate rhythm that is out of sync with the other speaker.

For voice, compare and contrast vocal qualities while reading simultaneously, or have the student try to match the pitch or vocal quality of the other reader.

King Bidgood's in the Bathtub

by Audrey Wood
San Diego, CA: Harcourt Brace Jovanovich, 1985, 1993

Suggested Grade and Interest Level: 1 through 3

Topic Exploration: Long ago and far away

Skill Builders:

Language literacy	Storytelling	**Articulation, *Th***
Sequencing	Problem solving	

Synopsis: An award-winning book about a fun-loving king who refuses to get out of his bathtub. Everyone in the court gets into the action, but it isn't until the page comes up with the obvious that the king finally dons his towel.

Method: For articulation, read the text, eliciting target words, including *bathtub* and *with*. For prediction, sequencing, and storytelling, invite children to predict what might be tried next to get the king out of his bathtub. Have the children retell the story of the king who wouldn't get out of his bathtub, recalling the schemes the people in the court tried. Provide scaffolding as necessary.

For problem solving, ask students to identify the problem. Ask questions such as these:

What facts can you state about it?
What happens because of the problem?
What attempts do the people of the court make to solve the problem?
How many other ways can you think of to coax the king out of the bathtub?
If you were living in the castle, who would you like to be and what would you do?

GRADES 1-5

Kites Sail High: A Book About Verbs

by Ruth Heller
New York: Grosset & Dunlap, 1988, 1991

Suggested Grade and Interest Level: 1 through 5

Skill Builders:

Vocabulary   **Grammar and syntax**
Semantics   Tenses, present and past
Categories
Synonyms

Synopsis: Another outstanding book in Ruth Heller's language series that explains and investigates all you'd ever want to know about "the most superb word you've ever heard"—a verb!

Method: Before the read-aloud, ask students to identify the verb in the title. Explain that the book gives a great deal of information about verbs. It can be enjoyable just to listen to words like *indicative mood* and *subjunctive mood,* but the important thing to learn is that our language has rules. We already know the rules because we use them when we speak. We just may not know them by name.

During the read-aloud, pause to identify the verb in each line of text. Brainstorm other verbs in its place. For example, read

> Horses *thunder* down the road.

Ask which word is the verb. What other words can be used in its place? Some ideas: Horses *gallop, trot, saunter,* or *prance* down the road. As another example, read, "These kings *have* gold." Substitute another verb: These kings *like, wear, desire, attain, acquire,* or *amass* gold. Expand the sentences to make them richer, for example,

> These kings wear gold, hold scepters, and dress in the elaborate style of past centuries.

Extended Activity: After the read-aloud, talk about verbs and other words as having roles to play in our language (and in all other languages). If we could put language on a stage, we would see a show in which certain words play particular parts.

Use the chalkboard to draw a stage (a large box with curtains across the top and along the sides). Divide the stage into two sections. Label the first section "Nouns" and the second section "Verbs." Or draw your own stage and create a transparency for an overhead projector.

Ask students to recall some of the animals, people, and objects in the book. If a student recalls the pelicans, for example, write *pelicans* beneath the heading "Nouns."

Tell the students that the things they named are going to be in a Word Show. Ask students what they want the pelicans to do on stage. They can choose the verb from the text or come up with their own. Perhaps they want the pelicans to dive. Write the word *dive* beneath the heading "Verbs." Read across, "Pelicans dive."

Repeat the process until you have written many activities taking place on the stage. Some students can act out the parts as if on a stage. Then have students create graphics by drawing an action taking place on the stage. They will write the verb phrase in a sentence beneath it, highlighting the verb with a different style of writing, a different color, or other distinctive feature. Mount the graphics on colored paper and display them in the classroom.

The Knight and the Dragon

by Tomie de Paola
New York: Putnam, 1980, 1992

Suggested Grade and Interest Level: 1 through 5

Topic Exploration: Long ago and far away

Skill Builders:

Vocabulary	**Language literacy**
Grammar and syntax	Storytelling
Tenses, present and past	**Articulation**
	Carryover for any sound

Synopsis: Neither the knight nor the dragon has ever fought a duel. So with the help of "how-to" books, they both prepare to fight each other. At times, just the artist's pictures tell the story, leading the children to talk about what's happening during the combatants' preparation.

Method: Read and interact to elicit target structures. Vocabulary includes

ancestors	armor	barbecue
cave	dragon	knight
rummage	swish	

For storytelling, encourage children to retell the story after the read-aloud. Show the pictures and talk about how the story happened long ago, in an age of kings and queens and knights and dragons. Prompt the children to begin the retelling with "once upon a time." Ask story grammar questions, such as who the story is about, what happened to start the story off, and so forth. Whether in a small group or full classroom, each child can have a chance to participate by adding details and dialog, as well as the essential story grammar elements.

The Legend of Bluebonnet

by Tomie de Paola
New York: Putnam, 1983

Suggested Grade and Interest Level: 1 through 4

Topic Explorations: Community; Culture and history, Native American; Folklore, Native American; Seasons, Spring

Skill Builders:

Vocabulary	**Language literacy**
Attributes	Storytelling
	Problem solving
	Compare and contrast

Synopsis: A Native American girl sacrifices her most precious possession in a burnt offering to save her tribe from drought and famine. She-Who-Is-Alone brings rain to the plains, and according to Comanche Indian lore, the Great Spirits still remember her sacrifice every spring when the land now called Texas is covered with beautiful blue flowers.

Method: Before the read-aloud, discuss what a drought is and how the absence of rain can affect people, particularly people such as the Comanches, who live closely tied to the earth. Also talk about Comanche beliefs and the ceremonies they performed to bring rain.

After the read-aloud, encourage children to retell the story. Ask questions to help them structure the narrative. For example,

> Where does the story take place?
> How did the girl feel about the draught?
> What did she want to do about it?

For problem solving, ask children to state the problem in the story. What happened because of the problem? Talk about different ways it might be solved.

Extended Activity: Describe She-Who-Is-Alone. Ask children to brainstorm words to describe what kind of a girl she was. Give examples based on her actions; for example, "She was brave because she sacrificed her doll." "She was a loving (caring) girl because she wanted to help the people of her tribe."

List ways She-Who-Is-Alone is like children in other cultures. How is she different?

Leo the Late Bloomer

by Robert Kraus
Old Tappan, NJ: Windmill Books, 1971, 1993

Suggested Grade and Interest Level: 1 through 4

Topic Explorations: School activities; Self-esteem

Skill Builders:
Vocabulary	Language literacy	Articulation, *L*
Idioms	Discussion	

Synopsis: Leo's parents come to the conclusion that Leo is a late bloomer because he can't seem to do anything right. And then, one day, "in his own good time, Leo bloomed." Excellent for a discussion of self-esteem.

Method: Before the read-aloud, ask children to explain the expression "late bloomer" and discuss its meaning.

After the read-aloud, discuss why Leo's parents called him a "late bloomer" and talk about other areas of life in which a person may be late in blooming. Also talk about the virtues of patience and becoming what you want to be "in your own good time."

For articulation, use the *L* words from the text for auditory bombardment before reading aloud. As you read, stress the *L* words and pause to model a word, phrase, or sentence for the child to repeat.

Lilly's Purple Plastic Purse

by Kevin Henkes
New York: Greenwillow Books, 1996

Suggested Grade and Interest Level: 1 through 3

Topic Exploration: School activities

Skill Builders:

Vocabulary	**Language literacy**
Adjectives	Cause-and-effect relationships
Grammar and syntax	Problem solving
Possessive nouns	Drawing inferences
Possessive pronouns	**Phonological awareness**
Past tense	Articulation—*L, L* blends; *R*

Synopsis: Lilly loves going to school wearing her red cowboy boots with the stars. She wants to be a teacher when she grows up, just like her adored Mr. Slinger. But when Mr. Slinger asks Lilly to wait until the appropriate time to share her new movie star sunglasses with the glittery diamonds and her purple plastic purse that plays music, Lilly becomes impatient. She writes her teacher an unkind note, for which she is very sorry for later, and both she, her parents, and Mr. Slinger must work to resolve the problem.

Method: Before reading what may be a familiar story to the children, obtain their background knowledge about the characters and events in the book. Ask who the story is about, where it take places, what happens to start the story off, and what the major events are in the story.

During the read-aloud, briefly pause to allow the children to elaborate on the meaning and expand on the descriptions and actions. Ask children to interpret the feelings of Lilly based on the text and illustrations and state what precipitated them. Model, shape, and recast target structures of grammar and syntax such as past tense. Use Lilly's cherished red cowgirl boots, movie star sunglasses, and purple plastic purse to elicit possessive forms of nouns and pronouns. Use the many adjectives in the text when describing her special articles of clothing. Also pause for the children to use the story's many adjectives in sentences of their own.

After the story, talk about what Lilly learned from her experience. Work on problem identification and problem-solving skills by asking children to state the problem in the story. When Lilly couldn't wait and interrupted Mr. Slinger's lesson, what happened? What are some of the things Mr. Slinger did in response to her problem? Talk about the way Lilly felt because of the problem. What things did she do to handle her problem? Draw inferences about how Lilly came to decide on these solutions. What did Lilly do together with her parents that helped solve the problem? What was the result? What did Mr. Slinger do then?

For cause-and-effect relationships, ask children to state what caused Lilly to write the unkind note that she sneaked into Mr. Slinger's bag. What effect did the note have on Lilly's relationship with Mr. Slinger? What effect did Mr. Slinger's note and the snack that he placed in her purple plastic purse have on Lilly? What did this cause her to do? What was the effect of her freshly baked snacks and her note of apology on her teacher? On her? As children respond to these questions, use scaffolding in helping them structure their responses with words such as *then, because, resulted in, caused, since,* and *the reason.*

Use the words of the text to play phonological awareness games. See the entry in the Pre-K catalog for activities that address earlier phonological awareness levels.

PLAY   **Say-It-Until-You-Hear-It.**

Children synthesize one-syllable words divided into onset-rime. Present the word with a clear pause between the onset and rime. Demonstrate how to elongate the parts to blend them together, saying them a little quicker each time until they are readily identified. Provide scaffolding until children are ready to do it on their own. For example, say

> Put these two parts together: *m–ad*.
> Say it until you hear it: *Mmmmm . . . aaad. Mmm . . . ad. Mad.*

Other words from the text beginning with a single sound include the following:

w-ait	s-ad	n-ote
n-ice	l-ab	s-ad
r-ead	l-ook	

Then demonstrate how to synthesize one-syllable words divided into onset-rime beginning with a two-consonant cluster, as in

sn-ack (snack)	cl-ap (clap)	st-ay (stay)
gr-ow (grow)	sn-eak (sneak)	sk-ool (school)
cl-ick (click)	dr-ew (drew)	st-ar (star)
sm-all (small)		

PLAY   **Roll-It-Out.**

Children synthesize a C–V–C word by blending each of its phonemes. Demonstrate by elongating the phonemes and blending them in faster and faster sequences until children can identify the word. For example, say

> w–ai–t
> What's the word? Roll it out. *Wwww . . . āāāā . . . t. Www . . . ait. Wait.*

Once children are successful, present each of the phonemes separately so they can "roll them out" on their own, in shorter and shorter sequences, to find the word. Use the one-syllable C–V–C word list provided above.

PLAY   **Break-It-Up.**

Children analyze one-syllable C–V–C words to identify the beginning, middle, and ending sounds. Begin activities with initial sounds, and then proceed to middle and ending sounds. For an example on how to demonstrate finding the middle sound in *wait*, ask

> What's the sound in the middle of *wait*?
> Break it up: *Wwwww . . . -āāāā . . . -t. . . . w-ā-t.*
> *ā* is the sound in the middle of *wait*.

Continue to present one-syllable C–V–C words provided in Say-It-Until-You-Hear-It so children can break them up and identify the sounds in each position.

(continues on next page)

PLAY Break-It-Up. *Continued*

In the last stage of the game, children identify all the sounds in the word. Demonstrate how to elongate the sounds and then break them up to identify each one. For example, ask

> What are all the sounds in the word *wait?*
> Roll it out and break it up: *Wwww . . . -āāāā . . . -t. . . . w-ā-t.*
> *W-ā-t* are all the sounds in *wait.*

PLAY Delete-It.

Children omit the first sound in one-syllable words from the text. Demonstrate by saying the word slowly, then leaving off the initial sound. To demonstrate using *wait,* for example, say

> Listen to how I can make *wait* become *ate.*
> I delete the first sound. *Wait. Ate.*
> Now you delete it. *Wait . . .*

Continue with the C–V–C words provided until children are successful. Then repeat the same task using Lilly's name. Present the name "Lilly" and demonstrate how to remove the first sound to make her name "Illy." Then ask the children to recall what her name was before you changed it for the response, "Lilly." Continue demonstrating with other names (in the book and in the classroom) until the children are ready to do it on their own.

PLAY Switch-It.

Children delete the initial sound of the word and exchange it with a new sound to make another word. Demonstrate first, then prompt with cues as necessary. For example,

> Say *wait.*
> Now say *wait,* only delete the *w* and switch it with *l.*
> What new word can you make? (late)

Continue with the list of C–V–C words until children experience success. Then play the game with Lilly's name. Begin by reviewing how you removed the first sound to get "Illy." Show how to switch the first sound from an *l* to a *b* to get "Billy." Then ask children to tell you what the name was before you changed it.

Some suggestions are to switch the *l* in Lilly to

> *m* (as in the name Millie)
> *w* (as in the name Willie)
> *d* (dilly)
> *h* (hilly)
> *s* (silly)
> *ch* (chilly)
> *fr* (frilly)

Continue to play Switch-It with other children's names in the same way.

For general articulation of any sound, read the story aloud and have children chime in, repeating their target sound at appropriate places in the text where they identify it. Children will no doubt enjoy identifying their target sound and repeating the word or phrase in which it appears because they are usually familiar with the text.

For articulation of *R*, use the text that is heavily loaded with the *L* phoneme in various target structures to give the practice words more meaning and interest. For example, practice using the target phoneme in Lilly's name at the syllable level, as in

> Lil-lil-lil
> ly-ly-ly
> li-ly, li-ly, li-ly

Words from the text include *Lilly, loves, lunchroom, milk, pencils, class, classmates, Wilson, purple, plastic, Mr. Slinger, encyclopedias, volunteered, clap, excellent, glittery, really, glasses, sunglasses, played excellent, look, looked,* and so on.

For sentence-level practice, use portions of the text for repetition by the children, as in

> Lilly loved school.
> Lilly loved the pointy pencils.
> Lilly loved the way her boots went clickety-clickety-click down the long, shiny hallways.
> Lilly loved . . . chocolate milk in the lunchroom.

Use carrier phrases with the words from the text, as in

> When Lilly went to school, she _____.
> Mr. Slinger was a nice teacher because _____.
> Lilly liked her purple plastic purse because _____.
> Lilly liked her movie star sunglasses because _____.

Have students use sentences of their own that reflect the story. Children can repeat the lines of the text that contain *L*, such as "Lilly loved school," "She had a brand new purple plastic purse," and "Lilly had a hard time listening."

This book is also available in a Spanish version, titled *Lily Y Su Bolso de Plastico,* translated by Teresa Malwer.

Liza Lou and the Yeller Belly Swamp

by Mercer Mayer
New York: Macmillan, 1976

Suggested Grade and Interest Level: 1 through 5

Topic Exploration: Trickster tales

Skill Builders:
  Language literacy   Articulation—*R, S,* and *Z*
  Problem solving
  Drawing inferences

Synopsis: Charming little Liza Lou won't be lured by the goblins, witches, and monsters of the Yeller Belly Swamp. She outwits them every time in this clever trickster tale.

Method: Before the read-aloud, discuss the cover and ask students to predict the setting for the story. Ask students what they know about bayous—marshy, riverine areas of the South where the water is slow moving and often stagnant. Discuss what it might be like to "pole" a boat.

Read aloud, pausing after each of Liza Lou's encounters with the intruder. Have the students state Liza Lou's goal and the problem she encountered in achieving it. Have them describe how she outsmarted the villain.

> Did she mean what she said?
> What did she really mean?
> What was she trying to do?
> What was the result?

For articulation of *L, S,* and *Z,* pause at appropriate places in the text to ask questions that elicit the target, as well as to have students provide the character's name, "Liza Lou," and the story's setting, the Yeller Belly Swamp.

London Bridge Is Falling Down

by Peter Spier
New York: Doubleday, 1967, 1985

Suggested Grade and Interest Level: 1 through 5

Topic Explorations: Culture and history, English; Folk songs; Long ago and far away

Skill Builders:

Grammar and syntax	Language literacy	Articulation, *L* and *J*
Present tense	Problem solving	Fluency
	Verbal expression	

Synopsis: The text is the familiar song. The illustrations are in the elaborate style of the author.

Method: For present progressive tense and verbal expression, the children can imitate sentence structures, describe the events in the pictures, and offer other solutions to the problem of repairing London Bridge.

For problem solving, ask what facts can be stated about the problem of London Bridge falling down.

> What caused this to happen?
> What happened because of the problem?
> What are some of the ways to solve the problem?
> What is the best solution?

For articulation, use the *L* and *J* words from the text for auditory bombardment before reading aloud. Then read the text, stressing the *L* and *J* words and pausing periodically to model a word, phrase, or sentence for the children to repeat. Use "London Bridge is falling down" as a carrier sentence before turning each page.

For fluency, stress the rhyme and meter as you read aloud. Encourage repetition of the verse, especially speaking in unison. Use the rhythmic, repetitive verse to have the child produce progressively longer phrases and sentences, maintaining airflow throughout phonation.

Lovable Lyle

by Bernard Waber
Boston: Houghton Mifflin, 1969

Suggested Grade and Interest Level: 1 through 5

Topic Exploration: Friendship

Skill Builders:
    Language literacy   **Articulation, L**
    Problem solving

Synopsis: Everyone loves Lyle the crocodile. Everyone! Then one day, a "I hate you" note is slipped under the door. Lyle sets out to prove how nice he really is, only to make matters worse.

Method: Before the read-aloud, use the words of the text printed below for auditory bombardment. Then read the text, stressing all the *L* sounds. After reading each page, ask questions to elicit sentences containing some of the many *L* words in the text. Some words to include are

children	play	troubles
Clover Sue Hipple	closed	
lifeguard	world	

Also have the child repeat a carrier phrase such as "Who hates Lovable Lyle?" or "Poor Lyle, the crocodile."

After the read-aloud, help children develop problem-solving skills by asking them to state the problem in the story. How did Lyle try to solve the problem? How was his problem finally resolved?

Note: Read also *Lyle, Lyle, Crocodile* by the same author.

Mammalabilia

by Douglas Florian
San Diego, CA: Harcourt Brace, 2000

Suggested Grade and Interest Level: 1 through 4

Topic Exploration: Animals

Skill Builders:

Vocabulary	**Grammar and syntax**	**Phonological awareness**
Associations	Advanced syntactic structures	**Articulation**
Morphological units		General caryover of all sounds

Synopsis: A collection of humorous short poems about mammals, including a tiger, gorilla, and rhebok, is presented in this clever little book.

Method: First read and enjoy one of the short poems. Then teach the meanings of the words as used in context. "The Beaver" provides a good example.

> Wood-chopper
> Tail-flopper
> Tree-dropper
> Stream-stopper

Have students explain the associations. For example,

> A beaver chops wood, so it is a wood chopper.
> A beaver "drops" trees by gnawing on the wood until the tree falls, or "drops" to the ground, so it is a tree dropper.
> A beaver has a tail that flops, so it is a tail flopper.
> A beaver stops up streams with the trees it chews on, so it is a stream stopper.

Teach morphological units by having students listen to the little word in the following words: *chopper, dropper, flopper,* and *stopper.* What little word can be heard when they are said slowly?

Explain one meaning of the suffix *-er.* It is used to differentiate between someone (or something, like a beaver) and what the someone (or something) does.

> A beaver who chops is a chopper.
> Choppers chop.
> A beaver who drops is a dropper.
> Droppers drop.

(PLAY) **Add-It-On with suffixes.**

Children put root word plus suffix together to make a two-syllable word. For example, say

> Put *-er* after *chop.*
> What word is it now? (chopper)

Another example:

> Put *-er* after *drop.*
> What word is it? (dropper)

And so on. Then show children what other words they can make with the root word *chop* (*chops, chopped, chopping, choppy, choppier, choppiest*) and use the words in sentences to create meaning.

(PLAY) **Leave-It-Out with suffixes.**

Children say a two-syllable word ending in *-y*, then leave out the suffix *-y* to reveal the root word. Demonstrate by saying, for example,

> Say *chopper* without saying *-er.*
> What little word is left? (chop)

Continue using the words in the text, including *flop, chop,* and *drop.*

> **PLAY** **Switch-It.**
>
> Children delete the initial sound of the word and exchange it with a new sound to make another word. Demonstrate first, then prompt with cues as necessary. For example,
>
> > Say *chopper.*
> > Now say *chopper,* only delete the *–er* and switch it with *–ing.*
> > What new word can you make? (chopping)
>
> Continue with the words from the text until children experience success. Then play the game with suffixes *-y, –ier,* and *–iest.*

Poems are great ways to teach advanced syntactical structures. Creating such sentences helps students understand the structures when they are heard or in written form. "The Coyote" provides a good example:

> I prowl
> I growl
> My howl
> Is throaty.
> I love a vowel
> For I am a coyoooote.

Brainstorm a few sentences about the coyote, such as

> The coyote prowls.
> The coyote howls.

Expand the sentences.

> The coyote prowls through the neighborhood.
> The coyote howls at the moon.

Choose one as the root sentence and turn the other into a verb phrase.

> Root sentence: The coyote howls at the moon.
> Verb phrase, beginning with the action: Prowling through the neighborhood,
> Combine them: Prowling through the neighborhood, the coyote howls at the moon.

Then vary the position of the phrase within the sentence for syntactical variety:

> Howling at the moon, the coyote prowls through the neighborhood.

You may need to use a connector word, like this:

> The coyote howls at the moon *while* prowling through the neighborhood.

Use the four-part method to create embedded sentences:

1. Begin a basic sentence. Create:

> The coyote is on the prowl.

2. Ask a *how* (*where, why, when*) question to expand the sentence. For example,

> *How* does the coyote prowl?
> *Howling hungrily.*

3. Pick a modifier to add to the subject.

> What kind of a coyote?
> Wild.

4. Show how to combine the elements using the modified subject, inserting the expander into the basic sentence, and finishing with the remainder of the basic sentence, as in

> A: The *wild* coyote, howling *hungrily,* is on the prowl.

The rhyming in these short verses is excellent for older students to increase phonological awareness. Here is the poem "The Mule":

> Voice of the mule: bray
> Hue of the mule: bay
> Fuel of the mule: hay
> Rule of the mule: stay

First teach vocabulary. For example, *bay* may be an unfamiliar word. Explain that the reddish-brown color of a horse or similar animal can be called *bay.*

(**PLAY**) **Rhyme-It-Again.**

After each rhyming set, children identify the rhyming word they just heard. For example, say

> *Bray* rhymes with _____. (bay)
> *Hay* rhymes with _____. (stay)
> *Fuel* rhymes with _____. (mule)

(**PLAY**) **Do-They-Rhyme?**

Children identify whether word pairs rhyme. Intersperse unmatched sets into the following rhyming word pairs:

Bray, hay—Do they rhyme?	*Hay, say*—Do they rhyme?	*Say, see*—Do they rhyme?
Stay, fuel—Do they rhyme?	*Fuel, mule*—Do they rhyme?	*Stay, bray*—Do they rhyme?

(**PLAY**) **Make-a-Rhyme.**

Children supply another rhyming word after a set of two are presented. Give an initial phoneme cue if needed. Accept any nonsense word. For example, ask

> What word rhymes with *say? Say, neigh* (mmmm . . . _____)

More rhyming words for *say* include *ray, day, gay, jay, lay, pay, stray, clay, tray, fray, gray, pray, play, sleigh, weigh,* and *yea!*

(**PLAY**) **Say-It-Until-You-Hear-It.**

Children synthesize one-syllable words divided into onset-rime. Present the word with a clear pause between the onset and rime. Start with words that begin with a continuous single consonant sound. Demonstrate how to elongate the onset part to blend the two parts together, saying them a little quicker each time until they are readily identified. For example,

(continues on next page)

PLAY **Say-It-Until-You-Hear-It.** *Continued*

Put these two parts together: *m-ule.*
Say it until you hear it. *Mmmmm . . . ule. Mm . . . ule. Mule.*

Continue with these words of the text:

s-ay	h-ay	f-uel
s-ee	r-ule	

PLAY **Roll-It-Out.**

Children synthesize a consonant-vowel-consonant (C-V-C) word by blending each of its phonemes. Demonstrate by elongating the phonemes and blending them together in shorter and shorter sequences until children can identify the word. For example, say

m–u–l
What's the word? Roll it out. *Mmmm . . . uuu . . . lll. Mule.*

Present each of the phonemes separately so children can "roll them out" on their own, in shorter and shorter sequences, to find the word. Use the one-syllable C-V-C words provided in Say-It-Until-You-Hear-It.

PLAY **Break-It-Up.**

Children analyze a one-syllable C-V-C word to identify all of the sounds. Begin with initial sounds, then proceed to middle and ending sounds. For an example of finding the middle sound in *mule,* ask

What's the sound in the middle of *mule*?
Break it up: *Mmmm . . . –ūūū . . . –lll. . . . M–ū–l.*
ū is the sound in the middle of *mule.*

Continue to present one-syllable words provided.

In the last stage of the game, children identify all the sounds in the word. Demonstrate how to elongate the sounds and then break them up to identify each one. For example, ask

What are all the sounds in the word *mule*?
Roll it out and break it up: *Mmmm . . . –uuu . . . –lll. . . . M–u–l.*
M–ū–l are all the sounds in the word *mule.*

Continue with the following words from the poem: *bay, rule,* and *fuel.*

Then play these phonological awareness games with all the short poems in the book.

For use in articulation therapy, the student can read the poems, maintaining almost any target phoneme production. For generalization, students can describe the animal of the poem using the words of the text.

The Man Who Could Call Down Owls

by Eve Bunting
New York: Macmillan, 1984

Suggested Grade and Interest Level: 3 through 6

Topic Explorations: Conservation; Owls

Skill Builders:

Vocabulary	**Language literacy**
Semantics	Predicting
Attributes	Cause-and-effect relationships
	Drawing inferences
	Critical thinking
	Discussion

Synopsis: A gifted man who befriends owls shows a young man, Con, his skills. Then a strange "distractor" becomes envious of the owl man and attempts to gain his power in an unacceptable way. The owls take swift revenge and, in the absence of the owl man, make Con their new friend. The story names many owl species, including barn owl, elf owl, screech owl, great horned owl, great snowy owl, hawk owl, and great gray owl.

Method: Before the read-aloud, elicit background information on owls. Talk about the special features of the species and the special sensitivity of people who work with a particular breed of animals or birds.

Pause briefly during the reading to encourage children to think critically and predict story events. Ask the children whether they think the stranger can obtain the owl man's power by taking his cloak and willow wand. What do they think will happen? Do they think the owls will come to him?

Have children make inferences about story events that are not explained in the text or pictures.

> What happened to the owl man?
> What makes you think so?
> Why is the stranger wearing his cloak and hat and carrying his willow wand?
> Is the stranger telling the truth when he says the owl man gave them to him?
> How did Con know how the stranger obtained them?

After the read-aloud, encourage the children to talk about the story's cause-and-effect relationships. Ask what the effect of the stranger's acts was on the owl man. What caused the owls to swoop down on the stranger? What effect will the owl man's absence have on the owls?

For attributes, talk about what the owl man was like. How can he be described? Brainstorm words such as *gentle, kind, intuitive, sensing, patient, intelligent, knowledgeable, dedicated,* and *insightful.* What happened because of his talent and power? What attributes can the students ascribe to the stranger and to Con?

For discussion, talk about what the author is saying about life and our planet, about protecting nature and its inhabitants. Ask questions such as these:

> Does the author have a lesson in mind for us to learn? What makes you think so?
> What might the stranger symbolize?
> What might the young man, Con, stand for?
> What do the owls stand for?
> What might the owl man symbolize?

Extended Activity: Break the students into groups and assign each group to report on one type of owl mentioned in the text. Encourage them to use dictionaries, encyclopedias, and other reference books from the school library in their research. Have each member of the group report on a particular aspect of the owl, such as its markings, habits, habitat, survival status, and more. Have each group create and present to the class a journal of interesting information about owls, along with illustrations, newspaper articles, and other odds and ends about owls.

Many Luscious Lollipops: A Book About Adjectives

by Ruth Heller
New York: Grosset & Dunlap, 1989, 1992

Suggested Grade and Interest Level: 1 through 5

Skill Builders:
> **Vocabulary**   **Articulation, *S* and *Z***
> Semantics
> Categories
> Morphological units

Synopsis: This book, one in Ruth Heller's entertaining language series, captivates young ones with its imaginative designs and expressive words. It also teaches comparatives and superlatives—*taller* and *tallest, more* and *most, less* and *least.*

Method: Before the read-aloud, discuss how descriptive words can make what we say more interesting. Show the difference between two sentences such as these, asking which sentence tells more:

> That's my cat.
> That big, gray, soft, cuddly cat is mine.

Define adjectives as "describing words" before introducing the book. Tell the children they will hear lots of information about these special words, but the important thing to remember is how descriptive they make our language sound.

Read aloud and have students practice expanding utterances using the adjectives presented. Talk about the meanings of the words, including the longer words such as *asteroidal* and *universal.* Then encourage the children to use the words in sentences they create themselves.

Also brainstorm other adjectives. For example, the text reads, "twelve large, beautiful, blue, gorgeous butterflies." Ask the children what other words they can think of to describe butterflies—*colorful, fluttery, pretty, small,* and *delicate,* for example. Continue to brainstorm other adjectives to describe the people, animals, objects, and ideas presented.

For categories, group objects shown in the book. For example, pause on the butterfly page and ask children if they can name some other pretty insects, such as ladybugs, grasshoppers, and moths.

For articulation, pause to model a target word or elicit a response containing the target sound with the heavily loaded *S* and *Z* words of the text.

Extended Activity: After the read-aloud, talk about adjectives and other words as having roles to play in our language (and in all languages). If we could put language on a stage, we would see a show in which certain words play particular parts.

Draw a stage on the chalkboard (a large box with curtains across the top and along the sides). Divide the stage into three sections. Label the first section "Adjectives," the middle section "Nouns," and the third section "Verbs." Or draw a stage on a separate piece of paper and make a transparency for an overhead projector.

Ask students to recall some of the animals, people, and objects in the book. Tell them you are going to put them in a "Word Show." If a student recalls the tennis player, for example, write *tennis player* on the stage beneath the heading "Nouns."

Ask what words can be used to describe the tennis player. Students can choose adjectives from the text or come up with their own. If a student offers *weary,* for example, write *weary* on the stage beneath the heading "Adjectives."

Ask students what they would like the weary tennis player to be doing on the stage. Perhaps they want the weary tennis player to collapse. Write across the stage, "a weary tennis player," and write the word *collapses* beneath the next heading, "Verbs."

Repeat the process until you have written in many descriptive phrases. Select students to role-play each entry on the stage. Ask the audience to identify which phrase each student is portraying. Then have students create graphics by drawing an event from the Word Show. They will write a sentence beneath the drawing, highlighting the adjective with a different style of writing, a different color, or some other distinctive feature. Mount the graphics on colored paper and display them in the classroom.

Martha Speaks

by Susan Meddaugh
Boston: Houghton Mifflin, 1992

Suggested Grade and Interest Level: 1 through 4

Topic Explorations: Animals, Dogs; Literacy; Pets; Speaking and communicating

Skill Builders:

Grammar and syntax	**Language literacy**	**Pragmatic language**
Tenses, present and past	Sequencing	
	Cause-and-effect relationships	
	Problem solving	

Synopsis: One day when Helen fed her dog alphabet soup, something amazing happened. Instead of the letters going down to Martha's stomach, they went up to her brain. As a result, Martha could speak—and speak she did. At first she answered the family's questions. Why didn't she come when they called her, had she always understood what they said, and why did she drink out of the toilet bowl? But as time went by, her loquaciousness got on everyone's nerves. She made embarrassing comments, telephoned large orders of barbecue beef to be delivered to the house, talked through everyone's TV shows, and caused all sorts of other problems. Fed up with her talking, the family gets angry and tells her to "shut up." This hurts Martha's feelings. As a result, she won't speak at all until her voice saves them from a robbery, and all is forgiven. This book makes a nice segue into using language appropriately in a variety of social situations. It also has made the top of various book lists, including the *New York Times, Horn Book Magazine, Parents Magazine,* and the American Library Association's *Booklist.*

Method: One suggestion for introducing the story is to ask children if they like alphabet soup. What do they like best about alphabet soup? Do they look to find the letters of their name? Do they know other people who like alphabet soup? Ask if anyone has a story to share about the time he or she had alphabet soup. Tell the children you have a special story to share with them about alphabet soup.

Pause during the story to "read" the expressions on the characters' faces as they react first in surprise to a talking dog and then in embarrassment and frustration as she continues to talk—a lot and inappropriately.

After the read-aloud, do a picture walk-through, and sequence the events of Martha's mischief. Assist children in expressing cause-and-effect relationships by having them connect Martha's actions of eating alphabet soup with her ability to talk. Model and shape sentences of correct grammar and syntax for target structures.

Have the children identify the problem in the story.

> Why didn't Martha's family stay proud and happy that their dog could talk?
> What was it about Martha's talking that the family didn't like?
> What did she do that wasn't appropriate?
> How could she have solved the problem so that the family would not have yelled at her?

For pragmatic language, discuss the rules for give-and-take of conversation. Also discuss the importance of politeness in social language. Ask the following questions:

> Why is it not a good idea to say what's on your mind to people if it isn't polite?
> How could Martha have been polite to the man at the bus stop? What might she have said instead?
> How could she have been more respectful of the family when they were watching their favorite TV show?
> Why is it important not to talk all the time and to let other people talk, too?
> What are some of the consequences when people don't use their talking appropriately?
> What effect did the words "shut up" have on Martha?
> What are some other ways her family could have dealt with the problem?

Note: Read also *Martha Calling, Martha Bla Bla,* and *Martha Walks the Dog* by the same author.

Meanwhile

by Jules Feiffer
New York: Michael di Capua Books, HarperCollins, 1997

Suggested Grade and Interest Level: 2 through 5

Topic Explorations: Cowboys and cowgirls; Literacy; Outer space; Pirates

Skill Builders:

Vocabulary	**Language literacy**
Semantics	Relating personal experiences
Higher-level concepts	Predicting
Grammar and syntax	Verbal expression
Tenses, present and past	**Articulation, General**

Synopsis: Raymond's mother is always calling him, and with Raymond's mother, it's always, "Right now!" and never "No big deal, you can do it next Tuesday, Raymond." That's when Raymond catches sight of a word on the page of his comic book: *meanwhile.* With Mom's escalating demands in the background, Raymond uses the useful trick of a quick change of scene to escape his own predicament. He creates his own "meanwhile," both literally, by scrawling it onto his wall in red pen, and figuratively, by instantly escaping onto a pirate ship. Follow Raymond on his action-packed, multi-phased, freewheeling adventures. The comic book style and subject matter can make this book suitable for all ages.

Method: Introduce the story by opening up a discussion about comics. Elicit prior knowledge of the word *meanwhile*. If needed, tell how it is used in comics as a transition device in escaping from one perilous scene into the next. Give a definition, explaining that something is going on in another place at the same time. Give examples within the context of students' own lives.

Read the story aloud. The cartoon-style balloon dialog reads easily from one to the next and gives listeners a sense of story. At each point where Raymond finds himself in a situation with dire consequences, ask students to predict how Raymond will escape. Students can supply the transition word *meanwhile*. The repetition of the words, "Raymond knew he had one last chance to save himself," is ideal to underscore and signal the predictable moments.

After the read-aloud, revisit the pages. The action sequences and verbs used in the text are ideal for encouraging retelling and facilitating verbal expression. Structure sentences to teach skills of grammar and syntax. Some examples in past tense include

> Ramond dueled the wicked pirates.
> He clenched a sword between his teeth.
> He switched on his backpack-autopower-vapor writer.
> He scratched out *meanwhile*.
> Raymond ducked the missiles in outer space.
> He shouted as loud as he could.

Use the vocabulary of the text to teach words within the context of the story:

> hopeless (the situation)
> fore
> aft

Multiple meaning words include

> reason (tried to)
> odds (evened out)

Continue to increase vocabulary usage and reinforce the concept of the simultaneousness of time by having students construct sentences about their own lives using the word *meanwhile*. Students can relate personal experiences (from made-up stories) about what is happening at that moment in time and what is happening at the same time in another location, such as a treehouse, a mountaintop, or an arcade. Also talk about the concept of time as it relates to the earth. For example, in your town it may be morning, but for students halfway around the world it would be nighttime.

For any articulation carryover, children can describe what is happening to Raymond in his adventures by using accurate target phonemes in connected speech or read the dialog in the cartoon balloons.

Mine, All Mine: A Book About Pronouns

by Ruth Heller
New York: Puffin Books, 1997

Suggested Grade and Interest Level: 1 through 5

Skill Builders:
 Grammar and syntax
 Pronouns—personal, possessive, and reflexive
 Advanced syntactic structures

Synopsis: Another in the Ruth Heller *World of Language* series that is just as stellar as the rest. Ms. Heller's creative way of looking at language makes the study of word usage an engaging activity. The book begins by showing what it would be like if we had no pronouns. For instance, "King Cole would call for King Cole's pipe. King Cole would call for King Cole's bowl and King Cole's fiddlers three. On and on . . ./it makes me yawn./It's awkward and wordy/The rhythm is gone." Despite the fact that the book's illustrations are geared toward younger children, older children will still learn about language because of the clever way the author presents the concept in the text.

Method: Begin by introducing the book and its author and illustrator. Show the cover illustrations of the beautifully and colorfully wrapped packages. Mine, all mine, hers, all hers, his, all his, or theirs, all theirs? Which is it? Talk about the fun you can have with words.

First, read a passage, such as the following, aloud:

 "Reflexive pronouns end in 'self.'
 This messy elf just helped
 himself."

Then, pause and assist children in recasting the text with another subject. Some suggestions include the following:

 This messy kangaroo just helped *himself* to the cookies.
 This greedy mouse just helped *herself* to the cheese.

Teach relative clauses by reading the lines of text about relative pronouns:

 "Relative pronouns make a connection.
 Here is Narcissus, who loved his reflection."

Pause so that children can recast the text with another subject:

 Here is the gnome who loves his books.
 Here is Cinderella who lost her glass slipper.

Continue pausing to expand on and clarify the text and illustrations. Also have children recast the text on pronouns for experience in the use of more complex sentence structures.

Read all the books in Ruth Heller's series, including *Behind the Mask: A Book About Prepositions*.

Ming Lo Moves the Mountain

by Arnold Lobel
New York: Greenwillow Books, 1982; Morrow, 1993

Suggested Grade and Interest Level: 2 through 5

Topic Explorations: Folklore, Chinese; Humor

Skill Builders:

Grammar and syntax
Past tense
Advanced syntactic structures

Language literacy
Predicting
Sequencing
Problem solving
Drawing inferences
Discussion

Synopsis: If only Ming Lo and his wife could get rid of the mountain in front of their house, they would be happy. When Ming Lo's wife decides he must move it, he goes to a wise man for help. This tongue-in-cheek story has many opportunities for language enrichment, plus a few reality checks along the way. Ming Lo achieves his goal, but how did he do it?

Method: Before the read-aloud, present the book and its title and ask students how one might move a mountain.

During the read-aloud, pause to use the text as a model for past-tense structures. Ask questions to elicit target structures.

For prediction, exercise children's logical thinking skills. Can Ming Lo really move the mountain by pushing a tree against it with all his might? Why or why not? Encourage students to predict the outcome, then turn the page and ask them to describe what happened. Were their predictions right?

For problem solving, pause to identify the problem in the story. Ask students to think of other ways Ming Lo might solve his problem.

After the read-aloud, ask children to infer what really happened when Ming Lo did the steps of the dance of the moving mountain. When he stepped back with one foot then the other, did the mountain move? Try acting out the dance.

For sequencing, ask students to recount the ways Ming Lo tried to move the mountain. What did he do first? What did he try next? What happened after that? What did he finally do to solve his problem?

For complex syntactic structures, assist students in structuring language by beginning sentences with adverbial phrases:

When Ming Lo went to the wise man, _____.
When Ming Lo returned home, _____.
When Ming Lo stepped backwards, _____.

Discuss the use of humor. Why is the story funny or ridiculous? Why do we enjoy stories such as this one?

Miss Fannie's Hat

by Jan Karon
Minneapolis, MN: Augsburg Fortress, 1998; New York: Puffin Books, 2001

Suggested Grade and Interest Level: 1 through 4

Topic Explorations: Clothing, Hats; Colors; Memory and remembering; Sharing

GRADES 1–5

Skill Builders:

Vocabulary	**Grammar and syntax**
Semantics	Tenses, present and past
Adjectives	**Language literacy**
Attributes	Problem solving
Similes and metaphors	Discussion
Morphological units	

Synopsis: Miss Fannie, at 99 years old, is faced with a tough decision: Which one of her fabulous hats should she donate to the church auction in time for Easter? As she takes time to think about each hat in her outstanding collection, she recalls the special events of her life. When she wore the green velour hat, for example, she experienced the great flood of 1914. When she wore another, she was milking her grandmother's cow, Flower. So it seems she can part with none of them, especially her favorite, the pink straw hat with the silk flowers. Eventually she decides to give away her favorite—the most famous of all her hats—which brings great joy to herself and others. This is a wonderfully touching story about care taking, gift giving, unselfishness, and love.

Method: Before the read-aloud, discuss vocabulary words *donate* and *auction*. Describe how auctions function, and explain that for charity auctions people donate, or give away, something so that others can buy it. The money from the sale goes toward a good cause. Describe an auction and how people "bid" on items they like and want. Elicit children's experiences, if possible. Review some of the words used in the text and other related words based on the story to build comprehension and meaning:

donate	auction	charity
bid	famous	unselfish
wardrobe		

During the read-aloud, encourage children to describe Miss Fannie's hats and thereby build their repertoire of adjectives and their ability to attach attributes to objects. Several delightfully illustrated pages depict a closet full of hats in all sizes, colors, and shapes. There is the red felt hat with the big feather, the green velour with the fancy pin, the pink straw with silk roses. Full-page illustrations leave plenty of room to pause for verbal descriptions. Orange, purple, peach, teal, yellow, orange, and pink. Polka dots, feathers, plumes, pins, ruffles and bows, wide brims, ruffled brims, and floppy brims.

Also, be sure to describe Miss Fannie's cats pictured impishly wearing her hats on many of the pages.

Use the text and illustrations to model and teach present and past tense as the children talk about what happens in the story. Also discuss the use of the simile, "Mama's hair, soft and gray like the feathers of a dove." What else can the children think of that is soft and gray? (For example, feathers, storm clouds, and kitten's fur.) Demonstrate how to make different similes with their associative words.

After the read-aloud, build skills in the comprehension and usage of morphological units by having children compare and contrast the words *selfish* and *unselfish*. What does each mean? Give some examples and have the children supply some from their own experiences.

Build a lesson using the word *unselfish* by using it as a cornerstone. First talk about words beginning with *un-* to demonstrate prefixes:

do, undo	tie, untie	plug, unplug
fold, unfold	lock, unlock	sure, unsure
block, unblock	kind, unkind	avoidable, unavoidable
cool, uncool	available, unavailable	
willing, unwilling	lace, unlace	

Then talk about the root word in *selfish* and *unselfish*. What little word can the children hear as you say it slowly, prolonging the phonemes? What little word is in *herself, himself, selfless, oneself,* and *self-control*?

Use the other word *selfish* to identify the suffix in other words such as

> bluish
> redish
> childish

Other words associated with the story in which to practice morphological markers include

> goodness
> kindness

Put *un* in front of *kind*. What word is it? Put *un* in front of *sure*. What word is it? And so on.

For problem solving, ask children to state the problem in the story.

> Why couldn't Miss Fannie decide on a hat to give away?
> What happened because of the problem?
> Did Miss Fannie enjoy thinking about the special times in her life?
> How was the problem solved?
> How did she feel about it?
> How would the story have been different if she had not given her hat for auction?
> What would you have done if you had been Miss Fannie?

Extended Activity: Make tissue paper hats. Have cardboard forms ready-made for children to choose from: baseball cap shapes, wide-brimmed sun hats, even bonnets. Children can cut various free-form shapes of different-colored tissue paper and glue them onto the cardboard. Display them on the wall or bulletin board with labels containing adjectives that the children write or dictate.

The class can also make collages of hats cut from magazines.

Miss Nelson Is Missing!

by Harry Allard and James Marshall
Boston: Houghton Mifflin, 1977, 1985

Suggested Grade and Interest Level:	1 through 5
Topic Explorations:	Careers; Humor; School activities; Trickster tales

Skill Builders:

Language literacy	**Articulation, S**
Cause-and-effect relationships	
Drawing inferences	
Discussion	

Synopsis: In this story, sweet Miss Nelson can't get control of her classroom. Enter the strict, wicked-looking substitute, Miss Viola Swamp. After several experiences with Miss Swamp, the children quickly learn to value the virtues of their gentler teacher. This is a story students of all ages can relate to.

Method: This "trickster tale" is excellent for facilitating comprehension and production of more complex narratives and the development of an oral-literate language style. Ask questions to elicit story grammar components, especially with regard to what the characters may be feeling and thinking and how this is different from the way they are acting.

After the read-aloud, assist children in retelling the story using language to express the cause-and-effect relationships, for example,

> The kids misbehaved. As a result, Miss Viola Swamp came to the classroom.
> Miss Swamp gave the kids lots of homework because they misbehaved.
> The kids missed Miss Nelson, so they went to her house.
> Because Miss Nelson was missing, the kids went to Detective McSmog.
> When the kids misbehaved, it caused the principal to come into the classroom.
> The kids thought Miss Swamp was very strict, so when Miss Nelson returned, they were on their best behavior.

For articulation, select target words from the text for auditory bombardment before reading. Then read the text, stressing *S* and *Z* sounds. After reading each page, shape sentences loaded with the target sound by asking questions to elicit the many *s* words in the text. Then watch how quickly the children will do this on their own.

Note: Read also *Miss Nelson Is Back* and *Miss Nelson Has a Field Day* by the same author.

Mr. Gumpy's Outing

by John Burningham
Orlando, FL: Holt, Rinehart & Winston, 1978, 1990

Suggested Grade and Interest Level: 1 through 3

Topic Explorations: Animals, Farm; Boats; Country life; Journeys; Sharing

Skill Builders:

Vocabulary	**Grammar and syntax**	**Articulation—*R, S,* and *Z***
Semantics	Possessive nouns	
	Negative structures	
	Question structures	
	Language literacy	
	Predicting	

Synopsis: Mr. Gumpy goes for a ride on the river in his boat. As he paddles along, various animal friends ask to come along. Mr. Gumpy agrees, but with stipulations. As the animals accumulate in the boat, the inevitable happens.

Method: To practice possessive nouns, pause while reading to ask whose boat the animals are in, whose house they are having tea at, and whose outing it was originally supposed to be.

To practice question structures, ask the children to repeat the animals' requests to come along. For negative structures, rephrase Mr. Gumpy's responses, for example,

> He can't squabble.
> He can't hop.
> Can the children predict the next mishap?

For *R, S,* and *Z,* pause to interact using the target words of the text. Encourage repetition of the phrase *down the river* or some other variation of it in response to questions about where the boat is.

GRADES 1–5

The Mitten: A Ukrainian Folktale

by Jan Brett
New York: Putnam, 1990

Suggested Grade and Interest Level: 1 through 2

Topic Explorations: Animals, Forest; Folklore, Ukrainian; Humor; Owls; Seasons, Winter

Skill Builders:

Vocabulary	Language literacy	Articulation—*L, S, and Z*
Attributes	Predicting	
	Verbal expression	
	Drawing inferences	
	Discussion	

Synopsis: Against her better judgment, Nicky's grandmother knits him white mittens. When Nicky takes off for the forest, one mitten falls on the snow and becomes home to an increasing number of animals. The border pictures build anticipation for the next approaching animal. They also show Nicky in the woods, unaware of his lost mitten. When an incredible number of increasingly larger animals share the cozy habitat, a surprising event reunites Nicky and his mitten—something on the order of a big sneeze and a lucky catch!

Method: Elicit children's prior knowledge before the read-aloud. Ask the children to name animals that live in the forest. Then introduce them to the names of animals in the story. Ask what the children know about hedgehogs. Talk about how their prickles are like those of porcupines. Ask what they know about owls. Talk about owls having talons, just like eagles. Discuss badgers and their passion for digging.

For predictions and verbal expression, pause to talk about the border pictures. They show what is happening to Nicky in a different part of the forest as his mitten is filling up. Once the pattern of the story is established, see whether children can predict, based on the border picture, which animal will come to the mitten next.

For drawing inferences, draw on prior knowledge to discuss the animals' reactions. Ask why the mole and the rabbit didn't want to argue with anyone that had prickles. What was it about the owl's "glinty talons" that made the other animals quickly let him inside? Why did they offer the thumb of the mitten to the badger after seeing his "diggers"?

For attributes, name the reasons the animals liked the mitten—it was white, good for camouflage, warm, soft, and so on.

Discuss the absurdities. What's funny about a mole and a rabbit being inside a boy's mitten? What's funny about a mole and a rabbit and a hedgehog being inside a mitten? What about a mole, a rabbit, a hedgehog, and an owl inside a mitten, and so on? Also ask what is funny about the grandmother's expression when she examines the stretched-out mitten. Do the children think she knows what happened? Do they think she can figure it out?

For articulation, capitalize on words such as *snow, forest, lost,* and *talons.* Pause to ask questions that elicit answers containing the target sounds.

The Mixed-Up Chameleon

by Eric Carle
New York: HarperCollins, 1975, 1984, 1988

Suggested Grade and Interest Level: 1 through 2

Topic Explorations: Animals, Zoo; Colors; Humor; Part–whole relationships; Self-esteem

Skill Builders:

Vocabulary	Grammar and syntax	Language literacy
Semantics	Possessive nouns	Cause-and-effect relationships
Associations		Verbal expression
Attributes		Discussion

Synopsis: Thinking its life is not that exciting, a chameleon goes to a zoo. Wishing it were more like the animals it sees, the chameleon begins to adopt their characteristics. It becomes an increasingly hilarious, mixed-up mess of different animal parts, losing its identity. Finally (and thankfully), it decides it likes itself better the way it is—a plain old chameleon.

Method: Begin by asking children what they know about chameleons. Discuss chameleons' characteristics and lead into the story by looking at the title and making story predictions.

For encouraging children to use language to compare and contrast, pause for children to identify the colors the chameleon turns. Then ask how the chameleon is like and unlike different things in the story.

For possessive nouns and for attributes, pause to have children identify each animal part the chameleon acquires. As the chameleon adds more parts (reindeer antlers, fish fins, a giraffe neck, etc.), pause to recall the animals the parts came from. The tabs on the left show the original animals. For example, look at the polar bear tab to recall how the chameleon became big and white. Next, look at the flamingo tab and recall how the chameleon got pink wings and stilt-like legs. Continue in this way as you tell the story of how the chameleon became so mixed up.

After the read-aloud, ask children to explain why the chameleon was so mixed up. What caused the chameleon to grow fins? What caused it to grow a giraffe's neck, and so on? Talk about what caused the chameleon to turn it-self back into a chameleon. Then hold a discussion about the importance of liking yourself the way you are. Have all the children share something unique about themselves.

Extended Activity: Make a "collage chameleon." Trace the outline of the chameleon from one of the pages in the book. Transfer it to a stencil or onto paper for each child. Gather pipe cleaners for reindeer antlers, cotton balls for polar bear fur, red yarn for the fox tail, orange tissue paper for fish fins, and purple tissue paper for seal flippers. Have children paste these parts onto the outline to make their own mixed-up chameleons.

Mouse Mess

by Linnea Riley
New York: Scholastic, 1997

Suggested Grade and Interest Level: 1 through 2

Topic Explorations: Colors; Food; Messes; Shapes and visual images

Skill Builders:

Vocabulary	Language literacy
Categories	Sequencing
Prepositions	**Phonological awareness**
Grammar and syntax	
Present tense	

Synopsis: A little mouse listens for the "all-clear" of human feet retreating up the stairs, then comes out of his cozy house for a midnight snack in the kitchen. Very shortly, Ritz crackers, Oreo cookies, and corn flakes spill onto and clutter the counter. They are soon joined by the cheese, olives, peanut butter, and fruit in the messiest, jumbled up kitchen counter you've ever seen. Short rhyming verse with plenty of sound effects—crunch-crunch, crackle-sweep— accompanies delectable pictures that take the reader through a sequence of rascally mouse actions. To finish his night's work, he turns on the faucet, takes a bath in a teacup, and leaves for home just before the family comes down for breakfast. This little sleeper is charming and rich with possibilities.

Method: Before the read-aloud, spend a few minutes identifying the mouse and all the different food items on the cover.

Read the story through without interruption while children connect with the pictures and with the rhythm and flow of the short, rhyming text.

After the read-aloud, do a picture walk-through and pause at every page to describe the mouse's actions. Elicit grammar and syntax constructions. Some suggestions for present-tense sentences (with optional prepositional phrases) include

> The mouse is building sandcastles with brown sugar.
> The mouse is raking corn flakes into piles with a fork.
> The mouse is spreading peanut butter and jam onto the bread.
> The mouse is popping the tops off the bottles.
> The mouse is soaking the jam between his toes.

During the picture walk-through, sequence the actions of the story, from the mouse asleep in his little house un- til he leaves the messy kitchen and goes back home to bed. Then have children take turns telling the action of the story from the illustrations.

Have children categorize all the food into food groups. For example, name all the snack foods. Name all the sandwich foods. Name all the breakfast foods. Present the names of several foods within a group, along with an odd item. Have the children pick out which food doesn't belong in the category.

For phonological awareness training, first reread the text. If necessary, review or begin with earlier levels of activ- ities in the Pre-K catalog. The following is a continuation of games at the phoneme level.

PLAY **Say-It-Until-You-Hear-It.**

Children synthesize one-syllable consonant–vowel–consonant (C–V–C) words divided into onset-rime. Present the word with a clear pause between the onset and rime. Demonstrate how to elongate the parts to blend them to- gether, saying them a little quicker each time until they are readily identified. Provide scaffolding until children are ready to do it on their own. For example, say

> Put these two parts together: *m–ess.*
> Say it until you hear it. *Mmmmmm . . . ess. Mmm . . . ess. Mess.*

Other words from the text beginning with a single sound include

m-ouse	f-eet	f-un
s-oak	t-oes	p-op
f-ed	f-ood	

Then demonstrate how to synthesize one-syllable words divided into onset-rime beginning with a two-consonant cluster, as in

sn-ack	fl-akes	sw-eep
sl-ip	sn-iff	br-ead
sm-ear	sp-ill	st-airs

PLAY Roll-It-Out.

Children synthesize a C-V-C word by blending each of its phonemes. Demonstrate by elongating the phonemes and blending them together in shorter and shorter sequences until children can identify the word. For example, say

> m-e-ss
> What's the word? Roll it out. *Mmmm-eee-sss. Mess.*

Once children are successful, present each of the phonemes separately so they can "roll them out" on their own, in shorter and shorter sequences, to find the word. Use the one-syllable C-V-C word list provided above.

PLAY Break-It-Up.

Children analyze one-syllable C-V-C words to identify the beginning, middle, and ending sounds. Begin activities with initial sounds, then proceed to middle and ending sounds. For an example on how to demonstrate finding the middle sound in *mess*, ask

> What's the sound in the middle of *mess*?
> Break it up: *Mmmmm . . . eee . . . ssss . . . m-e-ss.*
> ĕ is the sound in the middle of *mess*.

Continue to present one-syllable C-V-C words provided above so children can play Break-It-Up and identify the sounds in each of the positions.

In the last stage of the game, children identify all the sounds in the word. Demonstrate how to elongate the sounds and then break them up to identify each one. For example, ask

> What are all the sounds in the word *mess*?
> Roll it out and break it up: *Mmmm . . . eeee . . . sss. . . . M-e-ss.*
> *M-e-ss* are all the sounds in *mess*.

PLAY Delete-It.

Children omit the first sound in one-syllable words from the text. Demonstrate by saying the word slowly, then leaving off the initial sound. To demonstrate using *feet,* for example, say

> Listen to how I can make *feet* become *eat.*
> I delete the first sound. *Feet. Eat.*
> Now you delete it. *Feet . . .*

Use the list of one-syllable words provided above. Also practice with both words in the book's title. Present the words *Mouse Mess* and demonstrate how to remove the first sounds in the words to make *ouse ess.* Then ask the children to recall what the words were before you changed them. Continue demonstrating with other groups of words in the text until the children are ready to do it on their own.

PLAY **Add-It-On.**

Children insert a new sound into a word to make a new word. For example,

> Listen to how I can make *soak* become *smoke:*
> I start with *sss*, and then add on *mmmmm* to *oke*.
> Then I have *sssssssmmmmmooooooke. Sssmmmooooke. Smoke.*
> Now you try it.
> Say *soak*.
> Now add the *m* sound after *s*. What new word do you have? *sm . . .* (smoke).

Continue to make new words from the C–V–C words lists in Say-It-Until-You-Hear-It.

> For example, *pop* becomes *plop* and *prop*.
> *Fed* becomes *Fred* and *fled*.

PLAY **Switch-It.**

Children delete the initial sound of the word and exchange it with a new sound to make another word. Demonstrate first, then prompt with cues as necessary. For example,

> Say *mess*.
> Now say *mess*, only delete the *m* and switch it with *t*.
> What word can you make? (tess)

Continue with the one-syllable C–V–C words provided above. Then play the game with the book's title. Review how you removed the first sound in both words to get *_ouse_ess*. Show how to switch the first sound from *m* to *t* to get *Touse Tess*. Then ask children to tell you what the name was before you changed it. (If necessary, take one word at a time until children can produce the words on their own. Then combine the two words of the title.)

Some suggestions: Switch *m* in Mouse Mess to

> *n* (Nouse Ness)
> *f* (Fouse Fess)
> *p* (Pouse Pess)
> *ch* (Chouse Chess)

Continue to play Switch-It with some of the repetitive words from the text, such as

> hush, hush
> munch, munch

Also play Switch-It with food names and any other words from the text.

My Mama Says . . .

by Judith Viorst
New York: Atheneum, 1975, 1987

Suggested Grade and Interest Level: 1 through 5

Skill Builders:
Vocabulary	**Articulation, *S* and *Ch***
Adjectives	

Synopsis: Who says there isn't a mean-eyed monster with long shiny hair and pointy claws going scratchy-scratch, scritchy-scritchy-scratch outside the window? And so the fear of monsters persists despite Mama's reassurances.

Method: For *S*, pause to have children repeat target words. Point out one of the illustrated creatures and ask the children to name it. A ghost? A monster? A zombie?

Then structure responses to questions, for example,

> Q: How does the zombie walk up the stairs?
> A: Stiffly.

Also have children repeat on cue as you pause before turning each page: "Sometimes even mamas make mistakes."

For *Ch,* have the child repeat the phrase "scratchy-scratch, scritchy-scratch" before turning the page. Or structure responses to questions:

> Q: What does a demon do with its tail?
> A: Swishes it.

The Mysteries of Harris Burdick

by Chris Van Allsburg
Boston: Houghton Mifflin, 1984

Suggested Grade and Interest Level: 1 through 5

Skill Builders:
Grammar and syntax	**Language literacy**	**Articulation**
Tenses—present, past, and future	Cause-and-effect relationships	Carryover for any sound
Advanced syntactic structures	Storytelling	

Synopsis: A man named Harris Burdick once gave a series of mysterious pictures with provocative captions to a children's book publisher. Although he promised to produce the stories that went with them, he never returned. Thirty years later, Chris Van Allsburg reproduced the pictures and original captions, stimuli that can coax even the most unimaginative minds into some fascinating storytelling.

Method: For younger children, talk about present, past, and future in storytelling. Present the book, eliciting picture descriptions and ideas about what might have happened to start the story off. Ask children to think of a situation that might have come before the pictured event. What might have caused the event to happen? Have each child draw a picture of the idea, then share it with the class along with a verbal description. Assist them in expanding their descriptions to include adverbial clauses, beginning, for example, with *while, after, when, about the time, as,* or *because.*

Extended Activity: Help older children structure a story. Include setting in ⸺ ⸺ ⸺ers. (Suggest that perhaps some of the characters in the story are not seen in the author's ill⸺ ⸺en to think of an initiating event. Assist with suggestions if necessary. Then encourage them to devel⸺ y inventing a resolution to the problem. Children can write their stories and read them aloud. Encourage connective words such as *then, and,* and *because.*

Night in the Country

by Cynthia Rylant
New York: Bradbury Press, 1986; Macmillan, 1991

Suggested Grade and Interest Level: 1 through 5

Topic Explorations: Country life; Nighttime; Sounds and listening

Skill Builders:

Grammar and syntax	**Language literacy**	**Phonological awareness**
Tenses, present and past	Verbal expression	

Synopsis: The quiet sounds of a night in the country are soothing and evoke restful images. Ideal for developing listening skills and calming a group.

Method: Before the read-aloud, encourage children to recall some of the sounds they can hear at night. Snoring? Cars whizzing past? Clocks ticking? The refrigerator motor running? Present the book and title, having children make predictions before you begin the story.

During the read-aloud, encourage use of the verbs in the text, including *swoop, clink, patter,* and *nuzzle,* and help students to structure sentences in the present tense.

After the read-aloud, have children recall from the story all the sounds of a night in the country—the owls hooting, frogs croaking, cats purring, screen doors creaking, the house squeaking, and so on. Then assist students in structuring sentences using the words in the past tense.

Use the theme of the story to develop active listening skills. Encourage children to close their eyes and listen attentively to the sounds around them. What do they hear in the classroom? Is there any playground noise? Cars passing on the street? Bells ringing? Footsteps in the hall? Children's voices in the distance? Lights buzzing? Animals rustling in their cages?

PLAY   **The Listening game.**

Children must close their eyes while you provide a familiar sound. Children then guess what you did or what object made the sound. Some suggestions include

> Clap your hands
> Snip the scissors
> Ring a bell
> Open and close a drawer
> Rattle cellophane on a package
> Write on the board with chalk

Officer Buckle and Gloria

by Peggy Rathmann
New York: Putnam, 1995

Suggested Grade and Interest Level: 1 through 3

Topic Explorations: Animals, Dogs; Careers; Pets; Safety; School activities

Skill Builders:

Grammar and syntax	Language literacy
Pronouns, personal and possessive	Predicting
Tenses—present, past, and future	Sequencing
Negative structures	Cause-and-effect relationships
Question structures	
Advanced syntactic structures	

Synopsis: No one heeds the safety rules Officer Buckle so earnestly presents to the neighboring schools—until Gloria, the police dog, joins him onstage. The little dog is so extraordinarily entertaining that the children and teachers finally start observing the rules. Their performances become very popular, but when Office Buckle realizes it is Gloria that is the real attraction he is downhearted and sends her to the next assembly by herself. Feeling lonely without Officer Buckle, Gloria gets stage fright. Without anything to say, she is a flop. Because the children and teachers are back to their unsafe ways at the school, a set of calamitous events ensues, which leads to Officer Buckle's return with the pronouncement of Safety Tip 101: Always stick with your buddy. This Caldecott Medal winner is hilarious, endearing, and a good way to present safety issues—which says a great deal about the way children learn best, doesn't it?

Method: Before the read-aloud, elicit background knowledge about the word *safety* and have children recall some safety rules. Ask children to listen to see whether Officer Buckle says any of the ones they remembered.

During the read-aloud, keep interaction to a minimum, allowing the children to connect with the words and pictures of the story.

After the read-aloud, use the words and illustrations to help build grammar and syntax skills within the context of the story. For developing negative structures, use Officer Buckle's safety lessons, either from lines of the text or from those listed on the inside cover, to model for repetition, for instance,

> "Never stand on a swivel chair."
> "Never take other people's medicine."
> "Never play with matches."

For developing present-progressive tense structures, model and shape portions of the text as applicable. Pictures offer opportunities for describing Gloria's actions on stage. Read each of Officer Buckle's rules and have the children describe how Gloria demonstrates what happens when you don't follow each rule—for example,

> Rule: "Always wipe up spills before someone slips and falls."
> Possible sentences: Gloria is slipping; Gloria is sliding on her nose with her tail end in the air.

> Rule: "Never leave a thumbtack where you could sit on it."
> Possible sentence: Gloria is jumping up and grabbing her hind end.

> Rule: "Never go swimming during an electrical storm."
> Possible compound sentence: Gloria is jumping into the air (in shock) and her hair is standing on end.

Use the illustrations to structure sentences using the pronouns *he, she*, and *they* for Officer Buckle, Gloria, and the children.

On many pages there are illustrations of accidents about to happen. Shape and model future-tense structures—for example, Mrs. Toppel will (is going to) fall.

For producing question structures, have students play the part of Officer Buckle and ask questions, such as, "What could (can, would, might) happen if _____ ?"

Have another child use prediction strategies to express a possible effect.

For developing sequencing skills and expressing cause-and-effect relationships, retell the series of calamitous events at the school after Officer Buckle didn't come for the safety lesson. For example, prompt "It started when . . . "

> Someone left banana pudding on the floor. (Breaking a rule)
> What effect did that have?
> It caused everyone to slide into Mrs. Toppel.
>
> What effect did that have?
> She screamed and let go of the hammer.
>
> What effect did that have?
> She fell off her chair.
>
> What was Mrs. Topple doing that caused that to happen?
> She was standing on a swivel chair. (Breaking a rule)

Oh, Were They Ever Happy

by Peter Spier
New York: Doubleday, 1978, 1988

Suggested Grade and Interest Level: 1 through 5

Topic Explorations: Family relationships; Humor

Skill Builders:

Grammar and syntax	Language literacy	Articulation
Tenses, present and past	Relating personal experiences	Carryover for any sound
	Storytelling	

Synopsis: This book is a favorite that children of all ages can relate to. Mom and Dad go off on errands, telling their children that the baby-sitter will be coming in just a few minutes. When she doesn't arrive, the kids decide to help out by painting the house. The sight of their handiwork is something you must see to believe.

Method: Before the read-aloud, talk about ways children can be helpful around the house. Encourage children to describe some of the things they have done for their parents that they thought were helpful and how good they felt after having done them.

Present the book, encouraging picture descriptions on every page. Model and shape target structures. Pause to interject questions, such as

> What are the children doing now?
> What do you think their parents will say?
> Do you think the children are being naughty or trying to help?

After the read-aloud, encourage children to relate personal experiences. Begin by asking them whether they have ever done something they didn't realize would create a problem later. Or perhaps, like the children in the story, they thought they were being helpful, only to find out they actually made matters worse. Encourage children to talk about their experiences and draw parallels with the experiences of the characters in the book. You may even want to share an experience of your own.

Extended Activity: On a long piece of butcher paper, pencil in an outline of the house, complete with garage and fence. Go over the outline with a black marker. Then place the paper on the floor along with different colors of tempera paint, allowing students to paint the house. Afterward, have students retell the story. Provide scaffolding as necessary. Does their picture look better than the one they started with? Would they like to live in that house? Why or why not?

One Grain of Rice: A Mathematical Folktale

by Demi
New York: Scholastic, 1997

Suggested Grade and Interest Level: 1 through 5

Topic Explorations: Folklore, India; Number concepts; Sharing

Skill Builders:

Vocabulary	Grammar and syntax	Language literacy
Beginning concepts	Tenses, present and past	Sequencing
		Storytelling
		Problem solving

Synopsis: Exotic and beautiful, this "mathematical folktale," along with its evocative illustrations in gold-leaf detail, gives a sense of the atmosphere and culture of India. The story tells of a raja who, every year, keeps nearly all the rice the people of his country grow. In case of a famine, he says, he will feed everyone. But when a drought comes, he does not share, and the people go hungry. One day, Rani, a clever village girl, sees a load of the raja's rice go by and one grain fall to the ground. When she picks it up to give it back, the raja wishes to reward her. Rani requests just one grain of rice, doubled every day for 30 days. The raja foolishly thinks this won't amount to much, but in the end, Rani collects more than 1 billion grains—enough to feed all of the people who toiled so hard to grow it—and extracts a promise from the selfish ruler.

Method: Before the read-aloud, discuss the word *drought* and how the absence of rain can affect the people of a country. Discuss the word *raja,* a king or prince of India.

After the read-aloud, assist children in sequencing each exquisitely pictured delivery of rice, using the illustrations as a guide. Encourage the use of *first, next,* and *then* to connect the events:

> First a beautiful bird brought a single grain of rice.
> Then more grains were delivered in a small purse.
> The next day it came in a golden bag on a red cart.
> Then it came in a large drum delivered by a monkey.
> It continued to be brought in drums by deer, then oxen, then camels, then teams of camels, and finally

by herds of elephants until Rani had 536,870,912 grains of rice.

To build skills of grammar and syntax, shape target structures as children describe the animals and their movement in delivering the rice.

Encourage children's storytelling skills by asking questions to help them paraphrase words and structure the narrative—for example,

> Where does the story take place?
> Who were the characters?
> What did the raja do at the beginning of the story?
> What was the problem in the story?
> What did the people do about it?
> Who thought of a good idea to solve it?
> What did she do?
> What was the result?

For problem solving, ask students to state the problem in the story. What happened because of the problem? Talk about other ways it could have been solved. Ask students if they think Rani knew that she would end up with so much rice. Talk about why Rani was so clever and what math facts she had to know before she made her request. What did she know that the raja didn't?

Extended Activity: At the back of the book is a 30-day calendar. In each square is written the number of grains of rice received on that day, beginning with 1 grain and ending with 536,870,912. Conduct a class experiment using a calculator to prove the total figure is accurate. Introduce the word *square*, a quantity that is the second power of another, such as $4 \times 4 = 16$.

The Owl and the Pussycat

by Edward Lear
Illustrated by Jan Brett
New York: Putnam & Grosset, 1996

Suggested Grade and Interest Level: 1 through 3

Topic Explorations: Boats; Fairy tales and nursery rhymes; Folklore, English; Owls; Sea and the seashore

Skill Builders:

Vocabulary	Grammar and syntax	Phonological awareness
Semantics	Pronouns, personal and possessive	
	Tenses, present and past	

Synopsis: This is a Calypso, Caribbean-style version of the fanciful old tale of the owl who courts the pussycat in a beautiful pea green boat. Illustrations in this version are ideal for explaining some of the unusual words of the rhyme. They provide a great deal of opportunities for language expansion when the class discusses the items and characters and actions taking place around the lush, green tropical paradise. Included are the dapper owl and glamorous pussycat, hibiscus flowers, exotic fish, sea turtles, sea coral, and tropical fruit.

Method: Before the read-aloud, present the book's cover and elicit background knowledge about the nursery rhyme. See if children can recite portions of the rhyme and tell what the story is about. Introduce this version by talking about where the story takes place. Describe what the characters are wearing, what's in the boat, and the type of fish featured beneath the ocean.

During the read-aloud, pause to interact with children about the action taking place, shaping or modeling grammatical and syntactic structures at appropriate intervals throughout the rhyming text. Also clarify the meanings of several fun words the children can learn, for example,

> *a runcible spoon* (a fork-like utensil with wide prongs, as shown in the illustration)
> *a five-pound note* (like a five-dollar bill)
> *a shilling* (coin)
> *tarried* (stayed in one place; waited)
> *mince* (meaning mincemeat, as shown in the illustration)
> *quince* (a type of fruit)
> Define *elegant* and *charming* by pointing out the characters in the illustrations (mannerly, polite, and nice).

After the read-aloud, play phonological awareness games. First reread the text and make sure children understand the meanings of the words, especially those used in the following games. For earlier activities, see the same listing in the Pre-K catalog. Use any version of this tale that is available.

PLAY   **Say-the-Sound (initial).**

Children identify the beginning phoneme they hear in word pairs by saying the sound, for example,

> sea, sail
> What sound do you hear at the beginning of those words? *Sea, sail. Sea, sail.*
> Hear it, say it. (*s*)
> That's right. *s* is the sound at the beginning of these words.

Continue with the following words from the text:

sang, sea	love, look	hat, hand
ring, wrapped	fish, fowl	land, look
day, dined	danced, dined	moon, marry

PLAY   **Word-Search (initial).**

Children search the picture for a word that begins with a designated sound. Provide clues if needed. For example, say

> I'm thinking of a word that starts with *b.*
> What word starts with *b*? (Give phoneme/sound only.)
> *b . . . b . . . boat. Boat* starts with *b.*

Other words featured in this version include *basket, beads, banana,* and *beach.* More word sources for this sound and other sounds can be found on each page.

PLAY The Same-Sound (final) game.

Children identify whether word pairs end in the same sound. Say each pair of words, stressing final sounds. Then ask the children, "Do they end with the same sound?"

To make an unmatched pair, exchange one of the following words with another word from the text.

boat, cat	took, look	note, sweet
pound, wood	fish, splash	spoon, moon
plenty, honey	pound, land	nose, stars

PLAY Odd-One-Out (final).

From a string of words, children select the word that ends in a different sound. Stress final sounds. For example, say

> fish, splash, spoon
> Which word has a different ending sound? (spoon)
> That's right. *Spoon* is the odd one out.

Some four-word strings follow. Reduce to three-word strings as needed:

> owl, hill, fowl, hand
> honey, plenty, piggy, moon
> green, love, spoon, dine
> note, sweet, five, cat
> danced, fish, boat, wrapped
> end, hand, fish, pound
> tarried, turkey, married, sailed

PLAY Say-the-Sound (final).

Children listen to word pairs and produce the final sound that is common to each word. Using word pairs from the Same-Sound (ending) game provided above. Stress the final sounds. For example, ask

> What sound do you hear at the end of *boat* and *cat*?
> Hear it, say it.
> *Boat, cat. Boat, cat.* (t)
> That's right. *t* is the sound at the end of *boat* and *cat*.

PLAY Say-It-Until-You-Hear-It.

Children synthesize one-syllable words divided into onset-rime. Start with words that begin with a continuous single-consonant sound.

Demonstrate by presenting each part of the word separately. Show children how to elongate the onset part to blend the two parts together, saying them a little quicker each time until they are readily identified. For example,

> Put these two parts together: *m–oon.*
> Say it until you hear it. *Mmmm . . . oon. Moon.*

Other words from the text beginning with a single sound include

l-ight	f-ive	l-ove
n-ose	s-ail	sh-all

Then demonstrate how to synthesize one-syllable words divided into onset-rime beginning with a two-consonant cluster, as in

gr-een	tr-ee	st-ood
sl-ice	sm-all	st-ar
	sw-eet	sp-oon

PLAY Roll-It-Out.

Children synthesize a consonant-vowel-consonant (C-V-C) word by blending each of its phonemes. Demonstrate by elongating the phonemes and blending them together in shorter and shorter sequences until children can identify the word. For example, say

> m–oo–n
> What's the word? Roll it out. *Mmmm-ooo-n. Moon.*

Once children are successful, present each of the phonemes separately so they can "roll them out" on their own, in shorter and shorter sequences, to find the word. Use the one-syllable C-V-C word list provided in Say-It-Until-You-Hear-It.

PLAY Break-It-Up.

Children analyze one-syllable C-V-C words to identify the beginning, middle, and ending sounds. Begin activities with initial sounds, then proceed to middle and ending sounds. For an example on how to demonstrate finding the middle sound in *moon*, ask

> What's the sound in the middle of *moon*?
> Break it up: *mmmm-ooo-nnn-m-oo-n.*
> *oo* is the sound in the middle of *moon.*

Continue to present one-syllable C-V-C words provided in the Say-It-Until-You-Hear-It so children can "break them up" and identify the sounds in each of the positions.

In the last stage of the game, children identify all the sounds in the word. Demonstrate how to elongate the sounds and then break them up to identify each one. For example, ask

(continues on next page)

PLAY **Break-It-Up.** *Continued*

What are all the sounds in the word *five*?
Roll it out and break it up: *ffff-īīīī-vvv f-ī-v.*
F-ī-v are all the sounds in *five*.

PLAY **Delete-It.**

Children omit the first sound in one-syllable words from the text. Demonstrate by saying the word slowly, then leaving off the initial sound. To demonstrate using *boat*, for example, say

Listen to how I can make *boat* become *oat.*
I delete the first sound. *Boat. Oat.*
Now you delete it. *Boat. . .*

Use the list of one-syllable words provided in Say-It-Until-You-Hear-It. Once children experience success, use the words from the line, "by the light of the moon." Begin with the word *light* and build on each word until children can play Delete-It with the entire phrase. Their part will sound like this:

_y the _ight of the _oon

Extending the verse:

They _anced by the _ight of the _oon.

Extend the activity to four-sound words. For example,

Listen to how I can make *fowl* become *owl.*
I delete the first sound. *Fowl. Owl.*
What little word is left? (owl)

Continue with the following four-sound words:

land (and)
hand (and)
sand (and)

Continue with the one-syllable words beginning with a consonant cluster. Demonstrate how to delete a sound from the cluster, for example,

tr-ee becomes *tee*
sw-eet becomes *seat*
sl-ice becomes *lice*
st-ar becomes *tar*
sp-oon becomes *soon*

GRADES 1–5

> **◁ PLAY ▷**   **Add-To-It.**
>
> Children insert a new sound into a three-sound word to make a four-sound word, for example,
>
> > Listen to how I can make *owl* become *fowl.*
> > I add *f* to *owl. Fffff-owl. Fowl.*
> > *Owl, fowl. Owl, fowl.*
> > Now you try it.
>
> Continue with the three-sound words *land, hand,* and *sand,* and proceed to one-syllable words beginning with a consonant cluster, as done in Delete-It.
>
> Then play Switch-It. Children delete the initial sound of the word and exchange it with a new sound to make another word. Demonstrate first, then prompt with cues as necessary, for example,
>
> > Say *moon.*
> > Now say *moon,* only delete *m* and switch it with *t.*
> > What new word can you make? (*tune*)
>
> As children experience success, play the game using the phrase "They danced by the light of the moon." An example using the *t* sound would sound like this:
>
> > They *t*anced by the *t*ight of the *t*une.
>
> Continue switching initial phonemes to create humorous, nonsensical titles.

Note: Another recommended version: *The Owl and the Pussycat,* illustrated by James Marshall. The influence is "quite English," with a tuxedoed owl and a pussycat with some elaborate hats—only in this the pea green boat is a luxury liner. Illustrations provide for the same activities, with many good vocabulary words to discuss. Other versions are also available.

Pancakes for Breakfast

by Tomie de Paola
New York: Harcourt Brace Jovanovich, 1978

Suggested Grade and Interest Level: 1 through 4

Topic Exploration: Cooking

Skill Builders:

Grammar and syntax	**Language literacy**
Pronouns—personal, possessive, and reflexive	Relating personal experiences
Tenses, present and past	Sequencing
	Storytelling
	Problem solving
	Verbal expression
	Explaining processes in detail

Synopsis: A wordless book about a little old lady who awakens on a snowy day with the thought of pancakes for breakfast. The illustrations show her reaching for her recipe book and fetching the ingredients, besieged by difficulties at every step. Undaunted, she milks the cow, collects the eggs, and churns the butter, only to have her efforts foiled by her naughty dog and cat. The little old lady overcomes this, too, and ends her morning at the neighbor's breakfast table—with the satisfaction that only determination and comfort food can bring.

Method: Before presenting the book, ask the children what they know about pancakes. How are they made? How do the children like to eat them? Have several children relate their experiences of eating pancakes for breakfast:

> Who makes pancakes at their houses?
> Do they recall a special time when they had pancakes?
> What was the occasion?
> How did they feel?

Present the book, encouraging children's verbal expression as they tell the story from the pictures. Shape and model grammatical and syntactic structures as needed. Stress the use of the reflexive pronoun in sentences such as

> She's making pancakes for herself.
> She's going out to get the eggs by herself.

After the read-aloud, have children sequence the story events. What happened after the old lady woke up? What steps did she take to make her pancakes? Help children recall the order of events and explain the process of making pancakes out in the country where people don't always rely on grocery stores for their food.

For storytelling skills, ask story grammar questions, such as

> Who was the story about?
> Where did it take place?
> What happened to start the story off?
> What was the lady's plan?

Discuss the old lady's problems and how she solves them, for example,

> What did she do when she didn't have any eggs? Any butter? Any syrup?
> What did she do when the dog and cat ate up all the batter?
> What else could she have done?
> If you were the old lady, what would you have done?

Have children brainstorm other possibilities at this juncture.

> What if the little old lady didn't have any neighbors close by?
> What do you think she would do?
> If you were making pancakes and ran out of ingredients, what would you do?
> If your pets ate up all of your breakfast, what would you do?
> Do you like the little old lady? Why?

Extended Activities: Make a semantic web by diagramming children's questions related to pancakes. Start with the word *pancakes* circled on the board. As you talk about pancakes, write down associated ideas. What do the children want to know about them? For example, do they want to know how they're made or what ingredients are needed to make them? Write these questions near the circle, then draw a line connecting the circle to each question.

Then go back to the word *pancakes*. Have the children think of other types of questions. Do they want to know all the different types of toppings one can put on pancakes? Draw a line in the direction of another thought labeled "Toppings." Do they want to know where pancakes can be purchased? Draw a line in the direction of the thought labeled "Where to find." Help children look at statements and generate questions as you model self-learning strategies.

Then read the story, asking children to listen for the answers to some of their questions. Afterward, form collaborative groups. Help children answer the questions by generating statements about pancakes from the information presented, for example,

> Pancakes are made of _____.
> The best toppings for pancakes are _____.
> You can get pancakes by _____.

Vary the sentence structure:

> To eat a stack of pancakes, you must first _____.
> Making pancakes from scratch is a lot of work.
> The best way to make pancakes is to keep your cat and dog out of the kitchen.
> After making pancakes from scratch, you'll need to have a long rest.

For teaching sequencing, draw illustrations that show the basic story parts. Ask children to put the pages in the correct order to tell the story of *Pancakes for Breakfast*. Then have them retell the story from the new storybook pages. Children can write or dictate sentences for the text and color in the illustrations.

The Paper Crane

by Molly Bang
New York: Greenwillow, 1985; Morrow, 1987

Suggested Grade and Interest Level: 2 through 5

Topic Explorations: Community; Culture and history, Japanese

Skill Builders:

Grammar and syntax	**Language literacy**
Tenses, past and future	Predicting
	Storytelling
	Drawing inferences
	Discussion

Synopsis: An unusual man enters a restaurant whose owners are poor and in need of guests. Although the man has no money, the owners serve him as if he were a king. He pays the owners for his meal by making a paper crane from a napkin. The crane magically comes to life. Soon guests come to the restaurant from all around to see the dancing crane.

Method: Before the read-aloud, elicit background information on the art of origami. What sorts of things can one make out of folded paper?

During the read-aloud, pause to elicit past-tense structures. Have students repeat portions of the text at appropriate intervals. For predicting and future tense, ask students to predict events and phrase their predictions in future tense, as in these examples:

> The owners will go broke.
> They will lose their restaurant.
> He will do something magical.
> The boy will clap his hands.
> Their business will come back.

After the read-aloud, hold a discussion about the lesson the story has for the readers: What might have happened if the owners had refused to serve the poor old man or had not treated him as they would an honored guest? What are the benefits of honoring and respecting life and human beings? Ask what might become of the young boy in the story based on the illustration on the last page.

Extended Activity: Follow the read-aloud with an origami lesson to demonstrate this ancient Japanese art. Look for a book in your library. Origami makes a good lesson on following directions. It's also an activity children greatly enjoy. Many adults practice this craft as a hobby. If possible, arrange for a parent or visitor from the community to demonstrate origami to the class.

Be sure to discuss the history of this increasingly popular craft. Talk about how it dates back to the 12th century and that originally a strip of dried abalone was attached to the origami ornament. The intricate figure was made as a gift, which represented a wish of good fortune from the giver.

Peter's Chair

by Ezra Jack Keats
New York: Harper & Row, 1967, 1983

Suggested Grade and Interest Level: 1 through 3

Topic Explorations: Family relationships; Growing up

Skill Builders:

Vocabulary	**Grammar and syntax**	**Language literacy**
Semantics	Possessive nouns	Relating personal experiences
Adjectives	Pronouns—personal and possessive	Cause-and-effect relationships
	Tenses, present and past	Drawing inferences
		Critical thinking

Synopsis: This story about growing up with a new baby brings up many feelings. Warmly told with imaginative, colorful illustrations, it's little wonder this tale has become a classic.

Method: Before the read-aloud, talk about things in the children's lives that were once important to them but that they have since outgrown. Then lead into the book with a discussion about the arrival of a new baby in the family. What does it feel like to be a big brother or sister?

During the read-aloud, use adjectives from the story when talking about the events. They include

> *pink* chair
> *new* baby
> *little* chair
> *tall* building

Use the text and illustrations to shape or model other target structures at appropriate intervals.

After the read-aloud, encourage critical thinking by discussing the story, asking questions that underscore the story's meaning:

> Why do you think they painted Peter's crib pink?
> How do you think Peter feels about that?
> What reasons might he have had to run away?

Why do you think he took his baby pictures with him?
What is Peter doing when he puts his shoes under the curtain?
Why does he want to trick his mother?
What happened when he did?

Encourage children to use conjunctions such as *because* and *so* in answering the questions to express causal relationships between facts. Ask children what they would have done if they were Peter.

For relating personal experiences, have children talk about younger brothers and sisters in their homes. Converse about how difficult it is to give up something you love but have long since outgrown.

Pickle Things

by Marc Brown
New York: Parents Magazine Press, 1980

Suggested Grade and Interest Level: 1 through 3

Skill Builders:
  Vocabulary
  Categories
  Phonological awareness
  Articulation—*L, R,* and *S*

Synopsis: This rhyming book depicts "all the pickle things you never see":

  "A pickle ear,
  a pickle nose,
  pickle hair,
  and pickle toes."

Method: Begin by reading the book through. Then review the pages and ask the children to name "the pickle things you never see."

For phonological awareness training, take advantage of the rhyming text to play some of the earlier rhyming games on the phonological awareness continuum.

PLAY   **Finish-the-Rhyme.**

Children supply the rhyming word left out at the end of a verse. Teach children to use the meaningful clues in the pictures as well as the meter of the verse to rhyme the word. If necessary, prompt with the picture cue and with the initial phoneme. Then gradually remove scaffolding, for example,

  You never hear a pickle talk.
  You never see a pickle _____.
  You never hear a pickle sing.
  You never see a pickle leave a _____. (ring, as in bathtub ring)

(PLAY) **Rhyme-It-Again.**

Children identify the rhyming word just heard after a rhyming set is given:

> *Talk* rhymes with _____ (*walk*)
> *Sing* rhymes with _____ (*ring*)

(PLAY) **Make-a-Rhyme.**

Children supply another rhyming word after two are presented. Use the rhyming words from the text. For example,

> What rhymes with *boat* and *coat*? (moat)

If children have achieved earlier phonological awareness levels, play some games involving oddity tasks at the phoneme level using the words of the text.

(PLAY) **Odd-One-Out (initial).**

Children select from a string of alliterative words the one that does not belong. For example, say

> pickle, pie, flakes
> Which word has a different beginning sound? (flakes)
> That's right. *Flakes* is the odd one out.

More three-word strings:

ball, bat, pickle	down, donuts, boat
kite, cake, pie	bike, boat, cake

(PLAY) **Odd-One-Out (final).**

This time children select from a string of words (all but one containing the same ending sound) the one that doesn't belong. Stress final sounds. For example, say

> cake, bike, nose, flake
> Which word has a different ending sound?
> That's right. *Nose* is the odd one out.

More four-word strings:

kite, ball, bat, hat	toes, nose, candies, snow
cake, talk, sing, shake	slope, up, rope, feet

PLAY **Odd-One-Out (middle).**

This time children select from a string of consonant–vowel–consonant (C–V–C) words with the same middle sound the one that doesn't belong. Some three-word strings:

cake, rain, feet	feet, leave, nose	bike, kite, make
toes, boat, hat	make, moat, toes	kite, pike, cake

PLAY **Say-the-Sound (initial).**

Children say the sound they hear at the beginning of both words, for example,

> ball, bat
> What sound do you hear at the beginning of those words? *Ball, bat. Ball, bat.*
> Listen to the sound and say it. (*b*)

Use variations of the word strings provided above in Odd-One-Out for beginning sounds.

PLAY **Say-the-Sound (final).**

This time children say the sound they hear both words end with. Word pairs include

kite, bat	cake, talk
walk, shake	toes, candies
moat, feet	slope, up

PLAY **Say-It-Until-You-Hear-It.**

Children synthesize one-syllable C–V–C words divided into onset-rime. Present the word with a clear pause between the onset and rime. Demonstrate how to elongate the parts to blend them together, saying them a little quicker each time until they are readily identified. Provide scaffolding until children are ready to do it on their own. For example, say

> Put these two parts together: *w-alk.*
> Say it until you hear it. *Wwwww-alk. Www-alk. Walk.*

Continue with these words from the text:

f-eet	sh-ake	t-alk
n-ose	l-eave	c-ake

PLAY Roll-It-Out.

Children synthesize a C–V–C word by blending each of its phonemes. Demonstrate by elongating the phonemes and blending them together in shorter and shorter sequences until children can identify the word. For example, say

> w–a–l–k
> What's the word? Roll it out.
> *Wwww-aaa-k. Ww-aa-k Walk.*

Once children are successful, present each of the phonemes separately so they can "roll them out" on their own, in shorter and shorter sequences, to find the word. Use the one-syllable C–V–C word list provided in Say-It-Until-You-Hear-It.

PLAY Break-It-Up.

Children analyze one-syllable C–V–C words to identify the beginning, middle, and ending sounds. Begin activities with initial sounds, then proceed to middle and ending sounds. For an example on how to demonstrate finding the middle sound in the word *walk*, ask

> What's the sound in the middle of *walk*?
> Break it up: *Wwww-aaaa-kkkk . . . w-a-k.*
> *ä* is the sound in the middle of *walk*.

Continue to present one-syllable C–V–C words provided above so children can "break them up" and identify the sounds in each of the positions.

In the last stage of the game, children identify all the sounds in the word. Demonstrate how to elongate the sounds and then break them up to identify each one.

PLAY Pickle-Talk (Delete-It).

Children omit the first sound in one-syllable words from the text. Demonstrate by saying the word slowly, then leaving off the initial sound. To demonstrate using *talk*, for example, say

> Listen to how I can make *talk* become *awk*.
> I delete the first sound. *Talk. Awk.*
> Now you do it. *Talk . . .*

After practicing with more one-syllable C–V–C words provided in Say-It-Until-You-Hear-It, do Pickle-Talk with the word *talk* again, then demonstrate with the word *pickle*. Then put the two words together: "Ickle Awk."

More Pickle-Talk with Ickle-Things:

Pickle toes becomes *ickle oze.*	*Pickle nose* becomes *ickle oze.*
Pickle hair becomes *ickle air.*	*Pickle cake* becomes *ickle ake.*

and so on.

PLAY   Advanced Pickle-Talk (Switch-It).

While still talking Pickle-Talk, switch the initial sounds in the Pickle-Talk words to different sounds to make new and advanced words. For example,

> Switch to *m*: *Pickle toes* becomes *Mickle Moze.*
> Switch to *t*: *Pickle hair* becomes *Tickle Tair.*
> Switch to *f*: *Pickle cake* becomes *Fickle Fake.*

and so on.

Then switch the initial sound in the first word with the initial sound in the other word. For example, *pickle talk* becomes *tickle pawk.*

> Listen to how I can take the first sound in *pickle* and switch it with the first sound in *talk*:
> *pickle talk/tickle pawk*
> Now you do it. *pickle talk/*(t)_____ (p)_____

More Pickle-Talk:

> *Pickle toes* becomes *Tickle Poze.*
> *Pickle nose* becomes *Nickle Poze.*
> *Pickle cake* becomes *Cickle Pake.*

Extended Activity: Play a game of Pickle-Things-Around-You. Brainstorm pickle things, including pictures of pickle things. Then put them in a rhyme. It's easy.

> Pickle paper, pickle books, pickle glasses, pickle nooks.

> Pickle boxes, pickle bears, pickle pictures, pickle chairs.

Make up categories of things that are pickle-like (and that no one sees, of course). The categories can rhyme or not, as the children choose:

> Pickle hot dogs, pickle fries, pickle drumsticks, pickle thighs.
> Pickle lettuce, pickle beans, pickle broccoli, pickle greens.
> Pickle jump ropes, pickle bats, pickle rackets, pickle balls.

Make a list of pickle things that begin with the same sound:

> For *p*: Pickle pencils, pickle pens, pickle paper, pickle peanuts, pickle pipe cleaners, pickle pears, pickle pandas, and pickle passengers.
> For *r*: Pickle radios, pickle rowboats, pickle wristwatches, and pickle ratatouille.

Piggie Pie

by Margie Palatini
New York: Houghton Mifflin, 1995

Suggested Grade and Interest Level: 1 through 5

Topic Explorations: Animals, Farm; Cooking; Holidays, Halloween

Skill Builders:

Vocabulary	**Language literacy**
Attributes	Sequencing
Grammar and syntax	Storytelling
Pronouns, personal and possessive	Problem solving
Past tense	**Phonological awareness**
Advanced syntactic structures	

Synopsis: Here's a feast of delicious words with which to say and play. Trendy, high-powered Witch Gritch is in the mood for the most delicious meal ever—piggie pie. But when she goes to the shelf to pull out her *Old Hag Cookbook*—"PROBLEM!"—she's got no pigs. So she flies on her broom to Old McDonald's farm, but not without first giving herself away. As she arrives, she writes "Surrender Piggies!" in the sky with her broom, giving her victims enough time to problem solve. They disguise themselves as geese, chickens, cows, and even Old MacDonald himself. So when she arrives in pursuit of them, she can't find a single one of those little porkers. The tie-in to familiar nursery rhymes gives additional laughs, especially for the older students. This is a read-aloud for any time, not just Halloween.

Method: Read it the first time without pausing. Then do a picture walk-through. For developing expression with the use of attributes, children can have fun describing the witch, including her long green fingernails, warty face, big pointy hat, and gap-toothed grin. Encourage other descriptions such as hungry, greedy, and outrageously wicked.

Improve grammar and syntax by having children talk about the action sequences in the story. The text provides some interesting words from which to model and shape target structures. Some past-tense examples include

> She pulled down her *Old Hag Cookbook.*
> She looked up a recipe.
> Gritch stomped her feet.
> Gritch paced the floor.

To address advanced syntactic structures, brainstorm a few sentences for one of the illustrated actions. Write the sentences down. Use one as the root sentence and turn the other into a verb phrase. Combine the two sentences. Then vary the position of the phrase within the sentence for syntactic variety, for example,

> She is writing "Surrender Piggies" in the sky.
> The witch flies over the farm on her broom.
> The witch flies over the farm on her broom, writing "Surrender Piggies" in the sky.
> Writing "Surrender Piggies" in the sky, the witch flies over the farm on her broom.
> Flying over the farm on her broom, the witch writes "Surrender Piggies" in the sky.

To teach storytelling skills, an important skill for literacy, discuss the story grammars, for example,

> Who was the story about? (Witch Gritch)
> Where did the story start out? (Gritch's house)
> When? (in the morning when she woke up)
> What happened to start the story off? (She wanted piggie pie but didn't have any pigs.)
> What did the character do to solve her problem? (went to the Yellow Pages to look up farms)
> What was the result? (She found Old MacDonald's farm listed.)
> What was the next thing the character did? (She flew to the farm on her broom and wrote "Surrender Piggies!" in the sky.)
> What was the result? (The pigs disguised themselves so she couldn't find any of them.)
> How did the story end? (She found the wolf and invited him to dinner.)
> How did the characters feel then? (Gritch was happy because she was thinking of him for her meal, and the wolf was happy because he was thinking the same thing. The pigs were happy too because they didn't get eaten!)

Children can take turns retelling the story, prompted by features in the illustrations and by the scaffolding questions. Encourage use of the connective words *and, then, so,* and *because.* After the story has been retold, ask children to share their favorite part so that the details of the story can be elaborated.

Use the words of the text to play phonological awareness games. See the *Piggy Pie* entry in the Pre-K catalog for activities that address earlier levels.

(PLAY) **Word-Search.**

Children search an illustrated page for a word that begins with the same sound as a target sound. Give clues and prompts as necessary, for example, say

> I'm thinking of a word in the story that starts with *w.* (Give phoneme/sound only.)
> What word starts with *w . . . wwwww . . . ?*
> That's right. Witch. *Witch* starts with *wwwww.*

Word sources are plentiful in each illustration.

(PLAY) **Say-It-Until-You-Hear-It.**

Children synthesize one-syllable consonant–vowel–consonant (C–V–C) words divided into onset-rime. Present the word with a clear pause between the onset and rime. Demonstrate how to elongate the parts to blend them together, saying them a little quicker each time until they are readily identified. Provide scaffolding until children are ready to do it on their own. For example, say

> Put these two parts together: *w-itch.*
> Say it until you hear it. *Wwwww-itch.*
> Faster and faster. *Www-itch. Witch.*

Other C–V–C words beginning with a single sound include

f-eet	l-ook
h-eap	d-uck

Then demonstrate how to synthesize one-syllable words divided into onset-rime beginning with a two-consonant cluster, as in

Gr-itch	br-oom	st-ew
sm-ack	gr-ouch	sc-are
	gr-in	sp-ell

(PLAY) **Roll-It-Out.**

Children synthesize a C–V–C word by blending each of its phonemes. Demonstrate by elongating the phonemes and blending them together in shorter and shorter sequences until children can identify the word. For example, say

> w–i–tch
> What's the word? Roll it out. *Wwww-iii-tch. Witch.*

(continues on next page)

GRADES 1–5

PLAY **Roll-It-Out.** *Continued*

Once children are successful, present each of the phonemes separately so they can "roll them out" on their own, in shorter and shorter sequences, to find the word. Continue with the one-syllable C–V–C words in the lists provided in Say-It-Until-You-Hear-It.

PLAY **Break-It-Up.**

Children analyze one-syllable words to identify the beginning, middle, and ending sounds. Begin activities with initial sounds, then proceed to middle sounds and ending sounds. For an example on how to demonstrate finding the middle sound in *boom*, treat *br* as one unit, without breaking up the sounds, and ask

> What's the sound in the middle of *broom*?
> Break it up: *Brrrrrrr-ooo-mmm . . . br-oo-m.*
> *oo* is the sound in the middle of *broom.*

Continue using the words in the lists provided in Say-It-Until-You-Hear-It.

In the last stage of the game, children identify all the sounds in one-syllable C–V–C words. Demonstrate how to elongate the sounds and then break them up in order to identify each one. For example, ask

> What are all the sounds in the word *witch*?
> Roll it out and break it up: *Wwww-iiiii-tch . . . W-i-tch.*
> *W-i-tch* are the sounds in *witch.*

PLAY **Delete-It.**

Children omit the first sound in one-syllable words from the text. Demonstrate by saying the word slowly, then leaving off the initial sound. To demonstrate using *witch*, for example, say

> Listen to how I can make *witch* become *itch.*
> I delete the first sound. *Witch. Itch.*
> Now you delete it. *Witch . . .*

Use the words in the list of one-syllable words provided in Say-It-Until-You-Hear-It. Then play the game with the alliterative words of the title. Repeat the demonstration, leaving out the initial sounds in the words:

> Piggie Pie

to make

> Iggie Eye

Ask children to recall what the words were before you changed them. Continue until the children are able to leave out the initial sounds in both words of the title on their own.

Extend the activity to four-sound words, for example,

> Listen to how I can make *farm* become *arm.*
> I delete the first sound. *Farm. Arm.*
> What little word is left? (arm)
> That's right. *Farm. arm.*

(continues on next page)

PLAY **Delete-It.** *Continued*

Continue with the following three- and four-sound words:

> f-eet (eat)
> th-ump (ump, as in umpire)
> p-ink (ink)

Move to one-syllable words beginning with a consonant cluster. Demonstrate how to delete a sound from the cluster. For example,

> Listen to how I can make *smack* become *sack*.
> I roll out *smack*: *Sssssmmmmmaaaak*.
> Delete the *mmmmmmmmmm*, and now I have *sssssaaaaak*.
> *Smmmmaaack, sssssaaaaak*.
> *Smack, sack*. Now you try it.

Once students are successful, present the game as follows:

> Say *grouch*.
> Delete the *gr*. What word do you have? (ouch!)

More variations of three- and four-sound words:

gr-ouch (ouch!)	sm-ack (sack)	sc-are (care)
gr-in (in)	pl-ump (pump, lump)	sp-ell (sell)
	gr-ump (rump)	st-ew (Sue, to)

Use the lines of Witch Gritch that she borrows from "Old MacDonald Had a Farm," leaving off the initial sound from the *kw* words, for example,

> Listen to the words *quack, quack*.
> Listen to how I can make *quack, quack* become *ack, ack*.
> *Quack, ack. Quack, quack, ack, ack*.
> Now you try it.

Then show how to put the new words into Gritch's lines until the children are ready to do it on their own, for example,

With a ack ack here	Here a ack, there a ack
And a ack ack there	Everywhere it ack acked

PLAY **Switch-It.**

Children delete the initial sound of the word and exchange it with another sound to form a new word. First use the words in the title, for example,

> Say *piggie*.
> Now say *piggie*, only delete the *p* and switch it with *t*.
> What new word can you make? *Tiggie*

(continues on next page)

PLAY **Switch-It.** *Continued*

Continue until the children can switch Piggie Pie to Tiggie Tie. Other switches include

Siggie Sie	Shiggie Shy
Figgie Fie	Friggie Fry
Liggie Lie	Sliggie Sly

Next, use Gritch's lines that she borrowed from "Old MacDonald" to substitute the beginning sounds in the *quack* words with another sound. For example,

Say *quack, quack.*
Now say *quack, quack,* only delete the *kw* sounds and switch them with *m* sounds.
What new words can you make? (mack, mack)

Once children can produce the switch on their own, put the words into the verse, as in

With a mack-mack here
And a mack-mack there
Here a mack, there a mack
Everywhere it mack-macked,
"No Miggies!"

Also use Gritch's expressions, such as, "Hand over those hogs" and switch *h* with another phoneme. Some suggestions include

Band over those bogs.
Sand over those sogs.
Fand over those fogs.
Land over those logs.
Mand over those mogs.

Note: If you haven't got your fill of crazy witches, read *Zoom Broom* by the same author for more fun!

Piggybook

by Anthony Browne
New York: Knopf, 1986, 1990

Suggested Grade and Interest Level: 3 through 5

Topic Explorations: Careers; Family relationships

Skill Builders:

Vocabulary	Language literacy
Idioms	Cause-and-effect relationships
	Problem solving
	Drawing inferences
	Discussion

Synopsis: Mrs. Piggett has a very important husband and two very important sons. She makes them breakfast, washes the dishes, vacuums the floor, and then goes off to work. She comes home to make them dinner and do more chores—until one day, accusing them all of being pigs, she leaves. By making actual pigs of themselves, the Piggetts realize how much Mother did for them. All ends well when Mrs. Piggett returns and the household roles change.

Method: Before the read-aloud, introduce the cover and ask, "Why do you think this mother's family is on her back?" Introduce the idiom "on one's back" and ask students to think about the question as you read aloud.

As you read, pause to discuss all the nuances in the artist's illustrations, such as the pig wallpaper and mantel decorations. Have students describe what is happening in the Piggett home. Why did the artist render Mr. Piggett and the boys large and in bold colors, while Mrs. Piggett is rendered smaller and in sepia shades? Why is Mrs. Piggett's face hidden? What do you think she is thinking?

For problem solving, ask what facts can be stated about the problem. What events led to the problem? In what other ways could Mrs. Piggett have solved her problem?

For cause-and-effect relationships, ask what changes occurred because of Mrs. Piggett's decision to leave.

> How do you think she felt when she left home?
> Why did she come back?
> What did the Piggetts learn when they were on their own?

After the read-aloud, ask again why the family is on Mrs. Piggett's back. Discuss other idioms such as "the straw that broke the camel's back" and "at the end of one's rope."

Discuss what responsibilities the students have in their own homes and all that their mothers do for them. Discuss the importance of cooperating as a team at home just as they do in school.

Pigsty

by Mark Teague
New York: Scholastic, 1994

Suggested Grade and Interest Level: 1 through 4

Topic Exploration: Messes

Skill Builders:

Vocabulary	Grammar and syntax	Language literacy
Semantics	Possessive pronouns	Relating personal experiences
Categories	Tenses, present and past	Predicting
Prepositions		Sequencing
Idioms		
Synonyms		
Antonyms		

Synopsis: Wendell Fultz's mother has declared his room a "pigsty." After her failed attempts to get him to straighten it up, she leaves matters in Wendell's own hands. Soon several pigs are keeping residence with him, fat little porkers that jump on the trampoline, engage in pillow fights, and play Monopoly with him. The mess just grows and grows until Wendell comes up with an answer—and a thoughtful one at that.

Method: Before the read-aloud, elicit the children's background knowledge about the word *pigsty*. Talk about pigs and their "habitats," how they enjoy rolling in mud and eating slosh in a dirty, fenced-in pen called a pigsty. Because pigsties are so dirty, the word is often used to label other places that are considered very messy. Based on this, have the children predict what the story might be about.

During the read-aloud, pause briefly for the children to describe illustrations of some of the activity taking place in Wendell's room. Shape and model grammar and syntax structures in a limited amount, if it can be done without interrupting the flow of the story. Ask children to state how Wendell *really* feels when he finds hoof prints on his comic books and chew marks on his baseball cards. Based on those inferences, ask children to make predictions about what will happen next. Will Wendell want the pigs to stay? Why or why not?

After the read-aloud, do a picture walk-through. Sequence the events of the story. Elicit grammar and syntax structures from descriptions about what the pigs are doing in the illustrations. Use the items in Wendell's room to elicit possessive pronouns for Wendell's belongings (e.g., *his* baseball cards, *his* comic books, *his* train set, and the pigs'—that is, *their*—suitcases). Use the placement of his belongings for prepositional phrases.

Talk about figures of speech and the idiom, "many hooves make light work," that is used in the text. Ask the children if they can guess at an explanation. What might that mean? What has hooves in the text? How might the pigs make light work? Light work for whom? Did the boy have to do much work himself when the pigs straightened up his room? Was this a good way to solve his problem?

The boy's mother calls his room a pigsty. Brainstorm synonyms for the word, such as *dirty, filthy, messy, cluttered*, and antonyms such as *clean, tidy, neat*, and *organized*.

Play Clean-Up and categorize things in a child's room that need to be put away (e.g., games, books, stuffed animals, clothing, sports equipment, musical instruments, bedding). Name items in the picture that can fit into each category. Where might each belong? (For example, on a shelf, in a toy chest, in the closet.)

Have students relate personal experiences of room clean-ups. Perhaps they have a system, a way to do it, or a time of the week they need to do it, such as Saturday morning. Perhaps there are special rules at their house that they want to share or a story about a time they did clean up.

Push, Pull, Empty, Full: A Book of Opposites

by Tana Hoban
New York: Macmillan, 1972

Suggested Grade and Interest Level: 1 through 5

Skill Builders:
> **Vocabulary**
> Beginning concepts
> Antonyms

Synopsis: A series of black-and-white photographs illustrates 15 pairs of opposite concepts, including *push/pull, in/out*, and *first/last*.

Method: Use the book as you would any visual stimulus. Cover one side of the page and ask for the opposite concept. Make up a sentence for each concept from the illustrations. Discuss word meanings.

Extended Activity: Play the game of opposites with things around the room. Ask such questions as

What do you see that is empty?
What do you see that is full?
What do you see that is soft?
What do you see that is hard?

Then go outside and observe things in the surrounding environment. What do you see that is translucent? What do you see that is opaque? What do you see that is alive? What do you see that is dead?

Some additional antonym pairs include

moist/dry
vacant/occupied
temporary/permanent
necessary/useless
swift/slow
stationary/moveable
stiff/limp

Read also *Over, Under, and Through and Other Spatial Concepts; I Read Signs, Is It Larger? Is it Smaller?;* and other photographic concepts books by the same author.

Quick as a Cricket

by Don Wood
Swindon, England: Child's Play International, 1990

Suggested Grade and Interest Level: 1 through 3

Topic Exploration: Animals

Skill Builders:
   Vocabulary
   Semantics
   Adjectives
   Similes and metaphors

Synopsis: A series of animals brilliantly illustrated in Don Wood's exuberant style are portrayed by their most salient characteristic. A short simile for each illustration constitutes the simple text.

Method: Before the read-aloud, talk about the characteristics of different animals. How would the children describe an elephant? A giraffe? A bumblebee? Make up similes for each animal; then introduce the book, showing children how they can make their language more fun, colorful, and descriptive.

During the read-aloud, have children join in. Apply each simile to a real-life situation, for example, "When Carlos is on the playground, he is as quick as a cricket" or "When I get up in the morning, I'm as slow as a snail." Then give the first half of the sentence and let the children fill in the simile. Once you've established the pattern, see whether children can create their own phrases.

Extended Activities: Ask students each to think of four or five adjectives that describe themselves. List them as character traits. Then take each trait and make up a simile associating the trait with an animal, person, or object. Expand the simile with a verb or prepositional phrase, for example, "I'm as quiet as a mouse in a cupboard" or "I'm as wild as a monkey in a tree."

Cut 11″ × 14″ (legal-size) paper in half lengthwise and give each student a sheet of paper. Fold it in half and then in half again, making four lengthwise sections. In each of the four sections, have children illustrate their similes using colorful marking pens. Write the sentence to complete the graphic. Separate each section with colorful borders filled with designs. Label the work "All About Me."

Rain Makes Applesauce

by Julian Scheer and Marvin Bileck
New York: Holiday House, 1964

Suggested Grade and Interest Level: 1 through 3

Topic Explorations: Food; Fruit; Growing cycles and planting; Weather, Rain

Skill Builders:

Grammar and syntax	**Language literacy**	**Phonological awareness**
Present tense	Sequencing	Articulation, *R* and *S*

Synopsis: Nonsense verses join with the repeated phrase *"rain makes applesauce"* to make up the text of this whimsical book. If there has ever been a children's book with magic in it, it has to be this one. If there is only one choice for a picture book as a historical, cultural document, it must be this one. Published in the 1960s, it has remained in print for more than 30 years, has been an award and honor recipient, and has been listed on the *New York Times* 10 Best Illustrated Books. The words, although they do not make sense, encourage children to chime in and make their own "silly talk." Look closely at the illustrations to discover the real story, cleverly hidden within. Great for the fall season.

Method: Before the read-aloud, elicit children's background knowledge about where applesauce comes from and how it is made.

During the read-aloud, elaborate on the text and ask children to join in as you repeat the refrain, "rain makes applesauce" and the girl's response, "Oh, you're just talking silly talk."

After the read-aloud, go back to the first page and point out, in the illustration, where two children are buying seeds from a seed cart. Model, shape, and recast present-tense structures. Once the children have discovered the story on their own, have them review the illustrations and sequence the steps of making applesauce.

Use the words of the text to play phonological awareness games. See the entry in the Pre-K catalog for activities that address earlier phonological awareness levels.

PLAY **Word-Search.**

Children identify a word from the story that begins with a designated sound. Give clues and prompts as necessary. For example, say

> I'm thinking of a word in the story that starts with *s*. (Give phoneme/sound only.)
> What word starts with *s . . . sssss . . .*?
> It's something the children are buying at the cart.
> That's right. *Seed. Seed* starts with *s*.

Word sources are plentiful on each page.

PLAY **Odd-One-Out (middle).**

Children select from a string of words the one that does not have the same middle sound, for example, say

> rain, made, make, seed
> Which word has a different middle sound? (seed)
> That's right. *Seed* is the odd one out.

Some three-word strings for identifying middle sounds include

shoes, sauce, moon	walk, sauce, hide	rain, soap, hole
seed, like, night	talk, sauce, shoes	slide, like, walk

PLAY **Say-It-Until-You-Hear-It.**

Children synthesize one-syllable consonant–verb–consonant (C–V–C) words divided into onset-rime. Start with words that begin with a continuous single-consonant sound. Demonstrate by presenting each part of the word separately. Show children how to elongate the onset part to blend the two parts together, saying them a little quicker each time until they are readily identified, for example,

> Put these two parts together: *s-eed.*
> Say it until you hear it. *Sssss-eed. Sss-eed. Seed.*

Other words from the text beginning with a single sound include

r-ain	sh-oes	m-ade
w-alk	m-oon	n-ight
l-ong	l-ike	s-oap
h-ole		

Then demonstrate how to synthesize one-syllable words divided into onset-rime beginning with a two-consonant cluster, as in

> sm-oke (smoke)
> sn-oot (snoot)
> sl-eep (sleep)
> cl-oud (cloud)
> sl-ide (slide)

PLAY **Roll-It-Out.**

Children synthesize a C–V–C word by blending each of its phonemes. Demonstrate by elongating the phonemes and blending them together in shorter and shorter sequences until children can identify the word. For example, say

> r-ā-n
> What's the word? Roll it out. *Rrrrr-aaaaa-n. Rain.*

Once children are successful, present each of the phonemes separately so they can "roll them out" on their own, in shorter and shorter sequences, to find the word. Use the one-syllable C–V–C word list provided above.

PLAY **Break-It-Up.**

Children analyze one-syllable C–V–C words to identify the beginning, middle, and ending sounds. Begin activities with initial sounds, then proceed to middle and ending sounds. For an example on how to demonstrate finding the middle sound in *rain*, ask

> What's the sound in the middle of *rain*?
> Break it up: *Rrrr-āāāāā-nnn . . . r-ā-n.*
> *ā* is the sound in the middle of *rain*.

Continue to present one-syllable C–V–C words from above so children can "break them up" and identify the sounds in each of the positions.

In the last stage of the game, children identify all the sounds in the word. Demonstrate how to elongate the sounds and then break them up to identify each one. For example, ask

> What are all the sounds in the word *rain*?
> Roll it out and break it up: *rrrr-āāāā-nnn . . . R-ā-n.*
> *R-ā-n* are the sounds in the word *rain*.

PLAY **Silly-Talk (Delete-It).**

Children omit the first sound in one-syllable words from the text. Demonstrate by saying the word slowly, then leaving off the initial sound. To demonstrate using *make,* for example, say

> Listen to how I can make *make* become *ache*.
> I delete the first sound. *Make. Ache.*
> Now you delete it. *Make . . .*

Continue with the following one-syllable words:

> made
> sauce
> shoes
> house
> walk
> day
> moon
> night
> soap

Demonstrate how to leave out the beginning sound with each word, asking children to recall what the word was before you changed it. Once children are ready to delete the first phoneme in all the words, their part will sound like this:

> "Ain Akes Applesauce"

PLAY **Silly-Talk.**

Use the repetitive lines of the story, "Oh, you're just talking silly talk." Practice the phrase as it stands several times. Then demonstrate, one word at a time, how to delete the initial phonemes to make the following:

> Awking Illy Awk
> Oh, you're just _awking _illy _awk

Model the exercise until the children are ready to do it on their own.

PLAY **More Silly-Talk (Switch-It).**

Children delete the initial sound of the word and exchange it with a new sound to make another word. Demonstrate first, then prompt with cues as necessary, for example,

> Say *rain*.
> Now say *rain*, only delete the *r* and switch it with *t*.
> What funny word can you make? (tain)
> Listen: *Rain* switches to *tain*.

Continue with the list of one-syllable words provided until children experience success. Then make more silly talk with the title. Switching the initial phonemes to *t*, the title will sound like this:

> Tain takes tapplesauce.

Other Silly-Talk possibilities include

> Rain rakes rapplesauce   Shain shakes shapplesauce
> Fain fakes fapplesauce   Bain bakes bapplesauce

Also practice with the phrase, "talking silly talk." Demonstrate how to replace the *t* and *s* with another designated sound. Using *m*, the new words will sound like this, *Oh, you're just mawking milly mawk.*

Other possibilities include

> Oh, you're just walking willy walk.
> Oh, you're just nalking nilly nalk. (Sounds like "knocking nilly knock")

Use another line of verse, such as

> "Monkeys eat the chimney smoke"

Delete it: onkeys eat the imney oke
Switch it: Wonkeys wheat the wimney woke

Another line of verse:

> "Dolls go dancing on the moon"

Delete it: olls go ancing on the oon
Switch it: Golls go gancing on the goon

For articulation of *R*, *S*, and *S* blends, children can recite the lines of repetitive text, repeat the lines of text after you, use the target sound in sentences that describe the action in the illustrations, and use the target sounds in sequencing the steps in making applesauce.

The Rat and the Tiger

by Keiko Kasza
New York: Scholastic, 1993

Suggested Grade and Interest Level: 1 through 3

Topic Explorations: Friendship; Manners and etiquette; Sharing

Skill Builders:
    Language literacy   **Pragmatic language**
    Problem solving
    Drawing inferences

Synopsis: An incongruous pair, Rat and Tiger are best of friends, playing cowboys and sharing meals. Tiger is bigger, naturally, so when it comes to playing cowboys, he gets to be the good guy; when they share doughnuts, he gets the bigger half; and when he wants a flower at the bottom of a cliff, he has the right to push Rat off to get it for him. Rat says he's just a little rat and silently endures. One day Rat builds a castle and Tiger angrily kicks it to pieces. That was the last straw for Rat, who declares Tiger "a big mean bully" and no longer his friend. The rest of the story finds them on a new playing field as Rat shows Tiger what it's like to be on the receiving end of a "bullyship," rather than a friendship.

Method: Before the read-aloud, introduce the book by asking children to share some of the rules of playing together, such as turn-taking and sharing. Have children brainstorm ways they are kind to their friends. Introduce the story of two friends, Rat and Tiger, and have the children describe the cover illustration.

Read the story aloud, pausing to point out—and interpret, if necessary—the expressions of the characters.

After the read-aloud, ask children to tell how they felt about the story. What did they think about the way Tiger and Rat behaved? Help children learn to draw inferences by filling in what happened between the pictures and text. For example, after Tiger pushes Rat off the cliff, the next picture shows Rat with bandages. Ask, How did Rat come to have bandages on his shoulder and knee?

Continue to help children infer meaning by asking,

> What did Rat mean when he said, "What could I say? I'm just a tiny little rat?"
> Why couldn't Rat tell Tiger how he felt?
> How did Rat feel when Tiger didn't play fair?
> What did Tiger learn?
> What did Rat learn?

For problem-solving skills, ask children to state the problem in the story.

> Why didn't Rat tell Tiger how he felt when Tiger was a bully?
> How did Rat solve his problem?
> How did Tiger solve his problem?
> Are there other ways they could have solved their problems?
> What could they have done in the first place to keep from almost ruining their friendship?

For improving pragmatic language skills, go over the ideas children brainstormed before the read-aloud about playing with friends and talk about how they apply to Rat and Tiger and to each other in real life. Include how to

make polite requests,	express your feelings,	say things that give the
be a good listener,	take turns in conversations,	speaker feedback, and
		say you don't understand someone.

The Relatives Came

by Cynthia Rylant
New York: Bradbury Press, 1985, 1993

Suggested Grade and Interest Level: 1 through 4

Topic Explorations: Country life; Family relationships; Journeys; Seasons, Summer

Skill Builders:

Vocabulary	Grammar and syntax	Language literacy
Prepositions	Pronouns, personal and possessive	Relating personal experiences
	Tenses, present and past	Sequencing
		Compare and contrast

Synopsis: Many enjoyable events take place when a family takes off from Virginia in the summertime to visit their relatives. Descriptions of the warm and humorous episodes make this an enjoyable language experience that may trigger memories of your own family get-togethers. This book is a good one to read during the first few weeks after summer, when vacation time is often a topic of conversation.

Method: Introduce the book by asking students to define the word *relative.* Talk about family members who are living far away. Discuss what happens when family members come to visit and how the children's daily lives and household routines may change to accommodate them.

During the read-aloud, pause to describe the humorous, action-packed pictures. Shape and model target structures. What happens when the relatives arrive? (They knock down the picket fence, for one.) How does the family's life change because of the visit? Also discuss the expressions on the characters' faces and interpret how they feel about each event.

After the read-aloud and to elicit past-tense forms, ask what kinds of activities the relatives engaged in. (For example, they made music with their instruments, sang, mended the fence, went on picnics, took pictures, got haircuts, played games, and so on.)

Talk about what the relatives have in common and how they are different. Similarities can be based on ages, things they did, relationships, the mothers coming from the same family, and so on. Differences can be based on living in different places, liking to do different activities, and so on.

Also discuss the countryside on the family's trip home. Does it look like it did when they left?

How is it different?
What does the color of the grapes on the way to the relatives versus on the way home tell us about summertime in the hills of Virginia?
What does it tell us about the length of the trip?

Sequence the story parts. Include, for example, driving to the relatives' house, arriving, hugging, going in the house, having supper, sleeping, playing, and returning home.

Ask students to relate their own experiences of traveling to visit relatives during vacations.

> How did they travel? What was it like?
> What did they do to prepare for the trip?
> What did they bring along to entertain themselves during the drive?
> How was their experience like Virginia family's in the book? How was it different?
> How did they feel when they left for home?

Rotten Ralph

by Jack Gantos
Boston: Houghton Mifflin, 1976, 1980

Suggested Grade and Interest Level: 1 through 5

Topic Explorations: Animals, Cats; Pets

Skill Builder:
  Articulation, *R*

Synopsis: Ralph is Sarah's very naughty cat. Sarah loves him despite his rottenness. Her father, however, is fed up with Ralph's behavior and leaves him at the circus. Ralph struggles to get free, sleeps in a garbage can with the alley cats, and finds his way home to become a very good cat—for a while, anyway.

Method: Before the read-aloud, ask children to share experiences of times when their pets have done something naughty. Talk about how children still love their pets in spite of it and ways to help pets learn better behavior while still being kind to them.

During the read-aloud, stress the *R* words. Ask the children to practice the *R* sound in the phrase "rotten Ralph" before turning each page. Or ask questions that will elicit answers containing it, such as

> Q: What did he have to do at the circus?
> A: Water the camels

> Q: What else?
> A: Carry the barbells

After the read-aloud, have children retell parts of the story, maintaining accurate production of the target phonemes.

Note: Read also *Rotten Ralph's Trick or Treat* and *Worse Than Rotten Ralph,* all chock-full of the *R* sound.

Scary, Scary Halloween

by Eve Bunting
New York: Clarion, 1986

Suggested Grade and Interest Level: 1 through 3

Topic Explorations: Holidays, Halloween; Seasons, Autumn

GRADES 1–5

Skill Builders:

Vocabulary	**Grammar and syntax**	**Language literacy**
Semantics	Present tense	Verbal expression
Categories		Point of view
Attributes		**Articulation, *S* and *Z***

Synopsis: A spooky favorite, complete with a vampire, werewolf, skeleton, and plenty of action-packed illustrations. The nonthreatening, rhyming text is ideal for eliciting a variety of language skills.

Method: It's best to read this story without interruption the first time. This allows children to experience the mood of the story.

For categories and attributes, brainstorm all the Halloween creatures that fall into the scary-creature category. Then go back through the pages and give attributes to each. Read the text on the page to start the children off. For example,

> "A vampire and a werewolf prowl.
> One growls a growl, one howls a howl. . ."

For literacy development, discuss who is telling the story. Through whose eyes are we seeing Halloween night? Reread the first paragraph for a clue. Go through the rest of the pages to find where the cat and her kittens are hiding and whose green eyes are peering out from the dark beneath the stairs. Ask questions such as these:

> What do you think the cats are thinking about on Halloween?
> What else might the cats see on Halloween?
> What do you think your cat (or the neighborhood cat) sees on your street on Halloween night?

For syntax, go back over the illustrations to describe the action. Shape and model present tense and other syntactic forms.

For articulation of *S* and *Z*, shape and model target phonemes from the text. Words include the following:

outside	goblins
skeleton	gremlins
spikes	skip
ghost	scream
sunken	bones
fence	

Have children repeat the verse "scary, scary Halloween" before you turn each page. Also make a game of finding all the target words on each page of text.

Sector 7

by David Wiesner
New York: Clarion Books, 1999

Suggested Grade and Interest Level: 1 through 5

Topic Explorations: Cities, New York City; Clouds; Imagination; Weather

Skill Builders:

Vocabulary	**Language literacy**	**Pragmatic language**
Prepositions	Predicting	**Articulation**
Grammar and syntax	Sequencing	General articulation
Tenses, present and past	Storytelling	Carryover of all sounds
	Point of view	
	Explaining processes in detail	

Synopsis: In another wordless picture book by Caldecott Medal winner David Wiesner, a boy visits the Empire State Building on a class field trip. Finding the city obscured by cloud cover, the class is at a loss, but the boy makes friends with a unique cloud. It takes him up over the city until they reach Sector 7, a floating cloud factory, and the boy sees how cloud formations are made. (From machines!) He enters into an area reminiscent of a great railroad terminus such as what is now the Musee d'Orsay in Paris. There he watches clouds being sent out in tubes for various destinations by stuffy, official-looking workers. The clouds complain to him about their boring shapes, so the boy elaborates on their blueprints, creating a blue line drawing of an exotic, wide-mouthed fish. The officials become angry, rip up his drawing, and escort him out. When he arrives back at the Empire State Building, he joins his class, looks up in the sky, and finds an elaborate cloud display over Manhattan in the shape of fantastic aquatic creatures. Although the meaning of Weisner's works, especially his wordless books, are always subject to his audience's interpretation, there is no escaping this book's theme of taking one's talents and ideas and sharing them with the world to make a change.

Method: Share this book more than once, because each time through, children will notice something else in the illustrations that gives the story more meaning. Before the read-aloud, study the cover and ask prediction questions. Then share the book, asking various students to describe the illustrations. Scaffold as needed. Shape responses to build the syntactic forms of tenses and prepositional phrases (e.g., *outside on the street, inside the Empire State Building, on the observation deck, up in the sky, above the city, beyond the horizon*).

Because of the implied interaction between the characters in this wordless book, it is ideal for having children compose their own text, especially dialog. To develop pragmatic language skills, ask children to suggest what the cloud might say to the boy when it makes friends with him atop the Empire State Building. What are some appropriate ways to initiate conversation? What are some appropriate ways the boy can respond to the cloud? The whole class can brainstorm ideas. Continue to build on the dialog aspect of the story with suggestions for what the clouds in the factory might tell the boy about their boring shapes, what the officials might say to each other and the boy, and so forth.

For storytelling, hold a readers' theater. One child can act out the part of the boy and one child the part of the cloud. The audience plays the children on the field trip. The character of the boy retells the story of how he visited a fantastic place in the sky where clouds are made (perhaps to a very disbelieving class). To work on point of view, have different "characters" tell what happened that day from their perspective. The officials can tell what happened one day when a young boy came to view the factory and caused a serious commotion, explaining their actions of escorting him out. The factory clouds can tell the story from their perspective, that of talking with a talented young visitor who had wonderful ideas. Even the class of children on the field trip can tell the story from their point of view.

To work on sequencing skills and explaining a process in detail, have children explain how the process of making clouds works in Sector 7. Include in the sequential steps how they are made, the types of clouds made (listed in the illustrations), how they are sent out in different directions, and the decision-making process involved in sending them in different directions, according to the illustrations and the children's imaginations.

Extended Activities: Have children write dialog to portions of the story. Children can write the dialog in story form or in comic book style, using dialog balloons. If the group of children is small, each child can take a section of the book and create the entire text. If the group is larger, several children can write the dialog to one or two scenes and share their different versions with the other children.

For another written language activity, have children create a blueprint for an ordinary cloud on a large piece of paper. Then, in one corner of the blue line drawings, draw a rather large box and list in sequential order the process of creating the cloud, as it would occur in Sector 7. On another piece of paper, children can create a blueprint for a spectacular cloud in any formation they choose. Create the same box for the process, only vary the process as necessary to form the spectacular cloud.

Seven Blind Mice

by Ed Young
New York: Philomel, 1992

Suggested Grade and Interest Level: 1 through 3

Topic Explorations: Colors; Days of the week; Folklore, India; Part–whole relationships; Shapes and visual images

Skill Builders:
   Vocabulary
   Semantics
   Adjectives
   Similes and metaphors

Synopsis: Based on the ancient fable from India of the blind men and the elephant, this is a tale of six mice that disagree on what they see. Not until the seventh mouse resolves the dilemma do they learn a valuable lesson: The whole is bigger than its parts. Paper collage illustrations by Caldecott award winner Ed Young are captivating.

Method: Before the read-aloud, review the names of the days of the week and present the idea of giving each day a color. Also name the parts of some animals to see whether children can guess the whole animal. Talk about how sometimes when we look at a part of something, we may not know what it is. We try to find out in many ways, by turning it around and upside down, picking it up, and so on.

Read the story, explaining the meanings of words such as *pillar, spear, cliff,* and *whole.* When turning to the page showing the object, ask children to identify the color. Present part of the elephant as shown and ask children to pretend they are mice. What are they looking at?

For younger children, reinforce the days of the week by encouraging repetition. When the text says the mouse went on Wednesday, for example, have children recite the days of the week up to Wednesday. Repeat when the next mouse ventures out on the next day, until the children are reciting all the days of the week by the end of the story. Use the class calendar as a visual aid if necessary.

After the read-aloud, ask children why the story is called *Seven Blind Mice.* Recall some of the things the mice thought they were seeing when they saw only part of the elephant. Then give adjectives to those parts.

Extended Activities: Create your own similes on the same pattern as the author. For example,

> Word: *pillar*
> Q: How would you describe a pillar?
> A: strong
> Adjective phrase: *strong pillar*
> Simile: as strong as a pillar
>
> Word: *snake*
> Q: How would you describe a snake?

A: slithery
Adjective phrase: *slithery snake*
Simile: as slithery as a snake

Have students create their own tissue paper collages of an animal or object and write a matching simile beneath it. Embellish with borders and elaborate script.

Note: This book makes a nice sequel to *It Looked Like Spilt Milk, Quick As a Cricket, I Went Walking,* or any of Tana Hoban's books.

Seven Brave Women

by Betsy Gould Hearne
New York: Greenwillow, 1997

Suggested Grade and Interest Level: 4 through 5

Topic Explorations: History, American; Women's lives

Skill Builders:

Vocabulary	Grammar and syntax	Language literacy
Semantics	Past tense	Storytelling
Attributes		Point of view
Homonyms		Retelling events
Synonyms		Discussion

Synopsis: A young girl recalls her mother's stories "about the brave women in our family—stories I can keep forever and pass on to my children"—and puts them down in story form. The result is a rich tapestry of American history. Each page is one illustrated chapter, telling of one woman's life during a particular time in history. It begins with her great-great-great grandmother who, during the time of the Revolutionary War, crossed the ocean in a wooden sailboat. Each life of an ancestor is marked by a war, yet their making of America was not in fighting wars but by building homes, pursuing their dreams, and living out their lives in the times in which they lived. Students learn a great deal about the benefits of storytelling, a skill that can be handed down through the generations. The short stories provide many good ways to ask content questions, especially about the vivid details in each woman's life.

Method: Introduce the book by asking children to think of brave women in history. Elicit responses and encourage explanations for why they were brave. (Some starters: Amelia Earhart, Sally Ride, Mother Teresa, Harriet Tubman, and Rosa Parks.) Then ask whether they had brave women in their own family histories. What sorts of things are they aware of that their ancestors or living relatives did? For example, most everyone had a relative or ancestor who came from another country. How did they travel to get there? Help children imagine what the experience was like and describe it. How might the women have been brave? Talk about the meaning of the words *ancestors, heritage,* and *genealogy.*

Read each one-page story individually, developing it into a separate lesson. Pause briefly in the reading to clarify more vocabulary words, such as *Mennonite.*

After the read-aloud, ask story comprehension questions. For example, in the first story, ask what sorts of things the girl's great-great-great grandmother did in her lifetime. Scaffold as necessary to shape past-tense structures and retelling of events, as in

> She kept herds of sheep.
> She made blankets from their wool.
> She made medicine from herbs.

> She helped her neighbors have babies.
> She made candles, soap, bread, and butter.
> How might she have been brave?

The girl's grandmother, who lived during the time of World War II, experienced different things in her lifetime. For example,

> She took fencing lessons just for fun.
> She played basketball on a first girl's team.
> She traveled to France to take harp lessons.
> She enrolled in architecture school.

When she went to architecture school, "the men met her with a sign that said, NO DOGS, CHILDREN OR WOMEN ALLOWED." She also had to take tests in a room by herself because she was the only woman in the school. Hold a discussion about the difficulties that women often had to overcome in history. Talk about the word *pioneer*, which has multiple meanings, and talk about how people who are first to open a way often have to overcome many harsh, severe obstacles, but they lead the way for others to come after them. Have children use the word in sentences and extend the meaning to the adjective form, as in *pioneer method*. Brainstorm synonyms for the word, such as *leader, trailblazer*, and *pathfinder*. Find the root words in these terms and look for reasons why these words came to be.

When she was 80 years old, the girl's grandmother wrote a book about buildings, and at 89 she wrote another one about builders. Ask children what sorts of attributes can be used to describe this woman. In addition to being brave, what other qualities did she have (or could she have had)?

This young girl's family ancestry is similar to other families whose women lived through war times and did brave and remarkable things while living so-called ordinary lives. Ask the children if they know stories about the women in their own families. Encourage students to relate the events or describe the person. Scaffold as necessary by assisting children in giving the details they are aware of, such as the woman's name, the relation, the time in which she lived, where she lived, and what she did. Perhaps the family has a keepsake of hers that the child can describe.

Discuss the compound word *keepsake*. (*Sake* meaning purpose or end, as in "for the sake of _____." Hence, *keeping* the item for the *sake* of memories, heritage, and so forth.) Recall some of the keepsakes the girl had from her ancestors. Go back through the story and make a list, including

> The white handkerchief that Elizabeth embroidered with an *E;*
> The quilt that her great-great grandmother made;
> The plates, cups, and saucers that her great grandmother painted;
> The brass tea pot that belonged to her grandmother who lived in India; and
> Another grandmother's harp.

These keepsakes are excellent story starters. Pick an item from the list and tell the story of the woman to whom it belonged, for example,

> The girl in the story has the china that belonged to her great grandmother. It has flowers that her great grandmother painted on the plates, cups, and saucers. When she was young she worked on her mother's farm. There were no art teachers where they lived, so she rode on a horse to a nearby town for art lessons and rode back to do to her chores. When she married a preacher and raised a family, she had no more time to paint, so she painted the china her family ate on.

For another way to engage children in storytelling activities, talk about point of view. Then have children tell one woman's story from the woman's perspective. What sorts of things were going on in her lifetime? Encourage children to tell her story against the backdrop of the times. How would they have shaped her life?

Extended Activities: Encourage parents and their children to talk at home about relatives and ancestors, and discuss one brave woman in particular. Perhaps parents can share the story of a family keepsake. Children can relate the story of the family keepsake to the group or class and describe the person to whom it belonged. Once they have shared their description orally, have the children write a story about the woman and relate how they came to have the item that once belonged to her. (Allow children to make up a story if they are unable to retrieve any family history.) Follow the message of the story by requiring that the story be about a woman to show how women were brave even though they never fought in wars. Include story elements and character attributes.

The Seven Chinese Brothers

by Margaret Mahy
New York: Scholastic, 1990, 1992

Suggested Grade and Interest Level: 1 through 5

Topic Explorations: Culture and history, Chinese; Folklore, Chinese; Long ago and far away

Skill Builders:

Vocabulary	**Grammar and syntax**	**Language literacy**
Attributes	Possessive pronouns	Predicting
Similes and metaphors	Tenses, present and past	Cause-and-effect relationships
		Problem solving
		Compare and contrast

Synopsis: Unusual watercolor illustrations depict the striking details of ancient China during the reign of the first emperor. The tale begins when a hole in the Great Wall prompts one of seven brothers to cry for the hardworking laborers who are repairing it. Because the teardrops could drown a village, a powerful brother decides it is best to repair the wall himself. His great strength incites fear and jealousy in the emperor. When the emperor's armies try to execute him, a tale unfolds of how each brother, because of an extraordinary talent, saves another from execution.

Method: Before the read-aloud, set the scene of ancient China. Talk about the Great Wall and how a cruel emperor worked thousands of laborers to death to build the longest structure on earth. Explain that the wall is so long that astronauts can see it from space.

While reading, pause to interact about the details in the illustrations and to comment on life in China in 200 BC. Describe the armor, clothing, flags, and ships. Once the pattern of the brothers switching places with one another is established, invite students to predict events to come. (For example, when one brother cannot be beheaded and the emperor orders him drowned in the morning, what is likely to happen next?) Encourage children to describe each of the brothers, using personal and possessive pronouns. Describe the action using present or past tense.

After the read-aloud, review the attributes of the characters. How were they different? How were they alike? What similes and metaphors were used to depict the emperor? For developing critical thinking, describe what events led to each brother's impending execution. How was each predicament resolved?

Extended Activities: Have children create similes to describe the emperor and the brothers. First use adjectives to describe them, for example,

What adjective can you use to describe the third brother? (*strong*)

What visual images come to mind when you think of *strong*? (Hercules? The strong man at the circus with barbells? An ocean liner?)

Then create the simile: The third brother was as strong as a mighty ship at sea.

In the story, each brother had a special talent or characteristic. Ask children to describe their special talents or features. Help them think of adjectives and create similes to describe themselves.

Note: Read also *Anansi the Spider.* Compare and contrast these two famous stories from different cultures.

Sheep on a Ship

by Nancy Shaw
Boston: Houghton Mifflin, 1989, 1991

Suggested Grade and Interest Level: 1 through 2

Topic Explorations: Animals; Boats; Sheep; Weather, Storms

Skill Builders:

Vocabulary	**Language literacy**
Semantics	Cause-and-effect relationships
Grammar and syntax	Problem solving
Singular and plural nouns	**Phonological awareness**
Tenses, present and past	**Articulation, *S* and *Sh***

Synopsis: Short, playful text tells of sailing sheep that fall asleep before an oncoming storm. In the midst of a shipwreck they chop down the mast and make a raft that carries them safely (well, almost) into port.

Methods: Before the read-aloud, read the title and ask students to predict what the story will be about.

Read aloud and show the illustrations without interruption, so the words of the story stand alone.

During the second read-aloud, share talk about what happens in the story. To increase vocabulary and story comprehension, discuss the words of the text and their meanings to prepare for story comprehension and the phonological awareness games that follow. Some suggested words include

deep-sea	collide	deck
mast	drift	float
port	dock	

To build grammar and syntax skills, share talk using the grammatical forms of the text and expand on the forms to create target structures.

For regular and irregular plural forms, contrast the words *sheep on a ship* with similar stories about *monkeys on a ship, elephants on a ship, mice on a ship,* and so on.

For tenses, rephrase and reshape the short text into sentences for repetition (e.g., "The sheep are napping." "The sheep napped.").

After the read-aloud, build language literacy skills by talking about the problem the characters had and what they did to solve it. For example, ask

How did the sheep get into trouble? (They fell asleep.)
What did they do about it? (They chopped the mast.)
Was it a good idea to chop down the mast? Why? (Yes. They made it into a raft.)
How did they get back to port? (They floated on the raft until they saw land.)
What are some words to describe how the raft moved in the water? (floated, bobbed up and down, meandered)
What did the sheep load on board at the beginning of the story? (The treasure chest.)
Why did the sheep take the treasure chest on the raft? (They didn't want the treasure chest to sink with the ship.)

The words of the text are ideal for phonological awareness activities. After a picture walk-through of the story, play the following sound games, beginning at each student's appropriate developmental level.

PLAY **Can-You-Hear-It?**

Talk about the words from the story that sound like what they describe, and use those words in new sentences:

lap—"waves lap": A kitten laps up milk.
slosh—"waves slosh": A pig sloshes in mud.
flap—"sails flap": Flags flap in the wind.

PLAY **Word-Search.**

Children search the picture for a word that begins with a designated sound. Provide clues if needed. For example, say

I'm thinking of a word in the story that starts with *sh*.
What word starts with *sh . . . . . .*? (Give phoneme/sound only.)
That's right. *Sheep*. *Sheep* starts with *sh*.

(Also ship, shark, shake)

More word sources can be found on each page.

PLAY **Say-the-Sound (final).**

Children listen to word pairs and produce the final sound that is common to each word. Using word pairs from the Same-Sound (ending) game provided previously. Stress the final sounds. For example, ask

What sound do you hear at the end of *wash, rush, slosh*?
That's right. *sh* is the sound at the end of *wash, rush, slosh*.

More word strings include

sheep, jump, trip	whip, rip, ship
chop, slip, jump	nap, map, flap
hail, rail, sail	shake, wake, make
port, short, sort	raft, craft, mast
dark, shark, shake	form, storm, warm
slide, collide, wind	

PLAY **Say-It-Until-You-Hear-It.**

Children synthesize one-syllable consonant–verb–consonant (C–V–C) words divided into onset–rime. Present the word with a clear pause between the onset and rime. Demonstrate how to elongate the parts to blend them together, saying them a little quicker each time until they are readily identified. Provide scaffolding until children are ready to do it on their own. For example, say

> Put these two parts together: *sh-eep.*
> Say it until you hear it. *Shshshsheep. Sheep.*

Continue with these C–V–C words from the text beginning with a single sound (shortening two-syllable words where needed):

m-ap	n-ap	l-ap
sh-ip	sh-ake	s-ail
s-ide	w-ave	r-ain

Then demonstrate how to synthesize initial consonant blends and rime into words until children can do it on their own. Words include

Sl-ip (e.g., sssslllllllll-iiip)	sl-osh	sl-eep
sl-ide	tr-ip	gr-ab
fl-ap	cr-ash	bl-ow

PLAY **Roll-It-Out.**

Children synthesize a C–V–C word by blending each of its phonemes. Demonstrate by elongating the phonemes and blending them together in shorter and shorter sequences until children can identify the word. For example, say

> sh-ee-p
> What's the word? Roll it out.
> *Shshshsh-eeee-p. Shshsh-eee-p. Sheep.*

Continue with a new word, presenting each phoneme so the children can "roll them out" on their own to find the word. Use the one-syllable C–V–C word list provided in Say-It-Until-You-Hear-It.

PLAY **Break-It-Up.**

Children analyze one-syllable C–V–C words to identify the beginning, middle, and ending sounds. Begin activities with initial sounds, then proceed to middle and ending sounds. For an example on how to demonstrate finding the middle sound in *sheep*, ask

> What's the sound in the middle of *sheep*?
> Break it up: *Shshshsh-ēēēēp . . . sh-ēē-p.*
> *ē* is the sound in the middle of *sheep*.

Continue to present one-syllable C–V–C words provided above so children can "break them up" and identify the sounds in each of the positions.

(continues on next page)

PLAY **Break-It-Up.** *Continued*

In the last stage of the game, children identify all the sounds in the word. Demonstrate how to elongate the sounds and then break them up to identify each one. For example, ask

> What are all the sounds in the word *sail*?
> Roll it out and break it up: *ssss-āāāā-lll. S-ā-l.*
> *S-ā-l* are the sounds in the word *sail*.

PLAY **Delete-It.**

Children omit the first sound in one-syllable words from the text. Demonstrate by saying the word slowly, then leaving off the initial sound. To demonstrate using *sail*, for example, say

> Listen to how I can make *sail* become *ale*. (Like *ginger ale*)
> I delete the first sound: *Sail. Ale.*
> Now you delete it. *Sail . . .*

Use the words in the list of one-syllable words provided above. Then play the game with the alliterative words of the title. Repeat the demonstration, leaving out the initial sounds in the words:

> Sheep on a Ship

becomes

> Eep on a Ip

Ask children to recall what the words were before you changed them. Continue demonstrating until the children are able to delete the initial sounds in both words on their own.

Next, demonstrate how to delete the final sound in words.

> Listen to how I can make *sheep* become *she*.
> I roll out *sheep: Sssshhhhheeeeeeppppp.*
> Delete *p*, and now I have *sheeeeeeee.*
> *Sheep, she.* Now you try it.

Continue

> Say *sail* without the *l.* (say)
> Say *wave* without the *v.* (way)
> Say *side* without the *d.* (sigh)
> Say *rain* without the *n.* (ray)

Extend the activity to four-sound words, for example,

> Listen to how I can make *dark* become *ark*.
> I delete the first sound. *Dark. Ark.*
> What little word is left? (ark)
> That's right. *Dark, ark.*

(continues on next page)

PLAY | **Delete-It.** *Continued*

Continue with four-sound words beginning with a consonant cluster. Demonstrate how to delete a sound from the cluster. For example,

> Listen to how I can make *slip* become *lip*.
> I roll out *slip: Ssssslllllllliiiiiiippppp.*
> Delete the *s*, and now I have *lllllliiiiiipppppp. Lip.*
> *Ssssslllllliiiiiipppp, lllllliiiiiippppp.*
> *Slip, lip.* Now you try it.

> Now listen to how I can make *slip* become *sip*.
> I roll out *slip: Ssssslllliiiiippppp.*
> Delete the *l*, and now I have *sssssssiiiiiipppp.*
> *Sssssssslllllllliiiiiippppp, sssssssiiiiiiipppppp.*
> *Slip, sip.* Now you try it.

Once the children are successful, present the task as follows.

> Say *trip* but delete the *t*.
> Say *trip* but delete the *r*.

More variations of three- and four-sound words to present include

> *Grab* becomes *gab*   *Flap* becomes *lap*
> *Crash* becomes *rash* and *cash*   *Sleep* becomes *leep* and *seep*
> *Splash* becomes *lash*

PLAY | **Add-It-On.**

Children insert a new sound into a word to make a new word. For example,

> Listen to how I can make *lip* become *slip:*
> I start with *s*, and then roll out *lllliiiiip.*
> Then I have *sssssssslllllip. Slip.*

Once children experience success, present the task as follows.

> Say *sip*.
> Now add *l* after *s*. (sl . . .)
> What new word do you have? (slip)

Continue with the word list above. For example, *sip* becomes *slip*, *rip* becomes *trip*, *tip* becomes *rip*, *gab* becomes *grab*, and so on.

PLAY | **Switch-It.**

Children delete the initial sound of the word and replace it with a new sound to make another word. Demonstrate first, then prompt with cues as necessary. For example,

(continues on next page)

PLAY Switch-It. *Continued*

Say *sheep.*
Now say *sheep,* but delete *sh* to get *eep.*
And switch it with *d* to get *deep.*
What new word did I make from *sheep? Deep.*
Sheep, deep.

Continue with the one-syllable words until children experience success. Substitute the initial sound. More examples:

Hoe: Delete *h* and switch it with *t.* (*toe*)
Sheep: Delete *sh* and switch it with *p.* (*peep*)
Ship: Delete *sh* and switch it with *ch.* (*chip*)
Port: Delete *p* and switch it with *sh.* (*short*)
Sail: Delete *s* and switch it with *t.* (*tail*)
Nap: Delete *n* and switch it with *l.* (*lap*)
Lap: Delete *l* and switch it with *m.* (*map*)

Continue to play Switch-It with the words of the title, *Sheep on a Ship.* Switch initial sounds with the following:

d: Deep in a Dip
m: Meep in a Mip
b: Beep on a Bip

and so on. Then progress to a consonant blend, as in *Freep on a Frip* and *Sleep on a Slip.* Remember to go slowly!

For articulation, encourage repetition of the text, which is chock-full of *Sh* and *S* sounds. Interact about what's happening, using target words. For auditory bombardment before reading aloud, include these words:

sheep	sail
ship	sea
short	sagging
shark	storm
slosh	mast
fish	waves
wash	

Note: Read also *Sheep in a Jeep, Sheep in a Shop,* and *Sheep out to Eat.*

Sing, Sophie!

by Dayle Ann Dodds
Cambridge, MA: Candlewick Press, 1997, 1999

Topic Explorations:	Cowboys and cowgirls; Family relationships; Music, musicians and musical instruments; Sounds; Weather, Storms

Skill Builders:

Vocabulary	**Grammar and syntax**	**Phonological awareness**
Semantics	Present tense	
Adverbs	Advanced syntactic structures	**Articulation, *S* and *Z***
Attributes		
Synonyms		

Synopsis: Sophie is a hoot. She loves her guitar, and at any moment she may break into song—one of her own, unique songs, like

> "My dog ran off/My cat has fleas/My fish won't swim/and I hate peas."

However, no one in her family likes to listen to them—or to her loud voice. Then, during a fierce thunderstorm, Sophie's singing calms her baby brother, and her family puts a new spin on their little shining star. This is a great book to show children how to create songs or poems from their own experience and express their thoughts and their language! Yippie-ki-yo!

Method: Before the read-aloud, ask children what they know about cowboys and cowgirls. Elicit background knowledge about the term *caterwauling*. Draw children's attention to the syllables in the word as they practice saying it. Give a definition, such as long, loud, shrieking, wailing sounds that cats and other animals sometimes make. Then ask the children to listen to the story. As soon as they hear the word, they can all say it after you.

During the read-aloud, limit interaction so that the words and rhythm of Sophie's songs can be thoroughly enjoyed. Pause at the word *caterwauling,* and after the children all repeat it, ask what they think Sophie's brother means when he says that her "caterwauling will scare all the fish away."

After the read-aloud, describe Sophie, including her 20-gallon hat, cowboy boots, and trusty guitar. Review the story and include a list of her attributes. Is she

> Quiet or loud?
> Energetic or lively?
> Shy or bashful?
> Happy or bored?
> A bother or a hoot?

For building grammar and syntax skills, demonstrate how to use the words as adjectives and adverbs that describe how Sophie sings her songs and plays her guitar. Put the adjectives and adverbs into a short sentence, then expand the sentence with an adverbial phrase, for example,

> Sophie sings.
> Loud Sophie sings.
> Lively little Sophie sings loudly.
> Lively little Sophie sings her songs loudly.
> Sophie sings in the cornfield.
> Lively little Sophie sings songs in the cornfield.
> Happy Sophie plays.
> Sophie plays happily.
> Sophie plays her guitar.
> Sophie wails.
> Sophie caterwauls as she plays her guitar.
> Sophie wails when she is singing and playing her guitar.
> Sophie scares the fish, she sings so loudly.

For synonyms, brainstorm other words for noise, such as

> sound
> racket
> caterwauling
> clatter (as in the poem, "The Night before Christmas" ". . . there arose such a clatter . . .")
> clamor

commotion
din (as in ". . . they made such a din" in *Who Sank the Boat*)
hubbub
hullabaloo

Reread some of Sophie's songs and use portions of them in games for phonological awareness training, for example,

"I'm a cowgirl
Through and through
Yippie-ky-yee!
Yippie ky-yuu!"

"But I'm a cowgirl
Don't you know!
Yippie-ky-yee
Yippee-ky-yo!"

Review or begin at earlier levels provided in the entry in the Pre-K catalog if appropriate. The following is a continuation of games at the phoneme level.

PLAY **The Same-Sound game.**

Children identify whether word pairs end with the same sound. For example, say

kite, coat
Do they end in the same sound?

Intersperse a few unmatched pairs into the following list of matched pairs:

hen, ran	hop, bump	yippie, worry
leg, bug	lost, not	rooster, tiger
wet, fat	shoes, peas	thunder, cider

PLAY **Say-It-Until-You-Hear-It.**

Children synthesize one-syllable consonant–vowel–consonant (C–V–C) words divided into onset-rime. Present the word with a clear pause between the onset and rime. Demonstrate how to elongate the parts to blend them together, saying them a little quicker each time until they are readily identified. Provide scaffolding until children are ready to do it on their own. For example, say

Put these two parts together: *s-ing.*
Say it until you hear it. *Sssss-ing. Sing.*

Continue with these C–V–C words from the text beginning with a single sound:

s-ong	w-ail
s-ock	f-ish
r-ug	c-at
	c-ow

(continues on next page)

PLAY Say-It-Until-You-Hear-It. *Continued*

Then demonstrate how to synthesize initial consonant blends and rime into words until children can do it on their own. Words include

> fl-ees (flees)
> pl-ay (play)
> cr-ow (crow)
> fr-og (frog)
> sw-im (swim)

If success is achieved, continue with

> sk-y (sky)
> st-uck (stuck)
> sp-ill (spill)

PLAY Roll-It-Out.

Children synthesize a C–V–C word by blending each of its phonemes. Demonstrate by elongating the phonemes and blending them together in shorter and shorter sequences until children can identify the word. For example, say

> w-ā-l
> What's the word? Roll it out. *Wwwwww . . . āāā . . . lll. Wail.*

Continue with a new word, presenting each of the phonemes so children can "roll them out" on their own to find the word. Use the one-syllable C–V–C word list provided in Say-It-Until-You-Hear-It.

PLAY Break-It-Up.

Children analyze one-syllable C–V–C words to identify the beginning, middle, and ending sounds. Begin activities with initial sounds, then proceed to middle and ending sounds. For an example on how to demonstrate finding the middle sound in *wail*, ask

> What's the sound in the middle of *wail*?
> Break it up: Wwwwwww . . . āāāā . . . lllll. W-ā-l.
> ā is the sound in the middle of *wail*.

Continue to present one-syllable C–V–C words provided above so children can "break them up" and identify the sounds in each of the positions.

In the last stage of the game, children identify all the sounds in the word. Demonstrate how to elongate the sounds and then break them up to identify each one, as in the example above. Continue with the C–V–C word list provided in Say-It-Until-You-Hear-It.

PLAY **Delete-It.**

Children omit the first sound in one-syllable words from the text. Demonstrate by saying the word slowly, then leaving off the initial sound. To demonstrate using *peas*, for example, say

> Listen to how I can make *peas* become *ease*.
> I delete the first sound. *Peas, ease. Peas, ease.*
> Now you delete it. *Peas* . . . (ease).

Use the words in the list of one-syllable words provided above.

Extend the activity to four-sound words beginning with a consonant cluster. Demonstrate how to delete a sound from the cluster to make another word. Then delete another sound to make another word, for example,

> Listen to how I can make *play* become *lay*.
> I roll out *play: plllāāāāā*.
> Delete the *p*, and now I have *lll . . . . āāā*.
> *Plllāāā, lllāāā*.
> *Play, lay*. Now you try it.
> Say, *play* and delete *p*.

> Now listen to how I can make *play* become *pay*.
> I roll out *play: plllāāā*.
> Delete *l* and now I have *pāāā*.
> *Pllāāā, pāāā*.
> *Play, pay*. Now you try it.
> Say *play* and delete *l*.

More variations of three- and four-sound words to present:

> *spill* becomes *ill, pill,* and *sill*
> *flees* becomes *fees* and *lees*
> *crow* becomes *row*
> *frog* becomes *fog*
> *sky* becomes *sigh*
> *stuck* becomes *tuck*

Then play the game with the alliterative words of the title. Repeat the demonstration, leaving out the initial sounds in the title, *Sing, Sophie*, to make *Ing, Ophie*. Ask children to recall what the words were before you changed them. Continue until the children are able to leave out the initial sound in both of the words of the title on their own.

PLAY **Add-It-On.**

Children insert a new sound into a word to make a new word. For example,

> Listen to how I can make *fees* become *fleas*:
> I start with *ffff*, and then add *llll*,
> and then roll them out to make *ffflllleeeez*.
> Then I have *fleas*.
> *Fleas, fees*.

(continues on next page)

> **PLAY** **Add-It-On.** *Continued*
>
> Once children are successful, present the task as follows.
>
> > Say *fees*.
> > Now add *l* and after *f*.
> > *Fl* . . . (eas). *Fleas*.
>
> Continue with the word list in Delete-It, reversing the order. For example, *pay* becomes *play*, *pill* and *sill* become *spill*, and so on.

> **PLAY** **Switch-It.**
>
> Children delete the initial sound of the word and replace it with a new sound to make another word. Demonstrate first, then prompt with cues as necessary. For example,
>
> > Say *wail*.
> > Now say *wail*, only delete *w* and switch it with *t*.
> > What new word can you make? (tail)
>
> Continue with the one-syllable words beginning with a single sound until children experience success. For example,
>
> > Cow: Delete *c* (sounds like *k*) and switch it with *n* (now)
> > Song: Delete *s* and switch it with *b* (bong)
>
> Four-sound words:
>
> > Girl: Delete *g* and switch it with *wh* (*whirl*)
> > Sound: Delete *s* and switch it with *p* (pound)
>
> Then play the game with the words of the title. Begin with *sing*, switching the initial phoneme, for example, with *t* to make *ting*. Continue with the word *Sophie*, and put the words together for a new title,
>
> > Ting, Tophie!
>
> Other possibilities:
>
> > Ming, Mophie!
> > King, Kophie!
> > Bing, Bophie!
> > Ding, Dophie!
> > Ging, Gophie!
> > Fing, Fophie!
>
> Have, fun!

For articulation of *S* and *Z*, make use of the text heavily loaded with the target sounds in eliciting the child's responses and in maintaining interaction around the story.

Extended Activity: Have children make up their own cowgirl or cowboy songs. You may even want to accompany them with a guitar. First establish a pattern for children to simply fill in the ending words to the starter lines. The words don't necessarily have to rhyme or make sense! Some suggestions include

> My dog _____ (went meow)
> My cat _____ (wears jeans)

My fish _____ (ran off)
I hate _____ (beans)
But I'm a cowgirl or cowboy
Don't you know
Yippie-ky-yee
Yippie-ky-yo.

Six Creepy Sheep

by Judith R. Enderle and Stephanie G. Tessler
New York: Puffin Books, 1993

Suggested Grade and Interest Level: 1 through 5

Topic Explorations: Holidays, Halloween; Humor; Seasons, Autumn; Sheep

Skill Builders:
  Vocabulary   **Language literacy**
  Semantics   Cause-and-effect relationships
  Idioms   Drawing inferences
  Grammar and syntax   **Articulation, *S* and *Sh***
  Past tense

Synopsis: Here's a humorous tale about six sheep who parade as ghosts on Halloween night. One by one, they are scared away by other trick-or-treaters. Because the ending is told through the illustrations, it takes verbal participation to decipher the conclusion. It's a good book for language activities in October—or at any time of the year.

Method: Before the read-aloud, introduce the concept of a word that means a group of things. Ask students what a group of cows is called, and ask what a huge number of ants is called.

During the read-aloud, encourage children to join in on the repetitive words, "one creepy sheep turned tail with a shriek."

For vocabulary, pause to discuss the idiom *turned tail,* meaning running away from trouble or danger. Interpret the meaning of *shriek.* Also discuss collective nouns, including *passel, flock, herd, warren,* and *gaggle.*

For cause-and-effect relationships and past tense, pause to verbalize the events that transpire. For example, ask, "Why are there only five sheep? What happened?" (One was frightened away by the trick-or-treater.) Point out verbs like *whisked* and *glimpsed* and have children use them in their own sentences.

After the read-aloud, recall trick-or-treaters that the six creepy sheep encountered (pirates, fairies, hobos, etc.). Use the alliteration in the story to ask about the trick-or-treaters, such as "What word describes a group of pirates and starts with *p*?" (passel)

A Snake Is Totally Tail

by Judi Barrett
New York: Macmillan, 1983; Aladdin, 1987

Suggested Grade and Interest Level: 1 through 3

Topic Exploration: Animals, Zoo

Skill Builders:
> **Vocabulary**
> Semantics
> Attributes
> Synonyms

Synopsis: Pictures captioned with alliterative sentences show the essential characteristics of a series of animals, from a snake to a dinosaur.

Method: Present the book, pausing at each picture to describe the essential characteristic of the animal. Talk about the adjective that is used to describe the essential part, such as *noticeably, basically, largely, fundamentally,* or *conspicuously.* Brainstorm other synonyms in place of each adjective (e.g., "A snake is *entirely tail.*" or "A snake is *all* tail.").

Ask about other characteristics of each animal that are not highlighted. What are the other characteristics of a snake? (scales, tongue, eyes) What are the other parts of a bear? (fur, claws, snout)

Think of other animals not mentioned in the book. Make up descriptions based on the models in the book.

> What is an ape?
> An ape is basically big.
> How about a lion?
> A lion is marvelously maned.
> And a whale?
> A whale is essentially enormous.

Extended Activities: Extend the idea of giving attributes to other topics such as sports, occupations, or vehicles. What's the essential thing about baseball or homework, for example? After the students give their preliminary ideas, see if they can think of alliterative phrases to describe the items:

> Tennis is inevitably invigorating.
> Soccer is constantly kicks.
> Skiing is timing turns.

Then let each student draw a picture similar to the author's and label it with one of the alliterative sentences. Make a class book and vote on one of the captions to use for the title of the book.

The Snopp on the Sidewalk and Other Poems

by Jack Prelutsky
New York: Greenwillow, 1976, 1977

Suggested Grade and Interest Level: 1 through 5

Topic Exploration: Humor

Skill Builders:
> Articulation—*L, S,* and *Z*

Synopsis: Vignettes in rhyming verse are illustrated with imaginary creatures that are always a hit.

Method: Pick out rhyming words in these short verses—for example, *glum* and *thumb, roam* and *home*—and make up stories about the pictures.

For articulation of *L,* read "The Lurp Is on the Loose." For articulation of *S* and *Z,* read "The Snopp on the Sidewalk" and "The Wozzit." Have the children repeat all the things the Wozzit ate in the closet:

trousers	a dress	slippers
toys	dessert	

Extended Activity: Brainstorm other imaginary creatures and make up names for them. List these nonsense words on the chalkboard. Then ascribe attributes to the various creatures. What does a pleemblime do? Perhaps it cleans your room when your mom says it needs to be done or automatically corrects your homework papers. And what is a snundly for? Perhaps checking under the bed for monsters. What does it look like? Pale and ghostly or big and shaggy? Then have the children create their own poems and illustrate them with the imaginary creatures.

Snow

by Uri Shulevitz
New York: Farrar, Straus & Giroux, 1988, 1999

Suggested Grade and Interest Level: 1 through 3

Topic Exploration: Seasons, Winter

Skill Builders:

Vocabulary	**Grammar and syntax**	**Language literacy**
Semantics	Pronouns—personal, possessive,	Predicting
Adjectives	and reflexive	**Articulation, *S***
Morphological units	Present tense	
	Negative structures	

Synopsis: A young boy predicts a snowfall in his quaint European town, but none of the adults believe him. When the snow arrives, it covers the rooftops of the old village. The Mother Goose characters on the bookstore sign come to life and celebrate in the town square along with the boy, his dog, and the once disbelieving townspeople.

Method: Before the read-aloud, show the cover (or inside title page if your book does not have a jacket or illustrated cover) and describe the setting for the story. Compare the town in the story with the town in which the children live, and ask them where they think the story takes place.

The text is brief and ideal for interacting with the children while reading. Pause at natural places to talk about the scenes and the action taking place in the illustrations. Elaborate on the text and ask comprehension questions. Throughout the beginning of the story, talk about how the boy is predicting that it will snow. Ask children to make their own predictions about what will happen based on one snowflake, then two snowflakes, and so on.

After the read-aloud, talk about the message of the story. What is the author telling us about life? Can your predictions sometimes turn out to be correct even if an adult doesn't think so?

Then do a picture walk-through. There is plenty of action to describe in the illustrations to structure present-tense sentences. Characters are

> "circling and swirling
> spinning and twirling
> dancing, playing,
> there and there,
> floating, floating through the air,
> falling, falling everywhere."

For encouraging the use of adjectives, describe the interesting characters—characters that are stooped over, have long beards, tall hats, tiny umbrellas, oversized radios, and so on. To build skills for pronoun usage, include words such as *he, she, they, her, his, theirs,* and *himself* in the constructions such as

> He is talking to his dog.
> His grandfather has a long beard.
> His beard reaches his tummy.
> He is thinking to himself that it will snow.
> She is carrying her little red purse and her long, skinny umbrella.
> They are happy about the snow in their little town.

Talk about what the grandfather meant when he said, "It's only a snowflake." Does he think it means it's snowing when there is only one snowflake in the sky? Construct other sentences with *only,* such as

> It's *only* a speck.
> It's *only* one, and not a lot.

And rephrase, such as,

> It's *just* a little drop.

Talk about what the man in the tall hat meant when he said, "It's nothing." Does he think that two snowflakes means it's going to snow? Have children construct sentences using the negative *nothing,* as in

> It's *nothing.*
> *Nothing* is going to happen.
> There is *nothing* that will come of two snowflakes.

Then rephrase, using only one negative, as in

> There is *no* snow.
> One snowflake *doesn't* mean anything.
> Two snowflakes *don't* mean anything.
> One snowflake means *nothing.*
> It is *not* snowing when just two snowflakes fall (says the man).

When you reach the page where the text describes the rooftops growing lighter and lighter, use the morphological marker *-er* in the word *lighter* to talk about the root word and explore the meaning of the word *light* (light in color, light in weight, light in calories, etc.). Ask children to think of other words that can describe the rooftops as they get more and more snow (such as *whiter* and *whiter*). Describe the snowfall as *heavy* and *heavier* and the people in the town square as *happy* and *happier.*

For articulation of *S,* use the text that is heavily loaded with *s* phonemes to practice production in progressively larger linguistic units. Reread the story and pause before the target word, having students fill in the expected word using the correct production. For carryover, have students retell the story from the illustrations.

The Snowy Day

by Ezra Jack Keats
New York: Viking Press, 1962, 1976

Suggested Grade and Interest Level: 1 through 2

Topic Explorations: Seasons, Winter; Weather

Skill Builders:

Grammar and syntax	**Language literacy**	**Articulation, *S***
Past tense	Relating personal experiences	
	Sequencing	

Synopsis: A child's delight at winter's first snowfall is richly depicted by this award-winning author and illustrator.

Method: Before the read-aloud, ask children to relate their experiences of a snowy day. Direct children's attention to the story by asking them to look and listen to see if any of the boy's experiences are like their own.

After the read-aloud, have children sequence the story events by asking them what they think the boy will tell his mother about his adventures in the snow when he returns home. Model and shape grammatic and syntactic structures, for example,

> He saw snow outside when he woke up.
> He put on his snowsuit.
> He walked through the snow.
> He made tracks.
> He found a stick.

Ask children to recall again how this boy's adventure is like their own experiences in the snow. What's the first thing they do when they want to go outside and play in the snow? Then what do they do? Continue to elicit a complete series of events. Encourage children to share more stories about playing in the snow.

Someday

by Charlotte Zolotow
New York: Harper & Row, 1965, 1989

Suggested Grade and Interest Level: 1 through 4

Topic Exploration: Self-esteem

Skill Builders:

Grammar and syntax	**Language literacy**	**Articulation, *S***
Future tense	Discussion	

Synopsis: The heroine of this story imagines herself in self-validating situations that children can certainly relate to, such as having her brother introduce her as his sister instead of the family creep.

Method: For future tense, discuss the concept of future events. Then pose questions from the text that must be answered in future tense.

For *S*, stress the target words, asking children to repeat them before you turn each page. Ask, *When?* after reading each page of text to elicit the target word, *someday.*

For discussion and carryover of *S*, ask what things the children would like to have happen to them someday.

Extended Activity: Have the children fantasize about what they would like to see happen someday in the future, either in their own lives or somewhere in the world. Brainstorm ideas on the chalkboard. Ask each child to create a graphic depicting what she or he would like to see happen someday and write a caption beneath the drawing.

Suddenly!

by Colin McNaughton
San Diego, CA: Voyager, Harcourt Brace, 1998

Suggested Grade and Interest Level: 1 through 2

Skill Builders:

Vocabulary	Grammar and syntax	Language literacy
Semantics	Possessive nouns	Predicting
Adverbs	Tenses—present, past, and future	Sequencing
Morphological units	Advanced syntactic structures	Cause-and-effect relationships
		Drawing inferences

Synopsis: A charming little pig walks home from school while being pursued the whole way by a hungry, determined wolf. Time and again the wolf's plans are foiled as happy little Preston changes course, unknowingly eluding his captor and providing plenty of amusement. Suddenly he remembers he needs to go to the store, then suddenly he remembers he left his money in his desk at school, then suddenly he stops at the park to play, and so on. Each "suddenly" causes a calamitous event for the wolf, who fortunately never gets to have his dinner.

Method: Before the read-aloud, talk about the word *suddenly.* Ask children about their experiences of *suddenly* remembering something, like what their moms asked them to do. Talk about what happens when one moves *suddenly.* Ask a child to demonstrate, with a facial expression and body language, how something happens *suddenly!*

During the read-aloud, engage children in making predictions about what will happen next based on the pattern of Preston eluding the wolf. Ask children to explain the motives of the wolf and talk about the action in the pictures to elicit sentence structures, including present, past, and future tenses.

After the read-aloud, help children draw inferences with questions designed to have them explain why the wolf is covered in bandages and being carried on a stretcher. Where is the wolf? Why is he there? What happened to him? For sequencing skills, review the illustrations and have children sequence the events of the story using words such as *then* and *next.*

To address cause-and-effect relationships, ask children to explain what happened every time Preston suddenly remembered something. Encourage, shape, and model language that includes words such as *then, because, the reason, since,* and *caused* in their explanations. Shape and model compound sentences, using the wolf's and Preston's actions in a compound sentence joined with *and.*

To continue work on morphosyntactic skills, have children describe the action in the illustrations using possessives, such as Preston's backpack, Preston's slingshot, Preston's money, Preston's desk, the wolf's claws, the wolf's teeth, the wolf's mouth, and the wolf's big nose.

To teach morphological units, first have children use *suddenly* in generating complete sentences in their explanations of events. Use the word in other sentences that apply to the children's own experiences. Encourage sentences such as

> He turned suddenly, and I bumped into him.
> She suddenly hugged her mom.
> The car suddenly stopped.
> It happened so suddenly that I couldn't stop it.

Start sentences off for the children to finish using *suddenly,* for example,

> Lucy got up to go to the bookshelf when . . .

Explain that by sometimes adding *–ly,* a word enables us to use it in another way—the adverb way. For example,

> It happened all of a *sudden.*
> *Suddenly* it happened.

Show children other words that can be used to apply the rule and put them in sentences as above. Some suggestions include

fortunate	sad	dark
perfect	light	quiet
graceful	quick	
neat	glad	

Use the phonological awareness games to teach morphological units.

PLAY **Delete-It.**

Children delete the final part—or suffix—from the word, for example,

> Say *suddenly* without saying *– ly.*
> What little word is left? (sudden)

Continue using the previously provided lists.

PLAY **Add-It-On.**

Children add a suffix to a root word, for example,

> Put *–ly* after *sudden.*
> What word is it now? (suddenly)

Another example includes

> Put *–ly* after *fortunate.*
> What word is it now? (fortunately)

and so on.

Sun Flight

by Gerald McDermott
New York: Four Winds Press, 1980

Suggested Grade and Interest Level: 3 through 5

Topic Explorations: Folklore, Greek mythology; Journeys; Long ago and far away

Skill Builders:

Vocabulary	Language literacy	Articulation—*R, S,* and *Th*
Semantics	Storytelling	
	Problem solving	
	Critical thinking	

Synopsis: A retelling of the Greek myth about Daedalus and his son, Icarus, who escape the labyrinth of King Minos in Crete when Daedalus fashions wings from bird feathers. But as the two fly out over the blue Aegean, Icarus, ecstatic with the thrill of flight, fails to heed his father's warning about flying too close to the sun.

Method: Before the read-aloud, talk with children about folklore and how stories were once handed down through generations by storytellers without ever being written down. Ask children to listen for a moral to this story.

During the read-aloud, pause to ensure meaning and define new words. Vocabulary includes

despair	intricate	labyrinth
maze	perish	recess
isle	toil	vaults
wrath		

After the read-aloud, discuss basic story grammar components and assist students in retelling the story. Describe the range of emotions and actions of the characters.

Ask students to define the problem in the story. What facts can be stated about the problem? What events led to the problem?

For critical thinking, discuss what the myth is telling us about human nature and the best way to achieve success. Talk about how too much of an exciting thing often can be harmful. Ask students to think of ways the moral of this story can be applied to excesses in our modern-day culture.

For articulation, read and discuss words of the text and illustrations containing target sounds. Some examples for *Th* include *myth, mythology, three, wrath, author, thought,* and *labyrinth.*

Swimmy

by Leo Lionni
New York: Pantheon, 1963; Knopf, 1987

Suggested Grade and Interest Level: 1 through 2

Topic Explorations: Friendship; Sea and the seashore

Skill Builders:

Vocabulary	**Language literacy**
Semantics	Storytelling
Attributes	Problem solving
Morphological units	

Synopsis: Swimmy, who looks different from all the other fish, loses his family to a big tuna fish in the sea. Alone, he sets out to explore the underwater world until he finds a school of fish just like his old family. But they're afraid to play with Swimmy until he solves the big, old, scary fish problem. Using his own uniqueness and a clever ploy, he persuades them all to swim away together, happily ever after.

Method: For vocabulary, discuss the words in the text and name some of the other creatures found in the sea, including

Medusa	seaweed	jellyfish	eel
lobster	sea anemones	invisible	school (of fish)

After the read-aloud, teach morphological word endings and comparatives by discussing the concepts of *big, little, bigger than,* and *smaller than.* Encourage children to use the words in sentences about Swimmy, such as

> Swimmy was *smaller than* the big tuna fish.
> The tuna fish was *bigger than* all the other fish.

Also ask children to name something in the ocean that is bigger than they are. What is in the ocean that is smaller than they are?

For storytelling and problem solving, discuss the following story elements:

> Who is the story about?
> Where did it take place?
> What happened to start the story off?
> How did Swimmy feel about that? What did he do?
> What happened next?
> How did Swimmy "think things through" to solve his problem?
> How did the fish change?

Extended Activity: Gather an assortment of objects from the ocean (sand, starfish, sand dollars, etc.), some of which Swimmy may have seen on his underwater journey. Put them in a paper bag. Have children take turns feeling the items (without looking at them) and think of attributes to describe them, such as *rough, smooth, big,* and *prickly.* Then reveal the items, naming them along with their attributes.

Teeny Tiny

Retold by Jill Bennett
New York: Putnam, 1985, 1986 (out of print)

Suggested Grade and Interest Level: 1 through 2

Topic Exploration: Folklore, English

Skill Builders:

Vocabulary	**Grammar and syntax**	**Language literacy**
Adjectives	Past tense	Sequencing
	Question structures	

Synopsis: An old English ghost story is retold. Everything in this book is teeny tiny, including the woman, her clothes, her pets, and the voice in the teeny tiny cupboard. This is a favorite story among children.

Method: Before the read-aloud, talk about things that are teeny tiny, like buttons, doll house furniture, and happy face stickers. Look around the room and characterize things as teeny tiny, constructing sentences with the words.

During the read-aloud, pause to teach adjectives by asking the children what kind of house, hat, dog, cat, and so on the woman has, eliciting the response teeny tiny.

After the read-aloud, elicit question forms by reversing the method described previously. You supply the answers while the children do the questioning:

> What kind of dog does she have?
> What kind of cat does she have?
> What kind of house does she have?

Then ask children to retell the sequenced events as you turn the pages. Model and shape grammatic structures.

The Tenth Good Thing About Barney

by Judith Viorst
New York: Atheneum, 1971, 1987

Suggested Grade and Interest Level: 1 through 5

Topic Explorations: Death and dying; Family relationships; Pets

Skill Builders:

Vocabulary	**Language literacy**
Attributes	Relating personal experiences
Grammar and syntax	Storytelling
Past tense	Drawing inferences

Synopsis: The cycle of life and death is explored as a boy grieves for his cat, Barney. After a funeral where he tells 9 good things about Barney, he comes to the 10th much later, after pondering and questioning the concept of death. This book is particularly helpful for encouraging discussion when dealing with loss in any form.

Method: Before the read-aloud, ask whether any of the children have ever had a pet that died. What happened? How did they feel about it? Explain that this story is about a boy who is sad and missing his cat, Barney.

Read the story aloud without pausing for interaction. After the read-aloud, have children recall the words the boy used to describe his cat, such as *brave, smart, cuddly,* and *clean.* Ask children whether they can think of 10 good things about their pets, a class pet, a friend, or other people. Brainstorm as a class and record the adjectives on the board.

For past tense, recount the events of the story, structuring target sentences as necessary, for example,

> The boy went to bed.
> The boy did not watch TV.
> Mother wrapped Barney in a scarf.
> Father buried Barney.

For storytelling, encourage children to recount the story while you provide scaffolding as needed. Ask what the problem was. Draw inferences about the boy's behavior, for example,

> How did the boy resolve the problem?
> Was it enough just to bury Barney?
> What helped the boy feel better about his missing cat?

That's Good! That's Bad!

by Margery Cuyler
New York: Holt, 1991, 1993

Suggested Grade and Interest Level: 1 through 5

Topic Explorations: Animals, Jungle; Zoos

Skill Builders:

Vocabulary	Language literacy	Fluency
Antonyms	Relating personal experiences	
	Predicting	
	Sequencing	
	Cause-and-effect relationships	
	Verbal expression	

Synopsis: A little boy goes to the zoo, where his parents buy him a balloon. Suddenly, it lifts him into the sky. The balloon carries him into a jungle and bursts on a prickly tree, leading the boy to some good and bad adventures. The funny pictures and the "Oh, that's good! No, that's bad!" theme offer lots of opportunities for participation.

Method: Before the read-aloud, talk about antonyms and brainstorm a few (e.g., up/down, backward/forward).

Read aloud and interact by asking

> What's the bad thing about _____? (e.g., sliding down the neck of a giraffe and falling into quicksand)
> What's the good thing about _____? (e.g., falling into quicksand next to an elephant)

Point out and name other animals in the background, including the macaw, ladybug, aphid, kudu, and sable antelope.

For cause-and-effect relationships, build a predictable pattern of adventure and misadventure. Ask

> What happened when the giraffe bent down to take a drink?
> What caused this to happen?
> What do you think will happen next?
> What makes you think so?

If necessary, point out the clues presented in the pictures.

After the read-aloud, recall the events, emphasizing the cause-and-effect relationships that create the story sequence.

For fluency, have the child participate in repeating the predictable, repetitive verse. Use the "That's good! That's bad!" theme to shape progressively longer responses produced on a sustained breath stream.

There's an Alligator Under My Bed

by Mercer Mayer
New York: Dial Books for Young Readers, 1987

Suggested Grade and Interest Level: 1 through 4

Skill Builders:

Vocabulary	Language literacy	Articulation, *L* and *R*
Prepositions	Predicting	
Grammar and syntax	Sequencing	
Tenses, present and past	Cause-and-effect relationships	
	Storytelling	

Synopsis: A little boy insists there's an alligator living under his bed. He conquers his bedtime fears by coaxing an alligator out from under his bed, down the stairs, and into the garage, using some pretty clever thinking.

Method: Before the read-aloud, ask children to make predictions about the story based on the book's title and cover illustration. Could an alligator really be under the boy's bed? Why might he think so?

During the read-aloud, pause to teach verb tenses as you model or shape sentences from the illustrations.

After the read-aloud, review the pages and locate the alligator and the boy, modeling and shaping phrases based on the text and illustrations, such as

> under the bed
> in the refrigerator
> beside the bed
> on top of the board
> across the hall

For problem solving, ask the children to explain how the boy solved the problem of having an alligator under his bed. For sequencing and cause-and-effect relationships, ask children to recall the events that took place in order for him to get rid of the alligator. Help them connect the events with words, such as *because* and *so,* to express the causal relationships.

To teach storytelling, elaborate on the sequence of events by eliciting answers to questions about story grammar elements. Focus especially on the boy's plan to solve his problem and the outcome of the plan.

For articulation, encourage interaction around the target words as you read aloud.

Read also *There's a Nightmare in My Closet* and *There's Something in the Attic* by the same author.

The Thing That Bothered Farmer Brown

by Teri Sloat
New York: Orchard Books, 1995, 2001

Suggested Grade and Interest Level: 1 through 2

Topic Explorations: Animals, Farm; Farms; Sounds and listening

Skill Builders:

Vocabulary	Language literacy	Phonological awareness
Semantics	Relating personal experiences	
Synonyms	Predicting	
Grammar and syntax	Sequencing	
Past tense	Cause-and-effect relationships	
	Drawing inferences	

Synopsis: What makes that "tiny, whiny, humming sound" and prevents Farmer Brown from getting his sleep? Follow the pages of the amusing, rhyming, repetitive, and cumulative verse until the answer is revealed—or guessed! A fun book you will want to read again and again. It's easy to see why it is an American Bookseller Kids' Pick of the Lists book.

Method: Before the read-aloud, explore the book's cover. What can be said about Farmer Brown from his appearance? Talk about the dog and cat asleep in the bed behind the frazzled-looking farmer. Read the title and predict what might happen in the story.

During the read-aloud, ask prediction questions and pause briefly to clarify meaning.

GRADES 1–5

After the read-aloud, teach synonyms by talking about how the author uses several words to tell how Farmer Brown feels about the mosquito. Read the title and start with *bothered*. Ask, "What's another word for *bothered*?" Encourage children to use the word in another sentence. Review the text using synonyms *annoying* and *disturbing*. Brainstorm other synonyms, including *irritated* and *bugged*.

Have children relate personal experiences about a tiny (or not so tiny) insect sound. To build sequencing skills, do a picture walk-through and ask children to sequence the actions using past-tense structures.

For phonological awareness training, reread the story, focusing on the target words of the following activities at the phoneme level. If needed, review or begin at the earlier levels elaborated upon in the Pre-K catalog.

PLAY **The Same-Sound (final) game.**

Children identify whether word pairs end with the same sound. Intersperse some unmatched pairs into the following word pairs so that children can identify that they do not end in the same sound. Some words from the text include

feet, sheet	bread, cooed	tiny, whiny
sheet, goat	soup, snap	tail, curl
snap, sleep	tails, hens	round, bed

PLAY **Say-the-Sound (final).**

Children listen to word pairs and produce the final sound that is common to each word. Use word pairs from the Same-Sound (ending) game provided above. Stress the final sounds. For example, ask

What sound do you hear at the end of *feet* and *sheet*?
That's right. *t* is the sound at the end of *feet* and *sheet*.

PLAY **Say-It-Until-You-Hear-It.**

Children synthesize one-syllable words divided into onset-rime. Present the word with a clear pause between the onset and rime. Demonstrate how to elongate the parts to blend them together, saying them a little more quickly each time until they are readily identified. Provide scaffolding until children are ready to do it on their own. For example, say

Put these two parts together: *w–all*.
Say it until you hear it. *Wwwwww-all. Wall.*

Continue with these consonant–vowel–consonant (C–V–C) words from the text beginning with a single sound:

s-oup	h-it
sh-eet	g-oat
s-un	t-ail
wh-ack	d-og
f-eet	d-ove

(continues on next page)

GRADES 1–5

<PLAY> **Say-It-Until-You-Hear-It.** *Continued*

Then demonstrate how to synthesize initial consonant blends and rimes into words until children can do it on their own. Words include

sw-at (e.g., sssswwwwww . . . . . aaat) (swat)
sn-ap
sm-ack
sn-ore
sl-eep
cl-uck
br-ay
br-ead

<PLAY> **Roll-It-Out.**

Children synthesize a C–V–C word by blending each of its phonemes. Demonstrate by elongating the phonemes and blending them together in shorter and shorter sequences until children can identify the word, as in

s–oo–p
What's the word? Roll it out.
Ssss-ooo-p. Soup.

Continue with a new word, presenting each of the phonemes separately so the children can "roll them out" on their own to find the word. Use the one-syllable C–V–C word list provided in Say-It-Until-You-Hear-It.

<PLAY> **Break-It-Up.**

Children analyze one-syllable C–V–C words to identify the beginning, middle, and ending sounds. Begin activities with initial sounds, then proceed to middle and ending sounds. For example, to find the middle sound in *soup*, ask

What's the sound in the middle of *soup*?
Break it up: *Ssssss-ooooo-p . . . s-oo-p.*
oo is the sound in the middle of *soup*.

Continue to present one-syllable C–V–C words provided in Say-It-Until-You-Hear-It so children can "break them up" and identify the sounds in each of the positions.

In the last stage of the game, children identify all the sounds in the word. Demonstrate how to elongate the sounds and then break them up to identify each one. For example, ask

What are all the sounds in the word *soup*?
Roll it out and break it up: *Ssss-oooo-p . . . s-oo-p.*
S-oo-p are all the sounds in *soup*.

PLAY **Delete-It.**

Children omit the first sound in one-syllable words from the text. Demonstrate by saying the word slowly, then leaving off the initial sound. To demonstrate using *sheet*, for example, say

> Listen to how I can make *sheet* become *eat*.
> I delete the first sound. *Sheet. Eat.*
> Now you delete it. *Sheet . . .*

Use the list of one-syllable words provided in Say-It-Until-You-Hear-It.

Extend the activity to four-sound words. For example,

> Listen to how I can make *farm* become *arm*.
> I delete the first sound. *Fffff-arm. Arm.*
> What little word is left? (arm)
> That's right. *Farm, arm.*

Continue with the words *round* and *sound*.

Then demonstrate how to delete a sound from a one-syllable word beginning with a consonant cluster.

> Listen to how I can make *snore* become *ore*.
> I roll out snore: *Sssssnnnnnnnnnnnoooooorrrrrr.*
> Delete the *ssnnnn* and now I have *ore*.
> *Snnnooooorrrrr, oooooorr.*
> *Snore. Ore.* Now you try it.

> Now listen to how I can make *snore* become *sore*.
> I roll out snore: *Sssssnnnnnnnnnnnoooooorrrrrr.*
> Delete the *nnnn*, and now I have *sore*.
> *Snnnooooorrrrr, sssssssooooooorr.*
> *Snore. Sore.* Now you try it.
> Say *snore* and delete *n*.

> Now listen to how I can make *snore* become *nor*.
> I roll out snore: *Sssssnnnnnnnnnnnoooooorrrrrr.*
> Delete the *sssss*, and now I have *nor*.
> *Snnnooooorrrrr, nnnnnooooooorr.*
> *Snore. Nor.* Now you try it.
> Say *snore* and delete *s*.

Continue with the one-syllable words beginning with a consonant cluster.

br-ead becomes *red, bed*	*sn-ap* becomes *sap, nap*	*sm-ack* becomes *Mack, sack*
st-op becomes *top*	*br-ay* becomes *ray, bay*	*cl-uck* becomes *luck*
sl-ep becomes *seep, leap*	*br-own* becomes *brow, bow*	

Also use the repetitive phrase from the text, *round and round*. Demonstrate how to leave out the beginning sound to make *ound and ound* in preparation for the next activity. Then ask children to recall what the word was before you changed it. Demonstrate until the children are ready to do it on their own.

GRADES 1–5

PLAY **Switch-It.**

Children delete the initial sound of the word and exchange it with another sound to make a new word. Demonstrate first, then prompt with cues as necessary, for example,

> Say *sheet.*
> Now say *sheet,* only delete the *sh* and switch it with *f.*
> What new word did I get from *sheet? Feet.*
> *Sheet, feet.*

Continue with the one-syllable words until children experience success. Then switch the initial phoneme with a consonant cluster. For example, *feet* becomes *street.* Then play the game with the words of the title. Begin with *round,* switching the initial phoneme. For example, when using *SI,* their part will sound like this:

> Something slying slound and slound.

Other possibilities:

> Something trying tround and tround.
> Something frying fround and fround.
> Something crying cround and cround.
> Something prying pround and pround.

Remember to go slowly!

Things That Are Most in the World

by Judi Barrett
New York: Atheneum Books for Young Readers, Simon & Schuster, 1998; First Aladdin Paperbacks, 2001

Suggested Grade and Interest Level: 1 through 5

Skill Builders:
> **Vocabulary**
> Semantics
> Morphological units

Synopsis: "The wriggliest thing in the world is a snake ice-skating." "The silliest thing is a chicken in a frog costume." The quietest thing, the prickliest thing, the hottest thing, and more are all depicted on the pages of this wonderful book of superlatives. (From the author of *Cloudy with a Chance of Meatballs.*)

Method: Present the book by asking the children to explain what *most* means, soliciting any number of responses and examples. Then read the text aloud, pausing to comment on each of the illustrations, including things that are the

oddest	teensie-weensiest	longest
jumpiest	smelliest	nearest

Encourage children to make up their own examples for each superlative. Ask children to give a complete sentence to elicit the morphological ending. Use classroom objects for ideas and themes such as food and vehicles, for example,

> I think the silliest thing in the world is pizza with whipping cream.
> I think the oddest thing in the world is a giraffe on a motorcycle.

After the read-aloud, revisit the pages. Have children structure new sentences for repetition that include the root word, then the suffix -er and -est. Give examples from the book, such as,

> A quiet thing is a library.
> A quieter thing is a boy sleeping in a library.
> The quietest thing is a boy sleeping in a library when a worm is chewing on his peanut butter sandwich.

As the last page of the book invites, have children fill in what the _____est thing in the world is about themselves. Prompt with some beginning sentences, such as,

> The happiest thing about me is _____.
> The cutest thing about me is _____.
> The smartest thing about me is _____.
> The chewiest thing about me is my _____.
> The loudest thing about me is my _____.
> The softest thing about me is my _____.
> The silliest thing about me is _____.

Then have them repeat this sentence: The very best thing in the world about me is me!

Extended Activity: Have the children draw a picture showing something that is most in this world. Turn it into a graphic with a descriptive sentence written in any creative and imaginative way allowable. Include a border as a frame and have each child share with the rest of the class.

The Three Billy Goats Gruff

by Peter Asbjornsen
New York: Harcourt, Brace & World, 1957, 1991

Suggested Grade and Interest Level: 1 through 3

Skill Builders:

Vocabulary	Language literacy	Voice
Semantics	Predicting	
Morphological units	Sequencing	
	Storytelling	

Synopsis: This is the familiar tale of the three billy goats, in successive sizes and successively louder voices, who outsmart the troll under the bridge.

Method: Before the read-aloud, elicit background knowledge about the story to determine how much the children already know. Talk about the cover and make story predictions, especially pointing out the sizes of the three billy goats. Discuss vocabulary words—such as *hooves, butted,* and selected words from your version of the text—by using them to talk about the cover.

During the read-aloud, pause to make predictions, point out information, and briefly discuss words to help children understand the meaning of the story.

After the read-aloud, bring awareness to morphological units *-er, -ier,* and *-iest* in root words such as *gruff* and *heavy* by reviewing the billy goats' voices, sizes, and weights. Have children use the words in their own sentences, including some of the following:

> The smallest, tiniest quietest billy goat.
> The bigger, larger, heavier, louder, gruffer billy goat.
> The biggest, largest, loudest, heaviest, gruffest billy goat.

Have children sequence the episode of each goat's encounter with the troll, including some of the dialog. Provide scaffolding as necessary, progressively withdrawing support as children are able to supply their own words, for example,

> The first billy goat walked across the bridge.
> Trip, trap, trip trap!
> "Who's that crossing over my bridge?" roared the troll.
> "It is I," said the tiniest billy goat.
> The troll said he was going to gobble him up.
> The tiniest billy goat told him to wait for the second billy goat because he was much bigger.

Help children develop story schema by asking questions that elicit their storytelling skills. If necessary, revisit the text and illustrations. Some sample questions:

> Who is the story about? (three billy goats named *Gruff*)
> Where does the story take place? (in a valley, meadow, on a hillside, etc.)
> What happened to start the story off? (They wanted to go up to the hillside where there was grass to eat.)
> What was the problem? (They had to cross a bridge to get there, and a troll lived under the bridge.)
> What did the billy goats do about it? (repeat the sequenced episodes)
> What happened when the biggest billy goat came across the bridge?
> How did the story end?

For voice training, portray the billy goats' and troll's voices to demonstrate different vocal qualities. Demonstrate a "small" (very soft) voice for the first billy goat, a "not-so-small" voice for the second billy goat, and "an ugly hoarse voice" for the big billy goat, as described in the text. Compare and contrast the roaring troll's voice with those of all three billy goats and discuss how the child feels about the characters or people who have these different vocal qualities. Use the smallest or "not-so-small" billy goat's voice to target easy onset of voice in progressively larger linguistic units.

Extended Activities: This is an excellent story for children to retell on a felt board. Cut out felt pieces for the troll and the three billy goats. Use an illustration from the book and a photocopier to outline and create templates for three successively larger goats. Do the same with the troll. Attach bright orange frayed yarn to the felt troll's head. Cut out a mountain, some green grass, and a bridge, and you are all set. During the storytelling, one child can move a goat over the bridge and say the goat's lines while another child moves the troll out from under the bridge and says its lines. You might even take small green felt pieces to put in the billy goats' mouths as they come back from the hillside having found their grass to eat.

Note: There are several versions of this tale, written by authors such as Paul Galdone, and illustrated by artists such as Janet Stevens and Stephen Carpenter (latter version edited by Bruse Asbjornsen). Although Peter Asbjornsen's version is ideal to use for vocal awareness, it may not be available in your library. If using another version, change the text by reading "hoarse" for the third billy goat's voice, as well as for the troll's.

The Three Pigs

by David Wiesner
New York: Clarion Books, 2001

GRADES 1–5

Suggested Grade and Interest Level: 3 through 5

Topic Explorations: Creativity; Fairy tales and nursery rhymes

Skill Builders:

Vocabulary	**Language literacy**	**Articulation**
Higher-level concepts	Predicting	General articulation
Grammar and syntax	Point of view	
Tenses, present and past	Retelling events	

Synopsis: David Wiesner creates a "soaring" variation of *The Three Little Pigs*. As this story goes, the little pigs really didn't get eaten up when the big bad wolf came huffing and puffing his way in for dinner. The old wolf's blast of air actually forced the first little pig right out of the frame of the story's illustration. The bewildered wolf is left at the doorstep while the pigs enter another dimension (the literate dimension?) on a paper airplane folded from one of the pages of their own story. As they transcend the scenes of their little houses, they enter nursery rhyme scenes where a cat plays a fiddle and the cow jumps over the moon. After they befriend the cat, they rescue a dragon out of a folktale where it is about to be slain by the prince. When it is time to go back, they reassemble the pages of their own story, reenter it (bringing along their new friends), and find the wolf still standing at the door. The dragon gets rid of the wolf, returning the good deed, and the pigs rewrite their own fate. The text is sparse as the illustrations tell the story and convey the thought-provoking message to readers and viewers of all ages.

Method: Before the read-aloud, review the original story of *The Three Little Pigs* for background knowledge. (You may first want to read Jon Scieszka's *The True Story of the Three Little Pigs* to get the wolf's point of view on the story. See catalog entry in this section.) Then show the book's cover and ask children to predict what the story will be about. Ask them to take a good look at the pigs. Are they the typical pigs from the familiar story? How do they appear different and how might the story be different because of this? From whose point of view do they think the story will be told?

Read through the story once, pausing for comments, but mostly to allow the children time to think about and experience what's happening in the story.

After the read-aloud, do a picture walk-through to develop grammar and syntax and story retelling. The book's interrupted narrative is ideal for setting up two sections of storytellers to demonstrate story construction and enhance comprehension. One group tells the original tale as it transpires on the pages. The other group, called the "imagination," "paper airplane," "flight out of mind," or "meanwhile" storytellers, tells of the pigs' adventure. In this way, children build on the concept of time as they gain a better sense of two stories happening at once but in different places. The first group retells the story until the wolf huffs and puffs at the first pig's door. The second group begins with "and he blew the little pig right out of the story." The first group then continues with the familiar story shown on the first two panels of the double spread. At the third panel, the second group picks up the story again, in "meanwhile" fashion, and tells how the pig falls out of the third frame and continues until all the pigs take to the air. The first group picks up the story again when the pigs reenter. The second group finishes with the new ending. (Just follow the illustrations!)

Confirm predictions made before the read-aloud and follow up with another discussion on point of view. Encourage children to give their reasons based on information in the story. Compare the story with Jon Scieszka's *The True Story of the Three Little Pigs*. From whose point of view was that story told?

Ask the children to think about what the author is saying. For younger children, use the imagination aspect to discuss how sometimes we can imagine different ways to tell stories or solve problems. For older children, if necessary, lead the discussion into talking about the borders and boundaries of our own lives and how the words can be used figuratively, showing another meaning as it relates to our lives. Think about the ways we sometimes get locked into doing and seeing things in the same old way, like an old tale that never changes. How are the borders of our own lives like the borders in the beginning of the story? Can we be blown out of our own boundaries by seeing things in different ways and thinking about different solutions to problems?

The interrupted text also allows two groups of students working on articulating speech sounds (the same or different sounds) to go back and forth in retelling the story while using the correct production of their target phoneme(s) in discourse.

Extended Activity: After the story has been discussed, encourage children to take a "flight into fancy" for themselves. Explain that they can go beyond the words and illustrations of familiar stories and break away with a "meanwhile" so that the story has a different ending. For older children, pass out classic children's stories to get them started. Once they have an idea in mind, have them fold a paper in fourths and illustrate a different edition in four parts, putting dialog balloons for the character's words just as the author/illustrator did in *The Three Pigs*. Be sure to include the border and perhaps an opening in one border for the new story to "enter." Help children brainstorm and sequence ideas as necessary. After they title the story, have them share it with the rest of the class.

Time Flies

by Eric Rohmann
New York: Dragonfly Books, Crown, 1997

Suggested Grade and Interest Level: 1 through 5

Topic Explorations: Birds; Dinosaurs; Long ago and far away; Museums; Weather, Storms

Skill Builders:

Vocabulary	Grammar and syntax	Language literacy
Semantics	Tenses, present and past	Sequencing
Beginning concepts	Advanced syntactic structures	Storytelling
Adjectives		Drawing inferences

Synopsis: In this wordless tale, a bird flies into the dinosaur hall of a natural history museum on a stormy night. Beautiful illustrations give a sense of quiet in which the imagination can "take flight." In a journey back through the ages, dinosaur skeletons transform and come to life as the museum walls become a prehistoric landscape, the stone columns turn into trees, and the huge bones are covered with the flesh of living creatures. The bird is swallowed by one of the dinosaurs but it isn't contained long. As the dinosaur's bony framework begins to emerge again, so do the walls of the museum. The bird flies free again, out of the beast and out of the building. It is the effect of the atmospheric paintings that create this extraordinary and unforgettable piece and won it a Caldecott honor.

Method: As with all wordless picture books, the possibilities for language use are limitless. The opportunities afforded by the absence of words are especially good for inferring meaning from the illustrations and nuances of the story. Introduce the book by talking about the concept of time.

During the showing, ask children to take turns describing the pictures and telling the story, using scaffolding as needed. Point out details such as how the lightning outside casts shadows of the dinosaur bones on the wall. Look at how the colors change. Ask them to describe the background changes as the bird flies from dinosaur to dinosaur. Brainstorm adjectives to describe the scene. Some suggestions include *eerie, spooky, adventuresome, quiet, mysterious,* and *surreal.* Children can construct sentences with the words using the illustrations for ideas.

Children can continue to describe how the artist portrayed the bird to give the reader and viewer a sense of story and what the bird might be thinking and feeling. Observe the mouth, neck, head, and wings of the bird and describe what they portray in their various positions. Use words such as *fright, amazement, shock,* and *disbelief.* When the bird's beak opens as it sees the dinosaur come to life, what might it be thinking? Children can express its thoughts.

To help students conceptualize time and the prehistoric ages, talk about how artists have rendered the era in their drawings and paintings. Describe the scenery and the land in which they lived. How is the earth different today? Define the word *prehistoric* and ask students to use it in a sentence. See what dinosaurs the children can name, including the pterodactyl. Ask whether they think the little bird might be an descendant of the prehistoric flyer and offer that scientists have different theories.

To teach storytelling skills, which are necessary for literacy, and to enhance sequencing abilities, have children retell the beginning of the story as the little bird might have told it upon returning home to its family and friends. Begin by having children answer initial story grammar questions, for example,

> Who/what was the story about? (I . . .)
> When? (on a stormy night)
> Where did it take place? (flying inside a natural history museum)
> What happened to start the story off? (I flew into an open window to get out from the storm and I found myself in this strange place.)
> What happened next? (I flew around, fascinated by the dinosaur skeletons, until I noticed the dinosaurs change. They actually grew flesh, their eyes appeared, and they came to life.)
> How did the character(s) feel about it? (I thought I was seeing things or that the lightning was playing tricks on me.)

Encourage elaborate descriptions and free expression. Continue to help children sequence the events of the story, using words and phrases such as *so, and then,* and *the next thing.*

For increasing grammar and syntax skills, model and shape language for target structures, including present and past tense. For older children, help to structure sentences with more variety and complexity by using prepositional phrases, such as

> The bird flew within the museum walls, between the eerie structures of the dinosaur skeletons.

and by using adjective clauses, such as

> Spooky and surreal, the walls of the museum actually transformed before my eyes.

Extended Activity: As with many Dragonfly books, the inside front and back covers give suggestions for activities and present interesting facts on the subject.

"Dinosaurs ruled the world for 150 million years—and then suddenly disappeared, perhaps in a matter of months. The reason why is still a mystery." Older students can write a story about how a wise professor bird told its friend it must have dreamed the event because dinosaurs are now extinct. Have students write a detailed account of a plausible, but creatively embellished, account of professor bird's theory on how dinosaurs became extinct—throughout the entire world over a period of just *one month*! Encourage creativity in the voice of professor bird.

Too Many Tamales

by Gary Soto
New York: Putnam, 1993

Suggested Grade and Interest Level:	1 through 5
Topic Explorations:	Culture, Hispanic; Holidays, Christmas

Skill Builders:

Vocabulary	**Grammar and syntax**	**Language literacy**
Semantics	Tenses—present, past, and future	Relating personal experiences
	Pronouns, personal and possessive	Sequencing
	Advanced syntactic structures	Storytelling

Synopsis: Maria feels very grown-up as she kneads the *masa* for the tamales she and her mother are making before Christmas. So when Mother takes off her wedding ring to answer the phone, Maria tries it on. Later, when the relatives arrive, Maria remembers seeing the ring drop into the *masa,* and she never retrieved it. Worried she had lost her mother's ring, she convinces the other children to eat all the tamales until they find it.

After stuffing themselves with too many tamales, Maria believes the youngest has swallowed it and goes to tell her mother the bad news. A touching story of the all-too-familiar experiences of childhood and how a loving, nurturing family responds to its young.

Method: This is a great book to read at holiday time to discuss the activities and foods of differing cultures. Before the read-aloud, talk about family gatherings during the holidays. Have children relate their personal experiences making holiday food. What holidays do they celebrate and what special foods are made or eaten at their house?

During the read-aloud, pause briefly to discuss story content and vocabulary such as *masa,* the Spanish word for flour or dough made of dried, ground corn. Other words to discuss in the story include

dusk	kneading
husks	nudged
littered	

After the read-aloud, go back through the pictures and clarify expressions and language use for better comprehension. For example, what did it mean when "Maria moved her nose off the glass and came back to the counter"? (Maria had been looking out the window while her nose was touching the glass.) What did it mean when "Rosa nudged her with her elbow and said, 'Hey, nina, . . . everyone knows that the second batch of tamales always tastes better than the first, right?'" (They really don't taste any better; it was something to say to make the situation not so bad.)

Sequence the steps in making tamales, according to the text or children's own experiences. They include

Pouring corn flour in a bowl
Moistening it with water
Kneading the *masa* (or dough)
Spreading the *masa* onto corn husks
Plopping a spoonful of meat in the center
Folding the husk
Placing it in a large pot of boiling water
Taking the tamale out when done
Putting it on a plate to cool

Use the steps in making tamales to build grammar and syntax skills such as present, past, and future tenses; personal and possessive pronouns; and prepositional phrases. Then review the story and illustrations, asking questions and eliciting language for responses containing additional target structures. (For example, "She is wiping her hands on the towel." "They ate all the tamales that were piled on top of the plate." "She will tell her mother what happened.")

Discuss the story grammars in preparation for storytelling. The artist's paintings warmly reinforce this story, especially in the expressions of the characters. They are ideal for relating how the characters respond and feel about their actions, and they create memorable impressions as well. Some suggestions include

> Who was the story about? (Maria and her family)
> Where did it take place? (her house)
> When? (at Christmas time)
> What happened to start the story off? (Maria and her mother were making tamales. Her mother left and she tried on her ring.)
> What happened next? (Maria's family came for dinner, and she remembered she left the ring in the dough.)
> What did Maria try to do to solve her problem? (She had the children eat all the tamales to find the ring.)
> What was the result? (She didn't find the ring. She thought Danny ate it.)
> What was the next thing that Maria did? (She went to tell her mother.)
> How did the characters feel? (Maria was worried and the children were stuffed and feeling sick.)
> What was the result? (She realized Mother had found the ring and was wearing it on her finger the whole time.)
> How did the story end? (The whole family made more tamales.)
> How did the characters feel then? (At first Maria felt like crying, but when the family all laughed with her, she forgot about her tears and laughed too.)

Have students take turns retelling the story, prompting them with features in the illustrations and providing scaffolding as necessary. Encourage use of words and phrases such as *and then, so,* and *because.*

After the story has been retold, ask more probing questions.

> What could Maria have done to avoid having to eat up all the tamales?
> What could Maria have done to avoid feeling so bad?
> What is the lesson the author is telling us?

Tough Boris

by Mem Fox
San Diego, CA: Harcourt Brace, 1994

Suggested Grade and Interest Level: 1 through 4

Topic Explorations: Boats; Long ago and far away; Pirates; Sea and seashore

Skill Builders:

Vocabulary	Grammar and syntax	Language literacy
Adjectives	Possessive pronouns	Verbal expression
Attributes	Tenses, present and past	Drawing inferences
		Articulation
		Carryover of any sound

Synopsis: Although the simple lines of the text tell of a gloriously vilified pirate, it is the splendid watercolor illustrations that create the dramatic story-within-a-story. Massive, bold, and hideously mean, Boris sports a hoop earring in one ear, brandishes a cutlass in one hand, and carries a parrot perched on his shoulder. He is unaware of his small stowaway, a barefoot lad with a violin case, until he catches sight of him halfway through the story. Tough Boris makes the boy play his instrument, and the fierce-looking crew stands still and listens. When his parrot dies, big, tough Boris cries and cries, and the boy grieves with him. There is a lot of dichotomy in this story, which gives readers something to contemplate and share. But the reassuring message comes through loud and clear.

Method: Before the read-aloud, ask students to describe a stereotypical pirate. Encourage lots of descriptions and recall classic pirates such as Captain Hook. Then show the book's cover and introduce Boris von der Borch. Does their descriptions match? Before beginning the reading, point out the boy who is on the cliff overlooking the sea on the imprint page. Encourage predictions about what he may be thinking and what the story might be about.

During the read-aloud, have students fill in the details of the story from the illustrations. (Save pointing out the small stowaway unless noted by an observant student.) For present and past tense, elicit target structures by asking questions about what is happening. Model and shape responses. Pause to make inferences about what is happening in the story (e.g., "What does the illustration imply about Boris' thoughts of the violin? How can you tell?" "Who does he think might have taken the violin?" "What is the reaction of the other pirates?").

After the read-aloud, continue to build inferencing skills by asking questions about the story (e.g., "How did the violin case get onboard the pirate ship?"). Go back over the pages to discover where the boy is hiding in the beginning illustrations. Continue to ask questions that help fill in the untold events of the story (e.g., "At what point might the boy have boarded the ship?" "What does the boy see from his vantage point?").

For vocabulary, especially attributes and adjectives, ask, "What are some words used to describe Boris?" Revisit the illustrations and reread the lines of the text. Words include

> tough
> massive
> scruffy
> greedy
> fearless
> scary

Each descriptive word is vividly exemplified in a watercolor illustration. Continue to build grammar and syntax by eliciting explanations for the word usage (e.g., "What is Boris doing in the picture that makes him so tough?" Expect an answer such as, "He's lifting a heavy buried treasure from a sandy beach.").

The words of the text apply to the pirate. What words can be used to describe the boy?

For possessive pronouns, make a game of pointing out what belongs to Boris (e.g., his parrot, his earring, his cutlass, his beard, his hat, his scarf, his treasure). What belongs to the boy?

To continue to increase vocabulary and generalize the learning, have students use the adjective describing Boris—along with other words of the story—in their own sentences. Scaffold sentences as necessary. Discuss other words one might use in relating the story:

> swashbuckling
> motley
> unkempt
> mercenary
> stowaway
> grieve

Train Song

by Diane Siebert
New York: Crowell, 1981; HarperCollins Children's Books, 1993

Suggested Grade and Interest Level: 1 through 5

Topic Explorations: Trains; Transportation

Skill Builders:

Grammar and syntax	**Language literacy**
Advanced syntactic structures	Verbal expression
	Drawing inferences

Synopsis: Beautiful language rolls off the tongue when you read this rhyming text. It imparts the rhythm, grace, and power of the mighty railway.

Method: Before the read-aloud, brainstorm words associated with trains. Then read the story aloud, pausing to describe the action in the pictures.

After the read-aloud, go back through the pages of illustrations and reword this rhyming text.

> "rolling
> rolling
> into town
> toward the platform
> slowing down
> creaking
> clanking
> air breaks squeal
> moaning—groaning
> steel on steel."

Then create sentences with adverbial phrases, such as

> Squeaking and clanking, the train rolled toward the platform.
> As the train rolled toward the platform, the air brakes squealed.
> With air brakes squealing, the train rolled into town.

The text reads

> "engineers with striped hats
> head-of-the-line aristocrats
> up in front
> sitting high
> see them wave as they go by."

A possible sentence with an embedded phrase is

> The engineer, sitting high like an aristocrat, waves to the boy.

After the read-aloud, see how many new words students can recall from the story. Then help them create more sentences from this list and their recollection of the story.

The True Story of the Three Little Pigs

by Jon Scieszka
New York: Viking Kestrel, 1989

Suggested Grade and Interest Level: 1 through 5

Topic Explorations: Fairy tales and nursery rhymes; Humor; Trickster tales

Skill Builders:

Language literacy	**Articulation**
Storytelling	Carryover for any sound
Drawing inferences	
Point of view	
Discussion	

Synopsis: Do you know the *real* story of the three little pigs? Mr. Wolf, tired of his longstanding reputation, now brings the true story to light. He was just borrowing a cup of sugar from his neighbor when he sneezed at the doorway. It wasn't his fault the flimsy little houses fell down.

Method: Before the read-aloud, ask students to recall the original story of *The Three Little Pigs.* (You may want to reread it beforehand.) Break the story up into three parts, having one child tell about the pig with the house of straw, another about the pig with the house of sticks, and the third about the pig with the house of bricks. (Remind children of the line in the original story, "Little pig, little pig, let me come in, or I'll huff and puff and blow your house down.") Introduce the new book as Mr. Wolf's version of the story.

After the read-aloud, discuss from whose point of view the story is told. What was Mr. Wolf's view of the situation? From whose point of view was the original *Three Little Pigs* story told? What makes the children think so?

For storytelling, first ask whether the students believe the wolf is telling the truth. Then have them retell the wolf's story at each house he came to. Be sure they demonstrate the sneeze that blew the house down. Compare and contrast the two versions: the traditional tale and the wolf's story. Take a vote. Which story does the class believe? Why? What do they think really happened?

Extended Activities: Stage a prison interview with the wolf. Divide the class into discussion groups representing different news stations. Assign one person in the class to be the wolf and another person to be the prison guard. Each group should come up with a list of 5 to 10 questions for the wolf to answer. One person in each group is selected to be the reporter who interviews the wolf in prison. The reporter can choose the name of a famous reporter such as Larry King, Barbara Walters, or Peter Jennings. The job of the prison guard is to bring the wolf to the reporter and insist on a courteous, respectful interview. The reporter then goes back to the group. The group then selects a TV broadcaster to report the interview on the evening news. Then the class simulates the broadcasts of various local news stations.

Also hold a class discussion on media bias. Which news report presented the facts in the most unbiased way? Which news report appeared to slant the story toward the wolf's version? Which report seemed to slant the story toward the traditional version? What basis do the students have for these opinions?

Tuesday

by David Wiesner
New York: Clarion Books, 1991

Suggested Grade and Interest Level: 1 through 5

Topic Exploration: Careers

Skill Builders:

Grammar and syntax	**Language literacy**
Tenses, present and past	Storytelling
	Problem solving
	Verbal expression
	Drawing inferences

Synopsis: In this Caldecott winner, pictures tell most of the entertaining tale. As the sun sets on a marshy lake and the moon begins to rise, the stage is set for a curious event: hundreds of frogs flying atop lily pads! Follow their adventures over rooftops, into and out of houses, and down neighborhood streets. Then, when dawn breaks, the party's over. At least for the frog species it is. Next Tuesday, out by the old barn, something strange begins to happen again. Who can explain this phenomenon? This is a good book for encouraging students' imaginations to "take flight."

Method: Before the read-aloud, elicit background information on frogs and encourage children to relate their experiences. Talk about frogs and their association with lily pads.

Present the book, asking one child at a time to describe what is taking place in the illustrations. Model and shape target grammatic and syntactic structures.

Encourage children to draw inferences about the story based on the characters' expressions; for example, what might the detective be thinking as he scratches his head? What might the reporter be saying to the man being interviewed? What might the man in his pajamas be saying to the reporter?

Extended Activities: Younger children can draw follow-up pictures that show what might happen next in the story. Have each student write a sentence or two that describes what's happening in the picture. Students can present their drawings to the class and tell the ending they made up.

Older students can stage a "scene-of-the-crime" interview. Assign various students the roles of police officers, reporters, scientists, criminologists, and eyewitnesses. Conduct interviews and reconvene to solve the mystery. Is the criminal a mad scientist who spills chemicals into the nearby lake? Or maybe this is an experiment conducted by space aliens? Whatever the solution is, there must be a clue!

Tyler Toad and the Thunder

by Robert L. Crowe
New York: Dutton, 1980, 1986

Suggested Grade and Interest Level: 1 through 4

Skill Builder:
    Articulation, *Th*

Synopsis: Tyler's fear of thunder is not assuaged by his friend's fanciful explanations.

Method: During the read-aloud, stress *Th* sounds. Before turning each page, ask a question to elicit a response containing *Th:*

> What is Tyler afraid of?
> Why won't Tyler come out of his hole?
> What happens when a Great Toad shakes a piece of tin up in the sky?

Allow children to supply the word *thunder* wherever it appears in the text, for example,

> "A gigantic clap of . . ."

Up, Up and Away: A Book About Adverbs

by Ruth Heller
New York: Grosset & Dunlap, 1991

Suggested Grade and Interest Level: 2 through 5

Skill Builders:

Vocabulary	**Grammar and syntax**
Semantics	Advanced syntactic structures
Adverbs	
Morphological units	

Synopsis: In her illustrious style, Ruth Heller shows us how "adverbs work terrifically when answering specifically . . . 'How?' 'How often?' 'When?' and 'Where?'" And that's just the beginning.

Method: Before the read-aloud, present the book's cover, asking students where the balloons are flying so the children can supply the adverbs. Explain that the book gives a great deal of information about adverbs, but the important thing to learn is that our language (as well as all others) has rules. Using various words according to these rules can make the language you use richer.

During the read-aloud, pause to identify the adverbs in the text. For example, read, "Penguins all dress *decently.*" Ask which word is the adverb. Brainstorm other words that could be used in its place. Some ideas include Penguins all dress *elegantly,* Penguins all dress *formally,* and Penguins all dress *neatly.* Expand the sentences to make them richer, for example: Penguins all dress elegantly for a romantic evening on the ice.

Teach embedded sentences by having students practice using adverbial phrases, as in, "On Sunday, *when* hot-air balloons *are frequently* seen drifting *regally* in the sky, we like to take a drive into the country."

In addition to focusing on the *–ly* ending on adverbs, teach regular comparative endings (as in *soon, sooner,* and *soonest*) and some irregular forms (as in *bad, worse,* and *worst*).

Extended Activity: Play Word-Show. After the read-aloud, talk about adverbs and other words as having roles to play in our language (and in all other languages). If we could put language on a stage, we would see a show in which certain words play particular parts.

Use the chalkboard to draw a stage (a large box with curtains across the top and along the sides). Divide the stage into three sections. Label the first section "Nouns," the second section "Verbs," and the third section "Adverbs." Or create a transparency for the overhead projector.

Ask students to name animals, people, and objects they would like to have in the "Word Show." If a student recalls the snails from the book, for example, write *snails* beneath the heading "Nouns." Ask students what they want the snails to do on stage. They can choose a verb from the text or come up with their own. Perhaps they want the snails to slither. Write *slither* beneath the heading "Verbs." Then ask how they would like the snails to slither. If the response is *slowly,* write it in and read across, "Snails slither slowly."

Elicit other types of adverbs by asking different questions, such as "How often?" "When?" and "Where?" Once you have made several entries as examples, have students create graphics by drawing an action taking place on the stage. Students can write a sentence containing the adverbial phrase under the drawing and highlight the adverb with a different style of writing, a different color, or another distinctive feature. Mount the graphics on colored paper and display them in the classroom.

The Very Worst Monster

by Pat Hutchins
New York: Greenwillow, 1985, 1988

Suggested Grade and Interest Level:	1 through 3
Topic Exploration:	Family relationships

Skill Builders:

Vocabulary	**Grammar and syntax**
Semantics	Present tense
Adjectives	
Morphological units	

Synopsis: Hazel's sibling rivalry leads her to prove to her family that she is the worst monster. Her "bad," "worse," and "worst" behavior doesn't seem to get her any attention at all.

Method: Before the read-aloud, elicit predictions about what the story will be about based on its title.

During the read-aloud, emphasize the words *bad, worse,* and *worst* as they are used in the story. Encourage children to use the words in their own sentences, based on Hazel's bad, worse, and worst behavior. Use the story to structure other sentences with present and past tense, using the same morphological endings. Ask, for example,

> Would Hazel get more attention with a *loud* voice?
> What if she used a *louder* voice?
> What if she used her *loudest* voice?
> Would Hazel get her family to notice her if she made a *big* mess?
> What if she made a *bigger* mess?
> What if she made the *biggest* mess you ever saw?
> Would Hazel's family pay more attention to her if she made a *big* frown?
> What if she made a *bigger* frown?
> What if she made the *biggest* frown she could possibly make?

Other comparatives to use in structuring sentences include

> good, better, best
> some, more, most
> long, longer, longest
> short, shorter, shortest
> small, smaller, smallest
> warm, warmer, warmest
> cold, colder, coldest

Waffle

by Chris Raschka
New York: Athenium Books for Young Readers, Simon & Schuster, 2001

Suggested Grade and Interest Level: 1 through 5

Skill Builders:

Vocabulary	**Phonological awareness**
Idioms	**Articulation, *F* and *L***
Homonyms (multiple meanings)	

Synopsis: Waffle, an amorphous-looking figure, is in a predicament. He worries, wiggles, wonders "what if," wishes he would, wants to, and eventually works up the courage and does it. About all we can make of Waffle is a brush of color for a head, a whir of motion for his body, and his red-checked harlequin pants. We never know what he worries about, either. But what we do see, on two double-page spreads, are repeated renditions of the word *waffle* and how it splits off and merges into itself to become the word *flew*. Bold, bright happy faces, grinning from ear to ear, pose a series of designs on the facing pages to form a neat little book sure to capture attention.

Method: Begin this read-aloud with a discussion of the more recognizable form of the word *waffle,* as it relates to a breakfast item. Elicit ideas about what it might also mean, and explain its meaning as it is used in the text—to go back and forth without coming to any clear decision or giving any clear meaning on an issue. For example, if you are waffling on an important issue, it's possible that you may not be doing something you might otherwise like to do.

During the read-aloud, pause briefly to interject comments about the character that will add meaning to the word *waffle* and the humorous text. For example, while reading "Waffle worried./Waffle wiggled," ask children if they can relate to being worried about some impending event.

While reading "Waffle waffled. He felt awful. He was a waffler and wafflers waffle," ask, "Why might Waffle feel awful? What might transpire because of someone realizing his or her own actions?"

While reading, "Now Waffle flies. Still a little fearfully, but . . . ," ask, "What do you think Waffle did?"

After the read-aloud, discuss the idiom on the last page of text, "Waffle worked a wonder (within)." What does the expression mean? Did something unbelievable or unexpected happen?

Ask students if they can share a time when they were worried about doing something, stalled, stewed, and finally did it. How did they feel afterward?

For introducing more homonyms, discuss other *w* words with more than one meaning, such as *wave, well,* and *watch.*

For phonological awareness training, use the words of the text in the following games, beginning at the child's developmental level.

PLAY **Word-Search.**

Children recall the words that begin with the same sound as a target sound or target word. Begin with the target word *waffle* and see how many words the children can recall that begin with *w* (e.g., *worried, wondered, wished,* etc.).

PLAY Say-It-Until-You-Hear-It.

Children synthesize one-syllable consonant–vowel–consonant (C–V–C) words divided into onset-rime. Present the word with a clear pause between the onset and rime. Demonstrate how to elongate the parts to blend them together, saying them a little quicker each time until they are readily identified. Provide scaffolding until children are ready to do it on their own. For example, say

> Put these two parts together: *w-ish.*
> Say it until you hear it. *Wwwww-ish. Ww-ish. Wish.*

Continue with some other C–V–C words that start with *w* and that are not found in the text but might be related, such as

win	wall	wide
ways	wise	week

PLAY Roll-It-Out.

Children synthesize words in the story by listening to their phonemes. Demonstrate by elongating each sound of the word and presenting it in shorter and shorter sequences until children can identify it, as in

> Put these two parts together: *Wwwwaaaaa–fffflllllll.*
> Say it until you hear it. *Wwwaaafffll. Waffle.*

Use other words in the text, rolling them out for the children to identify, such as

> *Hhhhhhhhuuuurrrrrrrrrrryyyyyyyy. Hurry.*
> *Wwwwwwwwooooonnnnnnnddeeerrrrr. Wonder.*
> *Wwwwwwiiiiiiiiiishshshshshshsh. Wish.*

PLAY Break-It-Up.

Use the words in Say-It-Until-You-Hear-It to analyze the words of the story, identifying all the sounds. For example,

> What are all the sounds in the word *wish?*
> Roll it out and break it up.
> *Wwwwiiishshshsh. W-i-sh.*

More words include

fly	flew	think
flies	felt	

PLAY Delete-It.

Children omit the first sounds in the words of the text. Demonstrate by saying a word slowly, then leaving off the initial sound until they are ready to do it on their own. Then begin the next word until the child can delete the whole phrase. For example, *Waffle worried* becomes *affle urried.*

Their parts will sound like this:

> Awful iggled
> Awful undered, ut if
> Awful ished that he ud

Note that it may be necessary to practice one word at a time.

> **PLAY** **Switch-It.**
>
> Using the short lines of the text, children replace the *w* sounds in the words you say with another designated sound, for example,
>
> "Repeat my words, only when I say *waffle* or any other *w* word, you will switch the beginning *w* sound with an *h* sound." Practice one word at a time until children have success. Their part will sound like this:
>
> > Hawful hurried
> > Hawful higgled
> > Hawful hondered, hat if?
>
> Switching with *t*:
>
> > Tawful tobbled
> > Tawful turried
>
> Some harder phonemes include
>
> > *Sc* (Scawful scurried) and *Kw* (Kwawful kwurried)
>
> Have fun!

For articulation, the text is a great tongue twister in which to practice the *F* and *L* phonemes. Simply repeat the lines of the text, retell the story, and perhaps make up one of your own about a waffler.

When I Was Young in the Mountains

by Cynthia Rylant
New York: Dutton Children's Books, 1982

Suggested Grade and Interest Level: 1 through 4

Topic Explorations: Country life; Family relationships; Memories and remembering

Skill Builders:

Grammar and syntax	**Language literacy**
Past tense	Relating personal experiences
Advanced syntactic structures	Compare and contrast

Synopsis: This beautifully told story is written as a woman's remembrance of her youth living with her grandparents in the West Virginia Appalachian Mountains. Pages begin with, "When I was young in the mountains," and go on to tell of her memories of events such as jumping into the swimming hole, pumping water from the well, and swinging on the porch while Grandfather sharpened her pencils with his pocketknife. Warmly told, the lovely series of descriptions of life in rural Appalachia provide opportunities for descriptions and language-building activities. A Caldecott Honor book.

Method: Before the read-aloud, present the book's cover, then encourage children to predict what the story will be about. Elicit background information about living in the country and the types of experiences a child might have.

During the read-aloud, pause to clarify meaning and relate the events of the book to children's experiences doing similar things in their own homes and communities today.

After the read-aloud, talk about the events in the girl's childhood. Assist children in retelling the events beginning with the adverbial phrase used in the story and ending with a complete sentence, for example,

> When she was young in the mountains, she _____ (went swimming in a swimming hole with snakes; stood in front of an old black stove to get warm; used a johnny-house in the middle of the night).

Assist children in relating personal experiences using the *when* clause. Then brainstorm events they recall from their memories, especially with grandparents. Talk about where the students lived when they were young and experienced the memories. Whether or not students lived in another state, another country, or in the same town they are living in today, sentences can be formed beginning with the *when* clause, for example,

> When I was young in (West Virginia, Idaho, Maine, or Vermont; Sacramento, Boise, Charlotte, Houston, Los Angeles, etc.), I used to _____ .

Help children use language to compare and contrast the girl's experiences with similar experiences they have today, for example,

> The girl in the story has similar experiences to me because we both go swimming. She went swimming in a swimming hole with snakes and I go swimming in the ocean.

Where Once There Was a Wood

by Denise Fleming
New York: Holt, 1996

Suggested Grade and Interest Level:　1 through 2

Topic Explorations:　Animals; Animals, Endangered; Conservation; Woods

Skill Builders:

Vocabulary	**Language literacy**
Semantics	Cause-and-effect relationships
Grammar and syntax	Problem solving
Past tense	**Phonological awareness**

Synopsis: Once there was a wood, a meadow, and a creek, with wildlife creatures engaged in their usual activities. Exquisite illustrations made of handmade paper art depict the scenes, while the brief, lyrical verse eventually reveals what displaced them—a new housing development. This book encourages children to protect nature.

Method: Before the read-aloud, read the title and discuss the illustration on the cover. Talk about the meaning of the word *wood* and elicit children's background knowledge about and experience with woods and meadows. Have the children name creatures that live in the woods. Then discuss what the word *habitat* means, such as a home for creatures in their natural environment. Other vocabulary words include

wood	meadow	creek
habitat	unfurl	speared
glittering	slithered	slipped
rambled	rummaged	

During the read-aloud, pause briefly, if necessary, to supply definitions of vocabulary words, comment on a page of illustrations, or discuss a word in the text. Use the text to elicit past-tense structures.

After the read-aloud, discuss the meaning of the story. Talk about displacement and provide examples to assist children in understanding the concept of something being replaced by something else.

> What does the title, *Where Once There Was a Wood* mean?
> Where might the creatures go if they lost their homes?
> What might happen if there were already too many creatures at the spot where they moved?
> Would there be enough food?

Reread the story, pausing to interact and use the words of the verse in creative ways, continuing to generate oral language.

For phonological awareness training, reread the story, focusing on the target words in the following phoneme-level activities. If needed, review or begin earlier levels provided in the entry for this book in the Pre-K catalog.

(PLAY) The Same-Sound (final) game.

Children identify whether word pairs end with the same sound. Intersperse unmatched pairs into the following list of matched pairs:

nuts, once	horn, raccoon	violets, pheasants
slip, deep	brood, food	creek, woodchuck
feed, seed	night, roost	fished, slipped
side, food	snake, creek	

(PLAY) Say-the-Sound (final).

Children listen to word pairs and produce the final sound that is common to each word. Use word pairs from the Same-Sound (final) game provided above. Stress the final sounds. For example, ask

> What sound do you hear at the end of *nuts, once*?
> That's right. *s* is the sound at the end of those words.

(PLAY) Say-It-Until-You-Hear-It.

Children synthesize one-syllable consonant–vowel–consonant (C-V-C) words divided into onset-rime. Present the word with a clear pause between the onset and rime. Demonstrate how to elongate the parts to blend them together, saying them a little quicker each time until they are readily identified. Provide scaffolding until children are ready to do it on their own. For example, say

> Put these two parts together: *f-ox*.
> Say it until you hear it. *Fffffff-ox. Fox.*

(continues on next page)

Say-It-Until-You-Hear-It. *Continued*

Continue with these C-V-C words from the text, beginning with a single sound (shortening two-syllable words where needed):

w-as (was)	w-ood (wood)	w-ing (wing)
w-ax (wax)	f-ern (fern)	r-ed (red)
r-est (rest)	s-ight (sight)	s-eed (seed)

PLAY **Roll-It-Out.**

Children synthesize a C-V-C word by blending each of its phonemes. Demonstrate by elongating the phonemes and blending them together in shorter and shorter sequences until children can identify the word. For example, say

w–u–z
What's the word? Roll it out.
Wwww-uuuu-zzzz. Ww-uu-z. Was.

Continue with a new word, presenting each of the phonemes separately so the children can "roll them out" on their own to find the word. Use the one-syllable C-V-C word list provided in Say-It-Until-You-Hear-It as well as these words:

nut	feed	food
deep	fish	night
side	red	

PLAY **Break-It-Up.**

Children analyze one-syllable C-V-C words to identify the beginning, middle, and ending sounds. Begin activities with initial sounds, then proceed to middle and ending sounds. For example, to demonstrate finding the middle sound in *wood*, ask

What's the sound in the middle of *wood*?
Break it up: *Wwww-oooo-d, w-oo-d.*
ŏŏ is the sound in the middle of *wood*.

Continue to present one-syllable C-V-C words provided in the previous games so children can "break them up" and identify the sounds in each of the positions.

In the last stage of the game, children identify all the sounds in the word. Demonstrate how to elongate the sounds and then break them up to identify each one. For example, ask

What are all the sounds in the word *seed*?
Roll it out and break it up: *Ssss-eee-d, S-ee-d.*
S-ee-d are the sounds in *seed*.

GRADES 1–5

GRADES 1-5

> **PLAY** **Delete-It.**

Children omit the first sound in one-syllable words from the text. Demonstrate by saying the word slowly, then leaving off the initial sound. To demonstrate using *wax*, for example, say

> Listen to how I can make *wax* become *axe*.
> I delete the first sound: *Wax. Axe.*
> Now you delete it. *Wax . . .*

Use the list of one-syllable words provided above. Then play the game with the alliterative words of the title. For example,

> Say *where* and delete the first sound. (air)
> Say *once* and delete the first sound. (nonsense word *unts*)
> Say *was* and delete the first sound. (nonsense word *uz*)

Then have children delete all the first sounds in the title of the story, *Where Once There Was a Wood*. Their part will sound like this:

> Air untz there uz a ood.

> **PLAY** **Switch-It.**

Children delete the initial sound of the word and replace it with a new sound to make another word. Demonstrate first, then prompt with cues as necessary.

> Say *wood.*
> Now say *wood*, but delete the *w.*
> And switch it with *c.*
> And you get _____. (could)
> *Wood, could.*

Continue switching the first sound in *wood* to make *good*, for example. Practice until the children can produce the switch on their own. Then switch the new word into the title, as in

> Where Once There Was a Good.

Other possibilities for switching *w* in wood include

could	should
hood	stood

Then, one by one, switch all the initial *w* words in the title to the initial *m* or *t*. Eventually, their part will sound like this:

> Mare munts there muz a mood

> With *t:* Tare tunts there tuz a tood.
> With *fl:* Flare flunts flare fluz a flud.

Remember to go slowly!

Where the Wild Things Are

by Maurice Sendak
New York: Harper & Row, 1963, 1984, 1988

Suggested Age and Interest Level:	1 through 3	
Topic Explorations:	Feelings; Journeys	

Skill Builders:

Vocabulary	Language literacy	Articulation—*R, S,* and *Z*
Attributes	Sequencing	
Grammar and syntax	Storytelling	
Past tense	Discussion	

Synopsis: No book list would be complete without the classic that changed the course of children's literature. A little boy's fantasy about monsters helps him work through a range of feelings. He winds up with the reassurance of love and safety that all children seek.

Method: Before the read-aloud, elicit background knowledge about the well-known story. Ask children to tell what they know about it. If it is the children's first experience with the book, elicit story predictions based on the book's cover.

Read the story aloud, pausing briefly to clarify meaning if necessary. Model and shape target grammatic and syntactic structures.

After the read-aloud, talk about Max and what kind of boy he is. Brainstorm attributes. If you are working in a small-group setting, draw pictures representing several key pages of the story. Have children sequence the pictures and use them to tell the story. Children can dictate sentences for you to write in as text.

Ask, "When Max is through eating dinner in his room, what do you suppose he will tell his mother about his trip?" Have students take turns pretending they are Max, telling his mother the story.

For storytelling and articulation, encourage retelling of the story events. Provide scaffolding by asking questions that elicit story grammar elements. In the beginning, where does the story take place? What happens to start off the story? How do the students think Max felt when he

> made mischief?
> got sent to his room?
> started out on his trip?
> saw the wild things?
> tamed the wild things?
> saw his dinner waiting?

For articulation, pause during the reading and encourage children to repeat the target words within the text. For carryover, have children retell the story in their own words, maintaining accurate production of the target phoneme(s).

Note: This book is also available in a Spanish version titled *Donde viven los monstruos.*

Whiskers and Rhymes

by Arnold Lobel
New York: Greenwillow Books, 1985; William Morrow, 1988

Suggested Grade and Interest Level: 1 through 4

Skill Builders:
 Articulation—*L, R, Z, Sh,* and *Ch*

Synopsis: A superb series of short, wonderfully appealing poems involving felines, illustrated like fairy tales. Rhyming words abound.

Method: Read the rhymes, then talk about George brushing his teeth with pickle paste: "His mouth so clean, teeth so green." Encourage children to make up their own silly rhymes using everyday words.

For articulation, look up in the table of contents which poems are likely to be heavily loaded with the target sound(s). Assign each child in the group a poem to practice using his or her target phoneme accurately. Some examples include

> "Whiskers of Style"
> "It Rains and It Pours"
> "Andrew Was an Apple Thief"
> "Dressed All in Cheese"
> "Sing a Song of Succotash"

Here's a poem for *J:*

> "Boom, boom!
> My feet are large.
> Each shoe is like a garbage barge.
> Boom, boom!
> My poor head aches
> Wherever I step, the sidewalk breaks."

Then ask the child to identify his or her target words and explain their use in the poem.

Who Is the Beast?

by Keith Baker
New York: Harcourt Brace Jovanovich, 1990, 1991

Suggested Grade and Interest Level: 1 through 5

Topic Explorations: Animals, Jungle; Conservation

Skill Builders:

Vocabulary	**Language literacy**
Semantics	Cause-and-effect relationships
Categories	Problem solving
Attributes	Compare and contrast
	Discussion

Synopsis: In richly illustrated scenes, a tiger lumbers through the dense and colorful vegetation of the jungle. One by one, the animals flee from the tiger, who begins to suspect he is feared. So he returns to the animals to point out the things he has in common with each of them.

Method: Introduce the book by showing its cover and talking about the jungle and how it is similar to a rain forest. In rain forests, there are many lush plants and trees, so many that the forest becomes thick and dense. Because of this, the animals that live there are mostly hidden, just like the tiger on the cover of the book. Discuss how half of the world's rain forests have disappeared because of our need for materials and what is happening to the animals (and the earth) because of it. Introduce vocabulary such as *habitat, equator,* and *conservation.*

Then read the story and interact with the children. When the text suggests the similarities among the animals (e.g., "I see eyes, green and round. We both have eyes to look around."), ask in what other ways the animals (in this case, a tiger and a snake) are alike. What are some ways they are different?

After the read-aloud, talk about the parts of the tiger that were shown and discussed in the book—whiskers, eyes, tail, paws, stripes, legs, fur, and others—and help children describe the tiger's attributes.

After the read-aloud, discuss the similarities and differences between humans and animals. From whose perspective is the story told? Is it from another animal's? Could it be from a human's? Talk about what the book might be saying about our attitudes toward the rain forests and animals. Talk about ways we can change our attitudes to change this situation.

Also ask students to interpret the meaning of the story. Ask them what "Now I see. We all are beasts—you and me" means in the context of the story. Follow the read-aloud with materials on tropical deforestation. Discuss solutions to the problem.

For problem solving, discuss what is happening to our rain forests today and what their destruction is doing to the animals that live there. Talk about ways to solve this problem so no more of the rain forests are destroyed. Some examples are recycling, planting trees, making room for animals, and educating people.

Extended Activities: Play the Imagine game. Ask the children to close their eyes and imagine their bathrooms at home. Play the game something like this: Imagine that 80 different plants are in your bathroom. Put in 10 monkeys, 15 beautiful butterflies, 3 tigers, 7 frogs, 40 spiders, 2 snakes, and 3 bats. Turn on the shower and let your bathroom fill up with steam. Now open your eyes. What is the habitat like?

Elicit descriptive words such as *warm, sticky, crowded,* and *uncomfortable.* Ask how it would feel to be one of the animals in this situation.

Play the Category game: Discuss the products of rain forests that people want to have. Bring in samples (real or facsimiles) of items such as chewing gum, cocoa, bananas, cinnamon, cloves, ginger, tea, coffee, cashews, wood, eggplant, peanuts, guavas, oranges, and pineapples. Have a scavenger hunt and ask the students to find the products. When finished, have groups of children sort and categorize the products. Then have each group present their products to the class.

Who Sank the Boat?

by Pamela Allen
New York: Coward-McCann, 1982; Putnam, 1990

Suggested Grade and Interest Level: 1 through 3

Topic Explorations: Animals, Farm; Boats

Skill Builders:

Vocabulary	Grammar and syntax	Language literacy
Antonyms	Question structures	Predicting
		Cause-and-effect relationships

Synopsis: This is a book that teaches the principles of balance, plus expectation and prediction of story events. As a cow, donkey, sheep, pig, and little mouse get into a rowboat one by one, the author asks, "Do you know who sank the boat?" The text is overflowing with speculation and language stimulation as questions prepare the children for each successive event.

Method: Before the read-aloud, make story predictions based on the book's cover.

During the read-aloud, interact to encourage predictions and model question structures.

After the read-aloud, teach antonyms by discussing the opposite concepts of *sink* and *float*. Ask questions such as

> What makes a boat sink in water? (When the boat weighs more than the water it displaces.)
> What makes a boat float in water? (When the boat weighs less than the water it displaces.)
> Why did the boat in the story sink? What would have happened if the sheep had gotten into the boat *without* balancing its weight?
> What would have happened if the mouse had gotten into the boat and balanced its weight like the sheep did? Would the boat have sunk?

Wilfrid Gordon McDonald Partridge

by Mem Fox
New York: Kane/Miller, 1985, 1989

Suggested Grade and Interest Level: 1 through 5

Topic Explorations: Community; Feelings; Friendship; Memory and remembering

Skill Builders:

Vocabulary	Language literacy
Semantics	Relating personal experiences
Similes and metaphors	Storytelling
Grammar and syntax	Problem solving
Tenses, present and past	Verbal expression

Synopsis: This is a warm tale of a boy who lives next to a home for elderly people. His special friendship with one of the residents helps her regain her memory.

Method: Before the read-aloud, ask children what they know about memory. Give definitions. Briefly share experiences of long ago. Ask children what they know about elderly people and their memories. Have they ever had a special older friend or neighbor? Show the book cover and encourage predictions about the story.

During the read-aloud, pause to restate the problem in the story. Ask questions to elicit present-progressive and past-tense sentence structures.

After the read-aloud, have children recount all the ways the boy helped his elderly friend regain her memory. What were the things that triggered the memories?

The boy in the story found that a memory is something that makes you laugh, makes you cry, and is as precious as gold. Have the children come up with their own original definitions for memory. Have them finish the sentence, "A memory is something that _____" (you see in your mind, reminds you of what happened last summer, etc.). For similes, have students finish the sentence, "A memory is as precious as _____" (a new kitten, a snowflake, etc.) with as many different endings as they can think of.

Extended Activity: Create a memory basket. Find a large basket or a box. Label it "Our Memory Basket." Throughout the year, put in mementos of class or group activities, such as pictures of field trips, a favorite book or two that the class or group has read, sample art projects, or anything that can be used for recalling class or group activities. Several times during the year, share the contents of the memory basket with the children and encourage them to talk about their experiences.

The Wind Blew

by Pat Hutchins
New York: Puffin, 1974, 1986

Suggested Grade and Interest Level: 1 through 4

Topic Explorations: Careers; Community, Weather

Skill Builders:

Vocabulary	Grammar and syntax
Semantics	Possessive nouns
Synonyms	Pronouns, possessive and personal
	Past tense

Synopsis: The townspeople begin to form a parade as they chase belongings being blown away by the wind.

Method: For possessive nouns and pronouns, ask whose items have blown into the sky (e.g., "Whose handkerchief?" etc.).

The rhyming verse makes it easy to remember irregular past-tense forms, such as

"It plucked a hanky from a nose
and up and up and up it rose."

Past-tense verbs include

blew	swept
grabbed	tossed
lifted	turned
snatched	whipped
stole	whirled

After the read-aloud, review the illustrations and use the verbs in the story to create sentences, for example,

The wind blew the hanky up to the sky.

For vocabulary and synonyms, ask children to change the verb and use another word from the story that means almost the same thing, for example,

The wind *lifted* the hanky up to the sky.

The wind *swept* the hanky up to the sky.
The wind *tossed* the hanky up to the sky.

Extended Activity: Cut out pieces of felt to represent each of the items that was picked up by the wind. Have the children try to remember the first thing lost to the wind and place the corresponding item on the felt board. Make up sentences about the wind blowing the items using a variety of verbs. For example, "The wind blew the newspaper up into the sky" or "The wind lifted the judge's wig to the sky." The time you invest in making the felt items will be well worth it because you can use them year after year.

Would You Rather . . .

by John Burningham
New York: Crowell, 1978

Suggested Grade and Interest Level: 1 through 4

Skill Builders:

Grammar and syntax	**Language literacy**	**Articulation—*R, S, Z,* and *Th***
Question structures	Verbal expression	
Advanced syntactic structures	Compare and contrast	

Synopsis: Here's a good book to get conversation going or break the ice in a new setting. It presents some silly, fun, and scary choices that children deliberate over with great delight.

Method: Before the read-aloud, talk about the choices we often can make and give children a fun, hypothetical example. For example, you might ask the children if they would rather go to a birthday party with their best friends, a purring pussycat on a rhinestone leash, or a naughty alien with no manners. Explain that the book will offer children some make-believe choices and that they can choose which scenario they would prefer.

Then read the text and ask for a response. Ask children to give the reasons they selected the choice, using connecting words such as *so* and *because* to create conjunctive sentences and logical reasoning skills.

To teach question structures, once you have modeled the "would you rather . . . " phrase, ask a child to present a page to the group and ask another child the question.

For articulation, have the children repeat each of the choices for additional practice with their target sounds. For articulation of *Th,* ask the child to respond, "I'd rather ____."

After the read-aloud, give the child a setting (zoo, theme park, shopping mall, or McDonald's) and encourage children to think of choices they would present to another child, for example,

"Would you rather swing on the bars, slide down a slide, or sit on the curb?"

Then have children expand their choices with interesting actions, animals, and people. For example, say

"Would you rather swing on the bars with a chimpanzee, slide down a water slide with a porpoise, or sit on the curb and eat Chicken McNuggets?"

The Wreck of the Zephyr

by Chris Van Allsburg
Boston: Houghton Mifflin, 1983

Suggested Grade and Interest Level: 3 through 5

Topic Exploration: Boats

Skill Builders:

Vocabulary	**Language literacy**
Semantics	Storytelling
	Problem solving
	Drawing inferences
	Critical thinking

GRADES 1–5

Synopsis: A shipwrecked sailboat on cliffs high above the sea prompts a visitor to ask an old man sitting nearby how this wreck came about. He responds with a strange story about a boy who wanted to be the greatest sailor in the world. Despite strong warnings, the boy takes the boat out in a storm. After being shipwrecked, he wakes to find himself on an island where sailors sail their boats high above the waves. The boy demands to learn the technique before he returns home. When he misuses his new skill, he pays the consequences.

Method: Before the read-aloud, ask the students what they know about sailing. If applicable, encourage them to relate personal experiences of sailing. Discuss seafaring terminology, such as *boom, tack, cockpit, rigging,* and *tiller.* Then introduce the book. Present the story as a conversation between two men. Ask what the title implies and have students predict what the story will be about.

To improve storytelling skills, first read the story without showing the pictures. Afterward, show Van Allsburg's illustrations but cover the text. Have students retell the story, while you prompt them by asking about story grammar elements and pointing out features in the illustrations. Provide additional scaffolding if needed. After the story has been retold by several students, ask more probing questions.

> What were the consequences of the boy's behavior?
> What could the boy have done to avoid his problems?
> What is the author saying about life?
> Why is this lesson so important?
> Have there been famous people who, like the boy, had great ambitions but were ruined when they misused their power?
> What became of them?

Allow students to linger over the illustrations.

> What feelings do they evoke?
> How do they relate to the feelings evoked in the story?
> How does the artist achieve the mysterious quality of his paintings?
> Does the theme remain the same through all the illustrations?

For critical thinking skills, ask, "What if you were the visitor listening to the story of the old man? Would you believe his story? Does the story of the boy give you an indication of who the old man may be?"

Then ask, "What if you were the old man telling the story? What were you doing and thinking before the visitor came? Did you tell a true story, or did you tell a story you only imagined but wanted to believe? If you embellished a story, what might your prior experiences have been like to imagine such an embellishment?"

The Wretched Stone

by Chris Van Allsburg
Boston: Houghton Mifflin, 1991

Suggested Grade and Interest Level: 2 through 5

Topic Explorations: Boats; Journeys; Literacy

Skill Builders:
Language literacy
Cause-and-effect relationships   Drawing inferences
Storytelling   Point of view
Problem solving   Discussion

Synopsis: Van Allsburg presents a seagoing adventure in his mystical style. Who can explain the glowing stone the crew recovered from an eerie, uncharted island? Stranger still, who can explain its effect on the crew, who are slowly turning into hairy apes? And what makes them so transfixed by the stone? Maybe your students have the answer.

Method: Before the read-aloud, talk about a sea captain's log, what it contains, and how it's like a journal of events at sea. Introduce the story as excerpts from the log of the *Rita Anne.* Ask from whose point of view the story will be told.

During the read-aloud, pause to interact about the story elements. Ask students to describe the strange aspects of the story, for example, ask

> What is it like on board the *Rita Anne*?
> What is it like on the island?
> What's happening to the crew?

Draw inferences about what happened during the storm. For problem solving, pause to identify the facts of the problem.

For cause-and-effect relationships, pause to discuss the transformation of the characters. What were they like and what did they do before the stone was found? What were they like after they became transfixed? What caused these changes?

For storytelling, encourage students to retell the story, including all the story grammar components. Provide scaffolding as needed. For example,

> Setting: Onboard the *Rita Anne,* while the ship sails out of harbor
> Characters: Captain tells of happy crew, singing, dancing, reading
> Initiating Event: Voyage going well until uncharted island is spotted
> Response: Surprise
> Plan: Go ashore to find fresh supplies
> Consequences: Glowing stone is found
> Plan: Stone taken back to ship
> Consequences: Crew members become transfixed by stone
> Reaction: Behavior changes; lose interest in reading, singing
> Plan: Captain decides to throw rock overboard

Consequence: Too late; storm comes up and boat is shipwrecked

Reaction: Crew members on island chagrined, speak little but becoming themselves again

For discussion, ask whether students can think of anything in life that may have a strong enough effect on a person to change the person's behavior or character. Brainstorm ideas. Discuss addictions, if age appropriate. Ask what the symbolism of the stone is. What is the author saying about life?

Extended Activities: Have each student write a story, this time from a crew member's point of view. What was it that happened on board the *Rita Anne*? Describe how it felt. What was it like to become transfixed? Was it really so terrible?

Discuss the shipwreck and how the crew was saved. Describe how they recovered and agreed not to talk about the incident. What did they learn about life? Why do they still have a strange appetite for fruit? Is this a residual effect of the stone? Brainstorm various ideas. Then have students describe subsequent events in journal form. Have them limit their journal entries to 10, recorded over a period of 6 months to a year.

You Can't Take a Balloon Into the Metropolitan Museum

by Jacquiline Preiss Weitzman
New York: Dial Books for Young Readers, 1998

Suggested Age and Interest Level:	1 through 5

Topic Explorations:	Art, artists, and architecture; Cities, New York City; Museums

Skill Builders:

Vocabulary	**Grammar and syntax**	**Articulation, *L***
Semantics	Present tense	Carryover for any sound
Beginning concepts	**Language literacy**	
Categories	Predicting	
Adjectives	Sequencing	
	Cause-and-effect relationships	
	Storytelling	
	Verbal expression	
	Compare and contrast	

Synopsis: This beautifully conceived wordless book stands out as a winner, enthralling its "readers" with the excitement of famous New York City landmarks. It tells the tale of a little girl who, before entering New York City's Metropolitan Museum with her grandmother, must leave her balloon with a guard who ties it to a railing for safekeeping. When an impish pigeon unties the string, the balloon floats away, and the guard takes off in pursuit of it. A series of chaotic and hilarious scenes involving the balloon transpire around the city's famous landmarks, while the girl and her grandmother are inside the museum viewing great works of art. But look closely. The various forms of art viewed by the girl and her grandmother are all replicated in the resulting mishaps of the balloon. Eighteen famous paintings and sculptures are reproduced on the pages. Without any words, this lovely book that has won a string of well-deserved awards explores the interconnectedness of art and life.

Methods: Begin by asking children to predict what the story will be about by looking at the cover. Elicit background knowledge about New York City, the Metropolitan Museum, and museums in general. Use the book in conjunction with others in this catalog with New York City as their subject and setting.

During the presentation, ask children to describe what is taking place in the illustrations. Work on the concept of time by giving students a sense that two separate stories are unfolding. One group of narrators can talk about what is happening in the museum, and another group can tell of events that transpire on the balloon's journey, pointing out the cause-and-effect relationships and temporal sequences. Model and shape grammatical and syntactic target structures. Ask questions, such as

> What happened when the balloon crossed the path of the bride getting out of the limousine in front of the Plaza Hotel?
> How did the balloon find its way into the hotel?
> What happened because of this?
> What was the reaction of the people?

Pick out individual characters in the scene and describe their reactions and the commotion the balloon is making.

Pay particular attention to the characters' expressions. Encourage verbal expression by allowing children to interpret the expressions on the characters' faces.

> Why does the woman at the zoo have her head in her hands?
> How do you suppose the girl is feeling when the doorman tells her she can't bring the balloon into the museum?
> What might she be saying?
> What might the doorman be saying?
> What might her grandmother be saying?

After viewing the book, go back to view the famous works of art. Take time to explore each one, encouraging children to use adjectives in the descriptions. Place the different types of art in different categories. Suggestions for categories include costumes, paintings, sculpture, and artifacts.

Compare and contrast the following:

> Edgar Degas ballerina sculptures and the girl's posing in front of the exhibit for her grandmother
> The "Portrait of a Lady with a Dog" and the woman walking her dogs in her jogging shoes, T-shirt, and peace sign necklace
> John Singer Sargent's "Spanish Fountain" and the fountain in Central Park
> The museum's Egyptian temple entrances and opera sets of *Aida*
> The people chasing after the balloon who caught onto the horse's bridle and the green urns the girl and her grandmother are viewing

For storytelling, construct another two-part activity. Have one child begin with the story elements of setting, characters, and the initiating event. Have another child tell the cause-and-effect sequences that occur with the balloon in the city. Have another child tell the sequence of events inside the museum. Provide scaffolding as necessary.

Spend several days on this book. After the story has been reviewed, go back over the works of art and spend time discussing them. What would the girl and her grandmother enjoy about this piece of art? Bring in other material such as art books from the library about some of the famous artists and the sites in and around Central Park.

For articulation of *L*, children can describe the scenes using a carrier phrase about the balloon, such as "The balloon is now floating toward . . ."

Note: If there's no time for a quick brushup on art history, a list of the reproduced works on the back page will put you at ease. They include those of Monet, Homer, Degas, Cassatt, and Pollock.

You Forgot Your Skirt, Amelia Bloomer

by Shana Corey
New York: Scholastic Press, 2000

Suggested Grade and Interest Level: 2 through 5

Topic Explorations: Clothing; Culture and history, American; Women's lives

Skill Builders:

Vocabulary	**Language literacy**
Semantics	Cause-and-effect relationships
Idioms	Problem solving
Similes and metaphors	Compare and contrast
Morphological units	

Synopsis: This is a delightfully charming story about Amelia Bloomer, born in 1818, who lived in Seneca Falls, New York, and was influenced by the women's rights advocate, Elizabeth Cady Stanton. After hearing Stanton at a convention, Amelia launched a newspaper, *The Lily,* which influenced women's ideas of dress and helped them form new self-concepts during the mid-1800s. The drawings humorously capture the elaborate dress of the day and help demonstrate how cumbersome the fashions were to wear. For example, the author writes,

> "Their dresses were so long that proper ladies looked like walking broomsticks. They acted like broomsticks, too, because their skirts swept up all the mud and trash from the street. What was proper about that?"

The drawings also draw attention to people's attitudes and the new sense of freedom women experienced when wearing the bloomers Amelia had inspired. The last page provides a short biography about Amelia Bloomer and gives interesting details about the women's movement, *The Lily,* and how women coined the term *bloomers* after the woman who dared to change the thinking of the day.

Method: Before the read-aloud, elicit children's background knowledge about the word *proper* and discuss the style of women's dresses and expected behavior in the 1800s.

Vocabulary words to introduce include

improper	aghast
corset	balderdash
(a)shame	pattern

Teach morphological units by demonstrating how prefixes change the meaning of root words. For example, *im-* before a root word means "not." Therefore, *im-* before the word *proper* means "not proper." Other words with *im-* prefixes include

im-polite	im-possible	im-patient
im-partial	im-practical	im-perfect
im-mobile	im-probable	im-moral

During the read-aloud, pause to elaborate on the meaning of the text and point out the details. The drawings offer plenty of opportunities for discussion about ladies' dresses. For example, dresses are shown styled with bricks (visually demonstrating how heavy they were) and shown with elaborately styled hemlines sweeping the streets and collecting trash inside the petticoats. Other examples show women in their gowns being cinched tight in their corsets—so tight they lose oxygen and faint in their finery. "What was proper about that?" repeats the text.

Also, pause to discuss the idiom, "*at the drop of a hat*" (meaning "*at the slightest provocation*") and the use of the similes "*like carting around a dozen bricks*" and "*like walking broomsticks.*"

After the read-aloud, review the pages and discuss the story. Help children use complex syntactic structures while discussing the story. Some examples include

> Amelia thought ladies' dresses were silly because _____.
> Amelia wanted to change the style of dress because _____.
> Amelia thought women should work so _____.
> Amelia liked Libby's outfit so _____.
> When Amelia met Lilly, she _____.
> When Amelia sewed her new outfit, she _____.
> When Amelia went for a walk in her new outfit, she _____.
> After the women saw Amelia's new outfit, they _____.
> After a while, bloomers went out of style, but _____.

Help children express the cause-and-effect relationships that make up the story by asking questions, such as

> What happened because Amelia Bloomer thought it was silly that proper ladies were not supposed to work?
> What happened because Amelia Bloomer decided it was silly that proper ladies had to wear silly dresses?
> What happened when Amelia Bloomer went for a walk in her newly styled skirt over the baggy pantaloons?

Elicit structures containing words such as *caused, because,* and *as a result of.* Some examples include

> Women started wearing pantaloons because of Amelia Bloomer.
> Amelia thought it was silly for women not to work. As a result, she started her own newspaper.
> Amelia decided she didn't have to dress in big skirts and petticoats. This caused women to change their minds.
> Women changed their minds because of Amelia's attitude.

Assist children in using language to compare and contrast ladies' long skirts with the new bloomers. How were they different? How were they still similar? Then compare and contrast the styles of today (depicted on one of the last pages) with the styles of the 1800s. How are they different? How are they similar to the new concept of the bloomers?

Zin! Zin! Zin! A Violin

by Lloyd Moss
New York: Simon & Schuster Books for Young Readers, 1995

Suggested Grade and Interest Level: 1 through 5

Topic Explorations: Music, musicians, and musical instruments; Number concepts; Sounds and listening

Skill Builders:

Vocabulary	**Grammar and syntax**
Semantics	Advanced syntactic structures
Categories	**Phonological awareness**
Adjectives	

Attributes
Similes and metaphors
Homonyms (multiple meanings)

Synopsis: One by one, musicians are introduced practicing their musical performance until a 10-piece orchestra is formed. The text, a cleverly written counting book, is a literary feast of rhyming couplets that impart the sounds and soul of classical music. In addition to the descriptions of instruments, the text gives definitions of numerical groupings. The playful, flowing illustrations picturing eccentric musicians give the reader a sense of excitement about the music.

Method: Before the read-aloud, brainstorm words associated with a violin.

What does it sound like?
What does it look like?
What are its features?
Where does one hear a violin?
In music played where?
In what types of music can you hear a violin played—Country? Rock? Folk? Classical? Jazz?

Elicit childrens' background knowledge about music, musical instruments, orchestras, and classical music.

During the read-aloud, let the words of the text speak for themselves as they create (along with the illustrations) the unique musical quality of the book. See if students notice two cats, a mouse, and a dog enjoying the music along with the audience.

After the read-aloud, teach vocabulary words by going back over the pages to look for the words of musical groupings, which include

solo	sextet
duo	octet
trio	nonet
quartet	chamber group
quintet	orchestra

Review their meanings and ask the students to use the words in a sentence. (More methods are listed below.) Some possible sentences to shape or prompt are

A solo is one musician playing alone.
A duo is when two musicians play together.
A quintet is a musical group of five.
A chamber group is made up of 10 musicians.

To develop and elicit the use of adjectives, encourage students to use the words of the text in language that describes the sounds of the instruments. Distinguish between what the instrument looks like and what it sounds like. Use the text, illustrations, and students' background information, if possible, to describe the instruments and their sounds, for example,

What words can you use to describe a trombone?

shiny	gliding
sliding	long
elegant	

What words does the author use to describe the *sound* of a trombone?

"mournful moan"
"silken tone"

Expand the words and combine them into a sentence, making use of the similes, for example,

It sounds like a mournful moan.
It has a silken tone.
It sounds like a mournful moan with a silken tone.

To increase grammar and syntax skills, reread each page and recast the text. Use a pattern, beginning with a sentence that the children can finish with adjectives from the text. After hearing the entire sentence, have the children repeat it themselves. For example,

The musician is playing a ____ (gliding, sliding trombone).
The musician is playing a ____ (bright, brassy French horn).

Note that not all of the pages of text use adjectives that can be used in these sentence patterns. If the text does not supply one, encourage students to use some of their own words based on the illustrations and their imaginations:

The musician is playing a ____ (blaring trumpet).
The musician is playing a ____ (sleek, smooth violin).

Then vary the sentence pattern, using adjectives that relate to the instruments' sounds:

The sounds of the oboe can be ____ (gleeful).
The sounds of the cello can be ____ (mellow).
The ____ (gleeful) sounds of the oboe can be heard.
The ____ (mellow) sounds of the cello can be heard.

Begin a sentence using the adjectives of the text in an adverbial phrase. Have students finish the sentence using the word from the text that denotes a musical grouping. Examples include

With a mournful moan and silken tone, ____ (the trombone plays its solo).
Singing and stinging its swinging song, ____ (the trumpet sounds great in a duo).
Bright and brassy, with valves all oiled, ____ (the French horn joins the duo and makes a trio).
A mello friend with neck extended, ____ (the cello plays in a quintet).

Here's an example with a metaphor:

The bassoon, *the lazy clown of the orchestra,* sounds low down and grumpy.

Play with the words of the text to rearrange them, demonstrating sentence variety, for example,

How does the author describe the sound of an oboe?

gleeful   sobbing
bleating   pleading

Possible sentences include

The oboe, gleeful and bleating, joins the other instruments.
Gleeful and bleating, the oboe joins the other instruments.
Joining the other instruments, the oboe sounds gleeful and bleating.
In joining the other instruments, the oboe sounds gleeful and bleating.

For teaching homonyms, use homophone pairs (one of which can be associated with the musical theme) in sentences that express their meaning. Some are

> hear, here
> beat, beet
> rap, wrap
> chord, cord
> lyre, liar
> metal, meddle, medal (sound nearly alike)
> soul, sole

Also use the homographs of the musical theme, including

> **bow** (as in bow to the audience in recognition; the forward of a ship)
> **bow** (as in the bow of a violin; a bow tie)
> **key** (as in key in which it is played; something that goes in a lock)
> **band** (a group of instrumentalists; a ring such as a wedding band or material that binds, such as a band around carrots or lettuce. Also note that sound is referred to in bands, such as frequency bands. A set of radio frequencies is called a band.)
> **rock** (a style of music; rock a baby back and forth)
> **roll** (rolling motion; a breakfast item)
> **hand** (as in the audience gave him a hand; the hand on your arm)
> **note** (musical note; note to a friend)
> **jam** (a meeting of musicians to play for their own enjoyment, or an impromptu performance by a group of musicians who do not normally play together; a fruit preserve to eat on toast; to press or squeeze together, as people jammed into a room)
> **pick** (a small object used for plucking the strings of a stringed instrument; to select or choose)
> **scale** (a succession of musical notes according to fixed intervals; an instrument to measure weight)
> **pop** (form of music; a quick, loud noise; a drink)
> **wind** (category of musical instruments; the movement of air)
> **reed** (category of musical instruments; a long sheaf of grass)
> **strings** (category of musical instruments played with a bow; something with which to tie up a package; *to pull strings* means to use one's influence)

The book also teaches the categories into which the instruments fall: strings, reeds, and brasses. (See above for homonyms.) Help students group instruments, musical styles, musical performances, musical groups, musical events, and musical locations into different categories to develop organizational strategies. Write down the category headings and make entries under each column. Use the list to present two words found under a category, adding an additional word that does not belong. Ask students to tell which word doesn't belong and why. Some examples include

> violin, guitar, oboe, CD (CD doesn't belong because it is not a musical instrument.)
> jazz, country-western, Aerosmith, rap (Aerosmith, or the name of a popular group students will relate to, doesn't belong because it is a rock group, not a type of music.)
> grocery store, amphitheater, concert hall, auditorium (Grocery store doesn't belong because live music is not played there.)

For phonological awareness training, make music of your own with the names of the instruments. For students who have already worked with success on previous levels of phonological awareness, engage in the following activities.

PLAY **Find-the-Little-Words.**

Children listen for little words within two-syllable words of the text. Stress and elongate syllables when present-ing the word. For example, say

> trombone
> Can you hear any little words in *trombone*? (bone)

Continue to find the little word within the word by deleting the first syllable or first phoneme (if possible) in the names of the instruments (change the stress pattern if necessary). Words include

> trum-pet (pet)
> vi-o-lin (lin, as in *Lynn*)
> o-boe (boe, as in *bow*)
> ba-ssoon (soon)
> clar-i-net (net, also *Claire*)
> fl-ute (lute)
> str-ings (rings)

PLAY **Leave-It-Out.**

Children say the name of a two-syllable instrument or another two-syllable word in the text, leaving out the be-ginning or final part to find a smaller word within, for example,

> Say *trombone*.
> Now say *trombone* but leave out *trom*.
> What little word is left? (bone)

Reverse the order to get a nonsense word. For example,

> Now say *trombone* but leave out *bone*.
> What funny word is left? (trom)

Continue with the following two-syllable words:

> trum-pet
> ba-ssoon
> en-core (pronounced *awn-core*)
> con-cert
> no-net (pronounced like *no* and stress on *net*)
> de-light
> be-hold
> good-bye
> good-night

PLAY Add-It-On.

Children put two syllables together to make a two-syllable word. Demonstrate first. For example, say

> Listen to me say *trom.*
> Now listen to me say *trom* and add *bone.*
> *Trombone.*
> What bigger word did I make? (trombone)

Then reverse the order in which the words are presented, for example,

> Put *bone* at the end of *trom.* What word do you have? (trombone)

Beginning with the two-syllable words, say part of the word and have the children supply the rest, for example,

> Say *trom* and add on *bone.*
> What word do you have? (trombone)

Continue with the two-syllable words and instrument words provided in the previous games.

PLAY Turn-It-Around.

Children reverse the parts of the word. For example,

> Put the word *bone* at the beginning of *trom.*
> What silly word do you have then? (bonetrom)
> What was it before we turned it around? (trombone)

Continue with the two-syllable words provided in the previous games.

PLAY Say-It-Until-You-Hear-It.

Children synthesize one-syllable words divided into onset-rime. Present the word with a clear pause between the onset and rime. Demonstrate how to elongate the parts to blend them together, saying them a little quicker each time until they are readily identified. Provide scaffolding until children are ready to do it on their own. For example, say

> Put these two parts together: *m-oan.*
> Say it until you hear it. *Mmmmm-oan. Moan.*

Continue with these consonant–vowel–consonant (C–V–C) words from the text beginning with a single sound:

z-in	l-oud
f-ive	n-eck
n-ote	n-ine
s-oul	t-en
s-ob	t-one

(continues on next page)

GRADES 1-5

PLAY **Say-It-Until-You-Hear-It.** *Continued*

Then demonstrate how to synthesize initial consonant blends and rime into words until children can do it on their own. Words include

fl-ute (fffffllllllll-ute)	sl-eek	sm-ooth
sl-ide	fl-oor	cl-ick
cl-ap	bl-ack	gr-eat
		str-ings

PLAY **Roll-It-Out.**

Children synthesize a C–V–C word by blending each of its phonemes. Demonstrate by elongating the phonemes and blending them together in shorter and shorter sequences until children can identify the word. For example, say

m–ō–n
What's the word? Roll it out.
Mmm . . . ōōōōō . . . nnn. Mmm . . . ōōō . . . nnn. Moan.

Continue with a new word, presenting each of the phonemes separately so the children can "roll them out" on their own to find the word. First use the one-syllable C–V–C word list in Say-It-Until-You-Hear-It.

PLAY **Break-It-Up.**

Children analyze one-syllable C–V–C words to identify the beginning, middle, and ending sounds. Begin activities with initial sounds, then proceed to middle and ending sounds. For an example on how to demonstrate finding the middle sound in *moan*, ask

What's the sound in the middle of *moan*?
Break it up: *Mmmmmm-oooo-nnnn. M–ō–n.*
ō is the sound in the middle of *moan*.

Continue to present one-syllable C–V–C words provided above so children can "break them up" and identify the sounds in each of the positions.

In the last stage of the game, children identify all the sounds in the word. Demonstrate how to elongate the sounds and then break them up to identify each one, as in the example above.

PLAY **Delete-It.**

Children omit the first sound in a word from the text. Demonstrate by saying the word slowly, then leaving off the initial phoneme or cluster. To demonstrate using *flute*, for example, say

Listen to how I can make *flute* become *lute*.
First I roll it out: *fffffflllllll-uuuut.*
Then I delete the first sound: *llll-uuuuut. Lute.*
Now you delete it. *Flute . . .*

(continues on next page)

PLAY **Delete-It.** *Continued*

Proceed with one-syllable names of the instruments, deleting the first sound in the following words:

> harp (arp)
> french horn (ench orn)
> strings (rings or ings)

Then two-syllable instruments:

> trombone (ombone)
> trumpet (umpet)
> cello (ello)
> oboe (boe, as in *bow*)
> bassoon (assoon)

Then three-syllable instruments:

> violin (iolin)
> clarinet (arinet)

PLAY **Switch-It.**

Children delete the initial sounds of instruments featured in the book and replace them with another designated sound to make nonsense instruments. Demonstrate first, then prompt with cues as necessary, for example,

> Repeat my words, only when I say *trombone*, switch the beginning sound with *d*.

Their part will sound like this:

dombone	dumpet	dute
dello	diolin	darp
darinet	dassoon	
dings	dench dorn	

Then try a consonant cluster: *fl*

> flombone
> flumpet

and so on. Have fun!

Extended Activities: Put on a music appreciation week. First introduce other instruments not referred to in the book.

Listen to classical music, such as *Peter and the Wolf,* and identify the instruments referred to in the book. Introduce the music of groups such as the Moody Blues in the albums *Days of Future Past* or *Best of the Moody Blues,* or the Beatles's in the album *Sergeant Pepper's Lonely Hearts Club Band,* where symphonies play along with the band, group, or recording artist. Encourage students to bring in their instruments and share their classical music and books they may have on the subject. Then expand the classical musical genre to other forms of music. Use one day of the week for each category of music, depending on the interests of the students. Some suggestions are Country-Western Day, Jazz Day, Soul Day, Folk Day, and Oldies Day.

Section 3

Books Are for Talking with Students in Grades 6 Through 12

- Using Picture Books That Build Communication Skills and Literacy Achievement in Preadolescents and Adolescents

- Looking for Books That Help Build Communication Skills and Literacy Achievement in Preadolescents and Adolescents

- Hints for Introducing Picture Books to Preadolescents and Adolescents

- A Catalog of Picture Books for Preadolescents and Adolescents in Grades 6 Through 12

Using Picture Books That Build

Communication Skills and Literacy Achievement in Preadolescents and Adolescents

The most salient difference between intervention with younger children and older children is this: intervention with older children must have them think about their thinking, think about their talking, talk about their thinking, and talk about their talking. . . . The best intervention provides ample opportunity for this cognitive-linguistic focus.

—McKinley (2000, p. 8)

An appropriate and carefully selected picture book can be presented and used successfully with middle school and high school students for the following purposes:

Communicative Competency

To develop pragmatic usage of language. Learning how to engage in language for social purposes, honing conversational abilities, and understanding the rules of conversation are often the focus of preadolescent and adolescent communication skills. Snow et al. (1998) state, "One avenue for introducing and refining new pragmatic functions is through experience with books and other literacy activities" (p. 49). Stories in which characters use language to deceive and pretend (e.g., *The True Story of the Three Little Pigs*) and themes that center on the rules of relationships and friendships or highlight communication skills (e.g., *The Gentleman and the Kitchen Maid*) can be effective in addressing language pragmatics.

Literacy Development and Academic Success

To develop a sufficient lexicon base. Landauer and Dumais (1997) found that the acquisition of vocabulary knowledge from text adds not only new words to one's vocabulary but also alters and refines the semantic representations of words already acquired. "Effective teaching elaborates various connections among better-known and lesser-known words, deepens and enriches existing knowledge, and seeks to build a network of ideas around key concepts that are well elaborated" (Moats, 2000, p. 112).

Using words in context, discussing their meanings, and using them in association with other words can be facilitated through reading aloud, and talking, too! Areas to include in building vocabulary skills follow:

- Synonyms: Words that have the same meanings or are near-perfect substitutes.

- Antonyms: Words that have opposite meanings.

- Multiple-meaning words: Words that have more than one meaning.

- Categories of words: Words that share the same semantic class or network. For example, words that have to do with feelings include *intense, remorseful, gentle, hostile,* and *ambivalent.*

- Associating words: Words that share the same thematic associations.

- Compare and contrast: Words can be expressed and defined on the basis of their shared attributes and contrasted on the basis of their contrasting features.

- Figures of speech: Figures of speech include idioms (words used as a unit that convey a specific meaning, although not literally), similes (words used as a unit that make use of the words *like* or *as* to show an implied connection or comparison between an idea and an unusual referent), and metaphors (words that have an implied connection or comparison between an idea and an unusual referent that don't use *like* or *as*).

To develop advanced syntactic structures. To understand and use a variety of complex sentence structures appropriately. Westby (1999) identifies various complex syntactic sentence structures of a literate language style, which include, but are not limited to, the following:

- Connective words such as *so, then, when, as a result, however,* and *although*
- Subordinate clauses, using phrases with such words as *while, until, as,* and *although*
- Embedded clauses, using words such as *who* and *where*
- Elaboration of noun phrases

To develop a literate language style.

- Verbal expression. To explain meanings, express thoughts, and relate events in explicit and descriptive language.
- Sequencing. To organize and report events sequentially, such as in steps or a string of temporally related sequential events.
- Cause-and-effect relationships. To state the events that lead to a problem and what caused the problem to occur. *Voices of the Alamo,* by Sherry Garland, requires an understanding of how the land was different in the past but has similar landmarks today.
- Identify problems and solutions. To state facts about a problem, think of ways to solve the problem, and provide evidence to defend potential solutions to the problem. To comprehend and retell a goal-based story, students must be able to identify the problem and the attempts the character or characters make in responding to it. (*The River Ran Wild: An Environmental History,* by Lynne Cherry, requires an understanding of the problem and the characters' attempts at solving it.)
- Compare and contrast. Stories and literature can be used to explain how two concepts (e.g., situations, characters, or other features of the text) are the same and different. (*Amelia and Eleanor Go for a Ride,* by Pam Muñoz Ryan, can be used to compare and contrast two historical women with similar characteristics.)

To develop narrative schema. To produce narratives containing all the essential story grammar elements of an appropriate developmental level (Applebee, 1978). Preadolescent and adolescent students should be able to produce narrative structures that contain, hierarchically,

- complex episodes (a complete episode with obstacles to a goal and with multiple attempts to reach the goal),
- multiple sequential episodes (e.g., more than one chapter or episodes that extend over periods of time),

- interactive episodes (e.g., two or more characters with interactive goals), and
- embedded episodes (e.g., one narrative structure embedded within another; Westby, 1999).

To further develop literacy achievement.

- To identify the purpose, theme, plot, point of view, and moral of a story. *Seven Brave Women,* by Betsy Gould Hearne, is an excellent book in which to address these aspects of literature.
- To predict events or information to which the text is leading.
- To draw inferences (e.g., helping students see the clues about how characters' emotions help to facilitate inferencing skills).
- To summarize the main idea.
- To state beliefs, opinions, and experiences related to the text.

To develop metalingusitic skills. To talk about and analyze the language code. Any activities that require students to think about language and analyze the language code involve metalinguistic skills. Examples of metalinguistic skills that can be addressed with the use of literature include the following:

- Distinguishing between form and referent (as in the word itself, or the mental construct of the word, as opposed to that to which the word alludes)
- Defining words
- Understanding the use of morphological bases (Research indicates that when middle-school students are given lessons on prefixes, suffixes, and word stems, they become more proficient comprehenders of the material they are studying; Otterman, 1990)
- Understanding and expressing plays on words, such as riddles and puns

To develop metacognitive skills. How well students construct meaning from what they read depends in part on metacognition. The ability to think about and control the learning process involves planning, monitoring comprehension, and revising strategies for comprehension (Knuth & Jones, 2001). Metacognition and awareness of emotionality are required to both interpret narratives and monitor conversation. Helping to facilitate these skills is a worthwhile endeavor "for all older elementary and middle school and high school students" (Catts & Kamhi, 1999). To construct meaning and to understand what they read, students must formulate questions about the text as they read and comprehend. By asking appropriate questions, students gain a model, or schemata, to use in becoming independent readers and learners. Thinking about why a story was told in a certain way is one aspect of metacognition that can be addressed with literature activities.

Speech Production

To Improve Articulation

- To produce the target sound in words and structured phrases and sentences. After stressing the target sounds within the text and before turning each page, pause to have the student repeat words in the story that contain the target sound, say a carrier phrase appropriate to the story, or answer a question that elicits a word or words from the text.
- To produce the target sound in conversation. After reading, discuss story events in language that contain the target sound.

To Speak Fluently

Rhythmic verses can help students produce a more natural flow of speech production. Use lots of literature that calls for a rhythmic type of response, such as *This Land Is Your Land,* by Kathy Jacobsen, and *Voices of the Alamo,* by Sherry Garland. Use literature creatively to help students maintain airflow in responses that increase in length from a single word, to a short phrase, to a full sentence. Keep in mind that by using a picture book to systematically increase the length of fluent responses, book talk can incorporate other objectives such as improving eye contact and communication appearance.

To Improve Vocal Quality and Minimize Vocal Abuse

Use books for shaping vocal quality as you would for improving fluency (students use the optimal voice in progressively longer responses). Also, use the characters and the dialog of characters to demonstrate and contrast different manners of voice production (e.g., a harsh, strident voice versus a gentle, easy voice) that exemplify the elements of vocal quality and care.

Objectives in communication skills and literacy achievement can be facilitated through thoughtful planning and careful selection of a picture book found within the great and wondrous domain of children's literature. The key is in the selection and presentation, which are addressed in the following pages.

Looking for Books

That Help Build Communication Skills and Literacy Achievement in Preadolescents and Adolescents

The Catalog of Picture Books in this section and the Skills index provide an assortment of appropriate books from a variety of genres. In making additional selections for this unique age group, look for the following:

Books that you love. Sharing your love and enthusiasm for a variety of literature genres is invaluable in addressing language skills and literacy achievement.

A limited text. Although lengthier texts can provide outstanding stories, books with concise but creative texts afford greater opportunities for interaction during intervention that often must occur within certain time constraints. Many high-quality picture books have excellent, brief texts and are interesting and engaging for people of all ages. Look for books that have

- adult or young adult characters as subjects (e.g., *Mountain Men: True Grit and Tall Tales*, by Andrew Glass),
- interesting topics (e.g., the Italian Renaissance in *Starry Messenger*, by Peter Sís, depicting the life of the famous scientist, mathematician, astronomer, and philosopher, Galileo Galilei),
- famous individuals (e.g., *Amelia and Eleanor Go for a Ride*, by Pam Muñoz Ryan, and *Stephen Hawking: Understanding the Universe*, by Gail Sakurai)
- sports heroes (e.g., *Home Run*, by Robert Burleigh),
- humor (e.g., *George Washington's Cows*, by David Small),
- comic book style (e.g., *Meanwhile*, by Jules Feiffer), or
- new-age or high-tech applications (e.g., *Casey at the Bat: A Ballad of the Republic Sung in the Year 1888*, by Ernest Lawrence Thayer).

Picture opportunities. The illustrations should

- provide additional language opportunities (e.g., *The River Ran Wild: An Environmental History*, by Lynne Cherry),
- enlighten the text (*The Gettysburg Address*, by Abraham Lincoln, illustrated by Michael McCurdy), and
- appeal to older audiences, even adults.

Relevancy. The text and illustrations are most effective when they

- relate to the students' lives and personal experiences (e.g., *Big Talk: Poems for Four Voices*, by Paul Fleischman), and
- relate to topics covered in core curriculum (e.g., *This Land Is Your Land*, by Woody Guthrie, for the Great Depression of the 1930s).

Variety of Genres. Picture books can be found in many sections of a library or bookstore. Check the

- junior section (e.g., *Seven Brave Women*, by Betsy Gould Hearne),
- folklore section (e.g., *How the Stars Fell Into the Sky: A Navajo Legend*, by Jerrie Oughton),
- science section (e.g., *Cloud Dance*, by Thomas Locker),
- history section (e.g., *Harriet and the Promised Land*, by Jacob Lawrence),
- language section (e.g., *The King Who Rained*, by Fred Gwynne),
- sports section (e.g., *Casey at the Bat: A Ballad of the Republic Sung in the Year 1888*, by Ernest Lawrence Thayer),
- poetry section (e.g., *Big Talk: Poems for Four Voices*, by Paul Fleischman), and
- young adult section (*Chicken Soup for the Teenage Soul Journal*, by Jack Canfield, Mark Victor Hansen, and Kimberly Kirberger).

Hints for Introducing Picture Books

to Preadolescents and Adolescents

Older students may have varied reactions to using picture books as educational resources. The way students are introduced to the medium can bring about an appreciation of this genre and open a new avenue of learning and communicating. Many illustrated books combine a unique literary style with an unusual or sophisticated art form that clearly are not limited to young children. These books have value and interest for people of all ages, including adults. They can enhance and clarify classroom curriculum, provide entertainment, and become a bridge to discussion and development of oral communication skills and literacy achievement. Here are some points to consider when presenting picture books:

- **Great talent is ageless.** Discuss how many renowned writers and artists design picture books for people of all ages because their medium is their passion. For example, Jacob Lawrence, a university professor whose series of masterful works of art hang in museums, has created the picture book, *Harriet and the Promised Land.* There is nothing young or youthful about this book, a work to be admired by any aged individuals. Thomas Locker, author of *Cloud Dance,* is another example of a painter whose works are displayed in museums. Some writers and illustrators regularly create material for adults. Christopher Bing, creator and illustrator of the new-age version of *Casey at the Bat: A Ballad of the Republic Sung in the Year 1888,* is a political illustrator for the *Wall Street Journal, The New York Times,* and the *Washington Post.* The words of Abraham Lincoln's *Gettysburg Address,* translated into 29 languages for careful study of its beautifully written prose, has been illustrated in a book for people of all ages, capturing the era and lending meaning to its words.

- **Illustrations provide unique views.** Talk about the topic of the book you are about to read and how it relates to the theme you are exploring. Explain that you are reading and sharing the picture book because it treats the topic in a unique way. Ask students what they know about the topic before you begin. Talk about other books from other genres that deal with the same topic. *The River Ran Wild: An Environmental History,* by Lynne Cherry, treats the topic of Native Americans, pollution, and natural environments from the unique perspective of activists who led to the river's amazing environmental cleanup. Its beautiful prose and its strikingly memorable visual images are meant for all ages to learn from and enjoy.

- **Illustrations record our culture.** Pictures that accompany literature are an especially rich source of cultural material. Illustrations are an essential part of the literature because they instill in the reader and viewer a sense of values, customs, and aesthetics of that culture. *Big Talk: Poems for Four Voices,* by Paul Fleischman and illustrated by Italian artist Beppe Giacobbe, is an example of illustrations for our present culture; *How the Stars Fell Into the Sky: A Navajo Legend,* by Jerrie Oughton, is an example of illustrations depicting Native American culture; and *Meanwhile,* by Jules Feiffer, is an example of illustrations depicting comic book culture.

- **Be sensitive to the age group.** If the preadolescent or adolescent student feels uncomfortable having you read a picture book aloud for fear of being compared to his or her regular education peers, place a plain manila folder over the book so that visitors entering the room will be unaware of the type of book being read aloud. This conveys sensitivity to the students' feelings, may help certain students save face in front of their peers, and provides a feeling of safety and comfort for the individual in the particular setting.

- **Enthusiasm is contagious.** Present the book as one you love to read yourself and therefore want to share, particularly if you are concerned about students' initial reactions.

- **My story for the day.** Introduce your students to the saying, "Every day should contain at least one good story." Present the book as something you are sharing for your story of the day, which happens to be beautifully illustrated for everyone's enjoyment.

- **Let me entertain you.** Explain that one purpose of books is to entertain. What better way to entertain a class than to read the text and display the art in books such as *Mountain Men: True Grit and Tall Tales,* by Andrew Glass, especially when applying it to history curriculum on the opening of the American frontier.

- **It's relevant!** Openly communicate with preadolescents and adolescents about how various ways of learning classroom curriculum and spoken language skills can be beneficial. Once students understand that the material you've chosen can relate to their own lives and personal experiences and can help them to learn better ways of communicating, lessons will have a more positive impact.

A Catalog of Picture Books
for Preadolescents
and Adolescents
in Grades 6 Through 12

Amelia and Eleanor Go for a Ride

by Pam Muñoz Ryan
New York: Scholastic Press, 1999

Suggested Grade and Interest Level: 6 through 12

Topic Explorations: Famous people, Heroes; History, American; Women's lives

Skill Builders:

Vocabulary	**Grammar and syntax**	**Pragmatic language**
Semantics	Advanced syntactic structures	
Higher-level concepts	**Language literacy**	
Idioms	Compare and contrast	
Similes and metaphors	Drawing inferences	
Synonyms		

GRADES 6–12

Synopsis: On April 20, 1933, two heroes of American history, friends who shared much in common, dined together at the White House. The two women, Eleanor Roosevelt and Amelia Earhart, then took a rare night flight over Washington, D.C. Certain facts were embellished for this beautifully crafted, black-and-white picture book, but most are documented, including the food served for dinner and the White House china on which it was served! What is noteworthy about this story is how the author uses the nearly identical actions of the two women to underscore their similarities. It is also a stunning reminder that two great American women of the past continue to be role models to girls and women today.

Method: Before the read-aloud, present the book and take a moment to elicit the students' background knowledge of the two women and the era in which they lived. Describe the prevailing thought about a woman's place in the world. Describe the era of the Great Depression and its effect on all Americans. Read or relate the information in the back of the book about how the author came to write about this little-known event in history.

During the read-aloud, interject conversation where appropriate to share briefly about the story, especially where the illustrations provide a natural pause or where there is little or no text.

After the read-aloud, go back through the pictures and discuss what the students learned about the two women from the story. For teaching idioms, reread the opening lines, "Amelia and Eleanor were birds of a feather" (people with interests, opinions, or backgrounds in common). Explain the idiom and have students use it in their own sentences. Suggestions for sentence starters include the following:

> Amelia and Eleanor were birds of a feather because _____.
> Because Amelia and Eleanor both liked to do exciting and daring things, _____.
> Birds of a feather, like Amelia and Eleanor, _____.
> My friend and I _____.

The author states that Amelia and Eleanor were similar in nature and personality. To increase the students' ability to compare and contrast, ask them to compare the two women. Ask, for example, If you were writing a paper on the two famous women, how would you support that fact? What situations in the text demonstrate that they were similar? Where in the text is Amelia's character described? Where in the text are similar characteristics of Eleanor described?

Some suggestions:

> Amelia and Eleanor agreed there was nothing quite as exciting as flying. What could compare? Well, they admitted, maybe the closest thing would be driving a fast car on a straightaway road with the wind blowing against your face.

Many people did not understand why a woman would want to risk her life in a plane.

Many people thought it was too bold and dangerous for a woman to drive a car, especially for the First Lady of the United States.

Other ways they were similar:

Both were already famous.

Both were women in an era in which women were not considered equal to men.

In what ways were they different?

Eleanor was older.

Amelia had what was considered a man's career, whereas Eleanor had a woman's "place," which was not considered a career.

Discuss the concept of independence. Although both women were married to husbands with high-powered careers, they were independent in their own right—in many ways. Ask students to share what the concept of independence means to them and how it can be applied to the two women of the story, to other women in history, and to the women they know.

To teach the use of similes, find examples of how the author used similes and metaphors to enhance her writing. Some examples include the following:

And the enormous, light-drenched monuments looked like tiny miniatures.

And even though they knew it was not so, it seemed as if the plane crawled slowly through starstruck space.

Eleanor marveled, "It's like sitting on top of the world!"

To increase students' abilities to generate synonyms, turn to the double-page spread of the lights of Washington, D.C., as they flew over the Capitol. Tell the students that the author uses the word *exciting* in her book to describe the way the two women felt about flying. Brainstorm other words that can be used to describe what Eleanor might have felt on her first night in flight. Some suggestions include

thrilling	exhilarating	elated
stirring	moving	overjoyed
	awe inspiring	

Use the brainstormed words in sentences of various constructions to relate the experience of the plane ride.

At several places in the story, the reader/listener can infer meaning when words in the text are used to describe what happened. For example, when Amelia and Eleanor returned from their airplane ride, the author says,

"They walked up the steps to the White House. Eleanor whispered something to Amelia, and then they hesitated, letting the rest of the group walk ahead of them."

Point out the illustration depicting the action and ask questions such as,

Because we already know what happens next in the story, what do you think Eleanor actually said to Amelia?

What do you think is meant by the word *hesitate*?

Why did they let the rest of the group walk ahead?

At the beginning of the story, when Eleanor dresses for dinner, the text states that her brother, Hal, "would be escorting her this evening because the president had a meeting to attend." The next line reads, "But Eleanor was used to that." What can you infer about Eleanor Roosevelt's life from that short sentence?

Also ask students to think about why this event in history might have gone by without much notice until the author found it in her research, especially because the president was not present at the event.

To increase the students' understanding and usage of advanced syntactic structures, show them how to play with words using the paragraph that describes the sights above Washington, D.C. First list the sights. For instance, the author describes the Potomac River, the Capitol dome, and the monuments (Lincoln Memorial, Washington Memorial, and Jefferson Memorial). Have the students pick out the words the author uses to describe the sights and write the words next to the sights. (Note, for this exercise, it must be established what the sights actually are like from the ground as well as how they appear from the air.) For example,

> the Potomac River: glistening with moonshine
> the Capitol dome: reflecting a soft golden halo
> the monuments: enormous (from the ground), light-drenched tiny miniatures (from the air)

Then show students how to use the descriptive words in embedded sentences. Use the two-page spread as feedback for their constructions. Note that it may be necessary at first to provide the ending of their sentences. Once students catch on, scaffolding can be used to a minimum and students can become more creative with their constructions.

Some possible sentences are

> The Potomac River, glistening with moonshine, was seen through the window of Amelia's plane.
> The Capitol dome, reflecting a soft golden halo, was a thrilling sight.
> The monuments, like light-drenched tiny miniatures, were spectacular sights to see from the air.

Use the following paragraph of text for additional sentences. The full-page spread of the White House as seen between the cherry blossoms of spring is also an excellent page for structuring advanced syntactic structures.

For pragmatic language, point out how the two women started out sharing conversation. Ask students to recall what they talked about at dinner. How did they share conversation at the dinner table that would relate to everyone there, including the reporters and the photographer? What did Amelia joke about? Why was joking about George Washington's crab chowder a good way to share conversation at that time? Why is it good to put people at ease in social situations?

Have students act out the parts of Amelia, Eleanor, and the other guests. Then have students think of another president.

For example, name another president such as Thomas Jefferson or Ronald Reagan. Then think of another kind of dish, such as strawberry shortcake or Caesar salad. Combine the two, and in a pleasing tone, have students act the part of Amelia using their own words in the conversation.

"If *soup* at the White House has such a fancy name, I wonder what the *next* course will be?" Another person could offer, "Perhaps Ronald Reagan salad with ranch dressing?" Whatever the words, it is important to help students see that tone of voice should be lighthearted and fun.

Anno's Journey

by Mitsumasa Anno
New York: Philomel Books, 1977

Suggested Grade and Interest Level: 6 through 12

Topic Explorations: Community; History, European; Journeys; Long ago and far away

Skill Builders:

Grammar and syntax	**Language literacy**	**Articulation**
Advanced syntactic structures	Storytelling	General articulation
	Compare and contrast	

Synopsis: The pictures in this wordless picture book tell the story of a journey through northern Europe. Each full-page spread is a detailed illustration of people at work in different European cultures.

Method: Have students guess which country is depicted on each page. What landmarks give clues to the country? Then compare and contrast different European countries and cultures. Use words such as *same, similar, different, however, instead of, in contrast to,* and *compared to.*

Ask students to identify what the characters are doing. Model and shape advanced syntactic structures of coordinating conjunctions such as *and* and *but,* subordinating conjunctions such as *because* and *so,* adverbial clauses such as those using *while* and *although,* and adverbial clauses with connective functions such as those using *if–then* and *however.*

Extended Activity: Have students create a short story, complete with characters and plot, based on a scene. Outline the story as follows:

> What is the time, location, context, and mood of the story?
> Who is the main character?
> What problem sets off the action in the story?
> How does the character respond to the situation?
> What plan does the character devise?
> What steps does the character take to solve the problem?
> Are they successful or not?
> What are the consequences?
> What is the reaction of the main character?

Anno's Medieval World

by Mitsumasa Anno
New York: Philomel Books, 1979

Suggested Grade and Interest Level: 6 through 12

Topic Explorations: History, Medieval; Long ago and far away

Skill Builders:

Vocabulary	**Language literacy**
Attributes	Cause-and-effect relationships
Grammar and syntax	Compare and contrast
Advanced syntactic structures	**Articulation**
	Carryover for any sound

Synopsis: Fascinating pictures and poetic text document how medieval peoples viewed their world. For example, Copernicus and his courageous followers, who convinced people that the world was not flat and motionless but round and in constant rotation around the sun, are discussed. The transition to this point of view caused great suffering, but the evidence finally triumphed over people's long-held beliefs.

Method: To teach comparing and contrasting, pause to describe life in medieval times as Anno depicts it. Compare and contrast life then and now. Are there similarities? What are the differences? Compare the process of change in our society today with how it occurred in the Middle Ages. Use words such as *same, similar, different, however, instead of, in contrast to,* and *compared to.*

To teach cause-and-effect relationships, ask students questions such as

What caused the people in the Middle Ages not to believe the new theory of the universe?
What were some of the events that led to the next stage of civilization, the Age of Reason?
What factors cause change today?
What are the effects of a change of view on a civilization?

To teach attributes, talk about the characteristics of the people who lived during the Middle Ages. What did it take for them to change? What attributes can you use to describe the people who led the slow changes? (For example, brave, intelligent, truth seeking, curious, visionary.)

Model and shape advanced syntactic structures. Some examples include the following.

Dependant clauses:

In medieval times, there were scientists who believed the earth moved around the sun.
People could not believe a new theory because their religious beliefs were strong.
Although scientists believed the earth moved around the sun, the people could not accept it.

Embedded sentence:

A few brave scientists, who were not afraid to stand up for what they believed in, helped to change people's views.
Most people in medieval times, because they were afraid to change their beliefs, could not believe a new theory (about the world).

Extended Activity: To enhance critical thinking skills, ask students to visualize themselves living in medieval times. Would they believe that ships setting sail for the east would fall off the edge of the earth, or would they believe that the ships would return safely? Why? What would be the effect today if someone made a discovery that was contrary to our beliefs? How would people respond? How would the media and our communication systems play roles in shaping our responses?

Arrow to the Sun

by Gerald McDermott
New York: Puffin Books, 1984

Suggested Grade and Interest Level: 6 through 12

Topic Exploration: Folklore, Native American

Skill Builders:

Language literacy
Sequencing
Cause-and-effect relationships

Problem solving
Critical thinking

Articulation—*S* and *Z, R,* and *Th* (voiced and voiceless)

Synopsis: The universal hero myth is embodied in this story of a boy who is rejected because he does not have a father. So the boy leaves on a quest to find him. When he is sent to the Lord of the Sun, his true father, he is not acknowledged until he undergoes a series of trials to prove his identity. Having accomplished them, he returns to earth with his father's spirit, where everyone rejoices with the Dance of Life.

Method: Pause to identify the problem in the story, asking the following questions:

> What events caused the problem to happen?
> What facts can you state about the problem?
> How does the boy solve his problem?
> Recall the series of trials in order that the boy underwent to prove he was his father's son.
> What caused the people to celebrate the boy's return with the Dance of Life?

For discussion, bring in materials to familiarize the students with Pueblo art. Compare the book's illustrations to Pueblo art. What qualities do they have in common?

Also discuss elements that are common to the hero motif in folktales. What ingredients does the story have that fit with the hero motif? How is the story like other hero myths?

For articulation, pause to elicit target words found in the text. Have students use the words in sentences that reflect the story. *Th* words include

father	mother	earth
through	this	nothing

Big Talk: Poems for Four Voices

by Paul Fleischman
Cambridge, MA: Candlewick Press, 2000

Suggested Grade and Interest Level: 6 through 12

Skill Builders:

Vocabulary	**Language literacy**
Semantics	Drawing inferences
Homonyms (multiple meanings)	**Pragmatic language**
Grammar and syntax	**Articulation**
Advanced syntactic structures	General articulation

Synopsis: Directions to this book state, "Get ready: Find three other speakers. Get set: Pick a color. Go! Read the words for your color all the way through the poem. . . . You're ready to make Big Talk. Have some toe-tapping, tongue-flapping fun!"

The collection of poems includes "Seventh-Grade Soap Opera" and "Ghosts' Grace." The words and style of the poems can provide motivating subject matter for working with older students. Another fitting name for the collection might be "Word Music." If you have never heard poems read aloud by different speakers speaking their lines, both at intervals and at the same time, in a beautiful cacophony of sounds, get ready for an incredible sound experience!

The artwork is appealing to older students, both in design and subject matter, because it depicts scenes from teenagers' lives.

Side note: The author says on the book jacket that he recently joined his first string quartet: "What joy! I've tried to bring this bliss into these spoken quarters."

Method: For average to above-average readers, this can be a fun read-aloud activity. For low-average readers, the activity is achievable also; however, spending time rehearsing the proper names in the text is advised. The idea is to read slowly, which will give some students an advantage.

After the read-aloud, help students understand the meaning of text that uses advanced syntactic forms. Begin by picking out parts of the poem the students particularly liked or sentences that can be confusing to a student who is language impaired. The following is a humorous line from the poem "Seventh-Grade Soap Opera."

(*Note:* This also can be used with students in higher grades. Rename the poem "Tenth-Grade Soap Opera" or something similar, or ask students if the poem applies to their age group.)

> "Randy pays Nicholas not to tell / Mr. Blair what went wrong when / he helped Jeremy dye his hair."

First identify any words that pose difficulty in the sentence. In this excerpt, *pays* may be confusing. Ask, for example,

> Who is the sentence about?
> Who pays whom?
> Why does Randy pay Nicholas?

Look for clues in the next line. The text says Randy pays Nicholas not to tell. Help students draw inferences by actively constructing meaning.

Possible suggestion: Randy does not want Nicholas to tell on him so he pays him money to keep quiet. Discuss students' background knowledge of the word *bribe*.

Break the sentence up visually by writing it out (on a chalkboard or small handheld white board). Then ask,

> Who was Nicholas going to tell?
> What was Nicholas going to tell Mr. Blair?

Infer meaning again.

Stated: Something went wrong when he (Randy) helped his friend (Jeremy) dye his hair.

Elicit students' prior knowledge by inquiring what might have gone wrong. For example:

> Can anything drastic happen why you dye someone's hair?
> What might have gone wrong here?
> What might Randy have done to Nicholas's hair?
> Why did Randy pay Nicholas?

Stated: So he would not tell.

Inferred: So he would not tell Jeremy's dad that he was the one who helped Jeremy dye his hair.

Help students draw inferences by actively constructing meaning based on their own experiences. A suggested line from the text reads,

> "Sonya sneaks out of the house / gets her ears pierced with Lauren and Lynn / then bumps into her grandmother."

First ask *why* Sonya sneaked out of the house.

Stated: Because she wanted her ears pierced.

Inferred: Because she was not allowed to get her ears pierced.

Inferred: Because she was grounded.

Continue to draw inferences from the rest of the phrase.

Is bumping into her grandmother something Sonya wants to do at this time? Why or why not?

Help students construct advanced syntactic structures by using the language from the text. For sentences with subordinate clauses, choose a phrase to begin a sentence. One type of subordinate clause is the dependent clause that begins with an adverb, such as

> While sneaking out of the house, Sonya got her ears pierced.
> While sneaking out of the house, Sonya ran into her grandmother.
> After Sonya sneaked out of the house, she got her ears pierced.
> After Sonya sneaked out of the house, she ran into her grandmother.

Supply students with a sentence that begins with an adverbial phrase. Some examples include

> Because Sonya wanted to get her ears pierced, . . .
> Because Sonya was grounded, . . .

Have students complete the thought. For example,

> Because Sonya wanted her ears pierced, she sneaked out of the house.
> Because she wanted her ears pierced, Sonya sneaked out of the house to meet Lauren and Lynn.
> Because she was grounded, Sonya had to sneak out of the house to get her ears pierced.

Use the four-part method to create an embedded sentence:

1. Begin with a basic sentence.

   Create: Sonya got her ears pierced.

2. Ask a *when* (or *where, why, how*) question to expand the sentence.

   Question: When did she get her ears pierced?

   Answer: After she sneaked out of the house

3. Pick a modifier and add it to the subject.

   Question: What is a word to describe Sonya?

   Answer: *Risky.*

4. Show how to combine the elements using the modified subject, inserting the expander into the basic sentence, and finishing with the remainder of the basic sentence, as in

> Risky Sonya, after she sneaked out of the house, got her ears pierced.

Demonstrate how to combine more elements, as in

> Risky Sonya, while sneaking out of the house to get her ears pierced, ran into her grandmother.
> Sneaky Sonya, while out getting her ears pierced with Lauren and Lynn, ran into her grandmother.

Look at the paintings for "Seventh-Grade Soap Opera," for example. Infer what might be happening in the students' lives. For example,

> Brenda calls Gregory.
> Derek snubs Catherine.

Ingrid tells Beverly.
Jason eyes Jacqueline.
Rick gives his e-mail address to Penelope.
Faith invites Gwendolyn.

For articulation, have students read aloud, maintaining the target phoneme(s) in their speech production.

Bill Gates: Helping People Use Computers

by Charnan Simon
New York: Children's Press, Grolier, 1997

Suggested Grade and Interest Level: 6 through 12

Topic Explorations: Famous people; Motivation; Speaking and communicating

Skill Builders:

Vocabulary	Language literacy	Pragmatic language
Semantics	Discussion	
Attributes		

Synopsis: Although written for early readers, the material is suitable for reading aloud to older students with language impairments for generating interesting and motivating discussions. The 48-page biographical work with references tells some of the history of the richest man in the world, known as the "Software King," and clearly explains how he helped bring personal computers into people's lives around the world. It also gives a history of the early computers, "large and awkward behemoths," and includes some of Microsoft's philanthropic works. Of special note is Gates's style of communicating with his company's employees.

Methods: Define the vocabulary words in the context of the text, including

competitive
philanthropy
educate (If someone disagrees with Bill, he will say, "Educate me on that.")
whiz kid
corporation
revolution
CEO (chief executive officer)

The text states, "It is impossible to think of personal computers without thinking of Bill Gates and Microsoft Corporation." It also describes Mr. Gates's competitive nature and how he encourages employees to come to work every day with a positive can-do attitude. Not everyone likes Bill Gates, however, and as explained in the text, some people think he is too competitive. Have a discussion on the pros and cons of his competitive philosophy. What is the good thing about competition? What can be weighed in on the negative side?

Also talk about the concept of motivation. How does Bill Gates motivate his employees? What are some of the conditions that may exist in this company that motivate the employees to want to succeed?

The book states that one of Bill Gates's favorite projects is Microsoft's program to give computers to inner-city and rural libraries that do not have the advantage of buying a good selection of books that other libraries have. With computers, these schools can link up with the Internet and use the resources from libraries all around the world with just a click of a button. Have a discussion on philanthropic works. Name other donors who give to charity, perhaps in your community. What are the positive outcomes of large corporations or donors of any kind helping others? Talk about ways all people can demonstrate charity, no matter what their financial position is.

To generate attributes, help students elicit words that describe Bill Gates. On what information do students base their opinions?

To teach pragmatic language, discuss the way in which the founder and CEO of Microsoft Corporation (according to the limited information from the text) communicates with his employees.

> Are employees allowed to disagree with him?
> In what way do students think this is done?
> What does Bill Gates mean when he says, "Educate me on that."
> What might be the effect of those words?
> Might this be a good personal communication strategy as well?

Stage a mock theater consisting of executives in a roundtable discussion. Have Gates appropriately respond to an executive with an opinion. (Suggestions include a new software program that the executive believes would be a success because it would make studying, dating, and relationships with parents easier for teenagers, thus generating more sales in that marketplace.) Gates can respond by saying, "Educate me on that." After the executive expresses his or her views, another student can do the same, pro or con. Then stop the process. Role-play the same scenario again, only this time Gates responds by saying, "That's a ridiculous idea. The teenage market won't go for it. Forget it," and cut off conversations when other executives try to explain their views.

> What effect does an honest inquiry have on the communication process?
> How does it make the other person feel?
> What is the result?
> What is the result when Gates disagreed and did not allow other executives to state their opinions?
> How could another executive express disagreement appropriately?
> How could Gates express disagreement appropriately?

To generalize the learning, ask the following questions:

> What ways can students express disagreement with their peers? What words can be used?
> Are there other appropriate ways to express disagreement?
> In what situations does that apply?
> Are there examples of situations students can think of where they could use these skills at home or at school? Help students brainstorm list of applicable situations.

Casey at the Bat: A Ballad of the Republic Sung in the Year 1888

by Ernest Lawrence Thayer
Illustrated by Christopher Bing
New York: Handprint Books, 2000

Suggested Grade and Interest Level: 6 through 12

Topic Explorations: Baseball; Famous people, Heroes; Folk tales, North American; History, American

Skill Builders:

Vocabulary	**Language literacy**
Semantics	Compare and contrast
Higher-level concepts	Drawing inferences
Idioms	Discussion
Similes and metaphors	

Synopsis: In this remarkable book, an award–winning political illustrator of the *Wall Street Journal* and *New York Times* pays tribute to the game of baseball and its place in American history. The words to "Casey at Bat," the well-known ode to a fallen baseball hero who strikes out, loses the game, and bitterly disappoints his fans, are incorporated into what appears to be a newly discovered, 100-year-old scrapbook. Included on each two-page spread is a scene from the poem. The illustrations are large scratchboard drawings that are remarkably similar to the engravings of the time period. Included in the scrapbook are the *Mudville Monitor* clippings of the events of the day (Casey's ninth-inning strikeout and the Mudville nine's 4 to 2 defeat), artifacts, period baseball cards, tickets, advertisements, and the like. All the items combine to re-create the era and capture the drama and exhilaration of baseball, giving the reader the sense of an American past. The illustrations and graphics on every page offer great possibilities for discussion.

Some history: "Casey at Bat" was first published in the *San Francisco Examiner,* on June 3, 1988, under a pseudonym. The writer, Ernest Lawrence Thayer (1863–1940), a student of philosophy and manager of wool mills, gave the poem to his friend and classmate, William Randolph Hearst, owner of the newspaper empire. It was said that he would rather it had been forgotten. (Perhaps because he became known for penning it and not for the type of literary works he felt would have been more fitting for a gentleman of his day and caliber.)

The last stanza,

> And somewhere men are laughing,
> and somewhere children shout;
> But there is no joy in Mudville—
> Mighty Casey has struck out.

has been recited through the decades, becoming an immortal ballad and a piece of Americana. However, without prior knowledge, some readers and viewers may be surprised to know that there was no such place as Mudville, no such game, and no such newspaper as the *Mudville Monitor,* which reported it.

It is only with the use of sophisticated electronics and computer graphics that the images of the book could be rendered with such realism. Paradoxically, it says just as much about our culture and times today as it does about this bygone era.

Method: Use this work to accompany a history unit, poetry unit, or sports unit; during the World Series games; or simply for the sheer pleasure of enjoying an amazing phenomenon of a book.

Before the read-aloud, present the backdrop of late 19th-century America. Elicit background knowledge about the history of the game of baseball. Vocabulary words include

> visage ("Great Casey's visage shown . . .")
> sport (of the game)
> straggling few
> deep despair
> preceded ("Flynn preceded Casey")
> grim melancholy
> lusty yell
> dell ("it rattled in the dell")

recoiled ("recoiled upon the flat")
advancing (to the bat)
doffed (his hat)
ease
pride
writhing (pitcher)
defiance ("gleamed in Casey's eye")
haughty grandeur

Higher-level concepts:

humiliation   defeat

Idioms:

Died at first
Get a whack at that
lulu (the former was a lulu)
cake ("the latter was a cake")
"Getting to the bat"

Metaphor:

Five thousand tongues applauded

Simile:

(The roar of the crowd) ". . . like the beating of the storm-waves on a stern and distant shore."

What can you infer about the thoughts and feelings of the crowd and the era in which the ode was written?

The following can be discussion items:

Discuss heroes. What is it that makes a person become a hero? Brainstorm ideas. What do heroes have that the average person does not? Talk about the feasibility of always winning for most ordinary people and the apparent ease of winning for very few people. Compare the hero's status with current sports heroes.

Discuss the concept of an idol and others' expectations of a great hero.

Discuss the style of the day, such as the baseball uniforms with their square caps and more formal style of shirts. Talk about the derbies of the men in the crowd and handlebar mustaches.

Talk about the prevailing thoughts of the day. How were thoughts different? Read the fictional newspaper clippings, which give a sense of what the game was like and what the issues of the day were. For instance, on May 28, 1888, an article states that lifting the ban on overhand pitching was under consideration.

Also, on the spread where Jimmy Blake "tears the cover off the ball," an editorial decries the practice of using only one ball throughout a game.

Elsewhere, the illustrations depict an African American player, and the clipping addresses the soon-to-be-instituted color line.

" 'Given the almost lackadaisical pace of some games in recent memory, anything which will speed up these afternoon doldrums can only be welcomed.' National Sports Reporter"

The editor's note states, "Casey stands as a heroic reminder that the blurring of fact and fancy, reality and imagination, resides at the core of the American experience." Discuss the meaning of fact and fancy and reality and imagination. What other American icons (perhaps people of folklore) fit into this description?

Chicken Soup for the Teenage Soul III: More Stories of Life, Love and Learning

by Jack Canfield, Mark Victor Hansen, and Kimberly Kirberger
Deerfield Beach, FL: Health Communications, 2000

Suggested Grade and Interest Level: 7 through 12

Skill Builders:

Vocabulary	Language literacy
Semantics	Problem solving
Attributes	Discussion

Synopsis: To attest to the popularity of this series, more than 50,000 submissions were received for the making of this third book of *Chicken Soup for the Teenage Soul*. Each book in the series is excellent for short, inspirational read-alouds on subjects that matter most to teenagers, such as relationships, friendship, love, family, lessons, overcoming obstacles, self-discovery, and more.

Method: Preselect one of the many short stories in this series (or from any of the others) appropriate for the individual or group with whom you are working. Prepare a few questions to encourage discussion and motivate students to talk about situations that make us look deeper into the human soul, situations that help us empathize with others to develop our own inner strength. An example lesson follows:

Read "Owning the World," a four-page story about Lizzie, who, together with her parents, learns of her diagnosis of leukemia. She considers this a "temporary obstacle" and decides she must face matters with grace and maturity. Not wanting to be the victim of things that would happen to her over her course of treatment, she takes the perspective of understanding that those around her are helping.

She finds that painting is a therapeutic avenue, and she describes her chemotherapy and the unsuccessful bone marrow transplant from her brother. After more rounds of treatment and more chemotherapy, she writes that this time she is glad that there was no evidence of leukemia found. As she responds to treatment, she reminds herself—and us in turn—"how valuable and fragile *everybody* is."

Just 2 months later, the editors received a note from Lizzie's parents that she had relapsed for the last time and died at their home. They acknowledged her greatness and her wish for mankind: "Begin now to live your life to the fullest—it is possible."

Discuss with students how Lizzie faced life when she learned she had leukemia. What does it mean to face something with grace? How did she demonstrate her maturity? Lizzie was open about her feelings of sadness about not being able to meet her loved one's expectations. What would you tell Lizzie if she were here today and she expressed her disappointment with herself for not being able to overcome her disease?

How can each of us better learn to cope with our disappointments?
What can we learn from Lizzie?
What are her attributes?
To what situations in our own lives can we apply perseverance, bravery, and a positive attitude?

Chicken Soup for the Teenage Soul Journal

by Jack Canfield, Mark Victor Hansen, and Kimberly Kirberger
Deerfield Beach, FL: Health Communications, 1998

Suggested Grade and Interest Level: 7 through 12

Topic Exploration: Motivation

Skill Builders:

Vocabulary	**Language literacy**
Semantics	Explaining processes in detail
Higher-level concepts	Discussion
Categories	**Pragmatic language**
Attributes	**Articulation**
	General articulation

Synopsis: After receiving letters from young readers of *Chicken Soup for the Teenage Soul* concerning their heartaches, disorders, and feelings of despair, the editors conceived and produced a journal. Stories, poems, quotations, and creative spaces provide teenagers with ideas for creating their own expressions. Additional spaces are designated for parents and friends to fill in. The book is divided into sections such as loving yourself, relationships, learning lessons, following your dreams, and making a difference.

Method: For people who work with teenagers, sections of the journal can offer ideas for meaningful activities to develop language skills. For example, in "Making a Difference," spaces are offered to teenagers to fill in what they enjoy doing because of the efforts of other people. Brainstorm ideas for a discussion about how other people make a difference in their lives. See the following suggestion.

Going to movies can provide teenagers with something they enjoy doing. A motion picture is the result of many people's efforts. Ask students to think about what goes into the creation, production, and distribution of a motion picture. What needs to happen to produce a movie? How does it reach moviegoers to provide them with enjoyment? Brainstorm the steps in the process as much as possible from what you or the students know. Categorize the jobs, such as on-site production crew, behind-the-scenes crew, sound crew, and so on. You may want to show a movie and fast forward to the list of credits. Stop on a frame in the credits so students can copy the jobs of those listed. Ask students to think about what jobs belong in which categories. Bring the enjoyment of a movie closer to home by following the process into the neighborhood theaters. How do movies get to moviegoers? Whose efforts are responsible for making movie viewing possible? Think about those people and their jobs, no matter how small, and how all those individuals make a difference in the students' lives. What would it be like if there were no motion pictures or videos?

Ask students to recall a time when someone they knew personally made a difference in their lives. Perhaps someone performed a small kindness or gave a compliment instead of an expected put-down. Encourage teenagers to talk about how they may have made a difference in the life of another. Simple ways, such as being a good listener when a friend needed them, are just as important as heroic deeds. Use this as a way to practice pragmatic language, such as giving compliments, acknowledging the speaker, and closing a discussion on a personal note.

Have students tell what it means to make a difference, now that they have learned that in some way, large or small, we all make a difference in each other's lives. By our actions, we can make an even bigger difference. Use the make-a-difference theme to talk about the concept of dedication and the commitment it takes to achieve goals.

In the section, "Following Your Dreams," facts are listed about famous people and what they went through to make their dreams become reality. Walt Disney is one example. Facts are given about how he was fired from his newspaper job because he lacked ideas and about how he went through bankruptcy several times. Use the

GRADES 6-12

theme and other resources to brainstorm attributes about Walt Disney (or other people who followed their dreams). Some suggestions include the following:

> artistic
> risk taker
> innovator
> visionary
> resourceful (found a way to make things work)
> optimistic
> persistent (when life hit hard, he did not give up)
> delightful (brought joy to others)

Joseph Campbell, famous "mythologist," teacher, and storyteller, had a message: "Follow your bliss." This book suggests to readers that they define what *bliss* means to them. In what ways can students follow their bliss, dreams, and goals? How is this different than just staying in a feeling-good state?

Continue to look through the book and pick out tasks applicable to students and groups. Create activities around the ideas as you help students express their thoughts and feelings.

For articulation, use the lists, stories, and poems that students generate orally to practice articulation skills. Have students write in journals that you provide. Ask students to present them out aloud, repeating their own words and thoughts using their target sound(s).

A Chocolate Moose for Dinner

by Fred Gwynne
Englewood Cliffs, NJ: Prentice Hall, 1976

Suggested Grade and Interest Level: 6 through 9

Skill Builders:
> **Vocabulary**
> Semantics
> Idioms
> Homonyms (multiple meanings)

Synopsis: Here is a witty collection of homonyms shown from a child's bewildered perspective. Who else but a child would conceptualize Mommy having a chocolate moose for dinner? Or toasting Daddy? Or wanting a new wing on the house?

Method: Read the book and discuss each homonym. Also discuss the idioms presented and their meanings.

Extended Activity: Have students make up some ambiguous phrases of their own and illustrate them the way the author did. Start off by brainstorming other homonyms and mixing up their meanings. Here are a few ideas:

> *pair* and *pare:* A pare of shoes.
> *beau* and *bow:* Bring your bow to the party.
> *sole* and *soul:* Do you feel it in your sole?

Think of some idioms and decide how they could be interpreted literally. Examples include

Catch your breath	Cat got your tongue	Stick your neck out
Afraid of your shadow	The apple of your eye	

Have students draw pictures illustrating the literal interpretations of these idioms. Have them write the idiom on the back of the picture illustrating it. Display the completed pictures around the room. Have the class or group view the pictures and try to guess (or express) what idiom each one illustrates. Afterward, allow each student to present his or her picture, then turn it over to reveal the idiom written on the back.

Note: See *The King Who Rained* in this catalog section. Also read *The Sixteen Hand Horse* and *A Little Pigeon Toad* by the same author.

Cloud Dance

by Thomas Locker
San Diego, CA: Silver Whistle, Harcourt, 2000

Suggested Grade and Interest Level: 6 through 12

Topic Explorations: Clouds; Science; Weather

Skill Builders:

Vocabulary	**Grammar and syntax**
Semantics	Advanced syntactic structures
Adjectives	
Similes and metaphors	

Synopsis: Thomas Locker's oil on canvas illustrations are simply gorgeous, and combined with his extraordinarily simple, lyrical text, they make this an ideal book to understand and build advanced syntactic structures. The artist shows clouds of different shapes and sizes drifting and dancing across various seasonal skies. At the back of the book, there is factual information about the formation and different types of clouds. The book is justly deserving of its multiple award-winner status and is very suitable for individuals of any age.

Method: Begin by showing the paintings of cloud formations in different seasons and during different parts of the day.

On many of the pages, the verb stands alone in a line of verse, such as

High, wispy clouds	Fluffy summer clouds	Soft, rosy clouds
race	march	flow
in the autumn wind.	in the blue sky.	in the dawn light.

First, construct simple sentences with the verb, such as

Clouds *flow.*
Clouds *march.*

Identify the adjectives in the poem. How are the clouds described? Exchange the adjectives on one page with the adjectives on another. Does the sentence make sense? Check the illustration. For example,

Fluffy, summer clouds flow in the dawn light.
Soft, rosy clouds march in the blue sky.

Expand the simple constructions with the adjectives.

Soft, rosy clouds flow.
Fluffy, summer clouds march.

Identify the adverbial phrases. Where are the clouds? Then expand the sentences again, such as

Soft, rosy clouds flow *in the dawn light.*
Fluffy, summer clouds march *in the blue sky.*

Introduce a referent into the sentence: a person named Eleanor, or Jack, for example. Add the person as the subject of the sentence and what he or she did (watched the clouds) as the predicate, as in the following:

Eleanor watched the soft, rosy clouds flow in the dawn light.
Jack watched the fluffy, summer clouds march in the blue sky.

Expand the sentence by giving details about Eleanor or Jack. Where was Eleanor and what was she doing when she watched the clouds? Put the verb first in the description. Sitting, standing? Waiting for someone? Students can use their imaginations to come up with the phrases, such as

Sitting quietly on her front porch, Eleanor watched the soft rosy clouds flow in the dawn light.
Standing on the hillside, Jack watched the fluffy, summer clouds march in the blue sky.
Standing with his dog Spark, Jack watched the fluffy, summer clouds march in the blue sky.

Show students how versatile language can be. Rearrange the words by inserting the phrase after the subject of the sentence to make an embedded sentence, such as

Eleanor, *sitting quietly on her front porch,* watched the soft, rosy clouds flow in the dawn light.
Jack and Spark, *standing on the hillside,* watched the fluffy summer clouds march in the blue sky.

Point out the use of figurative language, such as clouds "marching," and brainstorm other words that can be used as metaphors or similes for the way clouds move. Use them in varying lengths of sentence constructions.

The Cremation of Sam McGee

by Robert W. Service
New York: Greenwillow Books, 1986

Suggested Grade and Interest Level: 6 through 12

Topic Explorations: Death and dying; Folk tales, North American; Friendship; Loyalty

Skill Builders:

Vocabulary	**Language literary**
Semantics	Storytelling
Higher-level concepts	Problem solving
Grammar and syntax	Drawing inferences
Advanced syntactic structures	Discussion

Synopsis: This ballad of the Yukon Gold Rush by Robert W. Service was first published in Canada in 1907 in *Songs of a Sourdough* (and in the United States in *The Spell of the Yukon and Other Verses*). It tells how Sam McGee succumbs to the arctic cold and requests that his friend cremate his remains. The verse is accompanied by the paintings of Ted Harrison, whose unconventional use of colors such as purples, pinks, blues, and golds creates an authentic aura for the turn-of-the-century Yukon. The *Merriam-Webster's Encyclopedia of Literature* states, "The ballad has remained a favorite recitation piece because of its internal rhymes, driving rhythms, and macabre irony."

Method: Before the read-aloud, elicit background knowledge from students about the Yukon Territory and the gold rush. Evaluate the book's cover, its use of unusual colors, and make story predictions.

During the read-aloud, pause briefly to discuss vocabulary, such as *moil,* and the problem of the main character.

After the read-aloud, discuss concepts such as loyalty and obligation. Ask questions to facilitate comprehension. For example,

> What facts can you state about the problem?
> Why was his friend's last request so difficult?
> Why do you think he felt he had to carry out his friend's request, even though Sam was dead?
> How did his sense of obligation trigger a desire to carry out the request?

For storytelling, discuss story grammar elements. Encourage the use of connective words such as *nevertheless, meanwhile, because,* and *when* to express causal relationships. Also ask questions about the personalities of the characters.

Discuss the artist's choice of colors. Identify which colors are warm and which are cool, and talk about how warm and cool colors are used to add emotional overtones to the illustrations.

Extended Activity: Conduct a semantic webbing activity around the concept of loyalty. Write the word *loyalty* in the center of the board or large piece of paper and circle it. Ask students what questions arise when they think of loyalty. What feelings come to mind?

Associate ideas as you talk about loyalty to give students a deeper meaning of the concept. What do the students want to discuss about it? How is loyalty earned? What personality traits or environmental circumstances generate it? Write these questions on the board or paper and draw lines connecting *loyalty* to each question.

Go back to the central word, *loyalty.* What other ideas do students associate with the concept? Do they want to give examples of loyalty in other literary characters? Draw a line in the direction of another thought labeled *literary examples.* Do they want to give personal examples? Draw a line in the direction of the thought labeled *personal experiences.* Then generate statements based on these labels. Help students generate questions about these statements as you model self-learning strategies.

Divide the class or group into collaborative teams. Help students generate questions about loyalty from the information presented. For example,

> What does loyalty feel like?
> What does a feeling of loyalty make a person want to do?
> How does loyalty manifest itself?
> Who are some literary characters who have shown loyalty?
> Who are the people you know who have shown you loyalty?

Have the group discuss and answer the questions. Encourage them to use a variety of complex sentence structures. For example,

> Loyalty feels like _____.
> People who are loyal do not gossip, make cruel remarks, or turn their backs on people.
> Although people say they are friends, they may not always be loyal to each other.
> Loyalty, an important part of friendship, is one way to show you respect and care about someone.

Dakota Dugout

by Ann Turner
New York: Macmillan, 1985, 1989

Suggested Grade and Interest Level: 6 through 12

Topic Exploration: History, American

Skill Builders:
    Vocabulary   **Language literacy**
    Semantics   Drawing inferences
                              Critical thinking

Synopsis: A woman tells her granddaughter about her life experiences on the Dakota prairie more than a century ago. Students can learn about the lives of the early settlers from the black-and-white sketches and short, poetic verses.

Method: Before the read-aloud, activate students' knowledge of pioneer life. Talk about what a prairie is like—a treeless expanse of flatland covered with tall grass—and ask students to imagine what the conditions were like for the first settlers. Lead into the story by having students predict what the story will be about based on the book's title.

Encourage critical thinking by asking what the author is implying about life on the prairie in various poetic passages. Encourage students to use conjunctions such as *so* and *because* to express causal relationships and adverbial phrases using *when* to express temporal relationships. For example,

> What does the woman mean when she talks about "the empty cries of the long grass"?
> What does *jabber* mean?
> Why did she jabber back to a sparrow?
> Why do you think the young woman left her family to journey to a land unknown?
> What kind of people must the pioneers have been to survive their hardships and achieve success?
> What does *pioneer spirit* mean?
> What techniques does the author use to get the reader to feel the isolation of the prairie?
> How do you think the woman feels about those experiences as she tells them to her granddaughter?

Dogteam

by Gary Paulsen and Ruth Wright Paulsen
New York: Delacorte Press, 1993

Suggested Grade and Interest Level: 6 through 12

Topic Exploration: Animals, dogs; Careers

Skill Builders:
    Vocabulary   **Language literacy**
    Attributes   Verbal expression
    Similes and metaphors   **Articulation, *S* and *R***

Synopsis: Three-time Newbery winner Gary Paulson, who twice ran the Iditarod across Alaska, portrays the excitement and danger of dog racing at night. The repetition and rhythm of this prose poem give the reader a sense of what it is these dogs love to do.

Method: Before the read-aloud, set the stage by asking students what they know about dog racing in Alaska. Elicit background knowledge about the Iditarod. If necessary, explain that dogs prepare and train all year for the Iditarod.

After the read-aloud, brainstorm words that describe dogsled racing at night. How do the students imagine the dogs experience the event? How would they experience it?

Discuss the author's use of similes and metaphors, such as

". . . small songs of excitement when the harnesses are put on . . ."
"Straining to join the snow and the moon and the night . . ."
"Frozen and flat and white as the moonlight we slip out of the woods."

For articulation, students can repeat the words of the text and respond to questions that elicit target phonemes.

Extended Activity: From the list of words that describe dogsled racing, have students write prose poems. Encourage them to use repetition and rhythm and to use a phrase for a topic heading, as the authors did. Have them include a metaphor and simile in each poem.

The Gentleman and the Kitchen Maid

by Diane Stanley
New York: Dial Books for Young Readers, 1994

Suggested Grade and Interest Level: 6 through 12

Topic Explorations: Art, artists, and architecture; Museums

Skill Builders:

Vocabulary	**Language literacy**
Semantics	Problem solving
Similes and metaphors	Drawing inferences
Grammar and syntax	Discussion
Advanced syntactic structures	**Pragmatic language**

Synopsis: A young woman named Rusty, an art student, goes to a famous museum "lugging an easel, a canvas, and a paint box." She intends to copy the works of great masters to learn the artists' techniques. She is captivated most by certain paintings that hang in Room 12. One is called *The Kitchen Maid*, painted by a Dutch master (Vermeer), which is of a young servant girl with a basket of fruit in her arm. She appears to be looking at a gentleman in another painting titled *Portrait of a Young Gentleman.* He appears to be returning the gaze of the kitchen maid. As the story continues, they fall in love and all the characters in the paintings of Room 12 begin talking about their attraction to each other. Rusty observes this too, as she paints the gentleman. But when she returns the next day to finish her work, the painting of kitchen maid had been moved. The gentleman looks sad to her, so Rusty devises a way to reunite the two in a painting of her own.

Method: Before the read-aloud, elicit background knowledge about museums and great painters (Picasso and Monet are some names from the text). Encourage students to share their experiences of viewing paintings at museums. Talk about the meaning of "Dutch master" as it relates to a great painter. Suggestions for questions to encourage discussion and enhance understanding of the concept of a museum include the following:

Where do the paintings come from?
Can a viewer buy one?
How does a museum get money to buy paintings?

What other ways do museums have of obtaining art?
What is the purpose of a museum?
Do the works of art always stay in one position in the museum or do they move from their locations?
If they move, why do they move and where do they go?

Talk about exhibitions and paintings on loan from other museums. Brainstorm the names of several famous artists. Talk about students of art and how art classes often meet in museums to draw, sketch, and paint the great works of art.

Also talk about the sensitive natures of artists. What does it mean when an artist sees her subject through "new eyes" and with a "unique perspective"?

Preview the following vocabulary words:

museum	lugging	critics
object (the object of criticism)	contentment	
criticism	rendered	

Read the short text, pausing to ask students to infer meaning. Some examples include the following:

Why would the stern man believe it was the servant girl's fault for looking over her shoulder?
What does the gentleman in the painting mean when he responds to the stern man in black in another painting that "She obviously has an eye for quality."
What did the duchess mean when she said that Rusty's painting was a "pretty good likeness" and that it was "better than the last one."
When the painting of the kitchen maid was removed from Room 12, what did the duchess in the painting mean when she glanced pointedly at the gentleman and said, "And that . . . is an end to that!"

After the read-aloud, talk about the problem in the story. What happened because the museum director moved the painting of the kitchen maid? How did Rusty solve the problem? What was the outcome?

Discuss the use of the simile "The artist . . . had painted him as if he had just stepped out from a shadow." What image does this convey? Discuss the use of the metaphor "trapped in their different worlds, frozen in time." What does this mean?

Ask students to create dependent clauses by finishing these sentences:

The kitchen maid that the gentleman was gazing at _____ (was moved from Room 12).
The gentleman that Rusty was painting _____ (gazed longingly at the kitchen maid).
The art student went to the museum where _____ (she copied a famous painting).

Have students create the first part of the sentence for others to fill in. Examples:

The kitchen maid that _____ was _____.
The gentleman that _____ was _____.
The art student that _____ was _____.
The art student _____ (what did she do?) _____ (where did she do it?).

For pragmatic language, talk about the way the characters in the paintings responded to the romance taking place in Room 12. Contrast their style and manner of speech with Rusty's style. What did each of them say? When Rusty said, "She *is* lovely. Just perfect for you!" what effect might that have had on the gentleman and the kitchen maid? How does it feel when other people validate your feelings? Why is this often a good thing to do with your peers? With what other feelings and in what other circumstances can validation be used as an effective way to communicate?

George Washington's Cows

by David Small
New York: Farrar, Straus & Giroux, 1994; Sunburst, 1997

Suggested Grade and Interest Level: 6 through 8

Topic Explorations: Famous people; History, American; Holidays, Presidents' Day

Skill Builders:

Vocabulary	**Grammar and syntax**	**Language literacy**
Semantics	Past tense	Compare and contrast
Adjectives	Advanced syntactic structures	
Adverbs		
Morphological units		

Synopsis: At George Washington's home of Mt. Vernon, it is the animals that take the upper hand. Dressed in historical garb, the anthropomorphic cows, hogs, and sheep provide the hilarity. The pampered cows will not give milk until they have been moved into the finest quarters of the house, outfitted in lavender gowns, sprayed with expensive cologne, and bedded on cushions of silk! The hogs, "on the other hand / Were a genteel and amiable group / Delighted to help with the household chores / If a servant had fever or croup." But it is the sheep, the scholars, who top it off with their academic lesson to the ladies and gentlemen of the day. The zany text, marvelous watercolors depicting the expressions and gestures of the characters, the impeccable details of the site, and George's response to it all make this book one of the most entertaining read-alouds on anyone's library shelf.

Method: For older students, present the book by explaining that it is a children's book that is created to offer enjoyment and entertainment to people of all ages. It also offers historical accuracy of Mt. Vernon, the customs and dress of the day, and some sophisticated vocabulary words to learn. It is an ideal February activity to accompany a Presidents' Day theme. The following vocabulary words are presented in the text:

scones	obsequious (tones)	genteel
amiable	croup	impeccably (dressed)
scholar	impressive	degrees
ferried	muttered	despair

Before the read-aloud, help students gain an understanding of colonial life by presenting historically accurate photographs of Mt. Vernon and George Washington. Gather students' background knowledge as you talk about the times, style of living, dress, manners, and occupations during the colonial days.

Read the book, pausing to point out a feature or two when appropriate. After the read-aloud, build a lesson around the vocabulary. For example, using the word *obsequious,* first define the word, explaining that if someone acts obsequiously, the person is acting as if he or she was inferior to another. Have students act out the word, saying, "Yes, whatever you say," fawning over a peer, and saying, "Oh, you are so _____ [a word students will relate to]. If only I were as good as you!" (Be sure to reverse the roles.) Use the word in a sentence. Talk about what it means within the context of the story. Ask questions such as

> Why is it funny that the servants at Mt. Vernon had to speak in obsequious tones to the cows?
> How might someone speak to a cow in an obsequious tone?
> What might the servants of Mt. Vernon be saying in their obsequious ways?

Increase grammar and syntax skills by developing a lesson around the words of the story.

For example, use the word *obsequious* as an adjective to describe the servants and to create the beginning of a past-tense sentence for the students to fill in. For example, say,

"The obsequious servants _____ " and ask the students to finish the thought by referring to the illustrations. Suggestions include

    _____ begged the cows (to give milk).
    _____ sprayed the cows (with perfume).
    _____ made the cows clothes (such as lavender gowns).
    _____ dressed the cows (in lavender gowns).
    _____ made the cows' beds (and fluffed up their pillows).

Have the students begin and end a few sentences on their own.

To teach adverbs, change the adjective *obsequious* by adding the *–ly* suffix. This time, *obsequious* will describe how the servants attended to the cows.

    The servants _____.

Suggestions include

    obsequiously attended the cows.
    obsequiously begged the cows to give milk.
    obsequiously made the cows' beds.

Note: Use the vocabulary word *impeccably* to illustrate an adverb here as well. *How* were the pigs dressed? *Impeccably*!

Show students how to create sentences in more complex syntactical forms. First, create a verb phrase or adverbial phrase. For example, ask *when* the servants attended the cows. Suggestions include

    when working at Mt. Vernon
    every morning

Turn these words into phrases with which students can begin a sentence. For example, state the adverbial phrase:

    When working at Mr. Vernon, _____.

Students can complete the thought using the previous sentences:

    When working at Mt. Vernon, the servants obsequiously attended the cows.
    Every morning, the servants obsequiously begged the cows to give their milk.

Use the four-part method of creating embedded sentences:

1. Begin with a basic sentence.

    Create: The servants begged the cows.

2. Ask a *how* (*when, why, where*) question to expand the sentence.

    Question: How did the servants beg the cows?

    Answer: *In far too obsequious tones*

3. Pick a modifier and add it to the subject.

> The *humble* servants

4. Show how to combine the elements using the modifier, inserting the expander into the basic sentence, and finishing with the remainder of the basic sentence.

Resulting sentence:

> The *humble* servants, in *far too obsequious tones,* begged the cows (to give milk).

Some variations:

> The servants, feeding the cows scones, begged them every hour.
> The servants, spraying the cows with expensive colognes, begged them in obsequious tones.

Compare and contrast George Washington's cows to his hogs. How were his cows and hogs alike? Suggestions include

> They both dressed up in fine clothes.
> They both acted like people.
> They both took control of his house.

What was different in the behavior of the cows and hogs? Suggestions include

> The cows had a bad attitude, but the hogs were pleasant.
> The cows did not work, but the hogs worked hard and enjoyed it.
> The cows did not socialize or communicate with anyone, but the pigs liked hosting parties.

The Gettysburg Address

by Abraham Lincoln
Illustrated by Michael McCurdy, foreword by Garry Wills
New York: Houghton Mifflin, 1995

Suggested Grade and Interest Level: 6 through 12

Topic Explorations: History, American; Holidays, Presidents' Day

Skills Builders

Vocabulary	**Grammar and syntax**	**Language literacy**
Semantics	Advanced syntactic structures	Drawing inferences
Similes and metaphors		

Synopsis: It is what lies within the art of Michael McCurdy's black-and-white line drawings in this book that illuminates the famous words of Abraham Lincoln. Nothing more than a few eloquent lines of the address, each coupled with powerful illustrations, is contained within the 32 oversized pages, making this a picture book suitable for individuals of all ages. And similarly, as scholars and historians note, it is the poetic imagery and rhythms of the English language that very likely have made the Gettysburg Address the most cherished document in American history. The delivery of the famous address of 1863 is illustrated in richly detailed scratchboard illustrations that impart a sense of the Civil War era. Lincoln's words are carefully arranged to accompany the illustrations, which makes them easier to comprehend and gives the viewer a sense of what the audience must have imagined when these famous words were first spoken.

Method: During the read-aloud, without interrupting the text, let the powerful words and images sink in for the listener to reflect upon. After the read-aloud, go back over each page to put into words what each of the artist's messages imparts. Vocabulary words include the following:

conceived	endure	brought forth
proposition	resting place	fitting
consecrate	dedicated	hallow
nobly	advanced	devotion

For students with language learning disabilities, advanced syntactic structures may be difficult to comprehend, thereby diminishing the meaning of the message. Jointly look at each of the more difficult structures in this address (and the accompanying illustration) to perform an analysis that can make the message clear. For example,

"It is for us the living, rather, to be dedicated here to the unfinished work which they who fought / here have thus far so nobly advanced."

Clarify pronouns such as *us* and *they,* define terms such as *unfinished work* and *nobly advanced,* and have students rephrase sentences in their own words, such as

The soldiers who died at Gettysburg were noble. They helped in trying to win the war so that all men (and women) in this country could be free. But Abraham Lincoln is talking to those who are living and dedicating the moment to them because it is the living who must continue to finish the work that the soldiers died for. The war was not yet won and freedom was not yet gained for everyone.

Help students infer what is meant by words in the address such as *unfinished work.* Discuss that the Battle of Gettysburg was not a decisive enough battle to conclude the North's victory. But the battle was a symbol of victory for democracy, and the speech was the metaphor that made it so. What is the work Abraham Lincoln referred to? What did Abraham Lincoln want the different members of the audience to do?

Continue to assist students with inferencing skills by addressing what the illustrator wanted to show in his drawings. Read the foreword by the illustrator. Ask what kind of meaning the illustrations in the book might have had for him.

Grandfather's Journey

by Allen Say
Boston: Houghton Mifflin, 1993

Suggested Grade and Interest Level: 6 through 9

Topic Explorations: Culture and history, Japanese; Family relationships; Journeys; Memory and remembering

Skill Builders:
   Vocabulary
   Attributes
   Language literacy   Drawing inferences
   Relating personal experiences   Problem solving   Point of view
   Cause-and-effect relationships   Compare and contrast   Discussion

Synopsis: A Japanese American man recounts his grandfather's journey to America, a journey that he retraces later. The 1994 Caldecott award–winning illustrations are highly evocative of America and Japan of the past—from the railways to the riverboats, storefronts of American towns, and rubble of war-torn Japan. The scenic landscapes splendidly contrast the two cultures and underscore the men's dual heritage as well as their love of two cultures.

Method: Before the read-aloud, ask students what they know about the word *journey.* In what ways do people travel, and why do people like to travel? Discuss ways two countries can be different and how both may have many good and beautiful things about them. Look at the cover and discuss the title of the story, asking questions such as

> What does the young man's dress imply?
> How old would you guess him to be?
> Where does he appear to be?
> What does the title mean?
> Based on this information, what do you think the story will be about?

To teach likenesses and differences, pause during the read-aloud to compare and contrast the two cultures. For example, on one page, the young man is shown in Japanese dress, whereas on the opposite page he is shown in European dress. Discuss how both men were torn between their love of two countries.

> What did the grandfather like about America when he was in Japan and missed America?
> What did the grandfather like about Japan when he was in America and missed Japan?
> What would you do if you were the grandfather in the story?
> How are Japan and America alike?
> How are Japan and America different?

To help students draw inferences, pause to elucidate the meanings implied by the words in the story. When he was in America, why did the grandfather surround himself with songbirds? What was their importance? When the grandfather was in Japan, why did he raise warblers and silvereyes? When he grew older, why didn't the grandfather keep songbirds anymore?

To teach students about relating personal experiences, ask if they ever have been anywhere where they felt homesick.

> What did they miss?
> How did they feel?
> What did they do?
> How was the experience like the grandfather's in the story?
> How was it like the grandson's experience?

To teach problem solving, ask what facts the students can state about the problem in the story. How did the grandfather attempt to solve the problem? Can they think of other solutions that might have helped the grandfather overcome the feeling of being torn between two countries?

To work on identifying cause-and-effect relationships, ask what happened because of the grandfather's internal conflict? What effect did it have on his daughter? What effect did it have on his grandson?

To work on attributes, elicit words to describe the grandfather. What words can be used to describe the grandson?

To teach students about point of view, ask from whose point of view the story is being told. How do the students think the grandson knew so much about his grandfather's journey? How do you suppose he came to learn about it?

Extended Activity: Encourage students to interview their family members about their heritages. Did the students' grandparents come from another state? Another city? Another country? What about their great-grandparents? Have each student put together a journal of his or her family history. Encourage students to share their journals and their backgrounds in oral presentations to the class.

The Great Kapok Tree: A Tale of the Amazon River Forest

by Lynne Cherry
San Diego, CA: Voyager Books, 1991, 2000

Suggested Grade and Interest Level: 6 through 9

Topic Exploration: Animals, jungle; Conservation

Skill Builders:

Vocabulary	Grammar and syntax	Language literacy
Semantics	Future tense	Cause-and-effect relationships
Morphological units	Advanced syntactic structures	Problem solving

GRADES 6–12

Synopsis: The various animals that live in a Kapok tree of the Brazilian rain forest try to convince a sleeping man, whose plan is to chop down the tree, the importance of not taking away their home. When the man, young and handsome, falls asleep in the midst of the beautiful lush colors of the Amazon, a monkey first comes to whisper in his ear. He says that if he chops down the tree, the roots "will wither and die and there will be nothing left to hold the earth in place." Next, a toucan, a macaw, and a cock-of-the-rock, a dramatic-looking bird, tell him they have flown over the forest and have seen what happens when trees are chopped down. "Life and beauty disappear into ruins." Other forest creatures continue to speak to the man's subconscious until he finally awakes. His conscience then speaks to him, as it speaks to us all, and he takes his axe and leaves the forest.

Method: Before the read-aloud, discuss the important social and environmental issue of deforestation, and talk about something of an ecological nature in current world events. Introduce the setting of the story by showing the Amazon River and environs on an atlas and in additional literature selections.

Introduce the word *deforestation*. Talk about its root word and the prefix *de-*, meaning "removal and separation," and the suffix *–ation*, a combination of *ate* and *ion*, that turns the word *deforest* into a noun, as in the act of deforestation. Talk about other words with the same suffixes, such as separation, maturation, and computation.

During the read-aloud, briefly pause to clarify meaning and point out features of interest.

After the read-aloud, talk about the message in the story. What is the author saying to us about life on the planet?

To help students with advanced syntactic structures, create sentences using future tense and the auxiliary form of the verb, such as

> If people continue to chop down trees, there will be no more natural habitats for animals.
> The effect of deforestation would be that animals would have nowhere to live.
> The effect of deforestation would be that animals would be forced into places that are already overcrowded.

To teach about expressing cause-and-effect relationships, ask students to tell about the effects of deforestation, as reported by the tropical birds from their flights over the jungle. Help structure the use of words such as *if, then, because, the reason, since,* and *the consequence* in students' responses. Scaffold structures as necessary, withdrawing assistance as students achieve production on their own.

> If humans continue to cut down trees, the effect will be that . . .
> If the man in the story cuts down the tree and more humans were to cut down trees in the rain forests, then . . .
> The reason the animals did not want the man to chop down the tree was because . . .

To teach problem solving, ask students to define the problem in the story and state the solution or solutions. Start sentences off with words such as

> The problem in the story is that . . .
> The way to solve the problem is . . .

Follow up with a discussion on what each person on the planet can do to preserve and be cognizant of our natural habitats and natural resources.

Note: This book also is available in a Spanish translation, titled *El gran capoquero.*

The Great Wall of China

by Leonard Everett Fisher
New York: Macmillan, 1986

Suggested Grade and Interest Level: 6 through 9

Topic Explorations: Culture and history, Chinese; Long ago and far away

Skill Builders:

Vocabulary	**Language literacy**
Attributes	Storytelling
	Problem solving
	Discussion

Synopsis: As the title suggests, this book tells the story and history of the Great Wall of China. Built 2,200 years ago to keep out the Mongol invaders, the wall took 10 years to complete. The brief text and majestically rendered black-and-white illustrations make this an ideal book for small-group instruction and a time-effective stimulus for conversation on the curriculum-based topic of ancient China.

Method: For storytelling instruction, this is a good book to show that truth can be stranger than fiction. Teach the elements of storytelling by asking scaffolding questions. Have students describe who the story is about, where it takes place, what happened to start the story, how the characters responded (what plan was devised), how the plan was completed (actions), and consequences of the actions.

For attributes, talk about Ch'in Shih Huang Ti as a colorful person, both good and bad, from ancient history. List his qualities and attributes. What actions support these attributes?

Extended Activities: To teach problem solving, have students divide into groups and discuss how the emperor went about protecting his people and land. First, state the problem (all aspects in their entirety). Then state the emperor's solution.

What other ways were there to solve the problem? Which one would have been the best and why? Would the results have been the same? After the small-group discussions, have the groups present their solutions to the class or larger group and share their thoughts and ideas.

Also make a class or group story map for each of the story elements. Assign one student or one group to each part. When the story maps are completed, draw a line connecting the pictures. Be sure to illustrate the details, such as what the people looked like and wore, what building tools and materials they used, the terrain of the country, the manner in which they were forced to work, and the extent of the wall upon completion. (Be sure to tell students that this wall is so long and so well defined it can be seen by astronauts in space.) Have the students or groups orally present their parts of the story and the supporting details.

Harriet and the Promised Land

by Jacob Lawrence
New York: Simon & Schuster, 1968, 1993

Suggested Grade and Interest Level: 6 through 12

Topic Explorations: Art, artists, and architecture; Creativity; Culture and history, African and African American; History, American; Journeys

Skill Builders:

Vocabulary	Grammar and syntax	Language literacy
Semantics	Past tense	Drawing inferences
Attributes	Advanced syntactic structures	Answering *why* questions
		Discussion

Synopsis: A celebrated American artist whose work has hung in museums around the world painted the illustrations in this book. Accompanying them are short verses that tell the story of Harriet Tubman, the slave who led people to freedom.

Method: This is an excellent book to use in conjunction with a classroom history lesson on the Civil War. Before the read-aloud, discuss the meaning of the word *underground.*

On each page, pause to reflect on the symbolism the artist uses to convey his message. For example, look at Harriet scrubbing the floor. Why did the artist exaggerate the floor and her hand over the rag? Why is her head down and her face hiding from view? Point out that the extraordinary nature of the book is that the illustrations are a series of paintings by a great American artist known for painting in series of works. Talk about an artist's perspective and the qualities that distinguish great art. Talk about how artists can often tell a story with pictures rather than words and create feelings in people that can help them understand the complexities of a situation.

To teach advanced syntactic structures, have students create sentences based on the phrases of the verses. For instance, when the young Harriet holds the infant in her arms, use the verse and painting to form sentences such as

> Harriet had to sweep.
> Harriet had to rock her master's baby to sleep.
> Harriet had to sweep and rock her master's baby to sleep.
> Although Harriet was a child, she had to sweep and rock her master's baby to sleep.
> When Harriet was a child, she had to sweep and take care of her master's baby.
> The child, Harriet, whose jobs were to sweep and rock her master's baby to sleep, was never allowed a childhood of her own.
> Harriet led her people to freedom.
> Harriet led her people through an underground escape route to freedom.
> Harriet led her people out of the South, and they eventually found freedom.
> Harriet led her people out of the South through an underground escape route, where they eventually found freedom.

Extended Activity: Brainstorm attributes to describe Harriet Tubman. Suggestions include *brave, inspired, intelligent, focused,* and *determined.* Have students give examples to justify why they selected each word. (For example, Harriet was inspired because she was aroused by great faith to lead people to freedom.) Ask students what else they want to know about Tubman's experiences as a child or as an adult.

Break into learning groups. Have students put together a list of questions they would ask if they could interview Harriet Tubman. (Read also *Aunt Harriet's Underground Railroad in the Sky,* listed in the Grades 1 through 5 catalog, and other background information.) Allow students time to research their questions in the library.

Each group can select a student to play the role of Harriet Tubman. Then go back in time and have Ms. Tubman answer the students' questions based on knowledge gained in other readings and awareness of the conditions at the time. Ask groups to present their interviews to the class.

Home Run

by Robert Burleigh
San Diego, CA: Silver Whistle, Harcourt Brace, 1998

Suggested Grade and Interest Level: 6 through 9

Topic Explorations: Baseball; Famous people, Heroes

Skill Builders:

Vocabulary	Grammar and syntax	Language literacy
Semantics	Advanced syntactic structures	Drawing inferences
Similes and metaphors		Retelling events
		Discussion

Synopsis: This is a poetic account of one of the world's greatest sports figures, the legendary Babe Ruth. The verses use imagery and figurative language to describe how the mighty player prepared to hit a home run. Superimposed on each page is a vintage-style baseball card with a short story included on it. Interesting facts are presented, not only about his hitting but about his excellent pitching record and his legendary breakfasts, which "might include a dozen eggs and half a loaf of toast."

Method: Before the read-aloud, elicit background information on the game of baseball and Babe Ruth. Provide meaning and establish connections to the story through personal experiences and knowledge of such players as Barry Bonds and Mark McGwire.

During the read-aloud, pause briefly to define a word, leaving interaction to a minimum so listeners gain a sense of the language used in the poetic text. Point out the use of metaphors, such as in the first line of the following verse:

> "The ball cracks off the bat.
> It soars far up in the air
> As it passes first base.
> Going, going."

Point out the "sound" reference in the use of the word *cracks*. Help students hear and visualize the scene. Establish the emotional connection of the game with the player.

Do a picture walk-through and pause to read the information on the baseball cards. Ask comprehension questions and discuss facts such as how the baseball great came to be called Babe. After a discussion, use the facts to encourage students to rephrase and retell the events.

To develop inferencing skills, reread the text to discuss the following verse:

> "The fans crane their necks to follow
> But Babe already knows.
> The perfectness.
> The feeling.
> The boy-fire inside the body of a man."

Ask students to think about what the author is saying and how he chooses words to express what Babe feels as he hits the ball. Draw inferences about what Babe already knows. How does Babe know he will hit a home run? Provide meaning through personal connections. Talk about what the author is referring to when he uses the word *perfectness*.

To work on morphological units and metalinguistic awareness, talk about the syllables in the word *perfectness*. Identify the root word and the suffix. Ask or demonstrate how many words can be generated from the word *perfect* (e.g., *perfectly, perfected, perfectedly, perfecter, imperfect, imperfectable,* and *imperfection*). Talk about the word's relationship with other words such as *complete* and *unique*. Generate lists of words that can be combined with the suffix *-ness* (e.g., *like, sad, happy, quiet, loud, neat, crooked, tart,* and so on). Use the word in combination with a unit on U.S. government while discussing the U.S. Constitution's words, "In order to form a more perfect union."

Discuss the similes used in other lines of text and draw inferences:

"Then it is as it should be"
"Smooth as silk"
"Easy as air on the face"
"Right as falling water"

Encourage students to use the similes to generate their own sentences as they work on advanced syntactic structures. Assist students by starting sentences with an adverbial phrase. Have students finish the sentence with a simile, such as

When Babe Ruth hit the ball with the bat, it was as smooth as silk.
When Babe Ruth hit a home run, it felt as right as falling water.
When Babe Ruth felt the ball hit the bat, it was as easy as air on the face.

Support sentence constructions with scaffolding and gradually withdraw as students' mastery increases.

How the Stars Fell Into the Sky: A Navajo Legend

by Jerrie Oughton
Boston: Houghton Mifflin, 1992

Suggested Grade and Interest Level: 6 through 12

Topic Explorations: Culture and history, Native American; Folklore, Native American

Skill Builders:

Vocabulary	Grammar and syntax	Language literacy
Higher-level concepts	Advanced syntactic structures	Storytelling
		Drawing inferences

Synopsis: A retelling of a Navajo creation legend tells how First Woman uses her "jewels" to write the laws in the sky for her people to see. Using stars from the blanket at her feet, she records the laws by "placing her jewels across the dome of night" in a careful pattern. However, she is observed by Coyote, and of course the ever trickster of Navajo lore comes to offer his help. He spoils her careful and noble efforts when he impatiently picks up the blanket and hurls the stars at the sky in "wild disarray, shattering First Woman's careful patterns" and leaving the world forever in confusion about exactly what the laws may be. The text is in a beautifully simple, lyrical verse. Because of the message, the Navajo folklore, the adult characters (First Man and First Woman), and the style of paintings that capture the mysteries of the night sky with jewel-like images, the book is suitable for preadolescents and adolescents.

Before the read-aloud, elicit background knowledge about Navajo folklore. Talk about the character of Coyote and his role in Navajo legends. Discuss the concept of confusion and its opposite, harmony. Survey the text and pick out words, images, and concepts that may be important to preview for better understanding. Also talk about the uses of folklore and its origins.

During the read-aloud, pause briefly to clarify meaning, but for the most part, let the lyrical verse and the illustrations help to focus the students' attention on the story.

After the read-aloud, begin by talking about the story elements. Who was the story about? What did First Woman want to do?

Ask factual questions, such as

Why didn't she write the laws on the sun, as First Man suggested?
Why didn't she write the laws on the water as he also suggested?

Help students draw inferences to answer why First Woman wanted to write down laws. What did the laws and First Woman's stars symbolize?

Talk about order and making lists to get things done. Talk about school rules to follow that help the school run better. Talk about traffic laws that enable people to drive in a manner like everyone else in order to prevent confusion on the road. Continue with questions such as

What attribute did First Woman possess that Coyote did not?
Why did Coyote randomly fling the stars?
What was the result?
What did Coyote destroy?
What is the story saying about the dream of universal harmony?

Iktomi and the Boulder

Retold by Paul Goble
New York: Orchard Books, 1988

Suggested Grade and Interest Level:	6 through 12
Topic Explorations:	Folklore, Native American; Humor; Trickster tales

Skill Builders:

Language literacy	**Articulation**
Verbal expression	Carryover for any sound
Drawing inferences	
Point of view	

Synopsis: The Indian trickster, Iktomi, incurs the wrath of a huge boulder when he takes away the gift he gave to it. The boulder pins him down by rolling onto his legs, and all the animals that try to help cannot push it off. When the bats appear, Iktomi enrages them by telling them that the boulder "has been saying rude things" about them. The bats attack the boulder and break it into little chips of rock. The legend says that is why bats have flattened faces and why there are rocks scattered all over the Great Plains.

Method: Iktomi stories are excellent for interaction because they are strongly rooted in the oral tradition from which the stories came. Where the text changes to italics, students are invited to comment on Iktomi's words, thoughts, and deeds. The small text that represents Iktomi's thoughts can be read by a student, especially one who is practicing carryover of articulation skills.

Ask students to draw inferences about what kind of man Iktomi is based on his thoughts (e.g., "I'm looking my very best today" and "I'll look great at the dance tonight"). Also have them draw inferences about what Iktomi really means when he tells the bats that the boulder has been saying rude things about them.

Discuss from whose point of view the story is told. Does the point of view change? What makes the students think so?

Note: Be sure to read and enjoy *Iktomi and the Berries, Iktomi and the Buffalo Skull,* and other Iktomi stories by the same author.

Joyful Noise: Poems for Two Voices

by Paul Fleischman
New York: Harper & Row, 1988

GRADES 6–12

Suggested Grade and Interest Level: 6 through 12

Topic Exploration: Insects and spiders

Skill Builders:

Vocabulary	**Language literacy**	**Fluency**
Semantics	Drawing inferences	**Voice**
Similes and metaphors	**Articulation**	
Grammar and syntax	Carryover for any sound	
Advanced syntactic structures		

Synopsis: Members of the insect world and their characteristics and activities are set to verse for two voices to read aloud. (Different words are spoken by each speaker simultaneously.) The resulting harmony of sounds is a remarkable vocal event. This book is unique and highly deserving of its Newbery Award status.

Method: For average to above-average readers, this can be a fun read-aloud activity. For low-average readers, the activity also is doable; however, it is advisable to spend time rehearsing the proper names in the text. The idea is to read slowly, which will give some students an advantage.

Before the read-aloud, review some of the vocabulary in the poem to make the reading easier and more meaningful.

After the read-aloud, have students create their own embedded sentences based on the short phrases and sentences in the book. For example, the poem "Book Lice" reads

> "I was born in a fine old edition of Schiller
> While I started life in a private eye thriller . . ."
> "Later I lodged in Scott's works - volume 50
> While I passed my youth in an Agatha Christie."

Use the words of the text to construct progressively more complex sentences, as in

> Book lice live in dusty bookshelves.
> Book lice may spend many days in an old novel.
> Book lice, because they live in dusty bookshelves, may spend many days in an old, forgotten novel.
> Because book lice live in dusty bookshelves, they may spend many days in an old, forgotten novel.

For fluency, have a student read one column of text while you read the other. The duet-like verse provides excellent practice for speaking in rhythm because each speaker must maintain a separate rhythm that is out of sync with the other speaker.

For voice, compare and contrast vocal qualities while reading simultaneously, or have the student try to match the pitch or vocal quality of the other reader.

The King Who Rained

by Fred Gwynne
New York: Simon & Schuster Books for Young Readers, 1970

Suggested Grade and Interest Level: 6 through 12

Skill Builders:
    Vocabulary
    Idioms
    Homonyms (multiple meanings)

Synopsis: A child pictures the things she hears adults talk about, such as a king who rained, bear feet, and having a frog in one's throat.

Method: Before the read-aloud, talk about idioms and expressions of speech and how they sometimes are easy to misunderstand and get confused if one has not heard them. This may be true especially when heard from a child's perspective or when one is learning a new language. Explain that although this may be a children's picture book, it explains to everyone, adults included, how bewildering language can be when the message is not understood by the listener.

Read the book and pause to discuss each of the homonyms. Define all meanings for words such as *bill*, *train*, and *present*. Also discuss the idiom presented, "Sometimes mommy says she has a frog in her throat" and its meaning.

Note: Also read *The Sixteen Hand Horse* and *A Little Pigeon Toad* by the same author.

Learning About Courage from the Life of Christopher Reeve

by Jane Kelly Kosek
New York: Rosen, 1999

Suggested Grade and Interest Level: 6 through 12

Topic Exploration: Famous people, Heroes

Skill Builders:

Vocabulary	**Language literacy**
Semantics	Compare and contrast
Higher-level concepts	Retelling events
Attributes	Discussion

Synopsis: The famous actor, best known for his role in the movie *Superman,* is presented from the perspective of his courage in the face of his paralyzing accident and subsequent rehabilitation. One of many in a series highlighting famous people, this small book's photographs show Christopher Reeve during various times of his career and enjoying his favorite pastime of horseback riding, which on one occasion resulted in a tragic fall. There are also pictures that depict his rehabilitation and what he has done with his life in spite of his paralysis. The text of the book is mainly written for early readers. It can easily be adapted as a read-aloud and viewed for its photographs of this remarkable individual.

Method: Before the read-aloud, talk about the concept of courage. Give examples of people, such as firefighters, police officers, and rescue workers. Talk about the acts that they perform. Then ask students to think about the concept of courage in relation to themselves and to their peers.

During the read-aloud, pause to clarify meanings of words. Vocabulary presented includes the following:

paralyzed	challenging
rehabilitation	justice

A glossary at the back of the book gives the definitions. When pausing to talk, relate the vocabulary words to Christopher Reeve and then to the students' own lives.

After the read-aloud, talk about Christopher Reeve having to live each day with not being able to move his body or even breathe on his own. Then talk about the concept of courage. Ask what courage means in the life of Christopher Reeve. Ask students to give examples of how he demonstrates courage. Other suggested questions include the following:

What are the feelings he must overcome? (fear, anger, depression)
How does he overcome them?
What other attributes can be brainstormed about Christopher Reeve?
What does he do with his life despite his condition? (still acts, directs, gives speeches)
What other people, famous or not, have shown courage in the face of debilitating circumstances?

Also talk about his most famous role in the movie *Superman.* How does this hero figure compare with the real life of Christopher Reeve? Compare and contrast the life of a fictitious superhero with that of a real person.

Encourage students to select one event from Christopher Reeve's life to retell, such as what happened on the day of his accident, and so on.

Note: Other books in this series include *Learning About Creativity from the Life of Steven Spielberg, Learning About Assertiveness from Oprah Winfrey, Learning About Justice from the Life of Cesar Chavez, Learning About Responsibility from the Life of Colin Powell,* and *Learning About Strength of Character from Mohammad Ali.*

Learning About Determination from the Life of Gloria Estefan

by Jeanne Strazzabosco
New York: Rosen, 1996

Suggested Grade and Interest Level: 6 through 12

Topic Exploration: Famous people, Heroes

Skill Builders:

Vocabulary	**Language literacy**
Semantics	Retelling events
Higher-level concepts	Discussion
Attributes	

Synopsis: Gloria Estefan, the famous entertainer and daughter of a Cuban soldier who escaped Fidel Castro's regime, is highlighted in this small but powerful book that looks at the concept of determination. One of many in a series, it contains large text for early readers, but the photographs and presentation of this matter are meant for older children and adolescents. A brief history of her life and how her determination helped her succeed in hard times is given. It includes her years growing up poor in Miami, knowing her father was imprisoned in Cuba, and helping her mom while she was in school. During this time, she received an award for her progress learning English after only 6 months and subsequently attained a scholarship. Her determination to overcome an injury as a result of an accident also is featured. Included is information about her career as a singer, songwriter, recording artist, and performer.

Method: Before the read-aloud, talk about the concept of determination. Give students some examples that show determination on the part of individuals and ask them to give examples from their own lives or from the life of someone they know. Then ask them to keep the concept in mind as you read the text.

During the read-aloud, pause to clarify meanings of words. Vocabulary presented includes the following:

determination	scholarship
excel	chemical

A glossary at the back of the book gives the definitions. When pausing to talk, encourage the students to use the words as they relate to Gloria Estefan and to others who demonstrate similar character traits.

After the read-aloud, talk about Gloria Estefan and what has made her successful. Recall the details of her life from the story. Why do the students believe Gloria was able to overcome these obstacles?

Other suggested questions include the following:

What are some of the feelings she may have experienced coming to America and having to learn English? How does it appear she overcame them?
What are some of her other attributes besides determination?
What has she done with her life despite her unfortunate early experiences?
What other people, famous or otherwise, have shown determination in their lives?

Encourage students to select one aspect of the story and have them each retell one event, such as what her life was like when she was in school, how her accident happened, and so on.

Note: Other books in this series include *Learning About Creativity from the Life of Steven Spielberg, Learning About Assertiveness from Oprah Winfrey, Learning About Justice from the Life of Cesar Chavez, Learning About Responsibility from the Life of Colin Powell,* and *Learning About Strength of Character from Mohammad Ali.*

Learning About Forgiveness from the Life of Nelson Mandela

by Jeanne Strazzabosco
New York: Rosen, 1996

Suggested Grade and Interest Level: 6 through 12

Skill Builders:

Vocabulary	Language literacy
Semantics	Retelling events
Higher-level concepts	Discussion
Attributes	

Synopsis: Nelson Rolihlahla Mandela, the champion of equal rights for Blacks in South Africa, is highlighted in this small but powerful book that looks at the concept of forgiveness. One of many in a series, it contains large text for early readers, but the photographs and presentation of this matter are meant for older children and adolescents. The text is ideal for a read-aloud. It gives a brief history of Mandela's life and his aspirations to do something about apartheid. The book tells how he become a lawyer and about his arrest for sabotage and treason. After 27 years of imprisonment for opposing apartheid, Nelson (whose middle name means "to stir up trouble") was released, apartheid ended, and in 1993 he was awarded the Nobel Peace Prize. He became known worldwide as a symbol of change and forgiveness.

Method: Before the read-aloud, talk about the concept of forgiveness. Give students some examples and ask them to give examples of their own. Then ask them to keep the concept in mind as you read the story.

During the read-aloud, pause to clarify meanings of words. Vocabulary presented includes the following:

apartheid	ban
sabotage	treason

A glossary at the back of the book gives the definitions. When pausing for talk, encourage the students to use the words as they relate to Nelson Mandela and to conditions and situations in South Africa.

After the read-aloud, talk about Nelson Mandela and why his given name from the Tembu people, which means to "to stir up trouble," came to actually characterize him. Ask students to think about the conditions in which he was forced to live, his 27 years of imprisonment, and his resulting beliefs. Ask what forgiveness means in the life of Nelson Mandela. Why do the students believe he chose to forgive his captors? What was the result? Other suggested questions include the following:

What are the feelings he had to (and may still have to) overcome? (anger, resentment)
How did and does he overcome them?
What has he done with his life despite his unfortunate experiences?
What other people, famous or not, have shown forgiveness and benefited from this act it in their lives?

List other attributes of Nelson Mandela. Then encourage students to select one aspect of the story and have them each retell one event, such as what Nelson Mandela's early life was like, how and why he was imprisoned, and so on.

Note: Other books in this series include *Learning About Creativity from the Life of Steven Spielberg, Learning About Assertiveness from Oprah Winfrey, Learning About Justice from the Life of Cesar Chavez, Learning About Responsibility from the Life of Colin Powell,* and *Learning About Strength of Character from Mohammad Ali.*

The Man Who Could Call Down Owls

by Eve Bunting
New York: Macmillan, 1984

Suggested Grade and Interest Level: 3 through 6

Topic Explorations: Conservation; Owls

Skill Builders:

Vocabulary	Language literacy	
Semantics	Predicting	Critical thinking
Higher-level concepts	Cause-and-effect relationships	Discussion
Attributes	Drawing inferences	

Synopsis: A gifted man who befriends owls shows a young man, Con, his skills. Then a strange "distracter" becomes envious of the owl man and attempts to gain his power in an unacceptable way. The owls take swift revenge and, in the absence of the owl man, make Con their new friend. The story names many owl species, including barn owl, elf owl, screech owl, great horned owl, great snowy owl, hawk owl, and great gray owl.

Method: Before the read-aloud, elicit background information on owls. Talk about the special features of the species and the special sensitivity of people who work with a particular breed of animals or birds. Then talk about the concept of envy. Ask students to give examples or talk about their experiences in relation to the concept.

Pause briefly during the read-aloud to encourage children to think critically and predict story events. Ask the children if they think the stranger can obtain the owl man's power by taking his cloak and willow wand. What do they think will happen? Do they think the owls will come to him?

Have children make inferences about story events that are not explained in the text or pictures.

> What happened to the owl man?
> What makes you think so?
> Why is the stranger wearing the owl man's cloak and hat and carrying his willow wand?
> Is the stranger telling the truth when he says the owl man gave them to him?
> How did Con know how the stranger obtained them?

After the read-aloud, encourage talk about the story that includes cause-and-effect relationships. Ask what the effect of the stranger's acts was on the owl man. What caused the owls to swoop down on the stranger? What effect will the owl man's absence have on the owls?

To work on attributes, talk about what the owl man was like. How can he be described? Brainstorm words such as *gentle, kind, intuitive, sensing, patient, intelligent, knowledgeable, dedicated,* and *insightful*. What happened because of his talent and power? What attributes can the students ascribe to the stranger and to Con?

For discussion, follow up on the concept of envy and ask students to describe what happened in the story because of the stranger's envy of the owl man. Talk about the extreme polarity between the concept of sensitivity the owl man possessed and the concept of the distracter's envy. Then talk about what the author is saying about life and our planet and about protecting nature and its inhabitants. Ask questions such as these:

> Does the author have a lesson in mind for us to learn? What makes you think so?
> What might the stranger symbolize?
> What might the young man Con stand for?
> What do the owls stand for?
> What might the owl man symbolize?

Extended Activity: Break the students into groups and assign each group to report on one type of owl mentioned in the text. Encourage them to use dictionaries, encyclopedias, and other reference books from the school library in their research. Have each member of the group report on a particular aspect of the owl, such as its markings, habits, habitat, survival status, and more. Have each group create and present to the class a journal of interesting information about owls, along with illustrations, newspaper articles, and other odds and ends about owls.

Meanwhile

by Jules Feiffer
New York: Michael di Capua Books, HarperCollins, 1997

Suggested Grade and Interest Level: 6 through 9

Topic Explorations: Cowboys and cowgirls; Literacy; Outer space; Pirates

Skill Builders:

Vocabulary	**Language literacy**
Semantics	Relating personal experiences
Higher-level concepts	Predicting
Grammar and syntax	Verbal expression
Tenses, present and past	**Articulation**
Advanced syntactic structures	General articulation

Synopsis: The comic book style and subject matter of this book make it suitable for individuals of all ages. Raymond's mother is always calling him, and with Raymond's mother, it's always, "Right now!" and never "No big deal, you can do it next Tuesday, Raymond." That's when Raymond catches sight of a word on the page of his comic book: *meanwhile*. With Mom's escalating demands in the background, Raymond uses the trick of a quick change of scene to escape his own predicament. He creates his own "meanwhile," both literally, by scrawling it onto his wall in red pen, and figuratively, by instantly escaping onto a pirate ship. Follow Raymond on his action-packed, multiphased, free-wheeling adventures.

Method: Introduce the story by opening up a discussion about comics. Elicit prior knowledge of the word *meanwhile*. If needed, tell how it is used in comics as a transition device in escaping from one perilous scene to the next. Give a definition, explaining that something is going on in another place at the same time. Give examples within the context of students' own lives.

Read the story aloud. Or, if appropriate, have the students take turns reading aloud each phase of Raymond's adventure. The cartoon-style balloon dialog reads easily, giving listeners a sense of the story. At each point where Raymond finds himself in a situation with dire consequences, ask students to predict how Raymond will escape. Students can supply the transition word *meanwhile*. The repetition of the words, "Raymond knew he had one last chance to save himself," is ideal to underscore and signal the predictable moments.

After the read-aloud, revisit the pages. The action sequences and verbs used in the text are ideal for encouraging retelling and facilitating verbal expression. Structure sentences to teach skills of grammar and syntax. Some examples in past tense include the following:

> Ramond dueled the wicked pirates.
> He clenched a sword between his teeth.
> He switched on his backpack-autopower-vapor writer.
> He scratched out *meanwhile*.
> Raymond ducked the missiles in outer space.
> He shouted as loud as he could.

Create sentences with subordinate clauses such as

> While Max was reading his comics, his mom was calling for him to come to dinner.
> Max kept reading his comics because he did not want to come when his mother called him.
> The missiles from outer space kept coming as Max dodged them.

Use the vocabulary of the text to teach words within the context of the story:

hopeless (the situation)	reason (tried to)
fore	aft

Multiple-meaning words include odds (evened off). Continue to increase vocabulary usage and reinforce the concept of the simultaneousness of time by having students construct sentences about their lives using the word *meanwhile*. Students can relate personal experiences (from made-up stories) about what is happening at that moment in time and what is happening at the same time in another location, such as a motorcycle race, a snowcapped mountaintop, or an arcade. Also talk about the concept of time as it relates to the Earth. For people in your town it may be morning, but for students halfway around the world it would be nighttime.

For any articulation carryover, children can describe what is happening to Raymond in his adventures using accurate target phonemes in connected speech or read the dialog in the cartoon balloons.

Side Note: In introducing a comic-style book to older students who are language delayed or with reading impairments, it may be helpful and motivating to students to relate the success story of Charles Schwab. The famous businessman who owns one of the world's largest stock brokerage houses had to overcome a severe reading disability as a youth. He has said on many occasions that the only books he could read were comic books and that they helped him in his struggle because he found them fun and exciting. He is currently a large supporter of the International Dyslexic Society. In the end, success is all about finding something that "turns you on" and sticking with it.

Mountain Men: True Grit and Tall Tales

by Andrew Glass
New York: Doubleday Book for Young Readers, 2001

Suggested Grade and Interest Level: 6 through 12

Topic Explorations: Clothing, Hats; Folk tales, North American; History, American

Skill Builders:

Vocabulary	Grammar and syntax	Language literacy
Semantics	Advanced syntactic structures	Storytelling
Homonyms (multiple meanings)		Drawing inferences

Synopsis: Seven profiles of North American mountain men who blazed the trails to the West are presented along with their tall tales that made them legends. Fur trappers and frontiersmen such as John Colter, Jim Bridger, and Kit Carson, the first explorers of the American West beyond the Rocky Mountains, are described in short, chapter-like vignettes. The earth-toned illustrations are in the gritty, rough-hewn style of the Old West. The author describes the era as "a fleeting phase of our national life." Gathering stories on these men and presenting them from the angle of their tall tales is a good way to capture the attention of preadolescents and adolescents. The focus on storytelling also highlights the importance of narrative abilities, the ability to infer meaning, and the entertaining, if not thought-provoking, uses of language. The author helps separate truth from fantasy (although a reader will need to infer a little more), while giving an excellent history lesson.

A Little History: In the 1800s, tall beaver hats were the rage in the big cities of America. Then in the 1830s, fur hats went out of fashion due to the China silk trade, and beaver pelts no longer procured a high price. Many fur trappers became army scouts for work in preparation for the railroads, and many became guides to settlers in opening up the West. The book's foreword illustrates the hats of the day, including the quaker, stovepipe, Tricorn, and a lady's bonnet. The inside cover illustrates a map of the United States from 1803 to 1840, highlighting the Louisiana Purchase, Spanish Territory, Oregon Territory, and New England states. A pictorial list of "mountain man necessaries" and a glossary of "mountain man lingo"—which explains such words as *hos* (person), *didins* (food), and *porkeater* (greenhorn)—are included at the back of the book.

Method: The book offers much in the way of subject matter for remediating and enhancing oral language skills, and it nicely ties in with classroom lessons in American history. Suggestions for activities include the following.

Read "Colter's Run." John Colter's famous footrace in 1808 resulted (according to Colter) from a quick-witted plea bargain with Blackfoot warriors. When caught, Colter tells the tale that he pleaded with the Indians. He would accept a scalping or live burial, but "Please don't make fun of my sad skinny legs by chasing me across the prairie. I am slow as a turtle and it would make sorry sport."

Although John Colter's desperate flight from the Indians actually occurred, sorting out fact from fantasy provides an interesting discussion and a high-interest story through which to teach the skills of inferencing. First, address vocabulary words with multiple meanings by having students look at what Colter really meant by his words, "sorry sport." For example,

> What is the meaning of the words *sorry sport*?
> Did the warriors consider his capture and the deathly ordeal they would put him through an athletic event?
> What else does *sport* mean besides athletic activity? (recreation, diversion, or pleasant pastime)
> What else does *sorry* mean besides an apology? (wretched and useless)

Therefore, according to Colter's plea, it would useless to get him to run from them and find any satisfaction from such a recreation. Besides, he cannot run very well.

The author writes, "His hideous pleading sealed his fate."

To help students with language disabilities understand the expression "sealed his fate," discuss the word *fate* and the homonym *seal*.

> What was Colter's fate? (escaping by way of a foot race)

There are several meanings for the word *seal*.

> What could it mean in this context?
> What sealed or closed off any further possibility of another fate? (his hideous pleading)
> Why was it hideous? (He wanted to be so convincing and make the idea of a footrace sound so fearful and agonizing to him that the Indians would want this for his punishment, as a way of revenge to humiliate him. Therefore, when the Indians said this would in fact be what he got, Colter's pleading sealed his fate.)

According to Colter's later tale, his pleading for what he did not want talked the Indians into doing exactly what he *did* want. Was that Colter's plan? Also according to Colter's later version of what happened, the Blackfoot Indians thought they would catch a man with skinny legs (legs that were not strong enough to run fast) try to outrun them, when in fact Colter knew his advantage in escaping would be his speed.

The story and illustration go on to tell of the rigors of his race to freedom across cactus needles while a Blackfoot was gaining distance close behind. But does anyone really know how it happened? Given the part that we know as fact, what part of the story do students think was embellished and exaggerated? What are their reasons? Use inferencing skills to try to sort through fact and fiction. Was it really Colter's trickster-style pleading that "sealed his fate"? Or did he enjoy telling that tale later, when he wanted to make himself seem even more the hero, cast a humorous light on his story, or infer that he masterminded his escape to freedom?

The remaining mountain men stories provide excellent material for building inferencing skills. They also provide opportunities to build understanding and usage of advanced syntactic structures, performing analyses of the sentence structure similar to the above examples in the area of word meanings and broader story comprehension.

After the read-aloud, have students look up mountain men words in the glossary. Students can give definitions and use the words in sentences that might have been said when talking with a mountain man. Although these words are not used in discourse today, they provide an excellent way to model a process that can be used to expand vocabulary and improve both oral and written (i.e., textbook) language comprehension in other academic arenas.

GRADES 6–12

The Mysteries of Harris Burdick

by Chris Van Allsburg
Boston: Houghton Mifflin, 1984

Suggested Grade and Interest Level: 6 through 9

Topic Exploration: Imagination

Skill Builders:

Grammar and syntax	**Language literacy**	**Articulation**
Tenses, past and present	Cause-and-effect relationships	Carryover for any sound
Advanced syntactic structures	Storytelling	

Synopsis: A man named Harris Burdick once gave a series of mysterious pictures with provocative captions to a children's book publisher. Although he promised to produce the stories that went with them, he never returned. Thirty years later, Chris Van Allsburg reproduced the pictures and original captions, stimuli that can coax even the most unimaginative minds into some fascinating storytelling.

Method: For each illustration, have students brainstorm several ideas for what might have happened before the pictured event. List these ideas to use in the Extended Activity. Ask what might have caused the event to happen. Encourage students to elaborate on their ideas by giving examples and supporting details.

Have students create narratives, using the pictured event as the initiating event of the story.

Extended Activity: Assist students in structuring a story, using one of the ideas on the brainstormed list as the initiating event. Have them use the illustration to fill in information about the setting and characters. (Suggest that perhaps some of the characters in the story are not seen in the author's illustrations.) Ask story grammar questions to help students outline the story:

> Who is the main character?
> What is the event that starts the story?
> What is the character's response to this initiating event? How does he or she feel about it? What does this cause the character to do or want to do?
> What steps does the character take to solve the problem?
> How is the problem resolved?
> Do the characters change in the process?
> What is the outcome?

The students can illustrate their stories if they desire to.

Note: This activity can be done in cooperative learning groups. Have each group create a story map on a large piece of butcher paper.

The River Ran Wild: An Environmental History

by Lynne Cherry
San Diego, CA: Gulliver Green, 1992

Suggested Grade and Interest Level: 6 through 12

Topic Explorations: Conservation; Culture and history, American; Culture and history, Native American; History, American; Speaking and communicating; Women's lives

Skill Builders:

Vocabulary	Language literacy	Pragmatic language
Semantics	Cause-and-effect relationships	
Higher-level concepts	Problem solving	
Categories	Compare and contrast	
Adjectives	Discussion	

Synopsis: The book begins with an introduction outlining the 7,000-year history of the Nashua River in what is now New Hampshire and Massachusetts. The river's history leads to its polluted waters from the factories of the Industrial Revolution and the cleanup project in the 1960s, led by activist Marion Stoddart. Each double spread that follows treats one period or topic throughout the river's history. A brief, informative text is framed with a series of miniature illustrations on one page. Featured are pictures of significant wildlife that live by the river, implements used by Native peoples, inventions of the Industrial Revolution, and small scenes of the area. The facing page is a full-page painting depicting the river at one particular stage in its history, rendered in richly hued and detailed watercolors. The illustrations give meaning to the events and to the era, offering endless language possibilities.

Method: Before the read-aloud, locate the area of the Nashua River on a map of the United States to give students a sense of where the story takes place. Talk about *pollution* and students' background knowledge about the word. Review specific vocabulary words as appropriate, such as *pulp, chemicals, plastic, ecology, ecological,* and *stench.* Then talk about the concept of restoration and what it means in an environmental sense. Draw parallels to restoring old cars or vintage clothes. Then present the book, telling students it is one of the most amazing environmental success stories of our time.

During the read-aloud, pause to identify the pictures in the borders that detail various topics, including Native American tools and items of manufacture during the Industrial Revolution. Pause briefly to clarify meaning and pose thoughtful questions about the story.

After the read-aloud, use the illustrations to elicit descriptions. Students can use adjectives found in the text to describe the river before the pollution (clean, clear, sparkling), when the river began to change (inhabited with sick fish and wildlife), when it was at its worst (smelly, stagnant, clogged with pulp, and red, yellow, or green from the dye of the mill), and when it improved (moving, running again). Students can describe the river as it is from the pictures of white-tailed deer running along the riverbank and people fishing and kayaking in the clear, clean, sparkling waters.

Elicit sentences from students that compare and contrast the lush valley of the Native Americans and its clean, clear sparkling waters to the dying river, stagnant with red dye and pulp from a paper mill. Facilitate the use of words such as *same, different, however, but, on the contrary, rather than, instead of, when compared to,* and *as contrasted with.*

To identify a problem and facilitate a discussion on problem solving, have students define what the problem was with the river and what the solution was to restore it. Define waste processing plants if necessary.

To work on expressing cause-and-effect relationships, encourage sentence generation about the problem in relation to its cause. For example,

> "The reason the Nashua River was polluted was because pulp, dye, and fiber from the factories were dumped into the river."

Scaffold sentences by providing the first part and having the students complete the thought.

> Cause: Because factories dumped pulp, fiber, and dye into the river, ___.

> Effect: ___ it became stagnant, did not flow, turned red, and had a bad odor.

Discuss the story in terms of the attempts or goals of the Oweana, Marion Stoddart, the environmentalists, and people who wanted to restore the river.

> Given: They wanted to _____.

> Possible response: _____ clean up the river and restore its wildlife.

Students can state two, three, or four steps that were taken to obtain the goal. Use steps as supporting details to the main point, such as

> They traveled to each town along the Nashua.
> They spoke about the river's history.
> They had people sign petitions and send letters.
> They convinced paper mills to build plants to process waste to stop factories from polluting.

Encourage words such as *first, next,* and *last.*

Point out Marion Stoddart's ability to communicate effectively to different groups of people to bring the issue into focus. How might she have been so persuasive in leading to the river cleanup? How might she have presented the topic to get positive results? What obstacles might she have encountered? What might she have done in spite of this? Why might she be considered an extraordinary woman, especially in the time in which she lived?

To work on categorization skills, review the miniature pictures in the borders that center on a theme. Each frame is a replica of an object that depicted the times. These illustrations give students the visual sense of what transpired during that era and how these items have transformed in today's times. For example, ask students to categorize some of the items from the Industrial Revolution, such as

> Inventions: sewing machine, light bulb, camera, clock, typewriter, and phonograph
> Means of transportation: airplane, locomotive, automobile
> Significant events in history: Wright brothers' first airplane, Charles Lindbergh's flight across the Atlantic
> Communication devices: typewriter, telegraph machine, movie projector

Students must describe a category and use sentences with words such as *group, set, for instance, another, an example of,* or *another example of _____ is.*

Discuss the message in the story. What is the author saying about our earth and what its inhabitants can do to save it? What qualifications does one need to begin such a project?

What does this story demonstrate about fighting for what you believe?

Extended Activities: Discuss what we can do in our own environments to preserve our natural resources. Talk about an environmental issue that is close to your surroundings and have students role-play a meeting where people express opposing views. Help students express their positions and simulate a town meeting at the edge of the Nashua River in the late 1950s. Assign students the roles of factory owners, factory workers, and Native American tribespeople.

Rome Antics

by David Macaulay
Boston: Houghton Mifflin, 1997

Suggested Grade and Interest Level: 8 through 12

Topic Explorations: Art, artists, and architecture; History, European; Journeys

Skill Builders:

Vocabulary	Grammar and syntax	Language literacy
Semantics	Advanced syntactic structures	Drawing inferences
		Discussion

Synopsis: A carrier pigeon is released from her cage somewhere in the Italian countryside and flies over the city of Rome with an important message. When she decides to take the scenic route rather than proceeding directly to the destination ("which is standard pigeon procedure"), she takes the reader on a scenic, aerial tour over the ancient, fascinating city. The pigeon finally arrives, and her receiver is most delighted to read the one-word message she delivers. The illustrations are pen and ink, on colossal-sized pages. The pigeon is rarely seen; only her path, sometimes dizzying, is shown in red. Information on the Roman sites is given at the back of the book.

Method: Before the read-aloud, elicit background information on the city of Rome, the capital of Italy and the ancient capital of the Roman Empire. Talk about some of the sites of the city, including the Colosseum, which was opened in the year 80. Stress the significance of Rome having more artistic and architectural masterpieces than any other city in the world.

Also elicit background knowledge on carrier (or "homing") pigeons, and talk about how they are trained to carry messages to specific destinations.

Vocabulary includes

discombobulated	(without) reservation
inedible	impede
imposing	antics

During the read-aloud, pause at each page to study and enjoy the drawings, architecture, details, and humor depicted. Also talk about the words that describe the sites of the city, such as

ancient tombs	surrounding brick wall
archways	abandoned gatehouse
Colosseum	amphitheater
chiming midday bells	sun-warmed, terra-cotta rooftops
market square	narrow streets
cobblestones	granite column
entablature	marble scroll

After the read-aloud, go back over the pages and describe the pigeon's flight. Talk about what the pigeon's visual perspective lends to the story. Clarify the events taking place that you may not have caught on the first read. Especially significant to point out are the famous wild cats shown in the illustration of the Forum, the various cultures represented at the outdoor café in Piazza Novona (including one man of ancient culture talking on a cell phone), and the excavation of buried archaeological treasures taking place beneath the cobblestone streets. Ask students to point out what details in the illustrations amaze them most.

When discussing the pages, help students comprehend and use advanced syntactic structures. Construct subordinate clauses by starting with the same words such as "The homing pigeon" and complete the sentence with words from each page of text. Some examples include the following:

The homing pigeon that was released in the hills flew over "the high brick wall that once surrounded the city."
The homing pigeon that took the scenic route "approached an abandoned gatehouse."
The homing pigeon that was released from her cage circled over "the most famous amphitheater in the world."

Teach dependent clauses beginning with the adverb *while* by starting with the same words, such as "The homing pigeon," and completing the sentence with a clause using words from a page of text. Some examples, include the following:

> The homing pigeon swooped through the city while the workers excavated below the streets.
> The homing pigeon swooped through the city while the mechanics worked in the garage.
> The homing pigeon swooped through the city while the cat on the terra-cotta rooftop watched her.

Use the sentence on one of the first pages to demonstrate an embedded sentence. Page 11 reads,

> "Instead of traveling directly to her destination, which is standard pigeon procedure, she decides to take the scenic route."

Then have students create embedded sentences of their own using the text as a template or guide.

Teach students to construct sentences with connectives. Some examples include the following:

> The homing pigeon took a different route *when* she wanted to see the sights of the city.
> The pigeon is sent reeling *as a result of* colliding with a soccer ball.
> The pigeon flies between the ancient buildings *and* wants to land on a rooftop until she sees another cat nearby.
> She finds a nice place to rest on an outdoor umbrella *but* leaves after "a cell phone rudely bleeps."

Upon completion, discuss the author's choice of title, *Rome Antics*. What is one meaning for the word *antics*? How does the definition of playful tricks or capers apply both to the sender and to the pigeon?

What other meaning comes to mind when thinking about the word *antic*? What other words have the same beginning (*antiques, antiquity*)? Talk about the word *antique* and the Italian word *antico*, meaning ancient, and *anticamente*, meaning old. How do they apply to the story? Might all of these meanings have been the author's intent?

Seven Brave Women

by Betsy Gould Hearne
New York: Greenwillow Books, 1997

Suggested Grade and Interest Level: 6 through 12

Topic Explorations: Culture and history, American; History, American; Women's lives

Skill Builders:

Vocabulary	Grammar and syntax	Language literacy
Higher-level concepts	Past tense	Storytelling
Attributes		Compare and contrast
Homonyms (multiple meanings)		Point of view
Synonyms		Retelling events
		Discussion

Synopsis: A young girl recalls her mother's stories "about the brave women in our family—stories I can keep forever and pass on to my children" and puts them down in story form. The result is a rich tapestry of American history. Each page is one illustrated chapter, telling of one woman's life during a particular time in history. It begins with the narrator's great-great-great grandmother who, during the time of the Revolutionary War, crossed the ocean in a wooden sailboat. Each life of an ancestor is marked by a war, yet their "making of America" was not done by fighting wars but by building families and homes, pursuing their dreams, and living out their lives in the times in which they lived. Students gain a great deal of knowledge about the benefits of storytelling, a skill that can be handed down through the generations. The short stories provide many good ways to ask content questions, especially about the vividly expressed details in each woman's life.

Method: Introduce the book by asking students to think of brave women in history. Elicit responses and encourage explanations for why they were brave. (Some starters: Amelia Earhart, Sally Ride, Mother Theresa, Harriet Tubman, and Rosa Parks.) Then ask if they have brave women in their own family histories. What sorts of things are the students aware of that their ancestors or living relatives did? For example, most everyone had a relative or ancestor who at one time came from another country. How did they travel to get here? Help students visualize and conceptualize the experience and then describe it. How might that woman have been brave? Talk about the meaning of the words *ancestors, heritage,* and *genealogy.*

Read each one-page story individually, developing it into a separate lesson. Pause briefly in the reading to clarify more vocabulary words, such as *Mennonite.*

After the read-aloud, ask story comprehension questions. For example, in the first story, ask what sorts of things the girl's great-great-great grandmother did in her lifetime. Scaffold as necessary to shape past-tense structures and retelling of events, as in

> She kept herds of sheep.
> She made blankets from their wool.
> She made medicine from herbs.
> She helped her neighbors by delivering their babies.
> She made candles, soap, bread, and butter.
> How might she have been brave?

The girl's grandmother, who lived during the time of World War II, experienced different things in her lifetime. For example,

> She took fencing lessons just for fun.
> She played basketball on a first girl's team.
> She traveled to France to take harp lessons.
> She enrolled in architecture school.

When she went to architecture school, "the men met her with a sign that said, NO DOGS, CHILDREN, OR WOMEN ALLOWED." She also had to take tests in a room by herself because she was the only woman in the school. Have a discussion about the difficulties that women often had to overcome in history. Talk about the word *pioneer,* which has multiple meanings, and how people who are first to open a way for the rest of the people often have to overcome harsh, severe obstacles before they can lead the way. Have students use the word in sentences and extend the meaning to the adjective form, such as a "pioneer method." Brainstorm synonyms for the word, such as *leader, trailblazer,* and *pathfinder,* the root words in these terms, and how those words came to be.

When she was 80 years old, the girl's grandmother wrote a book about buildings, and at 89 years old, she wrote another one about builders. Have students list the attributes of this woman. In addition to being brave, what other qualities might she have had?

Compare and contrast two of the women described in the book. Assist students with the activity by modeling or recasting sentences containing words such as *are different, are similar, are alike, rather than, instead of, compared to,* and *in contrast to.*

The narrator's family ancestry is similar to other families whose women lived through war times and did brave and remarkable things while living so-called ordinary lives. Ask students what they know about the women in their families. Encourage them to relate the events or describe the person. Scaffold as necessary by assisting them to give the details they are aware of, such as the woman's name, her relation to the student, the time in which she lived, where she lived, and what she did. Perhaps the family has a keepsake of hers they can describe.

Discuss the compound word *keepsake*. (*Sake,* meaning purpose or end, as in "for the sake of ____." Therefore, *keep* the item for the *sake* of memories creates the word *keepsake*.) Recall some of the keepsakes the girl had from her ancestors. Go back through the story and make a list, including

> the white handkerchief that Elizabeth embroidered with an *E;*
> the quilt that her great-great grandmother made;
> the plates, cups, and saucers that her great grandmother painted;
> the brass teapot that belonged to her grandmother who lived in India; and
> another grandmother's harp.

These keepsakes are excellent story starters. Pick an item from the list and tell the story about the woman to whom it belonged. For example,

The girl in the story has the china that belonged to her great grandmother. It has flowers on the plates, cups, and saucers that her great grandmother painted. When her grandmother was young, she worked on her mother's farm. There were no art teachers where they lived, so she rode on a horse to a nearby town for art lessons and rode back to do her chores. When she married a preacher and raised a family, she did not have time to paint pictures, so she painted the china off which her family ate.

For another way to engage students in storytelling activities, talk about point of view. Then have children tell one woman's story from her perspective. What sorts of things were going on in her lifetime? Encourage students to tell her story against the backdrop of the times. How would the events of the time in which she lived have shaped her life?

Extended Activities: Encourage students to talk with their parents about their relatives and ancestors, especially in connection with the concept of bravery. After conversations with their parents, encourage students to share a story of one brave woman in particular. Perhaps parents have a family keepsake to describe. Students can relate the story of the family keepsake to the group or class and describe the person to whom it belonged and how the concept of bravery can be illustrated with this invidivual. Once the student has shared the description orally, have the student write a story about the woman and relate how the student came to have the item that once belonged to her. (Allow children to make up a story if they are unable to retrieve any family history.) Follow the message of the story by limiting the relative to a woman. Include story elements and character attributes in the written work.

Shadow

by Blaise Cendrars
Translated by Marcia Brown
New York: Scribner's, 1982

Suggested Grade and Interest Level: 6 through 12

Topic Explorations: Folklore, African and African American; Shadows

Skill Builders:

Vocabulary	**Language literacy**
Semantics	Compare and contrast
Attributes	Drawing inferences
Grammar and syntax	Discussion
Advanced syntactic structures	**Articulation, *Sh***

Synopsis: An African tale about shadows, written in verse as it might have been told by ancient storytellers. A Caldecott award winner.

Method: After reading each page, talk about how the storyteller describes what a shadow does. Define and use the story's vocabulary in sentences from the context of the story. Then relate the words to the students' own lives and generate further sentences. Words include

embers	hearth	mute
perch	prowl	spark
squirm	stagger	trickster
vain		

Generate more vocabulary by listing attributes of a shadow. Then compare and contrast shadows and reflections. When comparing and contrasting, model or shape sentences using words such as *same, similar, different, however, instead of, in contrast to,* and *compared to.*

To teach articulation, use the text, heavily loaded with the *Sh* phoneme, to generate sentences and spontaneous speech on the topic of shadows. Then talk about reflections, comparing the meanings of the two words containing the target phoneme.

Extended Activity: Ask the students how they would describe a shadow. Do a semantic webbing activity by associating groups of words with *shadow* as it is used in the context of the story. What words come to mind? Students can then take the brainstormed words and arrange them, adding more only if necessary, to create their own poems. Demonstrate use of advanced syntactic structures with adjective and relative clauses, using the lines of verse as a beginning basis. Also use the list of previously generated attributes to build noun phrases with modifiers (e.g., *sleek, mute, darting shadow*). Build a hierarchy of syntactic structures, from one or two words (e.g., *prowling, pausing, perching, lingering*), to simple phrases (e.g., prowling in the alleys, pausing at the doors, perching on the railings, lingering on the floor), to temporal clauses (such as prowling when it moves so slow, perching when it stops to rest), and so on.

Starry Messenger

by Peter Sís
New York: Farrar, Straus & Giroux, 1996; Sunburst, 2001

Suggested Grade and Interest Level: 6 through 12

Topic Explorations: Famous people; History, European; Long ago and far away; Science

Skill Builders:

Vocabulary	**Language literacy**
Semantics	Storytelling
Higher-level concepts	Problem solving
Categories	Drawing inferences
Similes and mctaphors	Explaining processes in detail
Grammar and syntax	Discussion
Advanced syntactic structures	

Synopsis: A multiple award-winning book of rare quality. Set in the Italian Renaissance period, the life of the great scientist Galileo is told with brief text, glorious illustrations, and copies of his famous sketches. The picture book, named for Galileo's published work by the same name, chronicles his achievements of the telescope and his celestial discoveries. It goes on to tell of his celebrity status, fall from favor with the Catholic Church, and his tragic ending of being imprisoned in his own home. The thought-provoking and stirring illustrations provide opportunity for discovery and discussion. The lovely text is in script, like Galileo's own handwriting, with added quotes by Galileo translated from Italian. Share and experience this work over many readings and many days.

Method: Before the read-aloud, elicit background knowledge about Galileo and talk about one of the greatest scientists of all time. Also talk about the Italian Renaissance as a time of awakening. Preteach some of the vocabulary words that appear in the text, including

tradition	celebrity
spyglass	astronomical
telescope	argumentativeness
Aristotle	gazed
prominences	chasms
nebulae	gratifying
law of falling bodies, 1604	law of the pendulum, 1583
law of floating objects, 1611	

Pause during the read-aloud to clarify meaning and pose thoughtful questions about the story. For example, pause to talk about how Galileo proved that Aristotle's experiments were wrong. Ask students to infer what this says about Galileo. What words can be used to describe his character based on this information? How did people react to this?

At the end of the read-aloud, discuss the Shakespearean quote that accompanies the illustration of all the new-born infants of Pisa wrapped in blankets at the time Galileo was born.

> "Be not afraid of greatness: some are born great, some achieve greatness, and some have greatness thrust upon them" (*Twelfth-Night*, Act II, Scene V).

Have a discussion about the word *destiny*. What is the significance of the illustrations pictured on the newborn babies' blankets that they are wrapped in? Which one is Galileo? What is the significance of the stars shining brightly on the blanket he is wrapped in? Based on the illustrations, have the students predict what the babies' destinies were likely to be.

Have students verbalize the illustrations of the Ptolemaic System of the solar system and describe how all the planets were believed to revolve around the earth. Then describe the Copernican System, where the earth moved around the sun. Have students compare and contrast the two systems using words like *same, different, similar, yet, alike, rather than*, and *instead of*.

Describe the metaphor "Italy was a quilt of city-states," using the illustrated map of Renaissance Italy depicting the Kingdom of Naples, the Republic of Venice, the Duchy of Tuscany, and so on.

Another use of a metaphor: "The moon is not robed in a smooth and polished surface but is in fact rough and uneven . . ."

Study the illustration of the Leaning Tower of Pisa. After the students learn of Galileo's experiment that the tower depicts, have them describe Galileo's experiment in their own words.

Describe the insets on the illustration of the map depicting "News of the telescope reaches Galileo" (i.e., Galileo demonstrating his telescope to a large audience of viewers; Galileo working at his desk with his compass and instruments).

Galileo's telescope was described as an instrument that magnified things 1,000 times larger and 30 times closer than what one can see with natural vision. Categorize other scientific instruments depicted in the illustrations.

How does the author infer what was going on in the mind and emotions of Galileo? What techniques does the author use in telling about Galileo's inquisition? Why did the author depict his prison room with a snake encircling the floor and dragons emerging from the walls?

Talk about the reasons why Galileo's life ended the way it did. Talk about the quote "Condemned to spend the rest of his life locked in his house under guard for believing what he proved to be true."

What is the meaning of the following quote, especially in context with the illustration of Galileo imprisoned in his room?

"Why should I believe blindly and stupidly what I wish to believe, and subject the freedom of my intellect to someone else who is just as liable to error as I am?"

Another quote from Galileo:

"With regard to matters requiring thought: the less people know and understand about them, the more positively they attempt to argue concerning them."

Stephen Hawking: Understanding the Universe

by Gail Sakurai
New York: Children's Press, 1996

Suggested Grade and Interest Level: 6 through 12

Topic Explorations: Famous people; Science

Skill Builders:

Vocabulary	Language literacy
Semantics	Relating personal experiences
Higher-level concepts	Drawing inferences
Attributes	

Synopsis: Black holes were first theorized in 1971 by one of the most brilliant theoretical physicists since Einstein, Professor Stephen Hawking. Students will gain an introduction to the man and how he became severely disabled from amyotropic lateral sclerosis (Lou Gehrig's disease). Although the text is very simple and glosses over some of his hardships, the photograph from *Star Trek: The Next Generation* on the opening page provides the often-needed hook to gain the interest of adolescents. In the scene from the popular television show, Hawking is sitting in his wheelchair equipped with computer devices that help him speak, playing poker with Albert Einstein and Sir Isaac Newton (computer-generated images) in the costume of their day. The book also will be of great interest to students with similar disabilities.

Method: When reading this book aloud, it may be necessary to simply omit text with definitions of words commonly understood or obvious to listeners. For an even better narrative, students can find an autobiography of Stephen Hawking in the Disability and A Brief History of Mine links at his Web site: www.hawking.org.uk. It begins with an interesting fact on the date of his birth: "8 January 1942 (300 years after the death of Galileo) in Oxford, England." (See entry for *Starry Messenger* in this catalog section.)

When Stephen Hawking nearly lost his life from pneumonia, a tracheotomy saved him but left him without the ability to speak. A California computer expert, Walt Woltosz, sent him a computer program he had written called Equalizer. Connected to a computer, it helped him speak and write. (See his Web site for more information and his experience with a speech synthesizer by Speech Plus.) He then was able to continue writing research papers, give lectures, and finish his book *A Brief History of Time: From the Big Bang to Black Holes* published in 1988, which became an all-time best-seller and also was made into a Hollywood movie. Ask thought-provoking questions such as

How might Stephen Hawking's life have been different if there were not software, speech synthesizers, and other technological devices?
Why does Stephen Hawking say he has learned that one need not lose hope?

Discuss the concepts of motivation, influence, and inspiration.

What motivates Stephen Hawking?
Why has this man's disease not stopped him from participating in life, traveling to see the Great Wall of China, going to concerts and parties, enjoying his family, and continuing in his search to understand the heavens?
Why does he say his condition has not prevented him from doing much?
Who has influenced him?
How does he try to keep from feeling sorry for himself?
How is he an inspiration to others with disabilities?
How is he an inspiration to others without disabilities?

Draw inferences about Stephen Hawking based on the facts given about his childhood.

Why might he have liked taking things apart and not putting them back together?
Why might he have had difficulty in school as a child?
What might his childhood have been like because of these conditions?

Students may want to relate personal experiences about similarities in their own lives and what or who has motivated and inspired them. Talk about how every individual (to some degree) has obstacles to overcome in his or her life. Discuss the need for humans to share their stories with one another.

Further reading found in the juvenile category includes

Stephen Hawking: Revolutionary Physicist (Great Achievers: Lives of the Physically Challenged), by Melissa McDaniel, John F. Callahan, and Jerry Lewis (introduction)

Adult books to share include

Stephen Hawking's book, *A Brief History in Time*
Introducing Stephen Hawking, by J. P. McEvoy, Oscar Zarate (contributor), Richard Appignanesi (editor), and S. Hawking
Hawking and Black Holes (The Big Idea series) by Paul Strathern

Stickeen: John Muir and the Brave Little Dog

by John Muir   Retold by Donnell Rubay
Nevada City, CA: Dawn, 1998

www. DawnPub.com

Suggested Grade and Interest Level: 6 through 12

Topic Explorations: Animals, Dogs; History, American; Pets

Skill Builders:

Vocabulary	Grammar and syntax	Language literacy
Semantics	Advanced syntactic structures	Drawing inferences
Attributes		Point of view
Similes and metaphors		Explaining processes in detail

Synopsis: The true story of a dog named Stickeen who accompanied John Muir, the great explorer and environmentalist, on an exploration in Alaska in 1880. With a storm blowing in the distance, Muir set off one morning to explore the glaciers, ordering the little dog back. But Stickeen refused, insisting he follow Muir into the treacherous territory. Hours later, Muir and Stickeen find themselves surrounded by deep canyons of ice, unable to leap the huge crevasse that stood before them. Muir wrote that the adventure was his "most memorable in all my wild days." John Muir's own story plus the dramatic, gripping illustrations of Christopher Canyon make this book a fascinating read for people of all ages.

Method: Before the read-aloud, discuss John Muir, the famous 19th-century naturalist who loved to go to wild places and experience the wonders of nature. Alaska, like Yosemite in California, was one of Muir's favorite places to explore. As an adventurer, explorer, scientist, author, and visionary, Muir's legacy was monumental. He taught people the importance of experiencing and protecting the natural environment. He urged President Theodore Roosevelt to protect America's natural heritage under the authority of the Antiquities Act of 1906 and inspired what is today the National Parks and Conservation Movements. His life remains an inspiration to people everywhere who love the natural environment and want to preserve it. His sensitive spirit is captured in this story he wrote about a dog that once, against his protests, joined him on an expedition.

Although the text is not lengthy, it is sufficient enough to be savored as a read-aloud over a number of days, if desired. Present the book in sections, as you would a chapter book. Throughout the readings, pause to discuss vocabulary and the illustrations of Muir, Stickeen, and the Alaskan wildlife. Pose questions to ensure students' understanding of the story's meaning. Discuss the vocabulary in the context in which it is used. Some vocabulary include the following:

puzzling	independent	glacier
noodle (slang for *head*)	forbidding	crevasses
chasms	tottered	noble (mountain)
marooned		

Assist students in using the words in spontaneously generated sentences. Help students rephrase the part of the story in which the vocabulary word appears. Then use the word as it applies to the students' own lives, giving the word relevancy.

A great deal of imagery is used in the text. Help students understand its uses and meaning by discussing the similes and metaphors. For example, as Muir and Stickeen climbed the snowy mountains, they watched the storm from afar. Muir writes, "What a song this storm sang!" Discuss what Muir meant and the sounds he could hear from the wind against the ice. Other examples:

"The glacier rose before us—huge and forbidding—like a great evil creature guarding a place no man had ever gone."
"Death seemed to lie within these holes."
What does the author want the reader to sense about this place?

After the read-aloud, go back over the pages and ask questions to elicit meaning from what the author implied. For example, Muir states, "Everyone else in the camp was sleeping, but I hurried to explore the music and motion of the storm." Today, people do not (or should not) go on such expeditions alone. Why might Muir have wanted to hurry off alone in pursuit of a storm? What do we know about him that might suggest his reasons?

When Stickeen would not leave him and go back to the camp, the author writes, "I could not shake him, no more than the Earth can shake the Moon, so I pushed on."

When Stickeen's paws began to bleed, Muir states, "Though I knew he would not thank me, I made him four tiny moccasins out of my handkerchief." What does he mean by saying the dog would not thank him? What is the author implying?

GRADES 6–12

Help learners with language disabilities understand complex sentences by going back over more difficult parts of the text to ensure meaning. For example, the author writes,

> "Though the crevasses lay like bottomless holes before us, Stickeen showed neither caution nor curiosity, wonder nor fear."
>
> "I have often felt that to meet one's fate on a noble mountain, or in the heart of a crystal glacier, would be a blessed end to an adventurous life."

To help students explain processes in detail, have them retell the steps Muir took in crossing the thin ice bridge to safety. Reread the text and study the illustration to gain further understanding. First, use three or four steps in retelling the text, and then expand with explanations to give more detail. Scaffold as needed. Two sample explanations to enhance or modify include the following:

The first:
> First, he chipped steps in the glacier so he could get down.
> Then he straddled the ice bridge and cut a path for Stickeen.
> Next, he moved across until he got to the next glacier.
> Finally, he made steps in the next glacier and climbed up.

The second:
> First, he chipped steps in the side of the glacier with his ice axe so he could get down.
> To do this, he held on to a notch he made in the ice with one hand and chipped more steps below him using the other hand.
> Finally, he was able to reach the ice bridge.
> Then, he straddled the ice bridge and cut off the rough and jagged tops with his ice axe so they were about 4 inches wide.
> He did this so he could move forward without getting jabbed and so Stickeen would have a narrow path on which to walk.
> When he got across the ice bridge, he chipped away at the ice to make steps in the side of the next glacier and finally climbed to the top.

Brainstorm words to describe the attributes of Stickeen. What parts of the story come to mind when thinking of them?

Brainstorm the attributes of Muir. Recall what Muir was like with Stickeen at the beginning of the story and what his relationship with Stickeen was like at the end of the story.

From whose point of view is the story told? How do you know?

Discuss how the experience with Stickeen changed Muir. What did he learn? Go back to the beginning of the story and describe Stickeen. How did Stickeen's relationship with Muir change at the end of the story?

The Stinky Cheese Man and Other Fairly Stupid Tales

by Jon Scieszka
New York: Viking, 1992

Suggested Grade and Interest Level: 6 through 12

Topic Explorations: Fairy tales and nursery rhymes; Humor

Skill Builders:

Vocabulary	**Language literacy**
Attributes	Storytelling
Grammar and syntax	Point of view
Advanced syntactic structures	**Articulation**
	Carryover for any sound

Synopsis: Madcap revisions of familiar fairy tales—along the lines of "Chicken Licken," "Cinderrumpelstiltskin, or the Girl Who Really Blew It," and "Jack's Bean Problem"—and amusing illustrations provide unlimited language opportunities and numerous fun-filled activities. Each story is a page or two in length. This book is a Caldecott Honor Book.

Method: Before the read-aloud, elicit students' background knowledge of the fairy tale that will be introduced, such as "Chicken Little," "Cinderella," "Rumplestiltskin," or "Jack and the Beanstalk." If the tale is familiar, have students tell what they can remember of the tale.

During the read-aloud, pause briefly to clarify meaning. Refer back the original fairy tales if necessary.

After reading each story, discuss how the author changed the original fairy tale to make it amusing. If necessary, follow the reading with another reading of the original story from a volume of fairy tales. Talk about the story's point of view and how it is different from the fairy tale. List the characters' attributes in the revised story. How have the characters changed? How did their problems change?

To teach carryover of articulation, have students read the short stories and then retell them.

Extended Activity: Students can create their own madcap revisions to fairy tales. First, take the fairy tale and change the point of view. Ask questions such as these to guide the students:

> From whose perspective could the tale be told?
> How could the characters be changed?
> How could their attitudes and traits be changed to reflect modern life?
> How could their problems be different when they are living in modern times?
> How could the choices they have for solving their problems be different now?

Have students describe the newly created characters, their predicaments, and the resolutions to their predicaments. Ask students to identify what the newly created characters are doing. Model and shape advanced syntactic structures of coordinating conjunctions such as *and* and *but,* subordinating conjunctions such as *because* and *so,* adverbial clauses such as *while* and *although,* and adverbial clauses with connective functions such as *if-then* and *however.*

This Land Is Your Land

by Kathy Jacobsen (words and music by Woody Guthrie)
New York: Little, Brown, 1998

Suggested Grade and Interest level: 6 through 12

Topic Explorations: Art, artists, and architecture; Cities; Culture and history, American; Famous people; Folk songs; History, American; Journeys; Music, musicians, and musical instruments

Skill Builders:

    Vocabulary

Higher-level concepts	Idioms	**Language literacy**
Categories	Similes and metaphors	Drawing inferences
Synonyms		

Synopsis: Once you see this book you will understand why it has been called an American treasure. The familiar folk song, which is the main text of the book, was originally written by Woody Guthrie to call attention to the plight of those hit hardest by the Great Depression. It has become what is now a joyful tribute to the beautiful landscapes, diversity, and indomitable spirit of the American people. As the lines of the song unfold, a premier folk artist's unforgettable, meticulously rendered paintings present a rich tapestry of vignettes and majestic postcard vistas. (Ms. Jacobsen's work is featured in many museums, including the Smithsonian.) In this work, she re-creates the path taken by Guthrie across the country, from the deserts and wide-open prairies to the cities teaming with people, to architectural feats of Grand Coolie Dam to the Golden Gate Bridge. A tribute to Guthrie written by folksinger Pete Seeger is included in the back of the book. Also at the back of the book is a biographical scrapbook highlighting Guthrie's life and career, the history of the song, and the impact of the Depression era, which illuminates the importance and emotional appeal of "This Land Is Your Land."

Method: Use this book in conjunction with classroom lessons in American history and geography. Discuss the inside cover and the stream of old cars traveling across the map of the western states on Route 66. Talk about the significance of Route 66. What is the significance of the incoming stream of people? What does it say about the history of this country, especially in the early 20th century? What does it say about the people's hopes and desires?

Also talk about folk art, which is the style of art depicted in the book. Ask students why this type of art is a good complement to Woody Guthrie's song.

Special Note: In addition to teaching the message of Guthrie and higher-level concepts, be sure to take time to enjoy the illustrations and find Woody, wearing his checked shirt and carrying his guitar, within them.

To increase vocabulary and the understanding of higher-level concepts, discuss the words *hope* and *despair.* Build discussions around the pictures of the Dust Bowl era and the pictures of homelessness and hungry people in line for food. Talk about what it may have been like to be a farmer and have nothing to produce and lose your land, your farm, and have nothing to eat. What would it be like if you felt it would always be so terrible? What would it feel like if you felt life might be better in another part of the country?

Talk about the word *compassion,* the feeling of deep sympathy and sorrow for those stricken with misfortune. Talk about the human spirit and wanting to help lessen others' suffering. Ask what compassion can do for people and their country. What things and conditions could come of it? Discuss what kinds of things students can do to demonstrate their compassion for people less fortunate. What might be the result of such actions?

To develop inferencing skills and teach comprehension and use of metaphors, read the quotes by Woody Guthrie in the boxes at the corners of the inside pages. For example, "My eyes have been my camera taking pictures of the world and my songs have been messages that I tried to scatter across the back sides and along the steps of fire escapes and on the window sills and through the dark halls."

Point out the importance of the use of metaphors in songs and poems. What does Guthrie mean when he says, "My eyes have been my camera"? What do cameras do? What do we get from them? Ask students to infer meaning from the rest of the quote. What was Guthrie's purpose in songwriting? Ask students if they were songwriters, to whom would they speak? What would they want to convey? Like Guthrie, what observations can they make? What is important to them?

To teach categorization skills, discuss organizational strategies to identify the different aspects of America presented in "This Land Is Your Land." For example, a quilt might serve as a metaphor. Have students visualize a quilt, or even a series of quilts, with each square representing something about America. Sort each picture of

America into piles according to the category in which they belong. In a category of natural landscapes, you might include the desert, Niagara Falls, the Utah mountains, the Grand Canyon, and the Mississippi River. In another possible category of architectural structures, name items that are illustrated on the pages, like the Statue of Liberty, San Francisco's Chinatown, and Victorian townhouses. Other possible categories are farmlands, cities, types of labor forces, and people. Into which category would you put the Mississippi River? Into which category would you put Colorado's Mesa Verde, a Louisiana plantation, or the garment workers? (See the Extended Activities section below for a written language assignment.)

To further increase vocabulary and concept development, read the quote, "Stick up for what you know is right." Talk about the striking garment workers of the 1920s pictured in the illustrations and how women were forced to work for low wages and how they spoke out about it. Name instances in more recent history when people have taken a stand for what they believed in. Suggestions include the Vietnam War protests, the boycott on tuna that resulted in dolphin-safe tuna fishing, the protests of deforestation and other natural environment concerns that led to proliferation of many endangered species, and America's stand on human rights' violations taking place in countries around the world today. Ask students to share thoughts and opinions about things going on in their lives that they believe are not right. If they were songwriters, what would they want to convey to people?

Discuss the expression "speaking out" and what it means to be able to express your opinion and speak out about what you believe in. Brainstorm synonyms and idioms such as *outspoken, truthful, frank,* and *up front.*

Infer meaning from Guthrie's many quotes on the pages of the book. For example, read, "This world is your world and my world. Take it easy, but take it." What did Guthrie mean by these words? How can they be applied to one's own life? What is beautiful about this world to you? What can you do to, as Guthrie says, "take it"? What does the expression "take it" mean?

Read and study the pictures to find the meaning of the following lines:

> "As I went walking, I saw a sign there
> And on the sign it said 'No Trespassing,'
> But on the other side it didn't say nothing;
> That side was made for you and me."

Can that concept apply to our lives today? In what way?

More quotes include

> "I have room for one more friend and he is Everyman."
> "I'm going where the climate suits my clothes."

Also discuss other concepts presented in the book, such as beliefs, values, opportunity, and freedom.

Extended Activity: Play the song for students to hear, as well as other folk songs from a tape or CD. After categorizing the concepts and aspects of America depicted in the illustrations, write a paragraph on the topic of one category, using the items in each category to develop topic sentences. Use the illustrations to develop the supporting details. For example, students can write an essay or story about the places Guthrie walked. A possible title would be "As He Went Walking." Limit the topic to one of the categories, such as the people he encountered or the natural landscapes he saw. For the topic sentences, draw from the items that were placed in that particular category. For the supporting details, draw from the details in the illustrations.

To further develop writing skills, ask students to take a favorite quote of Guthrie's and develop it into an essay. What do they believe he meant, for example, by, "This world is your world and my world? Take it easy, but take it"? Have students state their belief and support it with examples from their lives. Share their essays during a folk song week, where various songs, including those of Woody Guthrie and those sung by Pete Seeger, are presented.

The Three Pigs

by David Wiesner
New York: Clarion Books, 2001

Suggested Grade and Interest Level: 6 through 12

Topic Explorations: Creativity; Fairy tales and nursery rhymes

Skill Builders:

Vocabulary	**Language literacy**
Higher-level concepts	Predicting
Similes and metaphors	Point of view
Grammar and syntax	Retelling events
Tenses, present and past	**Articulation**
	General articulation
	Carryover for any sound

Synopsis: David Wiesner creates a variation of *The Three Little Pigs* and brings a message suitable for individuals of all ages. In this version, the little pigs really did not get eaten up by the big bad wolf but blast right out of the frame of the story's illustration. The bewildered wolf is left at the doorstep while the pigs enter another dimension (the literate dimension?), a world they venture into via a paper airplane folded from one of the pages of their own story. After they rescue a dragon out of the pages of a folktale where it is about to be slain by the prince, it is time to go back. They reenter (bringing along their new friends) and find the wolf still standing at the door. The dragon returns a good deed, and the pigs rewrite their own fate. As the pigs transcend out of the confines of their stereotypical roles, Wiesner's illustrations change style into surreal, three-dimensional, new-age forms placed against the stark white background of open space (open mind?). The text is sparse, whereas the illustrations tell the story and convey the thought-provoking message to readers and viewers.

Method: Introduce the book to older students by explaining that the author has created this story in a particular way because he has a message. Ask students to look and listen to the way the story is put together. If appropriate for the audience, explain that the author's books (by no means only for children) access our unconscious, similar to a Rorschach test, and that they often reveal different things to different people or mean different things to different people. If necessary, ask a student to review aloud the original three little pigs story to ensure all students have the background information necessary to understand the story.

Read through the story once. Leave interaction to a minimum and allow time between pages for students to think about and experience what is happening in the story.

After the read-aloud, do a picture walk-through to develop grammar and syntax and retelling events. The book's interrupted narrative is ideal for setting up two storytellers to demonstrate story construction and enhance comprehension. One student tells the original tale as it transpires on the pages and the other student tells of the pigs' adventure.

Confirm predictions made before the read-aloud and follow up with another discussion on point of view. Encourage students to give their reasons based on information in the story. Compare the story with Jon Scieszka's book *The True Story of the Three Little Pigs*. (See entry in this catalog.) From whose point of view was that story told?

Have a discussion and ask the students to think about what the author is saying. If necessary, lead the discussion into talking about the borders and boundaries of our own lives and how the concept can be used figuratively when relating it to our own lives. Think about the ways we sometimes get locked into doing and seeing things in the same old way, like an old tale that never changes.

How are the borders of our own lives like the borders in the beginning of the story?

Can we be blown out of the boundaries of our own lives by seeing things in different ways and thinking about different solutions to problems?

The interrupted text also allows two groups of students to work on articulating speech sounds (the same or different sounds) and go back and forth retelling the story while using the correct production of their target phoneme(s) in discourse.

Extended Activity: After the story has been discussed, encourage students to take a "step into a new dimension" and create a different ending to a familiar story. If necessary, pass out classic children's stories to get them started. Once they have an idea in mind, encourage them to write a new edition to an old story. Some questions to consider in writing include the following:

How did the character(s) enter a new dimension?
What words are used to denote "meanwhile"?
What happens in the "meanwhile" to create a different ending?

The True Story of the Three Little Pigs

by Jon Scieszka
New York: Viking Kestrel, 1989

Suggested Grade and Interest Level: 6 through 12

Topic Explorations: Fairy tales and nursery rhymes; Humor; Trickster tales

Skill Builders:
Language literacy
Storytelling
Drawing inferences
Point of view
Discussion

Articulation
Carryover for any sound

Synopsis: Do you know the *real* story of the three little pigs? Mr. Wolf, tired of his longstanding reputation, now brings the true story to light. He just was borrowing a cup of sugar from his neighbor when he sneezed at the doorway. It was not his fault the flimsy little houses fell down.

Method: Before the read-aloud, ask students to recall the original story of *The Three Little Pigs*. (You may want to reread it beforehand.) Break the story into three parts and have one student tell about the pig with the house of straw, another about the pig with the house of sticks, and the third with the house of bricks. (Remind students of the line in the original story, "Little pig, little pig, open up or I'll blow your house down.") Introduce the new book as Mr. Wolf's version of the story.

After the read-aloud, discuss from whose point of view the story is told. What was Mr. Wolf's view of the situation? From whose point of view was the original three little pigs story told? What makes the students think so?

Extended Activity: Stage a prison interview with the wolf. Divide the class into discussion groups representing different news stations. Assign one person to be the wolf and another person to be the prison guard. Each group should come up with a list of 5 to 10 questions for the wolf to answer. One person in each group is selected to be the reporter who interviews the wolf in prison. The reporter can choose the name of a famous reporter such as Larry King, Barbara Walters, or Peter Jennings. The job of the prison guard is to bring the wolf to the reporter and insist on a courteous, respectful interview. The reporter then goes back to the group. The group selects a TV broadcaster to report the interview on the evening news. Then the class simulates the broadcasts of various local news stations.

Have a class discussion on media bias. Which news report presented the facts in the most unbiased way? Which news report appeared to slant the story toward the wolf's version? Which report seemed to slant the story toward the traditional version? What bases do the students have for these opinions?

Tuesday

by David Wiesner
New York: Clarion Books, 1991

Suggested Grade and Interest Level: 6 through 9

Topic Exploration: Careers

Skill Builders:

Grammar and syntax	**Language literacy**	
Advanced syntactic structures	Storytelling	Verbal expression
	Problem solving	Drawing inferences

Synopsis: In this Caldecott award-winning book, pictures tell most of the entertaining tale. As the sun sets on a marshy lake and the moon begins to rise, the stage is set for a curious event: hundreds of frogs atop flying lily pads! Follow their adventures over rooftops, into and out of houses, and down neighborhood streets. Then, when dawn breaks, the party is abruptly over. At least for the frog species it is. Next Tuesday, out by the old barn, something strange begins to happen again. Who can explain these phenomena? This is a good book for encouraging students' imaginations to take flight.

Method: Before the read-aloud, talk about phenomenological events. Elicit students' background knowledge on interesting world events that often are left unexplained. Talk about what happens when such events are discovered.

During the read-aloud, refrain from initiating much interaction if this is the students' first experience with the book. Allow students to quietly connect with the story and form their own thoughts. Then present the book again, asking students to describe what is taking place. Encourage students to draw inferences about the story based on the characters' expressions. For example,

> What might the detective be thinking as he scratches his head?
> What might the reporter be saying to the man being interviewed?
> What might the man in his pajamas be saying to the reporter?

Model and shape advanced syntactic structures. Some examples include

> Although the lily pads were far from the pond, _____ (the detective couldn't figure out how frogs could have flown them; there was no evidence that frogs had flown on them around the neighborhood).

> The man in his pajamas who saw the flying frogs _____ (was talking to the reporter; told the reporter his story).

> The man said, "While I was _____ (having a snack; looking out the window), I saw _____ (frogs flying on lily pads; these frogs fly past the house)."

Extended Activity: Stage a "scene of the crime" interview. Assign various students the roles of police officers, reporters, scientists, criminologists, and eyewitnesses. Conduct interviews and reconvene to solve the mystery. Is the criminal a mad scientist who spills chemicals into the nearby lake? Or maybe this is an experiment conducted by space aliens. Whatever the solution is, there must be a clue.

Up, Up and Away: A Book About Adverbs

by Ruth Heller
New York: Grosset and Dunlap, 1991

Suggested Grade and Interest Level: 6 through 12

Skill Builders:

Vocabulary	Grammar and syntax
Adverbs	Advanced syntactic structures
Morphological units	

Synopsis: In her illustrious style, Ruth Heller shows us how "adverbs work terrifically when answering specifically . . . 'How?' 'How often?' 'When' and 'Where?'" And that is just the beginning.

Method: Before the read-aloud, explain that although many picture books are designed for children, this book is meant for people of all ages because of the way it treats the subject of adverbs. Use the hot air balloons on the book's cover to lead into the topic. Ask students to imagine a hot air balloon. Ask them where such balloons fly, such as over the land, so they can identify some adverbs. Supply the response of "up, up and away," which is the title of the book. Explain that the book gives a great deal of information about adverbs, but the important thing to learn is that our language has rules. Using the various words according to these rules can make the language you use richer.

Read and pause to identify the adverbs in the text. For example, read, "Penguins all dress decently." Identify the adverb. Brainstorm other words that could be used in its place. Some ideas: Penguins all dress elegantly. Penguins all dress formally. Penguins all dress neatly. Expand the sentences to make them richer; for example, Penguins all dress elegantly for a romantic evening on the ice.

Teach embedded sentences by having students practice using adverbial phrases, such as, "On Sunday, when hot air balloons frequently are seen drifting regally into the sky, we like to take a drive to the country."

In addition to focusing on the *–ly* ending on adverbs, teach regular comparative endings (such as *soon, sooner,* and *soonest*) and some irregular forms (such as *bad, worse,* and *worst*).

Extended Activity: After the read-aloud, talk about the roles adverbs and other words play in our language (and in other languages). If we could put language on a stage, we would see a show in which certain words play particular parts.

Use the chalkboard to draw a stage (a large box with curtains across the top and along the sides). Divide the stage into three sections. Label the first section "Nouns," the second section "Verbs," and the third section "Adverbs."

Ask students to name famous people, rare animals, and unique objects they would cast in the "Word Show." They can set the show to background music of they wish. If a student names an entertainer, for example, write the entertainer's name (or group name such as *NSYNC) beneath the heading "Nouns." (Remind students a group is a singular noun.) Ask students what they want the entertainers to do on stage. They can choose a verb from a current magazine if they wish or come up with their own. For example, if they want *NSYNC to perform, write the word *performs* beneath the heading "Verbs." Ask *how* they would like to hear *NSYNC perform. If the response is *brilliantly,* write it beneath the heading "Adverbs" and read across, "*NSYNC performs brilliantly."

Elicit other types of adverbs by asking different questions, such as "How often?" "When?" and "Where?" Once you have made several entries as examples, have students create graphics by drawing an action taking place on the stage or an action they recall from the book. Students can write a sentence containing the adverbial phrase under the drawing and should highlight the adverb with a different style of writing, different color, or other distinctive feature.

Voices of the Alamo

by Sherry Garland
New York: Scholastic Press, 2000

Suggested Grade and Interest Level: 6 through 12

Topic Explorations: Culture and history, American; Culture and history, Native American; History, American

Skill Builders:

Vocabulary	**Language literacy**
Similes and metaphors	Drawing inferences
	Point of view

Synopsis: This picture book for older students gives a dramatic and impressive history of the Alamo from 16 different historical figures, going all the way back to the origins of its land in 1500 up through today. Each person is illustrated and accompanied with a poem in that person's voice, which effectively gives different perspectives on the land. It begins with a Payaya maiden gathering pecans beside the river. As she reflects on the beauty of the land, she intones, "But this earth does not belong to me, for who can own the wind or rain?" The pages leap through time until another person speaks. In 1745, the Spanish padre stands in bare feet and robe in front of the mission built for the Christian work of "saving the souls of the gentle natives here." Regardless of the picture book venue, the poems, subject matter, and style of illustrations make this work suitable for all ages. The author's method of bringing a chronology of historical years into focus by creating meaning from characters' life experiences can be highly effective for the more concrete language learners.

Method: To develop understanding and use of metaphors, point out their use on the pages of each poem and evaluate how effective they are to help understand the thoughts and feelings of the characters.

To build inferencing skills, discuss how the author uses words to imply, rather than state, each person's point of view.

> What caused this person to have this view?
> What is each person's purpose in connection with the land?
> Why is each person's perspective different?
> What has time done to change the pervading thought?
> Which characters do you empathize with and why?

Some suggestions include

In 1803, a Spanish soldier states, "We planted cannon where crosses used to stand."

> What is the significance of this statement?
> What can be inferred?

In 1836, Davy Crockett is featured, a volunteer from Tennessee who came to help his friend James Bowie fight the Mexican army. His poem adds the words, "And maybe get a few acres of land for all our troubles, too."

In 1904, Miss Clara Discoll is featured as she declares that she will buy the Alamo herself if the Daughters of the American Revolution cannot save it. Her reason: "We must never forget the lesson of the Alamo."

> What does Clara Discoll believe was the lesson of the Alamo?
> What does the Alamo stand for?
> What happened during the siege of March 6, 1836?
> What eventually happened after that?

Today, the Alamo reminds people that freedom came with a price and that not everything is won easily.

> To whom does it belong today?
> To whom do you think it rightfully belongs?
> In what parts of the world today do people struggle over rights and territory?
> How does looking at other individuals' unique points of view on an issue such as this give one better understanding and perhaps a different perspective than that which was previously held?

Wilfrid Gordon McDonald Partridge

by Mem Fox
New York: Kane/Miller, 1985, 1989

Suggested Grade and Interest Level: 6 through 12

Topic Explorations: Community; Feelings; Friendship; Memory and remembering

Skill Builders:

Vocabulary	**Language literacy**
Semantics	Relating personal experiences
Similes and metaphors	Storytelling
	Problem solving

Synopsis: This is a warm tale of a boy who lives next to a home for elderly people. Through his special friendship with one of the residents, he helps her regain her memory.

Method: Before the read-aloud, present the book by telling students you are presenting a children's picture book for them to analyze how the author treats the subject of aging. Ask students what they know about elderly people and their memories. Have students define the word *memory*. Briefly give examples of how memories evoke different feelings.

Read aloud, pausing to restate the problem in the story.

After the read-aloud, have students discuss how the author demonstrated the elderly people's unique characteristics in a caring way. Talk about some of the ways the boy helped his elderly friend regain her memory. What were the things that triggered the memories?

The boy in the story found that a memory is something that makes you laugh, makes you cry, and is as precious as gold. Brainstorm as a class other original definitions for *memory*. Ask what happens when you remember something. Have a student recall an experience of remembering something. What feeling did that memory evoke? Have students finish the sentence, "A memory is something that ____." For similes, finish the sentence, "A memory is as precious as ____," with as many different endings as they can think of.

Extended Activity: For high school students, explore the topic of memory and aging by reading aloud from *When I Am Old I Shall Wear Purple: An Anthology of Short Stories and Poetry* (Manhattan Beach, CA: Papier-Mache Press, 1987). Stories and poems that tie in with the theme include "Warning" by Jenny Joseph, "The Trouble with Meals" by Elizabeth Bennett, "Hurricane" by Edna J. Gruttag, "Oh, That Shoestore Used To Be Mine" by Randeane Doolittle Tetu, "Translations" by Margaret H. Carson, and "Litany for a Neighbor" by Ellin Carter.

You also may wish to share another children's picture book about the memories of the elderly, titled *Miss Fannie's Hat,* by well-known adult fiction writer Jan Karon. (See the catalog for Grades 1–5.)

Have students create short poems of their own to explain the essence of memory or aging. Encourage them to make use of similes and to express the feelings they have about experiences with the elderly people in their lives.

The Wretched Stone

by Chris Van Allsburg
Boston: Houghton Mifflin, 1991

Suggested Grade and Interest Level: 6 through 9

Topic Explorations: Boats; Journeys; Literacy

Skill Builders:
Language literacy
Cause-and-effect relationships	Drawing inferences
Storytelling	Point of view
Problem solving	Discussion

Synopsis: Van Allsburg presents a seagoing adventure in his mystical style. Who can explain the glowing stone the crew recovered from an eerie, uncharted island? Stranger still, who can explain its effect on the crew, who are slowly turning into hairy apes? And what makes them so transfixed by the stone? Maybe your students have the answer.

Method: Before the read-aloud, talk about a sea captain's log, what it contains, and how it is like a journal of events at sea. Introduce the story as excerpts from the log of the *Rita Anne.* Ask from whose point of view the story will be told.

Read aloud, pausing to interact about the story elements. Ask students to describe the strange aspects of the story. For example,

> What is it like on board the *Rita Anne*?
> What is it like on the island?
> What is happening to the crew?

Draw inferences about what happened during the storm.

To teach problem solving, pause to identify the facts of the problem.

To teach cause-and-effect relationships, pause to discuss the transformation of the characters. What were they like and what did they do before the stone was found? What were they like after they became transfixed? What caused these changes?

To teach storytelling, encourage students to retell the story, including all the story grammar components. Provide scaffolding as needed. For example,

> Setting: On board the *Rita Anne,* ship sails out of harbor
> Characters: Captain tells of happy crew, singing, dancing, and reading
> Initiating Event: Voyage going well until uncharted island is spotted
> Response: Surprise
> Plan: Go ashore to find fresh supplies
> Consequences: Glowing stone is found
> Plan: Stone taken back to ship
> Consequences: Crew members become transfixed by stone
> Reaction: Behavior changes; lose interest in reading, singing
> Plan: Captain decides to throw rock overboard
> Consequence: Too late; storm comes up and boat is shipwrecked
> Reaction: Crew members on island chagrined, speak little but become themselves again

For discussion, ask if students can think of anything in life that may have a strong enough effect on a person to change that person's behavior or character. Brainstorm ideas. Discuss addictions, if age appropriate. Ask what the symbolism of the stone is. What is the author saying about life?

Extended Activities: Have each student write a story, this time from a crew member's point of view. What was it that happened on board the *Rita Anne*? Describe how it felt. What was it like to become transfixed? Was it really so terrible?

Discuss the shipwreck and how the crew was saved. Describe how they recovered and agreed not to talk about the incident. What did they learn about life? Why do they still have a strange appetite for fruit? Is this a residual effect of the stone? Brainstorm various ideas. Then have students describe subsequent events in journal form. Have them limit their journal entries to 10, recorded over a period of 6 months to a year.

Zin! Zin! Zin! A Violin

by Lloyd Moss
New York: Simon & Schuster Books for Young Readers, 1995

Suggested Grade and Interest Level: 6 through 12

Topic Explorations: Music, musicians, and musical instruments; Number concepts

Skill Builders:

Vocabulary	Grammar and syntax
Semantics	Advanced syntactic structures
Categories	
Adjectives	
Attributes	
Similes and metaphors	
Homonyms (multiple meanings)	

Synopsis: Ten instruments are introduced, one by one, each practicing their musical performance until a 10-piece orchestra is formed. The text of this cleverly written counting book is a literary feast of rhyming couplets while imparting the sounds and soul of classical music. In addition to the descriptions of the instruments, the text gives definitions of numerical groupings. The playful, flowing illustrations that picture eccentric musicians give the reader a sense of excitement about the music that can almost be heard.

Method: Before the read-aloud, present the book, its title, and author, and brainstorm words associated with a violin (which is pictured on the cover). What does the violin sound like? What does it look like? What are its features? Where does one hear a violin? Where is its music played? In what types of music can you hear a violin played? Country? Rock? Folk? Classical? Jazz? Elicit students' background knowledge about music, musical instruments, orchestras, and classical music.

During the read-aloud, let the words of the text speak for themselves as they create (along with the illustrations) the beautiful musical quality of the book. See if students notice two cats, a mouse, and a dog enjoying the music along with the audience.

After the read-aloud, to enhance vocabulary, go back over the pages and look for the words of musical groupings, which include

solo	quintet	nonet
duo	sextet	chamber group
trio	octet	orchestra
quartet		

Review the meanings of the words and ask the students to use the words in a sentence. (More methods are listed below.) Some possible sentences to shape or prompt include

> A solo is when one musical instrument is played alone.
> A duo is when two musical instruments are played together.
> A quintet is a musical group of five.
> A chamber group is made up of 10 musicians.

To develop vocabulary, especially adjectives, encourage students to use the words from the text in language that describes the sounds of the instruments. Distinguish between what the instrument looks and sounds like. Use the text, illustrations, and students' background information, if possible, to describe the instruments and their sounds. For example,

What words can you use to describe a trombone?

> shiny   brassy
> long   elegant

What words does the author use to describe the *sound* of a trombone? (Reread the text if necessary.)

> mournful moan
> silken tone

Expand the words and combine them into a sentence, making use of the similes. For example,

> It sounds like a mournful moan.
> It has a silken tone.
> It sounds like a mournful moan with a silken tone.

Put words from the text into phrases and have the students finish the sentence, using a pattern at first. Have students create phrases out of the adjectives, and assist in developing embedded sentences and other advanced syntactic structures.

Use adjectives from the text in an adverbial phrase and have the students finish the sentence with the word for the numerical grouping from the text. Examples include

> With mournful moan and a silken tone, _____ (the trombone plays in a solo).
> Singing and stinging its swinging song, _____ (the trumpet plays in a duo).
> Bright and brassy, with valves all oiled, _____ (the French horn plays in a trio).

More possible constructions:

> A mellow friend with neck extended, the cello plays in a quintet.
> Soaring high and moving in, the violin plays in a quintet.
> The musician plays the slender, silver flute.
> Sending our soul a-shiver, the flute plays in a sextet.
> The musician plays the slender flute, sending our souls a-shiver.
> Sending our souls a-shiver, the musician plays the slender, silver flute in a sextet.

Here is an example with a metaphor:

> The bassoon, the lazy clown of the orchestra, sounds low-down and grumpy.

How does the author describe the sound of an oboe?

gleeful
sobbing

bleating
pleading

The oboe, gleeful and bleating, joined the other instruments.
Gleeful and bleating, the oboe joined the other instruments.
In joining the other instruments, the oboe sounded gleeful and bleating.

For teaching homonyms, first use homophone pairs, one of which can be associated with the musical theme. Make sentences that express their meaning. Some include

hear, here
rap, wrap
liar, lyre
sole, soul

beat, beet
chord, cord
metal, meddle, medal

Also use the homographs of the musical theme, including

bow (as in bow to the audience in recognition; the forward of a ship)
bow (as in the bow of a violin; a bow tie)
key (as in key in which it is played; something that goes in a lock)
band (a group of instrumentalists; a ring such as a wedding band or material that binds, such as a band around carrots or lettuce. Also note that sound is referred to in bands, such as frequency bands. A set of radio frequencies is called a band.)
rock (a style of music; rock a baby back and forth)
roll (rolling motion; a breakfast item)
hand (as in the audience gave him a hand; the hand at the end of your arm)
note (musical note; note to a friend)
jam (a meeting of musicians to play for their own enjoyment, or an impromptu performance by a group of musicians who do not normally play together; a fruit preserve to eat on toast; to press or squeeze together, such as people jammed into a room)
pick (a small object used for plucking the strings of a stringed instrument; to select or choose)
scale (a succession of musical notes according to fixed intervals; an instrument to measure weight)
pop (form of music; a quick, loud noise; a drink)
wind (category of musical instruments; the movement of air)
reed (category of musical instruments; a long sheaf of grass)
strings (category of musical instruments played with a bow; something with which to tie up a package; *to pull strings* means to use one's influence)

The book also teaches the categories into which the instruments are placed: strings, reeds, and brasses. (See above for homonyms.) Help students group instruments, musical styles, musical performances, musical groups, musical events, and musical locations into different categories to help develop organizational strategies. Then present lists of items in a category with an additional word that does not belong. Ask students to tell which word does not belong and why. Some examples:

violin, guitar, oboe, CD (CD does not belong because it is not a musical instrument.)
jazz, country western, Aerosmith, rap (Aerosmith does not belong because it is a rock group, not a type of music.)
grocery store, amphitheater, concert hall, auditorium (Grocery store does not belong because live music is not played there.)

For comprehension and usage of more complex syntactical forms, help students build embedded sentences and shape structures with their adjective phrases. Possible sentence variations include

> The shiny trombone, sounding like a mournful moan, was played by the musician.
> Sounding like a mournful moan, the shiny trombone was played by the musician.

On another page, the text reads,

> "Fine FRENCH HORN, its valves all oiled
> Bright and brassy, loops all coiled
> Golden yellow, joins its fellows
> TWO, now THREE-O, what a TRIO!"

Ask,

How does the author describe a French horn?

Possible responses are

> Golden yellow with coiled loops
> With valves all oiled

Prompt students with a beginning sentence, then have them use their descriptions to form embedded phrases. Two possible sentence are

> The fine French horn, golden yellow with coiled loops, was played by the musician.
> The bright, brassy French horn, with valves all oiled, joined the other instruments.

Use one complex sentence as a template and map words from other verses onto it, such as

> The steely keys of the clarinet, its breezy notes so darkly slick, joined the other instruments.

Section 4

Parent Conference and Inservice Handouts

60 Recommended Picture Books for Children in Preschool and Kindergarten

Abuela
by Arthur Dorros
New York: Puffin Books, 1991

Alfie Gets in First
by Shirley Hughes
New York: Lothrop, Lee & Shepard
    Books, 1981, 1987

*Anansi the Spider: A Tale from the
    Ashanti*
Retold by Gerald McDermott
New York: Henry Holt, 1972

Annie and the Wild Animals
by Jan Brett
Boston: Houghton Mifflin, 1985,
    1989

*Antarctic Antics: A Book of
    Penguin Poems*
by Judy Sierra
San Diego, CA: Gulliver Books,
    1998

Big Fat Hen
by Keith Baker
San Diego, CA: Harcourt, 1997

Big Red Barn
by Margaret Wise Brown
New York: Scott, 1956;
    HarperCollins, 1989 (rev. ed.);
    HarperCollins, 1991

*Brown Bear, Brown Bear, What Do
    You See?*
by Bill Martin Jr.
Orlando, FL: Holt, Rinehart &
    Winston, 1967, 1983

*Caps for Sale: A Tale of a Peddler,
    Some Monkeys and Their
    Monkey Business*
by Esphyr Slobodkina
New York: Harper & Row, 1940,
    1947, 1968; Scholastic, 1987

Chicka Chicka Boom Boom
by Bill Martin Jr. and John
    Archambault
New York: Simon & Schuster
    Books for Young Readers,
    1989

Chicken Soup with Rice
by Maurice Sendak
New York: Harper & Row, 1962;
    Scholastic, 1986, 1991

Click, Clack, Moo: Cows That Type
by Doreen Cronin
New York: Simon & Schuster
    Books for Young Readers,
    2000

Corduroy
by Don Freeman
New York: Viking, 1968, 1993

Counting Crocodiles
by Judy Sierra
New York: Scholastic, 1997

Cowboy Baby
by Sue Heap
Cambridge, MA: Candlewick Press,
    1998

A Dark, Dark Tale
by Ruth Brown
New York: Dial Books for Young
    Readers, 1981, 1984

Don't Forget the Bacon
by Pat Hutchins
New York: Greenwillow Books,
    1976

Each Peach Pear Plum
by Janet and Allan Ahlberg
New York: Viking Kestrel, 1978,
    1992

*Eating the Alphabet: Fruits and
    Vegetables from A to Z*
by Lois Ehlert
San Diego, CA: Harcourt, 1989

The Empty Pot
by Demi
New York: Henry Holt & Company,
    1990; Owlet, 1996

HANDOUTS

The Foolish Tortoise
by Richard Buckley
Saxonville, MA: Picture Book
    Studio, 1985

Frederick
by Leo Lionni
New York: Knopf, 1967; Dragonfly
    Books, 1995

Gabriella's Song
by Candace Fleming
New York: Simon & Schuster, 1997;
    Aladdin Paperbacks, 2001

Geraldine's Blanket
by Holly Keller
New York: Greenwillow Books,
    1984; Morrow, 1988

Good Night, Gorilla
by Peggy Rathmann
New York: Putnam, 1994

Good-Night, Owl!
by Pat Hutchins
New York: Macmillan, 1972;
    Aladdin, 1990

The Grouchy Ladybug
by Eric Carle
New York: Harper & Row, 1977;
    HarperCollins, 1986

Growing Vegetable Soup
by Lois Ehlert
New York: Harcourt Brace
    Jovanovich, 1987

The Gruffalo
by Julia Donaldson
New York: Dial Books for Young
    Readers, 1999

I Know an Old Lady Who Swallowed
    a Fly
Illustrated by Stephen Gulbis
New York: Scholastic, 2001

I Went Walking
by Sue Williams
New York: Gulliver Books, 1989,
    1991, 1992

The Important Book
by Margaret Wise Brown
New York: Harper & Row, 1949

Is Your Mama a Llama?
by Deborah Guarino
New York: Scholastic, 1989, 1991,
    1992

It Looked Like Spilt Milk
by Charles G. Shaw
New York: Harper & Row, 1947,
    1988

It's the Bear!
by Jez Alborough
Cambridge, MA: Candlewick Press,
    1994

Jamberry
by Bruce Degen
New York: Harper & Row, 1983;
    Scholastic, 1990, 1992

King Bidgood's in the Bathtub
by Audrey Wood
San Diego, CA: Harcourt Brace
    Jovanovich, 1985, 1993

Little Green
by Keith Baker
San Diego, CA: Harcourt,
    2001

Mama Cat Has Three Kittens
by Denise Fleming
New York: Henrt Holt & Company,
    1998

Mammalabilia
by Douglas Florian
San Diego, CA: Harcourt,
    2000

The Mixed-Up Chameleon
by Eric Carle
New York: HarperCollins, 1975,
    1984, 1988

The Napping House
by Audrey Wood
San Diego, CA: Harcourt Brace
    Jovanovich, 1984, 1991

Night in the Country
by Cynthia Rylant
New York: Bradbury Press, 1986;
    Macmillan, 1991

Peter's Chair
by Ezra Jack Keats
New York: Harper & Row, 1967,
    1983

Planting a Rainbow
by Lois Ehlert
New York: Harcourt Brace
    Jovanovich, 1988, 1992

Polar Bear, Polar Bear, What Do
    You Hear?
by Bill Martin Jr.
New York: Henry Holt, 1991;
    Scholastic, 1992, 1993

Quack and Count
by Keith Baker
San Diego, CA: Harcourt, 1999

Quick as a Cricket
by Don Wood
Swindon, England: Child's Play
    International, 1990

Rosie's Walk
by Pat Hutchins
New York: Macmillan, 1968, 1971

The Secret Birthday Message
by Eric Carle
New York: Crowell, 1971, 1986

Silly Sally
by Audrey Wood
San Diego, CA: Harcourt Brace,
    1992

The Snowy Day
by Ezra Jack Keats
New York: Viking, 1962, 1976

Suddenly!
by Colin McNaughton
San Diego, CA: Voyager Books,
    Harcourt Brace, 1998

Swimmy
by Leo Lionni
New York: Pantheon, 1963; Knopf,
    1987

Ten, Nine, Eight
by Molly Bang
New York: Greenwillow Books,
   1983, 1991

*The Thing That Bothered Farmer
   Brown*
by Teri Sloat
New York: Orchard Books, 1995;
   First Orchard Paperbacks, 2001

The Very Busy Spider
by Eric Carle
New York: Philomel Books,
   1984

The Very Lonely Firefly
by Eric Carle
New York: Philomel Books,
   1995

Where Once There Was a Wood
by Denise Fleming
New York: Henry Holt, 1996

Where's My Teddy?
by Jez Alborough
London: Walker Books, 1992;
   Cambridge, MA: Candlewick
   Press, 1994

50 Recommended Low-Text Picture Books for Children in Elementary School

The Adventures of Taxi Dog
by Debra and Sal Barracca
New York: Dial Books for Young
    Readers, 1990

A Bad Case of Stripes
by David Shannon
New York: Blue Sky Press, 1998

Barn Dance!
by Bill Martin Jr. and John
    Archambault
New York: Henry Holt, 1986

Beast Feast
by Douglas Florian
San Diego, CA: Harcourt, 1994

A Chair for My Mother
by Vera B. Williams
New York: Greenwillow Books,
    1982, 1988, 1993

Chato's Kitchen
by Gary Soto
New York: Putnam, 1995

Come On, Rain
by Karen Hesse
New York: Scholastic, 1999

The Dalai Lama
by Demi
New York: Holt, 1998

*Dog Breath: The Horrible Trouble
    with Hally Tosis*
by Dav Pilkey
New York: Scholastic, 1994

Dogteam
by Gary and Ruth Paulsen
New York: Delacorte Press,
    1993

Fortunately
by Remy Charlip
New York: Parents Magazine Press,
    1964; Aladdin, 1993

The Gardener
by Sarah Stewart
New York: Farrar, Straus & Giroux,
    1997; Sunburst, 2000

George and Martha: Back in Town
    (and others in the series)
by James Marshall
Boston: Houghton Mifflin, 1984

George Washington's Cows
by David Small
New York: Farrar, Straus & Giroux,
    1994; Sunburst, 1997

Grandfather's Journey
by Allen Say
Boston: Houghton Mifflin, 1993

Here Come the Aliens!
by Colin McNaughton
Cambridge, MA: Candlewick
    Press, 1995

Hey, Al
by Arthur Yorinks
New York: Farrar, Straus & Giroux,
    1986

Hey! Get Off Our Train
by John Burningham
New York: Crown, 1989, 1990

Home Run
by Robert Burleigh
San Diego, CA: Silver Whistle,
    Harcourt Brace, 1998

Imogene's Antlers
by David Small
New York: Dragonfly Books, 1985

Insectlopedia
by Douglas Florian
San Diego, CA: Harcourt, 1998

The Journey
by Sarah Stewart
New York: Farrar, Straus & Giroux,
    2001

The Legend of Indian Paintbrush
by Tomie de Paola
New York: Putnam, 1991

Martha Speaks (and others in the
    series)
by Susan Meddaugh
Boston: Houghton Mifflin, 1992

Meanwhile
by Jules Feiffer
New York: Michael di Capua Books,
    HarperCollins, 1997

Miss Fannie's Hat
by Jan Karon
Minneapolis, MN: Augsburg
    Fortress, 1998; New York:
    Puffin Books, 2001

Mr. Gumpy's Outing
by John Burningham
Orlando, FL: Holt, Rinehart &
    Winston, 1978, 1990

Officer Buckle and Gloria
by Peggy Rathmann
New York: Putnam, 1995

Owl Moon
by Jane Yolen
New York: Putnam, 1987

Piggie Pie
by Margie Palatini
New York: Houghton Mifflin, 1995

Pigsty
by Mark Teague
New York: Scholastic, 1994

The Rain Came Down
by David Shannon
New York: Scholastic, 2000

Rain Makes Applesauce
by Julian Scheer and Marvin Bileck
New York: Holiday House, 1964

The Relatives Came
by Cynthia Rylant
New York: Bradbury Press, 1985,
    1993

The Secret Shortcut
by David Shannon
New York: Scholastic, 1996

Sector 7
by David Wiesner
New York: Clarion Books, 1999

Seven Brave Women
by Betsy Gould Hearne
New York: Greenwillow Books,
    1997

Sheep in a Jeep (and others in the
    series)
by Nancy Shaw
Boston: Houghton Mifflin, 1986

*The Tenth Good Thing About
    Barney*
by Judith Viorst
New York: Atheneum, 1971, 1987

This Land Is Your Land
Words and music by Woody
    Guthrie
Illustrated by Kathy Jacobsen
New York: Little, Brown, 1998

The Three Pigs
by David Wiesner
New York: Clarion Books, 2001

Too Many Tamales
by Gary Soto
New York: Putnam, 1993

Tough Boris
by Mem Fox
San Diego, CA: Harcourt Brace,
    1994

When I Was Young in the Mountains
by Cynthia Rylant
New York: Dutton Children's
    Books, 1982

The Wind Blew
by Pat Hutchins
New York: Puffin Books, 1974,
    1986

Would You Rather . . .
by John Burningham
New York: Crowell, 1978

The Wretched Stone
by Chris Van Allsburg
Boston: Houghton Mifflin, 1991

*You Can't Take a Balloon Into the
    Metropolitan Museum*
by Jacquiline Preiss Weitzman
New York: Dial Books for Young
    Readers, 1998

*You Forgot Your Skirt, Amelia
    Bloomer*
by Shana Corey
New York: Scholastic Press, 2000

Zin! Zin! Zin! A Violin
by Lloyd Moss
New York: Simon & Schuster Books
    for Young Readers, 1995

HANDOUTS

Reading Aloud to Young Children To Promote Emergent Literacy

A child can begin the reading process long before entering school. Thanks to many research studies, it is now known that reading is a *process of development* that emerges very early in life. This period of early literacy development begins at birth and continues until the child enters school. Your child's experiences, both at home and in preschool, help to prepare him or her to read before formal instruction begins.

The Value of Parents and Caregivers

There are many things that parents and caregivers can do to promote a child's growth during the early literacy years, including the following:

Create rich language experiences. The American Speech-Language-Hearing Association (ASHA, 2001) states that spoken language provides an important foundation for the development of reading and writing. To encourage your child's language development, talk in short, simple sentences. Give objects names. Describe objects and things in the world around you and your child. Tell stories, sing songs, and recite lots of poems and nursery rhymes.

Encourage your child to talk with you. Responding to your baby's coos and efforts to communicate is important. As your baby continues to grow and learns to say new words, continue to engage him or her in the give-and-take play of conversation. As your young child continues to grow, engage in extended conversations and continue to discover and talk about new words.

Read aloud from day one. Reading stories to your baby will help him or her hear the sound of your voice, the sounds of speech, and the rhythms and intonations of words in print. The National Research Council (Snow, Burns, & Griffin, 1998) has shown that reading regularly to a child has a direct benefit on his or her eventual success in reading. Hall and Moats (1999) have stated that reading aloud helps your child to

- develop background knowledge on a variety of topics,
- build vocabulary skills,
- become knowledgeable about the language of literature and the characteristics of stories,
- become familiar with the reading process, and
- identify reading as an enjoyable pastime.

Keep reading material where it can be seen. Children develop an awareness of the world of print from seeing books, magazines, and other printed material in the home and from seeing their parents engage in their own reading activities. They learn that books are important to adults and that print carries meaning.

Joint Book Talk

Talking about what you read is one way to help your child develop language and thinking skills and to promote growth during the early literacy years. In 1985, the Commission on Reading of the National Academy of Education referred to reading aloud, coupled with the activity of talking and sharing the information in stories, as the "single most important activity for developing the knowledge required for eventual success in reading (Anderson, Hiebert, Scott & Wilkinson, 1985, p. 23). The American Speech-Language-Hearing Association (ASHA, 2001) endorses joint book reading as an activity that promotes opportunities for eventual success in spoken and written language. Here are some suggestions and guidelines for using books for talking, too:

Discuss unknown words. This helps to build vocabulary and background knowledge and also helps your child to connect the story to his or her own world. Here are some steps to follow, using an example from *The Adventures of Taxi Dog*. The text reads,

> "I roamed all around."

- Find out if your child knows the word in question. For example, ask

> "Do you know what *roam* means?"

- Look for clues in the sentence. For example, reread the text that tells about Maxi growing up in the city looking for food. Your child can guess the meaning.
- Define the word. For example, say

> "That's very close. It means *to wander*. He walked around with no aim to get anywhere."

- Use it in a sentence. For example, say

> "You could say, 'Maxi roamed the streets looking for food.'"

- Link it to your child's own life and experiences. For example, say

> "Our doggie has a home and her own dish, so she doesn't need to roam around the neighborhood."

Read slowly and pause now and then to think out loud about the story.

- Talk about actions taking place.

> "Look what Maxi is doing!"

- Point out details that add meaning to the story.

> "Maxi finished eating all the food on his plate. Look how he's licking Jim. He's glad Jim is taking care of him."

- Relate the meaning to your child's own experiences.

> "Look how Jim and Maxi are waiting at the airport for someone who needs a ride. Remember how we got grandma and grandpa at the airport? There were taxis there, too."

- Ask open-ended questions, such as

> "Maxi entertains the passengers in the back seat. How do you _____?"
>
> "How do we know Jim's boss likes Maxi?"

rather than questions that can only be answered with a *yes* or *no* response.

- Ask questions that encourage your child to predict what might come next, such as

HANDOUTS

"I wonder what's going to happen now?"

Answer your child's questions. Don't be afraid to have the child take the lead. Talking about the stories you read helps your child to learn new words, adds to his or her background information, and links stories to real things your child has experienced. It also helps your child to better understand the story you are reading together.

References

American Speech-Language-Hearing Association. (2001). *Roles and responsibilities of speech–language pathologists with respect to reading and writing in children and adolescents* (guidelines). Rockville, MD: Author.

Anderson, R. C., Hiebert, E. H., Scott, J. A., & Wilkinson, I. A. G. (1985). *Becoming a nation of readers: The report of the Commission on Reading.* Washington, DC: National Academy of Education, Commission on Education and Public Policy.

Hall, S. L., & Moats, L. C. (1999). *Straight talk about reading: How parents can make a difference during the early years.* Chicago: Contemporary Books.

Snow, C. E., Burns, M. S., & Griffin, P. (Eds.). (1998). *Preventing reading difficulties in young children.* Washington, DC: National Academy Press.

HANDOUTS

Using Picture Books To Practice Articulation

Many children mispronounce certain speech sounds. For instance, *rabbit* may sound like *wabbit,* and *lollipop* may sound like *yawyeepop.* Using picture books is a good way to help your child practice correct sounds while reading and discussing what's happening in the illustrations.

Be sure that your child has practiced enough with the speech-language pathologist that he or she can hear and easily correct speech-sound errors. You may want to read the text and have your child repeat particular words that contain his or her speech sound (patterned books are especially good for this). For instance, after becoming familiar with the repeated phrases in *Chicken Soup with Rice* ("Going once, going twice, going chicken soup with rice"), your child will be able to repeat the phrases automatically from memory. Or, have your child read the book to you using the new speech sound. If recommended by the speech-language pathologist, you can have your child use the sound while talking about the book and illustrations.

Most picture books that have long narratives are not as suitable for practicing articulation. Here is a list of books that will encourage lots of speech—wordless picture books, books with shorter texts, and books loaded with a particular sound.

For the *K* Sound

Caps for Sale: A Tale of a Peddler, Some Monkeys and Their Monkey Business
by Esphyr Slobodkina
New York: Harper & Row, 1940, 1947, 1968; Scholastic, 1987

The Carrot Seed
by Ruth Krauss
New York: Harper & Row, 1945, 1989; Scholastic, 1993

Chicka Chicka Boom Boom
by Bill Martin Jr. and John Archambault
New York: Simon & Schuster Books for Young Readers, 1989

Chicken Soup with Rice
by Maurice Sendak
New York: Harper & Row, 1962; Scholastic, 1986, 1991

Click, Clack, Moo: Cows That Type
by Doreen Cronin
New York: Simon & Schuster Books for Young Readers, 2000

Corduroy
by Don Freeman
New York: Viking, 1968, 1993

Counting Crocodiles
by Judy Sierra
New York: Scholastic, 1997

A Dark, Dark Tale
by Ruth Brown
New York: Dial Books for Young Readers, 1981, 1984

Don't Fidget a Feather!
by Erica Silverman
New York: Simon & Schuster Books for Young Readers, 1994

Don't Forget the Bacon
by Pat Hutchins
New York: Greenwillow Books, 1976

Farmer Duck
by Martin Waddell
Cambridge, MA: Candlewick Press, 1992

Good Dog, Carl (and others in the series)
by Alexandra Day
La Jolla, CA: Green Tiger Press, 1985

I Went Walking
by Sue Williams
New York: Gulliver Books, 1989, 1991, 1992

Is Your Mama a Llama?
by Deborah Guarino
New York: Scholastic, 1989, 1991, 1992

Jesse Bear, What Will You Wear?
by Nancy White Carlstrom
New York: Macmillan, 1986

King Bidgood's in the Bathtub
by Audrey Wood
San Diego, CA: Harcourt Brace Jovanovich, 1985, 1993

May I Bring a Friend?
by Beatrice Schenk de Regniers
New York: Atheneum, 1964, 1971, 1989

The Mitten: A Ukrainian Folktale
by Jan Brett
New York: Putnam, 1989, 1990

My Mama Says . . .
by Judith Viorst
New York: Atheneum, 1975, 1987

Pancakes for Breakfast
by Tomie de Paola
New York: Harcourt Brace Jovanovich, 1978

Rosie's Walk
by Pat Hutchins
New York: Macmillan, 1968, 1971

For the *F* Sound

Annie and the Wild Animals
by Jan Brett
Boston: Houghton Mifflin, 1985, 1989

Deep in the Forest
by Brinton Turkle
New York: Dutton, 1976

Don't Fidget a Feather!
by Erica Silverman
New York: Simon & Schuster Books for Young Readers, 1994

Don't Forget the Bacon
by Pat Hutchins
New York: Greenwillow Books, 1976

Farmer Duck
by Martin Waddell
Cambridge, MA: Candlewick Press, 1992

For Laughing Outloud: Poems To Tickle Your Funnybone
Compiled by Jack Prelutsky
New York: Knopf, 1991

Fortunately
by Remy Charlip
New York: Parents Magazine Press, 1964; Aladdin, 1993

Frederick
by Leo Lionni
New York: Knopf, 1967; Dragonfly Books, 1995

Frog on His Own
by Mercer Mayer
New York: Dial Books for Young Readers, 1973, 1980

The Grouchy Ladybug
by Eric Carle
New York: Harper & Row, 1977; HarperCollins, 1986

Old MacDonald Had a Farm (and other authors' versions of this tale)
by Colin Hawkins and Jacqui Hawkins
New York: Price, Stern, 1991

One Fine Day
by Nonny Hogrogian
New York: Macmillan, 1971, 1974

The Snopp on the Sidewalk and Other Poems
by Jack Prelutsky
New York: Greenwillow Books, 1976, 1977

For the *L* Sound

Good-Night, Owl!
by Pat Hutchins
New York: Macmillan, 1972; Aladdin, 1990

Here Come the Aliens!
by Colin McNaughton
Cambridge, MA: Candlewick Press, 1995

Leo the Late Bloomer
by Robert Kraus
Old Tappan, NJ: Windmill Books, 1971, 1993

Lilly's Purple Plastic Purse
by Kevin Henkes
New York: Greenwillow Books, 1996

Liza Lou and the Yeller Belly Swamp
by Mercer Mayer
New York: Macmillan, 1976

London Bridge Is Falling Down
by Peter Spier
New York: Doubleday, 1967, 1985

Lovable Lyle (and others in the series)
by Bernard Waber
Boston: Houghton Mifflin, 1969

Pickle Things
by Marc Brown
New York: Parents Magazine Press, 1980

The Snopp on the Sidewalk and Other Poems
by Jack Prelutsky
New York: Greenwillow Books, 1976, 1977

There's an Alligator Under My Bed
by Mercer Mayer
New York: Dial Books for Young Readers, 1987

You Can't Take a Balloon Into the Metropolitan Museum
by Jacquiline Preiss Weitzman
New York: Dial Books for Young Readers, 1998

For the *R* Sound

Animalia
by Graeme Base
New York: Abrams, 1986, 1987

Arthur's Nose (and others in the series)
by Marc Brown
Boston: Little, Brown, 1976, 1986

Chato's Kitchen
by Gary Soto
New York: Putnam, 1995

Chicken Soup with Rice
by Maurice Sendak
New York: Harper & Row, 1962; Scholastic, 1986, 1991

George and Martha: Back in Town (and others in the series)
by James Marshall
Boston: Houghton Mifflin, 1984

Grandfather's Journey
by Allen Say
Boston: Houghton Mifflin, 1993

Harry the Dirty Dog
by Gene Zion
New York: Harper & Row, 1956, 1976

Hester
by Byron Barton
New York: Greenwillow Books, 1975

Lilly's Purple Plastic Purse
by Kevin Henkes
New York: Greenwillow Books, 1996

The Paper Crane
by Molly Bang
New York: Greenwillow Books, 1985; Morrow, 1987

Rain Makes Applesauce
by Julian Scheer and Marvin Bileck
New York: Holiday House, 1964

The Rain Came Down
by David Shannon
New York: Scholastic, 2000

Robot-Bot-Bot
by Fernando Krahn
New York: Dutton, 1979

Rotten Ralph
by Jack Gantos
Boston: Houghton Mifflin, 1976, 1980

The Thing That Bothered Farmer Brown
by Teri Sloat
New York: Orchard Books, 1995; First Orchard Paperbacks, 2001

The Treasure
by Uri Shulevitz
New York: Farrar, Straus & Giroux, 1978, 1986

There's an Alligator Under My Bed
by Mercer Mayer
New York: Dial Books for Young Readers, 1987

You Forgot Your Skirt, Amelia Bloomer
by Shana Corey
New York: Scholastic Press, 2000

For the *S* and *Z* Sounds

Alexander and the Terrible, Horrible, No Good, Very Bad Day
by Judith Viorst
New York: Atheneum, 1972, 1987

Animalia
by Graeme Base
New York: Abrams, 1986, 1987

Anansi the Spider: A Tale from the Ashanti
Retold by Gerald McDermott
New York: Henry Holt, 1972

Arthur's Nose (and others in the series)
by Marc Brown
Boston: Little, Brown, 1976, 1986

Berlioz the Bear
by Jan Brett
New York: Putnam, 1991; Scholastic, 1992

Caps for Sale: A Tale of a Peddler, Some Monkeys and Their Monkey Business
by Esphyr Slobodkina
New York: Harper & Row, 1940, 1947, 1968; Scholastic, 1987

Chicken Soup with Rice
by Maurice Sendak
New York: Harper & Row, 1962; Scholastic, 1986, 1991

Frog on His Own (and others in the series)
by Mercer Mayer
New York: Dial Books for Young Readers, 1973, 1980

Here Come the Aliens!
by Colin McNaughton
Cambridge, MA: Candlewick Press, 1995

Miss Nelson Is Missing! (and others in the series)
by Harry Allard and James Marshall
Boston: Houghton Mifflin, 1977, 1985

The Mitten: A Ukrainian Folktale
by Jan Brett
New York: Putnam, 1989, 1990

HANDOUTS

My Mama Says . . .
by Judith Viorst
New York: Atheneum, 1975, 1987

Rain Makes Applesauce
by Julian Scheer and Marvin Bileck
New York: Holiday House, 1964

Scary, Scary Halloween
by Eve Bunting
New York: Clarion, 1986

Sing, Sophie!
by Dayle Ann Dodds
Cambridge, MA: Candlewick Press,
   1997, 1999

Six Creepy Sheep
by Judith R. Enderle and Stephanie
   G. Tessler
New York: Puffin Books, 1993

*The Snopp on the Sidewalk and
   Other Poems*
by Jack Prelutsky
New York: Greenwillow Books,
   1976, 1977

Snow
by Uri Shulevitz
New York: Farrar, Straus & Giroux,
   1988, 1999

The Snowy Day
by Ezra Jack Keats
New York: Viking, 1962, 1976

Someday
by Charlotte Zolotow
New York: Harper & Row, 1965,
   1989

Suddenly!
by Colin McNaughton
San Diego, CA: Voyager, Harcourt
   Brace, 1998

Swimmy
by Leo Lionni
New York: Pantheon, 1963; Knopf,
   1987

Would You Rather . . .
by John Burningham
New York: Crowell, 1978

Books Are for Talking, Too! • © 2003 by PRO-ED, Inc.

Using Picture Books
To Practice Present Tense
(with Examples from *Goodnight Moon*)

Present tense is the *is/am/are doing* part of a sentence. Many children omit the helping verb and say sentences such as, "Bunny going bed."

Parents can help their child develop spoken language skills by reading and talking about the activities taking place in the story. The American Speech-Language-Hearing Association (ASHA, 2001) endorses joint book reading as an activity that promotes a child's success in spoken language interactions. Researchers have found that when children actively participate in the story, their sentence length expands and their language expression improves (Arnold & Whitehurst, 1994; Hall & Moats, 1999; Snow, Burns, & Griffin, 1998). This includes, among other language skills, constructing sentences with present-tense forms.

The following are tips for practicing present tense:

1. Stress the helping verb to draw the child's attention to it (e.g., "That's right, the bunny *is* going to bed").

2. Encourage the child to repeat your sentence. (e.g., Can you say, The bunny *is* going to bed?) If you're practicing the *is doing* form, just try to get that form right. Don't worry about other mistakes in the child's sentence.

3. When you hear the child say a sentence correctly, repeat it and draw the child's attention to "good speech" (e.g., "Yes, I can see the bunny is going to bed").

4. Talk to communicate. Always respond first to what the child means, then to the form of the sentence. You can *model,* or give an example of, the correct sentence.

5. Let the child know that you are pleased when you hear good talking. Then the child will know that good talking is important to you.

6. Use open-ended questions. For example, if you ask, "Where's the mouse?" the child will probably answer, "Under the bed." But, if you say, "I can't see the mouse," the child is more likely to say, "It's hiding under the bed."

7. Shorten longer sentences if you want the child to repeat them.

8. Be sensitive to your child's interest in the story. For example, it may be appropriate to read without pausing for interaction, especially the first time reading a story with rhyming text. Then reread the story on another occasion and pause at appropriate places to model sentences and encourage participation.

9. Take the child's lead when it comes to conversation. Children learn best when the topic is of interest to them. Don't be afraid of getting sidetracked when reading the story if it means that you can use the opportunity to create new learning experiences.

10. If possible, model sentences based on the illustrations, so that the child can "see what you're talking about."

An Activity You Can Do

Read aloud *Goodnight Moon,* by Margaret Wise Brown. Because the illustrations are similar throughout the book (one green nursery room), the child will pay attention to all the activities in the room.

The text doesn't have *is doing* sentences. However, you will find it natural to use the *is doing* form as you talk about the pictures.

Read the text.

> "And two little kittens
>
> And a pair of mittens
>
> And a little toy house
>
> And a young mouse."

Have the child point out, name, and talk about the kittens and mittens, the toy house, and the mouse. Stress the rhyming words. Say, "Listen, *kitten* and *mitten* sound almost the same. *Kitten, mitten.*"

Then, talk about other things you can see in the picture. Here are some sentences you might use:

> The fire is burning.
>
> The clock is ticking.

Continue reading the text while the child listens. When you reach the next room scene, point out the things that have changed.

> The bunny is resting (in his bed).
>
> The old lady is rocking (in her chair).

Then, make a game of searching for the mouse in each of the green room scenes. Continue reading until the next scene, then model more *is doing* sentences like these:

> The fire is burning.
>
> The clock is ticking.
>
> The moon is rising.
>
> The bunny is saying "goodnight."

References

American Speech-Language-Hearing Association. (2001). *Roles and responsibilities of speech-language pathologists with respect to reading and writing in children and adolescents* (guidelines). Rockville, MD: Author.

Arnold, D. S., & Whitehurst, G. J. (1994). Accelerating language development through picture book reading: A summary of dialogic reading and its effects. In D. K. Dickinson (Ed.), *Bridges to literacy: Children, families, and schools* (pp. 103–128). Cambridge, MA: Basil Blackwell.

Hall, S. L., & Moats, L. C. (1999). *Straight talk about reading: How parents can make a difference during the early years.* Chicago: Contemporary Books.

Snow, C. E., Burns, M. S., & Griffin, P. (Eds.). (1998). *Preventing reading difficulties in young children.* Washington, DC: National Academy Press.

Using Picture Books To Practice Past Tense
(with Examples from
Where the Wild Things Are)

Past tense is the *–ed* form of verbs, as in *walked*. Many common verbs used every day have irregular past tenses, such as *sat, ran, ate,* and so on.

Parents can help their child develop spoken language skills by reading and talking about the activities taking place in the story. The American Speech-Language-Hearing Association (ASHA, 2001) endorses joint book reading as an activity that promotes a child's success in spoken language interactions. Researchers have found that when children actively participate in the story, their sentence length expands and their verbal expression improves (Arnold & Whitehurst, 1994; Hall & Moats, 1999; Snow, Burns, & Griffin, 1998). This includes, among other language skills, constructing sentences in the past-tense form.

The following are tips for practicing past tense:

1. As the child learns the *–ed* form, he or she may begin to say *eated* instead of *ate.* Don't worry; this is normal.

2. The *–ed* form is hard to hear. When helping your child to learn this verb form, stress the sound as you talk.

3. Stress the meaning of the *–ed* part to help the child become aware of it. (e.g., Look, the boy is all done planting the seed. He plant*ed* it.)

4. Encourage the child to repeat your sentence. (e.g., Can you say "He planted the seed"?) The child may not repeat all the words exactly; just try to get the verb right.

5. When you hear the child say a sentence correctly, try to repeat it and draw the child's attention to good talking. (e.g., Yes, the boy watered the carrot a lot.)

6. Talk to communicate. Always respond first to what the child means, and then repeat the sentence in a more complete form.

7. Let the child know that you are pleased when you hear good talking. Then the child will know that good talking is important to you.

8. Most stories are written in past tense, so you will find lots of sentences to practice. You may want to shorten the text, especially if you want the child to repeat it.

9. Take the child's lead when it comes to conversation. Children learn best when the topic is of interest to them. Don't be afraid of getting sidetracked when reading the story if it means you can use the opportunity to create new learning experiences.

10. Model sentences based on the illustrations so that the child can see what you're talking about.

An Activity You Can Do

Read the following aloud from *Where the Wild Things Are,* by Maurice Sendak:

"The night Max wore his wolf suit and made mischief of one kind and another."

Then, pause to practice. Say,

Look, Max *chased* the dog (because the picture shows "chased"). Now, you tell me about the picture.

(Child gives response.)

That's right. And he *chased* the dog down the stairs.

Read further, until you say,

"And an ocean tumbled by with a private boat for Max and he sailed off through night and day"

Then, pause to practice. Say,

He *sailed* off in his boat.

Now you tell me the story. Tell me what happened to Max.

That's right. He *sailed* away on his boat that night.

Then, read aloud. Say,

"And when he came to the place where the wild things are they roared their terrible roars and gnashed their terrible teeth and rolled their terrible eyes and showed their terrible claws"

Then, pause to practice. Say,

Look at the monsters. What did the monsters do?

That's right (elaborating on the action words), they *roared*. They *showed* their claws. They *gnashed* their teeth (demonstrating *gnashed*).

Read aloud, saying

"Till Max said 'BE STILL!' and tamed them with the magic trick . . ."

Then, pause to practice. Say,

What did Max do? Yes, he *tamed* the monsters. He *stared* into their eyes. He said, "Be still." Then the monsters *called* him the most wild thing of all.

And give positive feedback. Say,

I like the way you said it!

References

American Speech-Language-Hearing Association. (2001). *Roles and responsibilities of speech-language pathologists with respect to reading and writing in children and adolescents* (guidelines). Rockville, MD: Author.

Arnold, D. S., & Whitehurst, G. J. (1994). Accelerating language development through picture book reading: A summary of dialogic reading and its effects. In D. K. Dickinson (Ed.), *Bridges to literacy: Children, families, and schools* (pp. 103–128). Cambridge, MA: Basil Blackwell.

Hall, S. L., & Moats, L. C. (1999). *Straight talk about reading: How parents can make a difference during the early years.* Chicago: Contemporary Books.

Snow, C. E., Burns, M. S., & Griffin, P. (Eds.). (1998). *Preventing reading difficulties in young children.* Washington, DC: National Academy Press.

HANDOUTS

Using Picture Books To Teach the Meanings of Words

(with Examples from
The Important Book
and *The Grouchy Ladybug*)

It is known that reading to a young child helps build the child's vocabulary and better prepares him or her for learning to read. Learning about life through the stories of others and hearing the words used in telling those stories help the child to learn the language of books and to acquire background knowledge—an essential component in learning to read. Children who have background knowledge and who are familiar with the words used in stories and books become better readers (Snow, Burns, & Griffin, 1998).

Talking about the words in stories is as important as hearing them read aloud. Reading often and pausing to talk about what you read helps to develop a child's language and emerging literacy skills. The American Speech-Language-Hearing Association (2001) encourages parents to participate in joint book reading with their child to develop early literacy. This involves parents and caregivers interacting as they read and share stories. Talking about the pictures, the words of the story, and the meanings of the words helps to build a base of knowledge on which the children draw when learning new things in school. A child takes advantage of his or her conceptual knowledge, memory, and skills of oral language when learning to read.

It is important to remember that *meaning* is not found on the words of the page. A child must create meaning by activating his or her own thoughts about the word or concept (Knuth & Jones, 1991). You can help your child construct meaning by linking new information to knowledge your child already has. This can provide a model for when the child must construct meaning on his or her own.

There are several aspects of meaning that the child must learn. You can help your child by talking about the words in books and keeping in mind the following aspects:

Vocabulary. Talking about what's inside a picture book is a great way to learn new words. Talk about all the different words in the text and the illustrations, including names of things (insect, storm cloud), names of actions (leap, slither), and describing words (huge, squishy).

Concepts. Children are expected to know many abstract ideas when they start school (e.g., colors, sizes, shapes, quantities, same and different). The text and illustrations in picture books are a good way to show the child these different ideas. Remember to relate the concept to something in your child's world.

For example, when reading *The Grouchy Ladybug,* by Eric Carle, point out the clock on each page and show how it tells the time of day in the story. Then show how the changing colors of the illustrations also reflect the time of day—the growing warmth of the sun at noon and the growing coolness of the night. Talk about the time of day at the moment you are reading the story, and find the page that best corresponds to that time. Ask the child what the ladybug might be doing at the time of day you are experiencing.

Using words correctly. Children learn from experience how to use words correctly. For example, many young children call all animals *dogs* until they learn that dogs are only one kind of animal. When they learn new words and use them in ways they can relate their own experiences, they learn the words for other things, such as the names of other animals. Older children learn, for example, that people can think but that rocks can't.

Tips

1. The most important thing you can do is to encourage the child to talk about the story and pictures with you.

2. If possible, point out the meanings of words using the pictures (e.g., Look, here are the monster's claws.).

3. Try to relate new words to things the child already knows (e.g., This monster is *very big*. It's *huge*. See, it's even bigger than the house.).

4. Don't be afraid to teach the child big, long words. Many children enjoy learning words we think are hard, such as the names of dinosaurs.

5. Many books are designed to teach new words and concepts, and such books make excellent read-alouds. Examples are picture dictionaries, books of colors and numbers, and Ruth Heller's books of collective nouns, verbs, adjectives, and adverbs.

An Activity You Can Do

Read *The Important Book,* by Margaret Wise Brown. This classic book is available at most libraries and at bookstores in a softbound, low-priced edition. Read aloud.

> "The important thing about an apple is that it is round. It is red. You bite it, and it is white inside and the juice splashes in your face, and it tastes like an apple, and it falls off a tree. But the important thing about an apple is that it is round."

Now, put the words in context. Say,

> Show me how you eat an apple.
>
> Oh, you bite it.
>
> Did the juice splash on your face? Is your face wet now?
>
> Is your apple fresh and crunchy, or old and squishy?
>
> Tell me what you do when you've finished.
>
> Do you throw it away?
>
> Because you don't eat the seeds?
>
> The part you throw away is called the *core*. It has the seeds in it.
>
> Was your apple good?
>
> Now you give me one.
>
> What color is it?
>
> What should I do with it?

Then ask thinking questions, such as

> What do you think the important thing about an apple is?
>
> What other things are round like an apple?
>
> What else has juice in it?

Books Are for Talking, Too! • © 2003 by PRO-ED, Inc.

References

American Speech-Language-Hearing Association. (2001). *Roles and responsibilities of speech–language pathologists with respect to reading and writing in children and adolescents* (guidelines). Rockville, MD: Author.

Knuth, R. A., & Jones, B. F. (1991). *What does research say about reading?* Retrieved January 30, 2002, from North Central Regional Educational Laboratory. http://www.ncrel.org/sdrs/areas/stw_esys/str_read

Snow, C. E., Burns, M. S., & Griffin, P. (Eds.). (1998). *Preventing reading difficulties in young children.* Washington, DC: National Academy Press.

HANDOUTS

Using Picture Books To Develop Sequencing Skills
(with Examples from
Rosie's Walk and *Corduroy*)

Sequencing, or telling the order of events, is an important skill—it requires that children organize information in a time frame, it helps them to process spoken language, and it gives them a basis to begin telling their own stories. One way to help children develop sequencing skills is to talk about familiar, procedural activities. For instance, "Tell me what you do when you get up and get ready for school," or "Tell me how to wash a car," or "How do you make a peanut butter sandwich?" Sharing a picture book presents an opportunity to talk about the order of events in a story.

Tips

1. As you read the story aloud, pause briefly to talk about each event. Encourage your child to describe what's happening, even if it's just a word or two.

2. Many events have natural cause-and-effect sequences. When one event in the story leads to the next, use words such as *which caused* or *that made* to show the connection between events.

3. After the story, play a game of recalling the events in the story. Take turns talking about the events in the order they occurred.

4. Make it easy. If necessary, use the pictures in the book to assist your child in remembering. Encourage the use of words such as *first, second, next,* and *last* to make the order clear and to connect the events.

5. Remembering and telling every event isn't necessary. It's better to focus on the major events that create the thread of the story.

An Activity You Can Do

Read *Rosie's Walk*, by Pat Hutchins. In this story, a fox trails a hen around the farmyard. The hen is unaware of the fox, and each time the fox starts to pounce, something happens to foil its attempt.

On each two-page spread, talk about what's happening to the fox. For instance, when Rosie walks "across the yard," she walks past a rake. As the fox chases the hen, it steps on the prongs of the rake. This makes the handle of the rake come up and hit the fox in the nose so lucky Rosie can just keep on walking. Help your child tell how stepping on the rake caused it to hit the fox in the head.

In another sequence, as Rosie walks "past the mill," her foot catches a string, which disengages a sack of flour, which falls on top of the fox. Ask your child to tell what's happening in the picture. What caused the flour to fall down on top of the fox? Help your child explain what Rosie did that caused the sack of flour to fall on the fox.

After the read-aloud, recall the events that took place in the story, asking, for example,

> What was the first thing that happened in the story?
>
> What else did the fox do?
>
> What did that cause?

Help your child understand the story sequence by asking questions that give part of the information in the story.

Another Activity You Can Do

Here's an example from *Corduroy,* by Don Freeman. Pause to talk about the following:

> A bear is on the shelf of the department store.
>
> A little girl sees it.
>
> Her mother can't buy it and says it doesn't have a button, anyway.
>
> That night, the bear goes to the furniture department to find a button.
>
> The night watchman finds him and returns him to the shelf.
>
> The next day, the little girl comes back with her money.
>
> She buys the bear and takes it home—and it still doesn't have a button.

Help your child recall the order of events in the story by naming an event and asking what happens next. This helps your child see how events are connected. For example, ask,

> What happened when the little girl walked past the shelf and saw the bear?
>
> What happened when the mother said she didn't have any money and that the bear didn't have a button?
>
> What did that make the bear want to do?
>
> What happened when the bear went to look for a button?

Also, be sure to talk about how one event leads to another in real-life situations. This is another way to help your child develop sequencing skills.

Using Picture Books
To Develop Storytelling Skills

Most children learn to read in school by reading stories. Children who have heard many stories learn what to expect in a story, which helps them to guess at the words they don't yet know how to read. For example, many stories begin with "Once upon a time." There's usually one main character or a good character and a bad character (like the three little pigs and the wolf).

We all tell stories about things that happen to us every day. When you ask, What happened at school today? or How did you skin your knees? you are asking the child to tell a story. Developing the ability to tell stories is important groundwork for learning to read. It is also an important part of a child's social development. Children who don't know how to tell stories may seem shy and be ignored in school.

Tips

1. Your child will learn most by hearing many different stories read aloud and hearing you tell stories about things that happen during the day.

2. When looking at a book, encourage your child to talk about what is happening in the pictures. If your child knows the story well, encourage him or her to tell parts of the story.

3. Encouraging your child to predict what's going to happen in the story teaches storytelling skills and adds to the fun and suspense of the book. Ask,

   What do you think will happen? or What would you do if you were the little girl in the book?

   If your child can't answer these questions, you can give a *model*, or example:

   If I were the little girl, I would. . . . What would you do?

   Or give a choice:

   "Do you think she would . . . , or would she . . . ?"

   Think of creative answers and encourage the same from the child. There's no such thing as a wrong answer, as long as the response relates to the problem.

4. Another important part of telling a story is being able to tell the order of events. As you read or tell a story, stress words that put the story in order, such as *first, and then, after that,* and *at the end.*

Books Are for Talking, Too! • © 2003 by PRO-ED, Inc.

5. You can ask questions to help your child include all the important parts of a story. Here are a few to remember:

> Where is the story happening?
>
> Who are the characters in this book?
>
> What happened to start the story, or what problem did the character have?
>
> What did the character(s) decide to do about this?
>
> What happened next?
>
> How did the character(s) feel?
>
> What was the character thinking?
>
> How did the story end?

6. Encourage and praise your child so that he or she thinks that storytelling is easy. Your child doesn't have to recall all of the events; pick a few and tell them in the correct order. Begin by having your child remember one event, then build on that. Then have the child try to remember two events in the next story, and so on.

7. Above all, remember to make reading together an enjoyable experience.

HANDOUTS

Sharing Wordless Picture Books

Many good stories are found in books that have no words. They are not only fun to look at, but they also help children to expand their language skills and prepare them for learning to read.

There are two types of wordless picture books. Concept books show a series of pictures related to a particular idea, such as opposites or colors. An example is Tana Hoban's *Push, Pull, Empty, Full.*

Another type of wordless picture book has a story to tell. In these books, each picture shows actions that establish the plot. The reader tells the story by interpreting what the pictures are saying.

By the time children are 5 or 6 years old, they begin understanding the passage of time and the feelings of characters. This is a good time to help them structure stories on their own.

The pictures in *You Can't Take a Balloon Into the Metropolitan Museum,* by Jacquiline Preiss Weitzman, tell a story. This fictional story has action going on in two parts of New York City that take place at the same time, which goes like this:

When a girl and her grandmother enter New York's great museum, the doorman tells the girl she cannot take her balloon inside. She does not want to part with it, so the doorman suggests that if he ties it to the railing outside, the balloon will be there for her when she comes out. He promises he will watch it, so the girl and her grandmother go inside. While they view the paintings and other great works of art, a pigeon flies up to the railing and unties the balloon. Before the doorman can do anything, the balloon is carried through the streets of New York by the pigeon, causing all sorts of hilarious mishaps. The doorman runs after the balloon but can't seem to catch it. Meanwhile, the girl and her grandmother are unaware of the missing balloon and of the misadventures it creates. But when they exit the museum, the balloon has amazingly found its way back to the entrance and the exhausted doorman appears to have done his job.

As you share the book, describe what's happening in the pictures. Ask questions that clarify the plot, such as

Where does the story take place? Who is the story about? (setting)

What happens to start the story? (story starter)

How did the girl feel? (reaction)

What did the doorman suggest to take care of the problem? (plan)

How did the plan work? (consequences)

What happened in the meantime? (plan)

How does the story end? (resolution)

How does the girl feel now? (reaction)

Recommended Wordless Picture Books

(or near wordless) for you and your child to share

Ah-Choo
by Mercer Mayer
New York: Dial Books for Young
  Readers, 1976, 1977

Anno's Journey*
by Mitsumasa Anno
New York: Philomel Books, 1977;
  Putnam, 1981

*April Wilson's Magpie Magic: A
  Tale of Colorful Mischief*
by April Wilson
New York: Dial Books for Young
  Readers, 1999

Clementine's Cactus
by Ezra Jack Keats
New York: Viking Children's Books,
  1999

Clown
by Quentin Blake
New York: Holt, 1996

A Country Far Away
by Nigel Gray
New York: Orchard, 1989

The Creepy Thing
by Fernando Krahn
Boston: Houghton Mifflin, 1982

Deep in the Forest
by Brinton Turkle
New York: Dutton, 1976

Dinosaur!
by Peter Sís
New York: Greenwillow, 2000

Dreams
by Peter Spier
New York: Doubleday, 1986

Free Fall
by David Wiesner
New York: Lothrop, Lee & Shepard,
  1988

Frog on His Own**
by Mercer Mayer
New York: Dial Books for Young
  Readers, 1973, 1980

Good Dog, Carl†
by Alexandra Day
New York: Simon & Schuster, 1996

*The Grey Lady and the Strawberry
  Snatcher*
by Molly Bang
New York: Four Winds Press, 1980,
  1984

Have You Seen My Duckling?
by Nancy Tafuri
New York: Greenwillow Books,
  1984

Hiccup
by Mercer Mayer
New York: Dial Books for Young
  Readers, 1976, 1978

*The Hunter and the Animals: A
  Wordless Picture Book*
by Tomie de Paola
New York: Holiday House, 1988

Junglewalk
by Nancy Tafuri
New York: Greenwillow Books,
  1988

Oh, Were They Ever Happy
by Peter Spier
New York: Doubleday, 1978, 1988

Paddy Under Water††
by John S. Goodall
New York: Atheneum, 1984;
  Macmillan, 1991

Pancakes for Breakfast
by Tomie de Paola
New York: Harcourt Brace
  Jovanovich, 1978

Picnic
by Emily Arnold McCully
New York: HarperCollins, 1984,
  1989

The Ring
by Lisa Maizlish
New York: Greenwillow Books,
  1996

Robot-Bot-Bot
by Fernando Krahn
New York: Dutton, 1979

HANDOUTS

Sector 7
by David Wiesner
New York: Clarion Books, 1999

The Snowman
by Raymond Briggs
New York: Random House,
    1999

Time Flies
by Eric Rohmann
New York: Dragonfly Books,
    Crown, 1997

Truck
by Donald Crews
New York: Puffin, 1980, 1985

Tuesday
by David Wiesner
New York: Clarion Books, 1991

*You Can't Take a Balloon Into the
    Metropolitan Museum*[†††]
by Jacquiline Preiss Weitzman
New York: Dial Books for Young
    Readers, 1998

*Read also *Anno's Britain, Anno's Italy, Anno's Medieval World,* and *Anno's USA* by the same author.

**Read also the following wordless books by the same author: *A Boy, a Dog, a Frog, and a Friend; Frog Goes to Dinner; Frog, Where Are You?* and *One Frog Too Many.*

[†]Read also *Carl Goes Shopping, Carl's Afternoon in the Park, Carl's Christmas, Carl's Masquerade, Carl Makes a Scrapbook, Carl Goes to Day Care,* and *Follow Carl* by the same author.

[††]Read also *The Ballooning Adventures of Paddy Pork, Creepy Castle, Edwardian Christmas, Edwardian Holiday, Edwardian Summer, Jacko, Naughty Nancy, Paddy Pork's Holiday, Paddy's Evening Out,* and *The Surprise Picnic* by the same author. These books are out of print but may be available on a limited basis and may be found in your school or local libraries.

[†††]Read also *You Can't Take a Balloon Into the Fine Arts Museum* and *You Can't Take a Balloon Into the National Gallery* by the same author.

Reading Aloud in Your Child's First Language

If your child's first language is not English, your child can still become an excellent reader and writer of the English language. Reading to your child in his or her first language is an important activity. It will help your child know many words and concepts in stories by the time he or she is ready to read in English.

Early in your child's life, read aloud in your native language and talk about what you are reading. Point to the pictures, name them, and talk about what is happening in the story. Reading to your child will strengthen your child's first language and help him or her form concepts and develop the English language, too.

Here are some things to do:

- Point out the pictures, especially if they help tell the story.

- Share conversation about what's happening on the page of the story.

- If you think your child might not understand a word or phrase, pause and talk about it.

- Use the word in another sentence and relate it to something the child knows.

- Pause in the reading to talk about the story.

- Don't be afraid to have your child take the lead.

- Praise your child's responses and his or her efforts in communicating.

Talking with your child's teacher about what you are doing at home to strengthen your child's spoken language is also important. Let the teacher know that your child's language skills are important to you. Remember, nothing is more important in helping your child become a strong reader than reading aloud and sharing stories together (DeBruin-Parecki, 2000).

Resources for Families and Caregivers: http://www.ed.gov/pubs/parents/Reader/read.html

References

DeBruin-Parecki, A. (2000). *Helping your child become a reader.* Washington, DC: U.S. Department of Education.

HANDOUTS

Section 5

Indexes

Topic Explorations

Alphabet
Animals
Arts, Artists, and
   Architecture
Baseball
Bears
Birds
Boats
Careers
Cities
Clothing
Clouds
Colors
Community
Conservation
Construction and Building
Cooking
Country Life
Cowboys and Cowgirls
Creativity
Culture and History
Daily Activities
Days of the Week
Death and Dying
Dinosaurs
Fairy Tales and Nursery
   Rhymes
Family Relationships
Famous People
Farms

Feelings
Folk Songs
Folklore
Food
Friendship
Fruit
Gorillas
Growing Cycles and Planting
Growing Up
History
Hobbies
Holidays
Honesty
Humor
Imagination
Insects and Spiders
Journeys
Literacy
Long Ago and Far Away
Loyalty
Manners and Etiquette
Memory and Remembering
Messes
Money
Months of the Year
Motivation
Museums
Music, Musicians, and
   Musical Instruments

Nighttime
Number Concepts
Outer Space
Owls
Part–Whole Relationships
Pets
Pirates
Safety
School Activities
Science
Sea and the Seashore
Seasons
Self-Esteem
Shadows
Shapes and Visual Images
Sharing
Sheep
Sounds and Listening
Speaking and
   Communicating
Trains
Transportation
Trickster Tales
Vegetables
Weather
Women's Lives
Woods
Zoos

TOPIC

Alphabet

Base, Graeme
Animalia
Martin, Bill Jr., and John
Archambault
Chicka Chicka Boom Boom
Sendak, Maurice
Alligators All Around:
An Alphabet

Animals

Base, Graeme
Animalia
Dunrea, Olivier
Bear Noel
Fleming, Denise
Where Once There Was a Wood
Florian, Douglas
Mammalabilia
Martin, Bill Jr.
Brown Bear, Brown Bear,
What Do You See?
Numeroff, Laura
Chimps Don't Wear Glasses
Shaw, Nancy
Sheep on a Ship
Wood, Don
Quick as a Cricket

Animals, Cats

Brett, Jan
Annie and the Wild Animals
Fleming, Denise
Mama Cat Has Three Kittens
Gantos, Jack
Rotten Ralph
Soto, Gary
Chato's Kitchen

Animals, Dogs

Barracca, Debra, and Sal Barracca
The Adventures of Taxi Dog
Meddaugh, Susan
Martha Speaks
Muir, John
Stickeen: John Muir
and the Brave Little Dog
Paulsen, Gary, and Ruth Paulsen
Dogteam
Pilkey, Dav
Dog Breath: The Horrible
Trouble with Hally Tosis

The Hallo-wiener
Rathmann, Peggy
Officer Buckle and Gloria

Animals, Endangered

Burningham, John
Hey! Get Off Our Train
Cowcher, Helen
Antarctica
Fleming, Denise
Where Once There Was a Wood

Animals, Farm

Allen, Pamela
Who Sank the Boat?
Brown, Margaret Wise
Big Red Barn
Burningham, John
Mr. Gumpy's Outing
Carle, Eric
The Very Busy Spider
Cronin, Doreen
Click, Clack, Moo:
Cows That Type
Fox, Mem
Hattie and the Fox
Hawkins, Colin, and
Jacqui Hawkins
Old MacDonald Had a Farm
Hutchins, Pat
Rosie's Walk
Martin, Bill Jr., and
John Archambault
Barn Dance!
Palatini, Margie
Piggie Pie
Sloat, Teri
The Thing That Bothered
Farmer Brown
Waddell, Martin
Farmer Duck
Williams, Sue
I Went Walking

Animals, Forest

Berger, Barbara
Grandfather Twilight
Brett, Jan
Annie and the Wild Animals
The Mitten: A Ukrainian
Folktale

Animals, Jungle

Baker, Keith
Who Is the Beast?
Cherry, Lynne
The Great Kapok Tree: A Tale of
the Amazon River Forest
Cuyler, Margery
That's Good! That's Bad!

Animals, Zoo

Barrett, Judi
A Snake Is Totally Tail
Base, Graeme
Animalia
Carle, Eric
The Mixed-Up Chameleon
de Regniers, Beatrice Schenk
May I Bring a Friend?
Guarino, Deborah
Is Your Mama a Llama?
Martin, Bill Jr.
Polar Bear, Polar Bear,
What Do You Hear?
Massie, Diane Redfield
The Baby Beebee Bird
Rathmann, Peggy
Good Night, Gorilla

Art, Artists, and Architecture

Jacobsen, Kathy
(words and music by Woody Guthrie)
This Land Is Your Land
Lawrence, Jacob
Harriet and the Promised Land
Macaulay, David
Rome Antics
Stanley, Diane
The Gentleman and
the Kitchen Maid
Weitzman, Jacquiline Preiss
You Can't Take a Balloon
Into the Metropolitan
Museum

Baseball

Burleigh, Robert
Home Run
Thayer, Ernest Lawrence
Casey at the Bat: A Ballad
of the Republic Sung
in the Year 1888

Bears

Alborough, Jez
  It's the Bear!
  Where's My Teddy?
Brett, Jan
  Berlioz the Bear
Carlstrom, Nancy White
  Jesse Bear, What Will You Wear?
Degen, Bruce
  Jamberry
Dunrea, Olivier
  Bear Noel
Freeman, Don
  Corduroy
McPhail, David
  Emma's Pet
Turkle, Brinton
  Deep in the Forest

Birds

Baker, Keith
  Little Green
Ehlert, Lois
  Cucú: Un cuento folklórico mexicano/Cuckoo: A Mexican Folktale
Massie, Diane Redfield
  The Baby Beebee Bird
Rohmann, Eric
  Time Flies
Tafuri, Nancy
  Snowy Flowy Blowy: A Twelve Months Rhyme

Boats

Allen, Pamela
  Who Sank the Boat?
Burningham, John
  Come Away from the Water, Shirley
  Mr. Gumpy's Outing
Crews, Donald
  Sail Away
Fleming, Candace
  Gabriella's Song
Fox, Mem
  Tough Boris
Lear, Edward
  The Owl and the Pussycat
Shaw, Nancy
  Sheep on a Ship

Van Allsburg, Chris
  The Wreck of the Zephyr
  The Wretched Stone

Careers

Allard, Harry, and James Marshall
  Miss Nelson Is Missing!
  (and other books in the series)
Barracca, Debra, and Sal Barracca
  The Adventures of Taxi Dog
Barton, Byron
  Airport
Brett, Jan
  Berlioz the Bear
Brown, Marc
  Arthur's Nose
Browne, Anthony
  Gorilla
  Piggybook
Fleming, Candace
  Gabriella's Song
Freeman, Don
  Corduroy
Hughes, Shirley
  Alfie Gets in First
Hutchins, Pat
  The Wind Blew
Paulsen, Gary, and Ruth Paulsen
  Dogteam
Rathmann, Peggy
  Officer Buckle and Gloria
Stewart, Sarah
  The Gardener
Wiesner, David
  Tuesday
Williams, Vera B.
  A Chair for My Mother
Yorinks, Arthur
  Hey, Al

Cities

Burton, Virginia Lee
  Mike Mulligan and His Steam Shovel
Jacobsen, Kathy
  (song by Woody Guthrie)
  This Land Is Your Land
Stewart, Sarah
  The Gardener

Cities, New York City

Barracca, Debra, and Sal Barracca
  The Adventures of Taxi Dog

Dorros, Arthur
  Abuela
Weitzman, Jacquiline Preiss
  You Can't Take a Balloon Into the Metropolitan Museum
Wiesner, David
  Sector 7

Clothing

Corey, Shana
  You Forgot Your Skirt, Amelia Bloomer
de Paola, Tomie
  Charlie Needs a Cloak

Clothing, Hats

Glass, Andrew
  Mountain Men: True Grit and Tall Tales
Karon, Jan
  Miss Fannie's Hat
Slobodkina, Esphyr
  Caps for Sale: A Tale of a Peddler, Some Monkeys and Their Monkey Business
Small, David
  Imogene's Antlers

Clouds

Locker, Thomas
  Cloud Dance
Shaw, Charles G.
  It Looked Like Spilt Milk
Spier, Peter
  Dreams
Wiesner, David
  Sector 7

Colors

Bang, Molly
  Ten, Nine, Eight
Brown, Margaret Wise
  Big Red Barn
Carle, Eric
  The Mixed-Up Chameleon
Crews, Donald
  Freight Train
Ehlert, Lois
  Planting a Rainbow

Karon, Jan
  Miss Fannie's Hat
Martin, Bill Jr.
  Brown Bear, Brown Bear,
  What Do You See?
Peek, Merle
  Mary Wore Her Red Dress and
  Henry Wore His Green Sneakers
Riley, Linnea
  Mouse Mess
Slobodkina, Esphyr
  Caps for Sale: A Tale
  of a Peddler, Some Monkeys
  and Their Monkey Business
Williams, Sue
  I Went Walking
Young, Ed
  Seven Blind Mice

Community

Anno, Mitsumasa
  Anno's Journey
Bang, Molly
  The Paper Crane
Barracca, Debra, and Sal Barracca
  The Adventures of Taxi Dog
Brett, Jan
  Berlioz the Bear
Burton, Virginia Lee
  Mike Mulligan and His
  Steam Shovel
de Paola, Tomie
  The Legend of the
  Bluebonnet
Fleming, Candace
  Gabriella's Song
Fox, Mem
  Wilfrid Gordon
  McDonald Partridge
Gray, Nigel
  A Country Far Away
Hoban, Tana
  I Read Signs
Hort, Lenny
  The Boy Who Held Back
  the Sea
Hughes, Shirley
  Alfie Gets in First
Hutchins, Pat
  The Wind Blew
Leaf, Margaret
  The Eyes of the Dragon
Pinkwater, Daniel Manus
  The Big Orange Splot

Williams, Vera B.
  A Chair for My Mother
Zion, Gene
  Harry the Dirty Dog

Conservation

Baker, Keith
  Who Is the Beast?
Bunting, Eve
  The Man Who Could
  Call Down Owls
Burningham, John
  Hey! Get Off Our Train
Cherry, Lynne
  The Great Kapok Tree: A Tale of
  the Amazon River Forest

  The River Ran Wild:
  An Environmental History
Cowcher, Helen
  Antarctica
Fleming, Denise
  Where Once There Was a Wood

Construction and Building

Burton, Virginia Lee
  Mike Mulligan and His Steam
  Shovel

Cooking

de Paola, Tomie
  Pancakes for Breakfast
Ehlert, Lois
  Growing Vegetable Soup
Palatini, Margie
  Piggie Pie

Country Life

Burningham, John
  Mr. Gumpy's Outing
Martin, Bill Jr., and John
  Archambault
  Barn Dance!
Rylant, Cynthia
  Night in the Country

  The Relatives Came

  When I Was Young
  in the Mountains

Cowboys and Cowgirls

Dodds, Dayle Ann
  Sing, Sophie!
Feiffer, Jules
  Meanwhile

Creativity

Baker, Keith
  Little Green
Lawrence, Jacob
  Harriet and the Promised
  Land
Lionni, Leo
  Frederick
Wiesner, David
  The Three Pigs

Culture and History, African and African American

Feelings, Muriel
  Jambo Means Hello:
  Swahili Alphabet Book
Gray, Nigel
  A Country Far Away
Lawrence, Jacob
  Harriet and the Promised
  Land
Ringgold, Faith
  Aunt Harriet's Underground
  Railroad in the Sky

  If a Bus Could Talk:
  The Story of Rosa Parks

Culture and History, American

Cherry, Lynne
  The River Ran Wild: An
  Environmental History
Corey, Shana
  You Forgot Your Skirt, Amelia
  Bloomer
Garland, Sherry
  Voices of the Alamo
Hearne, Betsy Gould
  Seven Brave Women
Jacobsen, Kathy
  (song by Woody Guthrie)
  This Land Is Your Land

TOPIC

Culture and History, Chinese

Fisher, Leonard Everett
The Great Wall of China
Leaf, Margaret
The Eyes of the Dragon
Mahy, Margaret
The Seven Chinese Brothers

Culture and History, English

Spier, Peter
London Bridge Is Falling Down

Culture and History, Hispanic

Dorros, Arthur
Abuela
Soto, Gary
Chato's Kitchen
Too Many Tamales

Culture and History, Japanese

Bang, Molly
The Paper Crane
Say, Allen
Grandfather's Journey

Culture and History, Native American

de Paola, Tomie
The Legend of Bluebonnet
Cherry, Lynne
The River Ran Wild: An Environmental History
Garland, Sherry
Voices of the Alamo
Goble, Paul
Iktomi and the Boulder
Oughton, Jerrie
How the Stars Fell Into the Sky: A Navajo Legend

Daily Activities

Carlstrom, Nancy White
Jesse Bear, What Will You Wear?
Gray, Nigel
A Country Far Away

Hines, Anna Grossnickle
Daddy Makes the Best Spaghetti
Small, David
Imogene's Antlers
Viorst, Judith
Alexander and the Terrible, Horrible, No Good, Very Bad Day

Days of the Week

Carle, Eric
The Very Hungry Caterpillar
Young, Ed
Seven Blind Mice

Death and Dying

Buscaglia, Leo F.
The Fall of Freddie the Leaf
Cazet, Denys
A Fish in His Pocket
Service, Robert W.
The Cremation of Sam McGee
Viorst, Judith
The Tenth Good Thing About Barney

Dinosaurs

Barton, Byron
Dinosaurs, Dinosaurs
Rohmann, Eric
Time Flies

Fairy Tales and Nursery Rhymes

Adams, Pam
This Is the House That Jack Built
Ahlberg, Janet, and Allan Ahlberg
Each Peach Pear Plum
Lear, Edward
The Owl and the Pussycat
Miranda, Anne
To Market, To Market
Prelutsky, Jack
Ride a Purple Pelican
Scieszka, Jon
The Stinky Cheese Man and Other Fairly Stupid Tales
The True Story of the Three Little Pigs

Turkle, Brinton
Deep in the Forest
Wiesner, David
The Three Pigs

Family Relationships

Browne, Anthony
Gorilla
Piggybook
Carlstrom, Nancy White
Jesse Bear, What Will You Wear?
Dodds, Dayle Ann
Sing, Sophie!
Freeman, Don
Corduroy
Guarino, Deborah
Is Your Mama a Llama?
Hines, Anna Grossnickle
Daddy Makes the Best Spaghetti
Hughes, Shirley
Alfie Gets in First
Hutchins, Pat
The Very Worst Monster
Keats, Ezra Jack
Peter's Chair
Pilkey, Dav
Dog Breath: The Horrible Trouble with Hally Tosis
Ringgold, Faith
Aunt Harriet's Underground Railroad in the Sky
Rylant, Cynthia
The Relatives Came
When I Was Young in the Mountains
Say, Allen
Grandfather's Journey
Spier, Peter
Oh, Were They Ever Happy
Small, David
Imogene's Antlers
Viorst, Judith
Alexander and the Terrible, Horrible, No Good, Very Bad Day
The Tenth Good Thing About Barney
Wells, Rosemary
Noisy Nora
Williams, Vera B.
A Chair for My Mother

Famous People

Jacobsen, Kathy
(song by Woody Guthrie)
This Land Is Your Land
Sakurai, Gail
Stephen Hawking:
Understanding the Universe
Simon, Charnan
Bill Gates: Helping People
Use Computers
Sís, Peter
Starry Messenger
Small, David
George Washington's Cows

Famous People, Heroes

Burleigh, Robert
Home Run
Kosek, Jane Kelly
Learning About Courage
from the Life of Christopher
Reeve
Ringgold, Faith
If a Bus Could Talk:
The Story of Rosa Parks
Ryan, Pam Muñoz
Amelia and Eleanor
Go for a Ride
Strazzabosco, Jeanne
Learning About Determination
from the Life of
Gloria Estefan
Learning About Forgiveness
from the Life of
Nelson Mandela
Thayer, Ernest Lawrence
Casey at the Bat: A Ballad
of the Republic Sung in the
Year 1888

Farms

Cronin, Doreen
Click, Clack, Moo: Cows That
Type
Hawkins, Colin,
and Jacqui Hawkins
Old MacDonald Had a Farm
Hutchins, Pat
Rosie's Walk
Sloat, Teri
The Thing That Bothered
Farmer Brown

Feelings

Brett, Jan
Annie and the Wild
Animals
Burningham, John
Aldo
Cazet, Denys
A Fish in His Pocket
Demi
The Empty Pot
Fox, Mem
Wilfrid Gordon
McDonald Partridge
Howe, James
I Wish I Were a Butterfly
Sendak, Maurice
Where the Wild Things Are
Viorst, Judith
Alexander and the Terrible,
Horrible, No Good,
Very Bad Day
Waddell, Martin
Farmer Duck

Folk Songs

Hawkins, Colin, and
Jacqui Hawkins
Old MacDonald Had
a Farm
Jacobsen, Kathy
(song by Woody Guthrie)
This Land Is Your Land
Langstaff, John
Oh, A-Hunting We Will Go
Peek, Merle
Mary Wore Her Red Dress
and Henry Wore His
Green Sneakers
Spier, Peter
London Bridge Is Falling
Down

Folk Tales, North American

Glass, Andrew
Mountain Men: True Grit
and Tall Tales
Service, Robert W.
The Cremation of
Sam McGee
Thayer, Ernest Lawrence
Casey at the Bat:
A Ballad of the Republic
Sung in the Year 1888

Folklore, African and African American

Cendrars, Blaise
Shadow
McDermott, Gerald
Anansi the Spider:
A Tale from the Ashanti

Folklore, Armenian

Hogrogian, Nonny
One Fine Day

Folklore, Chinese

Demi
The Empty Pot
Leaf, Margaret
The Eyes of the Dragon
Lobel, Arnold
Ming Lo Moves the Mountain
Mahy, Margaret
The Seven Chinese Brothers

Folklore, English

Bennett, Jill
Teeny Tiny
Lear, Edward
The Owl and the Pussycat

Folklore, Greek Mythology

McDermott, Gerald
Sun Flight

Folklore, India

Demi
One Grain of Rice:
A Mathematical Folktale
Young, Ed
Seven Blind Mice

Folklore, Mexican

Ehlert, Lois
Cucú: Un cuento folklórico
mexicano/Cuckoo: A Mexican
Folktale

Folklore, Native American

de Paola, Tomie
The Legend of Bluebonnet

TOPIC

Goble, Paul
Iktomi and the Boulder
(and other books in the series)
McDermott, Gerald
Arrow to the Sun
Oughton, Jerrie
*How the Stars Fell Into the Sky:
A Navajo Legend*

Folklore, Pan Asian

Sierra, Judy
Counting Crocodiles

Folklore, Ukrainian

Brett, Jan
*The Mitten: A Ukrainian
Folktale*

Food

Alborough, Jez
It's the Bear!
Degen, Bruce
Jamberry
Miranda, Anne
To Market, To Market
Riley, Linnea
Mouse Mess
Scheer, Julian and Marvin Bileck
Rain Makes Applesauce
Soto, Gary
Chato's Kitchen

Friendship

Brown, Marc
Arthur's Nose
Burningham, John
Aldo
de Regniers, Beatrice Schenk
May I Bring a Friend?
Fox, Mem
*Wilfrid Gordon McDonald
Partridge*
Howe, James
I Wish I Were a Butterfly
Kasza, Keiko
The Rat and the Tiger
Lionni, Leo
Swimmy
Marshall, James
George and Martha
(and other books in the
series)

Service, Robert W.
The Cremation of Sam McGee
Waber, Bernard
Lovable Lyle

Fruit

Carle, Eric
The Very Hungry Caterpillar
Scheer, Julian, and Marvin Bileck
Rain Makes Applesauce

Gorillas

Browne, Anthony
Gorilla
Rathmann, Peggy
Good Night, Gorilla

Growing Cycles and Planting

Demi
The Empty Pot
Ehlert, Lois
Growing Vegetable Soup
Planting a Rainbow
Krauss, Ruth
The Carrot Seed
Scheer, Julian, and Marvin Bileck
Rain Makes Applesauce
Stewart, Sarah
The Gardener

Growing Up

Keats, Ezra Jack
Peter's Chair
Keller, Holly
Geraldine's Blanket

History, American

Cherry, Lynne
*The River Ran Wild: An
Environmental History*
Garland, Sherry
Voices of the Alamo
Glass, Andrew
*Mountain Men: True Grit
and Tall Tales*
Hearne, Betsy Gould
Seven Brave Women
Jacobsen, Kathy
(song by Woody Guthrie)
This Land Is Your Land

Lawrence, Jacob
Harriet and the Promised Land
Lincoln, Abraham
The Gettysburg Address
Muir, John
*Stickeen: John Muir
and the Brave Little Dog*
Ringgold, Faith
*If a Bus Could Talk:
The Story of Rosa Parks*
Ryan, Pam Muñoz
*Amelia and Eleanor
Go for a Ride*
Small, David
George Washington's Cows
Stewart, Sarah
The Gardener
Thayer, Ernest Lawrence
*Casey at the Bat:
A Ballad of the Republic
Sung in the Year 1888*
Turner, Ann
Dakota Dugout

History, European

Anno, Mitsumasa
Anno's Journey
Macaulay, David
Rome Antics
Sís, Peter
Starry Messenger

History, Medieval

Anno, Mitsumasa
Anno's Medieval World

Hobbies

Stewart, Sarah
The Gardener

Holidays, Christmas

Dunrea, Olivier
Bear Noel
Soto, Gary
Too Many Tamales

Holidays, Halloween

Barton, Byron
Hester
Brown, Ruth
A Dark, Dark Tale

TOPIC

Bunting, Eve
In the Haunted House
Scary, Scary Halloween
Enderle, Judith R., and
Stephanie G. Tesslen
Six Creepy Sheep
Palatini, Margie
Piggie Pie
Pilkey, Dav
The Hallo-wiener
Silverman, Erica
Big Pumpkin

Holidays, Martin Luther King Jr. Day

Ringgold, Faith
If a Bus Could Talk: The Story of Rosa Parks

Holidays, Presidents' Day

Lincoln, Abraham
The Gettysburg Address
Small, David
George Washington's Cows

Honesty

Demi
The Empty Pot

Humor

Allard, Harry, and James Marshall
Miss Nelson Is Missing!
(and other books in the series)
Brett, Jan
The Mitten: A Ukrainian Folktale
Carle, Eric
The Mixed-Up Chameleon
Day, Alexandra
Good Dog, Carl
(and other books in the series)
de Regniers, Beatrice Schenk
May I Bring a Friend?
Enderle, Judith R., and
Stephanie G. Tesslen
Six Creepy Sheep
Goble, Paul
Iktomi and the Boulder
(and other books in the series)

Gulbis, Stephen
I Know an Old Lady Who Swallowed a Fly
Hutchins, Pat
Don't Forget the Bacon
Lobel, Arnold
Ming Lo Moves the Mountain
McNaughton, Colin
Here Come the Aliens!
Marshall, James
George and Martha: Back in Town (and other books in the series)
Prelutsky, Jack
The Baby Uggs Are Hatching!
For Laughing Outloud: Poems To Tickle Your Funnybone
The Snopp on the Sidewalk and Other Poems
Scieszka, Jon
The Stinky Cheese Man and Other Fairly Stupid Tales
The True Story of the Three Little Pigs
Small, David
Imogene's Antlers
Spier, Peter
Oh, Were They Ever Happy
Waddell, Martin
Farmer Duck

Imagination

Numeroff, Laura
Chimps Don't Wear Glasses
Van Allsburg, Chris
The Mysteries of Harris Burdick
Wiesner, David
Sector 7

Insects and Spiders

Carle, Eric
The Grouchy Ladybug
The Very Busy Spider
The Very Hungry Caterpillar
Finn, Isabel, and Jack Tickle
The Very Lazy Ladybug
Fleischman, Paul
Joyful Noise: Poems for Two Voices
Gulbis, Stephen
I Know an Old Lady

Who Swallowed a Fly
Howe, James
I Wish I Were a Butterfly
McDermott, Gerald
Anansi the Spider: A Tale from the Ashanti
Trapani, Iza
The Itsy Bitsy Spider

Journeys

Anno, Mitsumasa
Anno's Journey
Burningham, John
Hey! Get Off Our Train
Mr. Gumpy's Outing
Charlip, Remy
Fortunately
Crews, Donald
Sail Away
Truck
Jacobsen, Kathy
(song by Woody Guthrie)
This Land Is Your Land
Lawrence, Jacob
Harriet and the Promised Land
Macaulay, David
Rome Antics
McDermott, Gerald
Sun Flight
Ringgold, Faith
Aunt Harriet's Underground Railroad in the Sky
Rylant, Cynthia
The Relatives Came
Say, Allen
Grandfather's Journey
Sendak, Maurice
Where the Wild Things Are
Van Allsburg, Chris
The Wretched Stone
Yorinks, Arthur
Hey, Al

Literacy

Cronin, Doreen
Click, Clack, Moo: Cows That Type
Feiffer, Jules
Meanwhile
Meddaugh, Susan
Martha Speaks
Soto, Gary
Chato's Kitchen

TOPIC

Stewart, Sarah
The Gardener
Van Allsburg, Chris
The Wretched Stone

Long Ago and Far Away

Anno, Mitsumasa
Anno's Journey
Anno's Medieval World
de Paola, Tomie
The Knight and the Dragon
Fisher, Leonard Everett
The Great Wall of China
Fox, Mem
Tough Boris
Hort, Lenny
The Boy Who Held Back the Sea
McDermott, Gerald
Sun Flight
Mahy, Margaret
The Seven Chinese Brothers
Rohmann, Eric
Time Flies
Sís, Peter
Starry Messenger
Spier, Peter
London Bridge Is Falling Down
Wood, Audrey
King Bidgood's in the Bathtub

Loyalty

Day, Alexandra
Good Dog, Carl
Service, Robert W.
The Cremation of Sam McGee

Manners and Etiquette

de Regniers, Beatrice Shenk
May I Bring a Friend?
Buehner, Caralyn
It's a Spoon, Not a Shovel
Kaszka, Keiko
The Rat and the Tiger

Memory and Remembering

Fox, Mem
Wilfrid Gordon McDonald Partridge
Karon, Jan
Miss Fannie's Hat

Hutchins, Pat
Don't Forget the Bacon
Rylant, Cynthia
When I Was Young in the Mountains
Say, Allen
Grandfather's Journey

Messes

Browne, Anthony
Piggybook
Riley, Linnea
Mouse Mess
Teague, Mark
Pigsty

Money

Freeman, Don
Corduroy
Williams, Vera B.
A Chair for My Mother

Months of the Year

Sendak, Maurice
Chicken Soup with Rice
Tafuri, Nancy
Snowy Flowy Blowy: A Twelve Months Rhyme

Motivation

Canfield, Jack, Mark Victor Hansen, and Kimberly Kirberger
Chicken Soup for the Teenage Soul Journal
Simon, Charnan
Bill Gates: Helping People Use Computers

Museums

Rohmann, Eric
Time Flies
Stanley, Diane
The Gentleman and the Kitchen Maid
Weitzman, Jacquiline Preiss
You Can't Take a Balloon Into the Metropolitan Museum

Music, Musicians, and Musical Instruments

Brett, Jan
Berlioz the Bear

Dodds, Dayle Ann
Sing, Sophie!
Dorros, Arthur
Ten Go Tango
Fleming, Candace
Gabriella's Song
Jacobsen, Kathy
(song by Woody Guthrie)
This Land Is Your Land,
Martin, Bill Jr.,
and John Archambault
Barn Dance!
Moss, Lloyd
Zin! Zin! Zin! A Violin

Nighttime

Berger, Barbara
Grandfather Twilight
Brown, Margaret Wise
Goodnight Moon
Hutchins, Pat
Good-Night, Owl!
Martin, Bill Jr.,
and John Archambault
Barn Dance!
Massie, Diane Redfield
The Baby Beebee Bird
Rathmann, Peggy
Good Night, Gorilla
Rylant, Cynthia
Night in the Country
Wildsmith, Brian
What the Moon Saw

Number Concepts

Bang, Molly
Ten, Nine, Eight
Demi
One Grain of Rice: A Mathematical Folktale
Moss, Lloyd
Zin! Zin! Zin! A Violin
Sierra, Judy
Counting Crocodiles

Outer Space

Feiffer, Jules
Meanwhile
McNaughton, Colin
Here Come the Aliens!

Owls

Brett, Jan
The Mitten: A Ukrainian Folktale

TOPIC

Bunting, Eve
  The Man Who Could Call Down Owls
Hutchins, Pat
  Good-Night, Owl!
Lear, Edward
  The Owl and the Pussycat
Martin, Bill Jr., and John Archambault
  Barn Dance!

Part–Whole Relationships

Carle, Eric
  The Mixed-Up Chameleon
Young, Ed
  Seven Blind Mice

Pets

Brett, Jan
  Annie and the Wild Animals
Day, Alexandra
  Good Dog, Carl
Gantos, Jack
  Rotten Ralph
McPhail, David
  Emma's Pet
Mayer, Mencer
  Frog on His Own
Meddaugh, Susan
  Martha Speaks
Muir, John
  Stickeen: John Muir and the Brave Little Dog
Rathmann, Peggy
  Officer Buckle and Gloria
Viorst, Judith
  The Tenth Good Thing About Barney
Yorinks, Arthur
  Hey, Al
Zion, Gene
  Harry the Dirty Dog

Pirates

Burningham, John
  Come Away from the Water, Shirley
Feiffer, Jules
  Meanwhile
Fox, Mem
  Tough Boris

Safety

Rathmann, Peggy
  Officer Buckle and Gloria

School Activities

Allard, Harry, and James Marshall
  Miss Nelson Is Missing!
Cazet, Denys
  A Fish in His Pocket
Crews, Donald
  School Bus
Henkes, Kevin
  Lilly's Purple Plastic Purse
Kraus, Robert
  Leo the Late Bloomer
Rathmann, Peggy
  Officer Buckle and Gloria

Science

Locker, Thomas
  Cloud Dance
Sakurai, Gail
  Stephen Hawking: Understanding the Universe
Sís, Peter
  Starry Messenger

Sea and the Seashore

Burningham, John
  Come Away from the Water, Shirley
Cowcher, Helen
  Antarctica
Fox, Mem
  Tough Boris
Lear, Edward
  (Illustrated by Jan Brett)
  The Owl and the Pussycat
Lionni, Leo
  Swimmy
Rockwell, Anne
  At the Beach

Seasons

Buscaglia, Leo F.
  The Fall of Freddie the Leaf
Lionni, Leo
  Frederick
Sendak, Maurice
  Chicken Soup with Rice

Tafuri, Nancy
  Snowy Flowy Blowy: A Twelve Months Rhyme

Seasons, Autumn

Bunting, Eve
  Scary, Scary Halloween
Cazet, Denys
  A Fish in His Pocket
Enderle, Judith R., and Stephanie G. Tessler
  Six Creepy Sheep
Martin, Bill Jr., and John Archambault
  Barn Dance!
Scheer, Julian, and Marvin Bileck
  Rain Makes Applesauce

Seasons, Spring

de Paola, Tomie
  The Legend of Bluebonnet

Seasons, Summer

Rylant, Cynthia
  The Relatives Came

Seasons, Winter

Brett, Jan
  Annie and the Wild Animals
  The Mitten: A Ukrainian Folktale
Dunrea, Olivier
  Bear Noel
Keats, Ezra Jack
  The Snowy Day
Shulevitz, Uri
  Snow

Self-Esteem

Brown, Marc
  Arthur's Nose
Brown, Margaret Wise
  The Important Book
Buckley, Richard
  The Foolish Tortoise
Carle, Eric
  The Mixed-Up Chameleon
Demi
  The Empty Pot
Howe, James
  I Wish I Were a Butterfly

TOPIC

Kraus, Robert
   Leo the Late Bloomer
Lionni, Leo
   Frederick
Small, David
   Imogene's Antlers
Zolotow, Charlotte
   Someday

Shadows

Cendrars, Blaise
   Shadow
Hoban, Tana
   Shadows and Reflections

Shapes and Visual Images

Bang, Molly
   Ten, Nine, Eight
Carle, Eric
   The Secret Birthday Message
Hoban, Tana
   Is It Larger? Is It Smaller?
   Shadows and Reflections
Riley, Linnea
   Mouse Mess
Shaw, Charles G.
   It Looked Like Spilt Milk
Spier, Peter
   Dreams
Young, Ed
   Seven Blind Mice

Sharing

Burningham, John
   Mr. Gumpy's Outing
Carle, Eric
   The Grouchy Ladybug
Demi
   One Grain of Rice: A Mathematical Folktale
Karon, Jan
   Miss Fannie's Hat
Kasza, Keiko
   The Rat and the Tiger
Riley, Linnea
   Mouse Mess

Sheep

de Paola, Tomie
   Charlie Needs a Cloak

Enderle, Judith R., and Stephanie G. Tessler
   Six Creepy Sheep
Shaw, Nancy
   Sheep on a Ship

Sounds and Listening

Cronin, Doreen
   Click, Clack, Moo: Cows That Type
Dodds, Dayle Ann
   Sing, Sophie!
Dunrea, Olivier
   Bear Noel
Fleming, Candace
   Gabriella's Song
Martin, Bill Jr.
   Polar Bear, Polar Bear, What Do You Hear?
Martin, Bill Jr., and John Archambault
   Barn Dance!
Massie, Diane Redfield
   The Baby Beebee Bird
Moss, Lloyd
   Zin! Zin! Zin! A Violin
Rylant, Cynthia
   Night in the Country
Sloat, Teri
   The Thing That Bothered Farmer Brown

Speaking and Communicating

Cherry, Lynne
   The River Ran Wild: An Environmental History
Marshall, James
   George and Martha: Back in Town
Meddaugh, Susan
   Martha Speaks
Simon, Charnan
   Bill Gates: Helping People Use Computers
Waddell, Martin
   Farmer Duck

Trains

Burningham, John
   Hey! Get Off Our Train
Crews, Donald
   Freight Train
Siebert, Diane
   Train Song

Transportation

Barracca, Debra, and Sal Barracca
   The Adventures of Taxi Dog
Barton, Byron
   Airport
Burningham, John
   Hey! Get Off Our Train
Crews, Donald
   Freight Train
   Sail Away
   School Bus
   Truck
Siebert, Diane
   Train Song

Trickster Tales

Allard, Harry, and James Marshall
   Miss Nelson Is Missing!
Goble, Paul
   Iktomi and the Boulder
   (and other books in the series)
Mayer, Mercer
   Liza Lou and the Yeller Belly Swamp
Scieszka, Jon
   The True Story of the Three Little Pigs
Sierra, Judy
   Counting Crocodiles

Vegetables

Ehlert, Lois
   Growing Vegetable Soup
Krauss, Ruth
   The Carrot Seed
Miranda, Anne
   To Market, To Market

Weather

Crews, Donald
   Sail Away
Hutchins, Pat
   The Wind Blew
Keats, Ezra Jack
   The Snowy Day
Locker, Thomas
   Cloud Dance
Scheer, Julian, and Marvin Bileck
   Rain Makes Applesauce

TOPIC

Spier, Peter
Dreams
Tafuri, Nancy
Snowy Flowy Blowy:
A Twelve Months Rhyme
Wiesner, David
Sector 7
Wood, Audrey
The Napping House

Weather, Rain

Scheer, Julian, and Marvin Bileck
Rain Makes Applesauce

Weather, Storms

Dodds, Dayle Ann
Sing, Sophie!
Rohmann, Eric
Time Flies

Shaw, Nancy
Sheep on a Ship

Women's Lives

Cherry, Lynne
The River Ran Wild:
An Environmental History
Corey, Shana
You Forgot Your Skirt,
Amelia Bloomer
Hearne, Betsy Gould
Seven Brave Women
Ryan, Pam Muñoz
Amelia and Eleanor
Go for a Ride

Woods

Alborough, Jez
It's the Bear!

Where's My Teddy?
Fleming, Denise
Where Once There Was
a Wood

Zoos

Browne, Anthony
Gorilla
Cuyler, Margery
That's Good! That's Bad!
Martin, Bill Jr.
Polar Bear, Polar Bear,
What Do You Hear?
Massie, Diane Redfield
The Baby Beebee Bird
Rathmann, Peggy
Good Night, Gorilla

Skills

Vocabulary

SKILLS

Grammar and Syntax

Language Literacy

Relating Personal Experiences, 15, 21, 22, 28, 30, 47, 64, 69, 76, 78, 80, 81, 88, 97, 117, 138, 141, 156, 171, 172, 177, 189, 191, 205, 213, 214, 216, 263, 264, 299, 303, 312, 313, 317, 334, 343, 347, 349, 355, 382, 397, 404, 407, 418, 426, 449, 454, 455, 456, 466, 476, 484, 537, 551, 563, 575

Predicting, 22, 28, 40, 43, 78, 88, 104, 105, 110, 111, 112, 131, 138, 142, 146, 147, 155, 160, 214, 215, 216, 222, 230, 244, 268, 285, 308, 311, 317, 323, 345, 346, 347, 351, 379, 382, 385, 388, 389, 396, 406, 418, 429, 433, 447, 450, 455, 456, 461, 463, 484, 489, 549, 551, 570

Sequencing, 15, 21, 30, 40, 43, 47, 70, 75, 76, 78, 81, 84, 98, 101, 102, 103, 107, 112, 113, 131, 149, 155, 160, 163, 171, 173, 179, 186, 190, 205, 214, 215, 216, 222, 224, 227, 228, 230, 263, 264, 268, 274, 285, 289, 302, 308, 312, 323, 331, 345, 351, 355, 365, 381, 385, 390, 396, 398, 404, 413, 418, 421, 426, 429, 449, 450, 453, 455, 456, 461, 464, 466, 481, 489, 517

Cause-and-Effect Relationships, 39, 75, 90, 107, 111, 129, 132, 148, 155, 160, 163, 186, 214, 215, 216, 227, 228, 230, 243, 244, 268, 274, 276, 282, 283, 311, 313, 323, 334, 349, 350, 363, 369, 379, 381, 387, 390, 394, 396, 407, 417, 433, 434, 445, 450, 455, 456, 477, 482, 484, 488, 489, 491, 516, 517, 537, 539, 549, 554, 555, 576

Storytelling, 22, 29, 69, 83, 84, 100, 112, 156, 171, 207, 213, 222, 268, 269, 283, 289, 302, 303, 308, 312, 323, 326, 328, 331, 332, 343, 347, 351, 352, 353, 365, 367, 394, 397, 398, 404, 406, 413, 429, 431, 451, 452, 454, 455, 461, 464, 466, 470, 471, 481, 484, 487, 488, 489, 516, 529, 540, 543, 552, 554, 558, 561, 567, 571, 572, 575, 576

Problem Solving, 22, 39, 64, 83, 111, 131, 132, 163, 171, 185, 192, 207, 215, 243, 268, 274, 275, 282, 283, 284, 299, 311, 312, 313, 326, 334, 342, 349, 365, 367, 369, 372, 373, 374, 381, 385, 386, 398, 404, 413, 417, 425, 433, 434, 451, 452, 471, 477, 482, 484, 487, 488, 491, 517, 525, 529, 532, 537, 539, 540, 555, 561, 572, 575, 576

Verbal Expression, 22, 28, 31, 39, 41, 64, 88, 101, 106, 110, 117, 119, 141, 147, 148, 155, 188, 191, 214, 226, 269, 278, 282, 299, 307, 310, 312, 317, 331, 352, 355, 363, 373, 382, 389, 390, 395, 404, 428, 455, 467, 469, 471, 484, 486, 489, 531, 544, 551, 572

Compare and Contrast, 94, 102, 148, 191, 227, 243, 273, 290, 307, 308, 324, 329, 334, 363, 367, 426, 433, 476, 482, 486, 489, 491, 513, 516, 523, 534, 537, 546, 555, 558, 560

Drawing Inferences, 21, 40, 70, 75, 83, 100, 104, 111, 123, 132, 147, 156, 172, 185, 186, 213, 216, 268, 269, 276, 283, 284, 288, 290, 302, 303, 312, 313, 326, 328, 332, 333, 334, 341, 342, 345, 347, 349, 352, 364, 369, 372, 379, 385, 387, 389, 406, 407, 417, 425, 445, 450, 454, 456, 464, 467, 469, 470, 471, 487, 488, 513, 518, 529, 531, 532, 536, 537, 541, 542, 543, 544, 545, 549, 552, 557, 560, 561, 563, 564, 568, 571, 572, 574, 576

Point of View, 264, 331, 334, 352, 428, 429, 431, 463, 470, 488, 537, 544, 558, 564, 567, 570, 571, 574, 576

Critical Thinking, 172, 274, 275, 284, 333, 379, 407, 451, 487, 517, 531, 549

Answering *Why* Questions, 341, 345, 541

Retelling Events, 290, 326, 347, 431, 463, 542, 546, 547, 548, 558, 570

Explaining Processes in Detail, 404, 429, 526, 561, 564

Discussion, 15, 21, 84, 90, 100, 147, 148, 188, 243, 264, 273, 307, 311, 312, 332, 334, 341, 343, 345, 347, 368, 379, 385, 386, 387, 389, 390, 406, 417, 431, 449, 470, 481, 482, 488, 521, 523, 525, 526, 529, 532, 537, 540, 541, 542, 546, 547, 548, 549, 555, 557, 558, 560, 561, 571, 576

SKILLS

Pragmatic Language

SKILLS INDEX

The *Section* column indicates the section of a library in which the book is likely to be shelved, according to Library of Congress recommendations. Your library may use a different system.

E = Easy Fiction

N = Nonfiction

F = Folklore

P = Poetry

J = Juvenile Fiction

YA = Young Adult

VOCABULARY SEMANTICS

	Section	PK-K	1-5	6-12
Allen, Pamela				
Who Sank the Boat?	E	√	—	—
Asbjornsen, Peter				
The Three Billy Goats Gruff	F	√	√	—
Baker, Keith				
Who Is the Beast?	E	√	√	—
Bang, Molly				
Ten, Nine, Eight	E	√	—	—
Barracca, Debra, and Sal Barracca				
The Adventures of Taxi Dog	E	√	√	—
Barrett, Judi				
A Snake Is Totally Tail	E	—	√	—
Things That Are Most in the World	E	—	√	—
Barton, Byron				
Airport	E	√	—	—
Dinosaurs, Dinosaurs	E	√	—	—
Base, Graeme				
Animalia	E	√	√	—
Berger, Barbara				
Grandfather Twilight	E	√	—	—

	Section	PK-K	1-5	6-12
Brett, Jan				
The Mitten: A Ukrainian Folktale	F	√	√	—
Brown, Margaret Wise				
Goodnight Moon	E	√	—	—
The Important Book	E	√	√	—
Brown, Ruth				
A Dark, Dark Tale	E	√	—	—
Bunting, Eve				
The Man Who Could Call Down Owls	E	—	√	√
Scary, Scary Halloween	E	√	—	—
Burleigh, Robert				
Home Run	J	—	√	√
Burningham, John				
Mr. Gumpy's Outing	E	√	—	—
Hey! Get Off Our Train	E	√	—	—
Burton, Virginia Lee				
Mike Mulligan and His Steam Shovel	E	√	—	—
Canfield, Jack; Hansen, Mark Victor; and Kirberger, Kimberly (Eds.)				
Chicken Soup for the Teenage Soul Journal	YA	—	—	√

SKILLS

Vocabulary

	Section	PK–K	1–5	6–12
Carle, Eric				
The Grouchy Ladybug	E	√	—	—
The Mixed-Up Chameleon	E	√	√	—
The Secret Birthday Message	E	√	—	—
The Very Busy Spider	E	√	—	—
The Very Hungry Caterpillar	E	√	—	—
Cendrars, Blaise				
Shadow	P	—	—	√
Charlip, Remy				
Fortunately	E	√	—	—
Cherry, Lynne				
The Great Kapok Tree: A Tale of the Amazon River Forest	J	—	—	√
The River Ran Wild: An Environmental History	N	—	—	√
Cleary, Brian P.				
Hairy, Scary, Ordinary: What Is an Adjective?	E	—	√	—
Corey, Shana				
You Forgot Your Skirt, Amelia Bloomer	E	—	√	—
Cowcher, Helen				
Antarctica	N	—	√	—
Crews, Donald				
Freight Train	E	√	—	—
Sail Away	E	√	—	—
School Bus	E	√	—	—
Cronin, Doreen				
Click, Clack, Moo: Cows That Type	E	√	√	—
de Paola, Tomie				
Charlie Needs a Cloak	E	—	√	—
The Knight and the Dragon	E	—	√	—
Degan, Bruce				
Jamberry	E	√	—	—
Demi				
The Empty Pot	F	√	—	—
One Grain of Rice: A Mathematical Folktale	F	—	√	—

	Section	PK–K	1–5	6–12
Dodds, Dayle Ann				
Sing, Sophie!	E	√	√	—
Dorros, Arthur				
Abuela	E	—	√	—
Dunrea, Oliver				
Bear Noel	E	√	√	—
Enderle, Judith R., and Stephanie G. Tessler				
Six Creepy Sheep	E	—	√	—
Ehlert, Lois				
Cucú: Un cuento folklórico mexicano/Cuckoo: A Mexican Folktale	E	√	—	—
Growing Vegetable Soup	E	√	—	—
Planting a Rainbow	E	√	—	—
Feelings, Muriel				
Jambo Means Hello: Swahili Alphabet Book	E	—	√	—
Feiffer, Jules				
Meanwhile	E	—	√	√
Finn, Isabel, and Jack Tickle				
The Very Lazy Ladybug	E	√	—	—
Fleischman, Paul				
Big Talk: Poems for Four Voices	P	—	—	√
Joyful Noise: Poems for Two Voices	P	—	√	√
Fleming, Candace				
Gabriella's Song	E	—	√	—
Fleming, Denise				
Mama Cat Has Three Kittens	E	√	—	—
Where Once There Was a Wood	E	√	√	—
Fox, Mem				
Hattie and the Fox	E	√	—	—
Tough Boris	E	—	√	—
Wilfrid Gordon McDonald Partridge	E	—	—	√
Freeman, Don				
Corduroy	E	√	√	—

SKILLS

	Section	PK–K	1–5	6–12
Raschka, Chris *Waffle*	E	—	✓	—
Ringgold, Faith *If a Bus Could Talk: The Story of Rosa Parks*	N	—	✓	—
Rockwell, Anne *At the Beach*	E	✓	—	—
Rohmann, Eric *Time Flies*	E	—	✓	—
Ryan, Pam Muñoz *Amelia and Eleanor Go for a Ride*	N	—	—	✓
Sakurai, Gail *Stephen Hawking: Understanding the Universe*	N	—	—	✓
Service, Robert W. *The Cremation of Sam McGee*	P	—	—	✓
Shaw, Nancy *Sheep on a Ship*	E	✓	✓	—
Shulevitz, Uri *Snow*	E	—	✓	—
Sierra, Judy *Counting Crocodiles*	E	✓	✓	—
Simon, Charnan *Bill Gates: Helping People Use Computers*	N	—	—	✓
Sís, Peter *Starry Messenger*	N	—	—	✓
Sloat, Teri *The Thing That Bothered Farmer Brown*	E	✓	✓	—
Soto, Gary *Chato's Kitchen*	E	—	✓	—
Too Many Tamales	E	—	✓	—
Small, David *George Washington's Cows*	E	—	✓	✓
Imogene's Antlers	E	—	✓	—
Stanley, Diane *The Gentleman and the Kitchen Maid*	J	—	—	✓

	Section	PK–K	1–5	6–12
Stewart, Sarah *The Gardener*	E	—	✓	—
Strazzabosco, Jeanne *Learing About Determination from the Life of Gloria Estefan*	J	—	—	✓
Learning About Forgiveness from the Life of Nelson Mandela	J	—	—	✓
Teague, Mark *Pigsty*	E	—	✓	—
Thayer, Ernest Lawrence (Illustrated by Christopher Bing) *Casey at the Bat: A Ballad of the Republic Sung in the Year 1888*	F	—	—	✓
Turner, Ann *Dakota Dugout*	J	—	—	✓
Van Allsburg, Chris *The Wreck of the Zephyr*	E	—	✓	—
Weitzman, Jacquiline Preiss *You Can't Take a Balloon Into the Metropolitan Museum*	E	—	✓	—
Wiesner, David *Sector 7*	E	—	✓	—
Wood, Audrey *The Napping House*	E	✓	—	—
Wood, Don *Quick as a Cricket*	E	✓	—	—
Yorinks, Arthur *Hey, Al*	E	—	✓	—
Young, Ed *Seven Blind Mice*	E	✓	✓	—

Beginning Concepts

(Spatial)

	Section	PK–K	1–5	6–12
Burton, Virginia Lee *Mike Mulligan and His Steam Shovel*	E	✓	—	—

	Section	PK–K	1–5	6–12
Carle, Eric *The Very Hungry Caterpillar*	E	√	—	—
Hoban, Tana *Push, Pull, Empty, Full: A Book of Opposites*	E	—	√	—

(Time)

	Section	PK–K	1–5	6–12
Rohmann, Eric *Time Flies*	E	—	√	—
Weitzman, Jacquiline Preiss *You Can't Take a Balloon Into the Metropolitan Museum*	E	—	√	—

(Sizes, colors, and shapes)

	Section	PK–K	1–5	6–12
Carle, Eric *The Very Hungry Caterpillar*	E	√	—	—
Riley, Linnea *Mouse Mess*	E	√	—	—

(Quantity)

	Section	PK–K	1–5	6–12
Carle, Eric *The Very Hungry Caterpillar*				
Demi *One Grain of Rice: A Mathematical Folktale*	F	—	√	—

Higher-Level Concepts

	Section	PK–K	1–5	6–12
Bunting, Eve *The Man Who Could Call Down Owls*	E	—	√	√
Canfield, Jack; Hansen, Mark Victor; and Kirberger, Kimberly (Eds.) *Chicken Soup for the Teenage Soul Journal*	YA	—	—	√

	Section	PK–K	1–5	6–12
Cherry, Lynne *A River Ran Wild: An Environmental History*	N	—	—	√
Feiffer, Jules *Meanwhile*	E	—	√	—
Gray, Nigel *A Country Far Away*	E	—	√	—
Hearne, Betsy Gould *Seven Brave Women*	J	—	—	√
Jacobsen, Kathy (music and words by Woody Guthrie) *This Land Is Your Land*	F	—	—	√
Kosek, Jane Kelly *Learning About Courage from the Life of Christopher Reeve*	J	—	—	√
Oughton, Jerrie *How the Stars Fell Into the Sky: A Navajo Legend*	F	—	—	√
Ringgold, Faith *If a Bus Could Talk: The Story of Rosa Parks*	N	—	√	—
Ryan, Pam Muñoz *Amelia and Eleanor Go for a Ride*	N	—	—	√
Sakurai, Gail *Stephen Hawking: Understanding the Universe*	N	—	—	√
Service, Robert W. *The Cremation of Sam McGee*	F	—	—	√
Sís, Peter *Starry Messenger*	N	—	—	√
Stewart, Sarah *The Gardener*	E	—	√	—
Strazzabosco, Jeanne *Learning About Determination from the Life of Gloria Estefan*	J	—	—	√
Learning About Forgiveness from the Life of Nelson Mandela	J	—	—	√

SKILLS

	Section	PK–K	1–5	6–12
Thayer, Ernest Lawrence (Illustrated by Christopher Bing)				
Casey at the Bat: A Ballad of the Republic Sung in the Year 1888	F	—	—	√
Wiesner, David				
The Three Pigs	E	—	√	√

Categories

	Section	PK–K	1–5	6–12
Alborough, Jez				
It's the Bear!	E	√	—	—
Baker, Keith				
Who Is the Beast?	E	√	√	—
Barton, Byron				
Airport	E	√	—	—
Brett, Jan				
Berlioz the Bear	E	√	√	—
Brown, Marc				
Pickle Things	P	—	√	—
Brown, Margaret Wise				
The Important Book	E	√	√	—
Bunting, Eve				
Scary, Scary Halloween	E	√	√	—
Burningham, John				
Hey! Get Off Our Train	E	√	√	—
Burton, Virginia Lee				
Mike Mulligan and His Steam Shovel	E	√	—	—
Canfield, Jack; Hansen, Mark Victor; and Kirberger, Kimberly (Eds.)				
Chicken Soup for the Teenage Soul Journal	YA	—	—	√
Carle, Eric				
The Grouchy Ladybug	E	√	—	—
The Very Hungry Caterpillar	E	√	—	—
Cherry, Lynne				
The River Ran Wild:				
An Environmental History	N	—	—	√
Cleary, Brian P.				
Hairy, Scary, Ordinary: What Is an Adjective?	E	—	√	—
Crews, Donald				
Freight Train	E	√	—	—
School Bus	E	√	—	—
Truck	E	√	—	—
Degen, Bruce				
Jamberry	E	√	—	—
Ehlert, Lois				
Growing Vegetable Soup	E	√	—	—
Planting a Rainbow	E	√	—	—
Fleming, Candace				
Gabriella's Song	E	√	√	—
Freeman, Don				
Corduroy	E	√	√	—
Heller, Ruth				
A Cache of Jewels and Other Collective Nouns	N	—	√	—
Kites Sail High: A Book About Verbs	N	√	—	—
Many Luscious Lollipops: A Book About Adjectives	N	√	√	—
Hoban, Tana				
Is It Larger? Is It Smaller?	E	√	—	—
Hutchins, Pat				
Good-Night, Owl!	E	√	√	—
Jacobsen, Kathy (song by Woody Guthrie)				
This Land Is Your Land	F	—	—	√
McPhail, David				
Emma's Pet	E	√	—	—
Martin, Bill Jr.				
Brown Bear, Brown Bear, What Do You See?	E	√	—	—
Martin, Bill Jr., and John Archambault				
Barn Dance!	E	√	√	—

	Section	PK–K	1–5	6–12
Moss, Lloyd *Zin! Zin! Zin! A Violin*	E	—	✓	✓
Riley, Linnea *Mouse Mess*	E	✓	✓	—
Sís, Peter *Starry Messenger*	N	—	—	✓
Slobodkina, Esphyr *Caps for Sale: A Tale of a Peddler, Some Monkeys and Their Monkey Business*	E	✓	—	—
Teague, Mark *Pigsty*	E	—	✓	—
Weitzman, Jacquiline Preiss *You Can't Take a Balloon Into the Metropolitan Museum*	E	—	✓	—

Associations

	Section	PK–K	1–5	6–12
Brown, Magaret Wise *The Important Book*	E	✓	✓	—
Carle, Eric *The Mixed-Up Chameleon*	E	✓	✓	—
The Very Busy Spider	E	✓	—	—
Florian, Douglas *Mammalabilia*	P	—	✓	—
Numeroff, Laura *If You Give a Mouse a Cookie*	E	✓	✓	—
Silverman, Erica *Big Pumpkin*	E	✓	—	—

Adjectives

	Section	PK–K	1–5	6–12
Bang, Molly *Ten, Nine, Eight*	E	✓	—	—
Barton, Byron *Dinosaurs, Dinosaurs*	E	✓	—	—
Bennett, Jill *Teeny Tiny*	F	—	✓	—
Brown, Margaret Wise *Big Red Barn*	E	✓	—	—

	Section	PK–K	1–5	6–12
Brown, Ruth *A Dark, Dark Tale*	E	✓	—	—
Carle, Eric *The Very Busy Spider*	E	✓	—	—
The Very Hungry Caterpillar	E	✓	—	—
Cherry, Lynne *The River Ran Wild: An Environmental History*	N	—	—	✓
Cleary, Brian P. *Hairy, Scary, Ordinary: What Is an Adjective?*	E	—	✓	—
Cowcher, Helen *Antarctica*	N	—	✓	—
Fox, Mem *Tough Boris*	E	—	✓	—
Gackenbach, Dick *Harry and the Terrible Whatzit*	E	—	✓	—
Henkes, Kevin *Lilly's Purple Plastic Purse*	E	✓	✓	—
Heller, Ruth *Many Luscious Lollipops: A Book About Adjectives*	E	✓	—	—
Hoban, Tana *Is It Rough, Is It Smooth, Is It Shiny?*	E	—	✓	—
Shadows and Reflections	E	✓	—	—
Hutchins, Pat *The Very Worst Monster*	E	✓	✓	—
Karon, Jan *Miss Fannie's Hat*	E	—	✓	—
Keats, Ezra Jack *Peter's Chair*	E	✓	✓	—
Lionni, Leo *Frederick*	E	—	✓	—
Locker, Thomas *Cloud Dance*	N	—	—	✓
McPhail, David *Emma's Pet*	E	✓	—	—

SKILLS

Vocabulary

	Section	PK-K	1-5	6-12
Martin, Bill Jr. *Brown Bear, Brown Bear, What Do You See?*	E	√	—	—
Moss, Lloyd *Zin! Zin! Zin! A Violin*	E	—	√	√
Prelutsky, Jack *The Baby Uggs Are Hatching!*	P	—	√	—
Rohmann, Eric *Time Flies*	E	—	√	—
Shulevitz, Uri *Snow*	E	—	√	—
Slobodkina, Esphyr *Caps for Sale: A Tale of a Peddler, Some Monkeys and Their Monkey Business*	E	—	√	—
Small, David *George Washington's Cows*	E	—	√	√
Stewart, Sarah *The Gardener*	E	—	√	—
Tafuri, Nancy *Snowy Flowy Blowy: A Twelve Months Rhyme*	E	√	—	—
Trapani, Iza *The Itsy Bitsy Spider*	E	√	—	—
Viorst, Judith *My Mama Says . . .*	E	—	√	—
Weitzman, Jacquiline Preiss *You Can't Take a Balloon Into the Metropolitan Museum*	E	—	√	—
Wood, Audrey *The Napping House*	E	√	—	—
Silly Sally	E	√	—	—
Wood, Don *Quick as a Cricket*	E	√	√	—
Young, Ed *Seven Blind Mice*	E	√	√	—

Adverbs

	Section	PK-K	1-5	6-12
Charlip, Remy *Fortunately*	E	√	√	—
Dodds, Dayle Ann *Sing, Sophie!*	E	—	√	—
Heller, Ruth *Up, Up and Away: A Book About Adverbs*	E	—	√	√
McNaughton, Colin *Suddenly!*	E	—	√	—
Small, David *George Washington's Cows*	E	—	√	√
Stanley, Diane *The Gentleman and the Kitchen Maid*	J	—	—	√

Attributes

	Section	PK-K	1-5	6-12
Anno, Mitsumasa *Anno's Medieval World*	E	—	—	√
Baker, Keith *Who Is the Beast?*	E	√	√	—
Barrett, Judi *A Snake Is Totally Tail*	E	—	√	—
Barton, Byron *Dinosaurs, Dinosaurs*	E	√	—	—
Brett, Jan *The Mitten: A Ukrainian Folktale*	F	√	√	—
Bunting, Eve *Scary, Scary Halloween*	E	√	√	—
The Man Who Could Call Down Owls	E	—	√	√
Canfield, Jack; Hansen, Mark Victor; and Kirberger, Kimberly (Eds.) *Chicken Soup for the Teenage Soul III: More Stories of Life, Love and Learning*	YA	—	—	√

	Section	PK-K	1-5	6-12
Chicken Soup for the Teenage Soul Journal	YA	—	—	✓
Carle, Eric				
The Grouchy Ladybug	E	✓	—	—
The Mixed-Up Chameleon	E	✓	✓	—
Cendrars, Blaise				
Shadow	P	—	—	✓
de Paola, Tomie				
The Legend of Bluebonnet	F	—	✓	—
Dodds, Dayle Ann				
Sing, Sophie!	E	✓	✓	—
Ehlert, Lois				
Cucú: Un cuento folklórico mexicano/Cuckoo: A Mexican Folktale	E	✓	—	—
Fisher, Leonard Everett				
The Great Wall of China	E	—	—	✓
Fox, Mem				
Tough Boris	E	—	✓	—
Guarino, Deborah				
Is Your Mama a Llama?	E	✓	✓	—
Hearne, Betsy Gould				
Seven Brave Women	J	—	✓	✓
Howe, James				
I Wish I Were a Butterfly	E	✓	✓	—
Karon, Jan				
Miss Fannie's Hat	E	—	✓	—
Kosek, Jane Kelly				
Learning About Courage from the Life of Christopher Reeve	J	—	—	✓
Lawrence, Jacob				
Harriet and the Promised Land	F	—	✓	✓
Lionni, Leo				
Swimmy	E	✓	✓	—
McDermott, Gerald				
Anansi the Spider: A Tale from the Ashanti	F	—	✓	—

	Section	PK-K	1-5	6-12
Mahy, Margaret				
The Seven Chinese Brothers	F	—	✓	—
Martin, Bill Jr., and John Archambault				
Barn Dance!	E	✓	✓	—
McNaughton, Colin				
Here Come the Aliens!	E	—	✓	—
Moss, Lloyd				
Zin! Zin! Zin! A Violin	E	—	✓	✓
Muir, John (Retold by Donnell Rubay)				
Stickeen: John Muir and the Brave Little Dog	N	—	—	✓
Palatini, Margie				
Piggie Pie	E	✓	✓	—
Paulsen, Gary, and Ruth Paulsen				
Dogteam	E	—	✓	✓
Prelutsky, Jack				
The Baby Uggs Are Hatching!	P	—	✓	—
Ringgold, Faith				
If a Bus Could Talk: The Story of Rosa Parks	N	—	✓	—
Sakurai, Gail				
Stephen Hawking: Understanding the Universe	N	—	—	✓
Say, Allen				
Grandfather's Journey	E	—	✓	✓
Scieszka, Jon				
The Stinky Cheese Man and Other Fairly Stupid Tales	E	—	—	✓
Sendak, Maurice				
Where the Wild Things Are	E	—	✓	—
Simon, Charnan				
Bill Gates: Helping People Use Computers	N	—	—	✓
Strazzabosco, Jeanne				
Learning About Determination from the Life of Gloria Estefan	J	—	—	✓

Vocabulary

	Section	PK–K	1–5	6–12
Learning About Forgiveness from the Life of Nelson Mandela	J	—	—	✓
Viorst, Judith *The Tenth Good Thing About Barney*	E	✓	✓	—

Prepositions

	Section	PK–K	1–5	6–12
Ahlberg, Janet, and Allan Ahlberg *Each Peach Pear Plum*	E	✓	—	—
Alborough, Jez *It's the Bear!*	E	✓	—	—
Baker, Keith *Little Green*	E	✓	—	—
Bang, Molly *Ten, Nine, Eight*	E	✓	—	—
Brown, Ruth *A Dark, Dark Tale*	E	✓	—	—
Bunting, Eve *In the Haunted House*	E	✓	✓	—
Burton, Virginia Lee *Mike Mulligan and His Steam Shovel*	E	✓	—	—
Carle, Eric *The Secret Birthday Message*	E	✓	—	—
The Very Hungry Caterpillar	E	✓	—	—
Crews, Donald *Freight Train*	E	✓	—	—
Sail Away	E	✓	—	—
Day, Alexandra *Good Dog, Carl*	E	—	✓	—
de Regniers, Beatrice Schenk *May I Bring a Friend?*	E	✓	—	—
Degen, Bruce *Jamberry*	E	✓	—	—
Freeman, Don *Corduroy*	E	✓	✓	—

	Section	PK–K	1–5	6–12
Gackenbach, Dick *Harry and the Terrible Whatzit*	E	—	✓	—
Hill, Eric *Spot's Birthday Party*	E	✓	—	—
Hutchins, Pat *Rosie's Walk*	E	✓	—	—
Keller, Holly *Geraldine's Blanket*	E	✓	—	—
Mayer, Mercer *There's an Alligator Under My Bed*	E	✓	✓	—
Miranda, Anne *To Market, To Market*	E	✓	—	—
Palatini, Margie *Piggie Pie*	E	✓	—	—
Peek, Merle *Mary Wore Her Red Dress and Henry Wore His Green Sneakers*	E	✓	—	—
Pilkey, Dav *The Hallo-wiener*	E	✓	✓	—
Rylant, Cynthia *The Relatives Came*	E	—	✓	—
Slobodkina, Esphyr *Caps for Sale: A Tale of a Peddler, Some Monkeys and Their Monkey Business*	E	✓	✓	—
Small, David *Imogene's Antlers*	E	—	✓	—
Teague, Mark *Pigsty*	E	—	✓	—
Trapani, Iza *The Itsy Bitsy Spider*	E	✓	✓	—
Waddell, Martin *Farmer Duck*	E	✓	✓	—
Wiesner, David *Sector 7*	E	—	✓	—
Wood, Audrey *Silly Sally*	E	✓	—	—

SKILLS

Idioms

	Section	PK–K	1–5	6–12
Barracca, Debra, and Sal Barracca *The Adventures of Taxi Dog*	E	√	√	—
Browne, Anthony *Piggybook*	E	—	√	—
Corey, Shana *You Forgot Your Skirt, Amelia Bloomer*	E	—	√	—
Enderle, Judith R., and Stephanie G. Tessler *Six Creepy Sheep*	E	—	√	—
Fleming, Candace *Gabriella's Song*	E	√	√	—
Fox, Mem *Hattie and the Fox*	E	√	—	—
Gwynne, Fred *A Chocolate Moose for Dinner*	E	—	√	√
The King Who Rained	E	—	—	√
Jacobsen, Kathy (song by Woody Guthrie) *This Land Is Your Land*	F	—	—	√
Kraus, Robert *Leo the Late Bloomer*	E	—	√	—
Pinkwater, Daniel Manus *The Big Orange Splot*	E	—	√	—
Raschka, Chris *Waffle*	E	—	√	—
Ryan, Pam Muñoz *Amelia and Eleanor Go for a Ride*	N	—	—	√
Soto, Gary *Chato's Kitchen*	E	—	√	—
Stewart, Sarah *The Gardener*	E	—	√	—
Teague, Mark *Pigsty*	E	—	√	—

	Section	PK–K	1–5	6–12
Thayer, Ernest Lawrence (Illustrated by Christopher Bing) *Casey at the Bat: A Ballad of the Republic Sung in the Year 1888*	F	—	—	√

Similes and Metaphors

	Section	PK–K	1–5	6–12
Barracca, Debra, and Sal Barracca *The Adventures of Taxi Dog*	E	√	√	—
Burleigh, Robert *Home Run*	J	—	√	√
Corey, Shana *You Forgot Your Skirt, Amelia Bloomer*	E	—	√	—
Dunrea, Olivier *Bear Noel*	E	√	√	—
Fleischman, Paul *Joyful Noise: Poems for Two Voices*	P	—	√	√
Fox, Mem *Wilfrid Gordon McDonald Partridge*	E	—	√	√
Garland, Sherry *Voices of the Alamo*	J	—	—	√
Jacobsen, Kathy (song by Woody Guthrie) *This Land Is Your Land*	F	—	—	√
Karon, Jan *Miss Fannie's Hat*	E	—	√	—
Lincoln, Abraham (Illustrated by Michael McCurdy) *The Gettysburg Address*	N	—	—	√
Locker, Thomas *Cloud Dance*	N	—	—	√
Mahy, Margaret *The Seven Chinese Brothers*	F	—	√	—

SKILLS

	Section	PK–K	1–5	6–12
Moss, Lloyd *Zin! Zin! Zin!* *A Violin*	E	—	✓	✓
Muir, John (Retold by Donnell Rubay) *Stickeen: John Muir and* *the Brave Little Dog*	N	—	—	✓
Paulsen, Gary, and Ruth Paulsen *Dogteam*	E	—	✓	✓
Ringgold, Faith *Aunt Harriet's* *Underground Railroad* *in the Sky*	E	—	✓	—
Ryan, Pam Muñoz *Amelia and Eleanor* *Go for a Ride*	N	—	—	✓
Sís, Peter *Starry Messenger*	N	—	—	✓
Soto, Gary *Chato's Kitchen*	E	—	✓	—
Stanley, Diane *The Gentleman and the* *Kitchen Maid*	J	—	—	✓
Thayer, Ernest Lawrence (Illustrated by Christopher Bing) *Casey at the Bat: A* *Ballad of the Republic* *Sung in the Year 1888*	F	—	—	✓
Wiesner, David *The Three Pigs*	E	—	—	✓
Williams, Vera B. *A Chair for* *My Mother*	E	—	✓	—
Wood, Don *Quick as a Cricket*	E	✓	✓	—
Yorinks, Arthur *Hey, Al*	E	—	✓	—
Young, Ed *Seven Blind Mice*	F	—	✓	—

Proverbs

	Section	PK–K	1–5	6–12
Ehlert, Lois *Cucú: Un cuento* *folklórico mexicano/* *Cuckoo: A Mexican* *Folktale*	E	✓	—	—
Stewart, Sarah *The Gardener*	E	—	✓	—

Homonyms (Multiple Meanings)

	Section	PK–K	1–5	6–12
Allen, Pamela *Who Sank the Boat?*	E	✓	—	—
Fleischman, Paul *Big Talk: Poems for* *Four Voices*	P	—	—	✓
Fleming, Candace *Gabriella's Song*	E	✓	✓	—
Glass, Andrew *Mountain Men: True Grit* *and Tall Tales*	J	—	—	✓
Gwynne, Fred *A Chocolate Moose* *for Dinner*	E	—	✓	✓
The King Who Rained	E	—	—	✓
Hearne, Betsy Gould *Seven Brave Women*	J	—	✓	✓
Moss, Lloyd *Zin! Zin! Zin! A Violin*	E	—	✓	✓
Pilkey, Dav *Dog Breath: The Horrible* *Trouble with Hally Tosis*	E	—	✓	—
The Hallo-wiener	E	✓	✓	—
Raschka, Chris *Waffle*	E	—	✓	—
Slobodkina, Esphyr *Caps for Sale: A Tale of a* *Peddler, Some Monkeys* *and Their Monkey* *Business*	E	✓	—	—

SKILLS

	Section	PK–K	1–5	6–12
Small, David				
Imogene's Antlers	E	—	√	—

Synonyms

	Section	PK–K	1–5	6–12
Barrett, Judi				
A Snake Is Totally Tail	E	—	√	—
Dodds, Dayle Ann				
Sing, Sophie!	E	√	√	—
Finn, Isabel, and Jack Tickle				
The Very Lazy Ladybug	E	√	—	—
Fleischman, Paul				
Joyful Noise: Poems for Two Voices	P	—	√	—
Hearne, Betsy Gould				
Seven Brave Women	J	—	√	√
Heller, Ruth				
Kites Sail High: A Book About Verbs	E	—	√	—
Hoban, Tana				
Exactly the Opposite	E	√	—	—
Hutchins, Pat				
The Wind Blew	E	—	√	—
Jacobsen, Kathy (music and words by Woody Guthrie)				
This Land Is Your Land	F	—	—	√
Ryan, Pam Muñoz				
Amelia and Eleanor Go for a Ride	N	—	—	√
Sloat, Teri				
The Thing That Bothered Farmer Brown	E	√	√	—
Teague, Mark				
Pigsty	E	—	√	—

Antonyms

	Section	PK–K	1–5	6–12
Allen, Pamela				
Who Sank the Boat?	E	√	√	—

	Section	PK–K	1–5	6–12
Charlip, Remy				
Fortunately	E	√	—	—
Crews, Donald				
School Bus	E	√	—	—
Cuyler, Margery				
That's Good! That's Bad!	E	√	√	—
Hoban, Tana				
Exactly the Opposite	E	√	—	—
Is It Rough, Is It Smooth, Is It Shiny?	E	—	√	—
Push, Pull, Empty, Full: A Book of Opposites	E	—	√	—
Howe, James				
I Wish I Were a Butterfly	E	√	√	—
Teague, Mark				
Pigsty	E	—	√	—
Wildsmith, Brian				
What the Moon Saw	E	√	—	—
Wood, Audrey				
Silly Sally	E	√	—	—

Morphological Units

	Section	PK–K	1–5	6–12
Alborough, Jez				
Where's My Teddy?	E	√	—	—
Asbjornsen, Peter				
The Three Billy Goats Gruff	F	√	√	—
Baker, Keith				
Little Green	E	√	—	—
Barrett, Judi				
Things That Are Most in the World	E	√	√	—
Burleigh, Robert				
Home Run	J	—	√	√
Burton, Virginia Lee				
Mike Mulligan and His Steam Shovel	E	√	—	—
Carle, Eric				
The Grouchy Ladybug	E	√	—	—
The Very Hungry Caterpillar	E	√	—	—

SKILLS

Vocabulary

	Section	PK–K	1–5	6–12
Charlip, Remy *Fortunately*	E	✓	✓	—
Cherry, Lynne *The Great Kapok Tree: A Tale of the Amazon River Forest*	J	—	—	✓
Cleary, Brian P. *Hairy, Scary, Ordinary: What Is an Adjective?*	E	—	✓	—
Corey, Shana *You Forgot Your Skirt, Amelia Bloomer*	E	—	✓	—
Demi *The Empty Pot*	F	✓	—	—
Dorros, Arthur *Abuela*	E	—	✓	—
Florian, Douglas *Mammalabilia*	E	—	✓	—
Heller, Ruth *Many Luscious Lollipops: A Book About Adjectives*	E	✓	✓	—
Up, Up and Away: A Book About Adverbs	E	—	✓	—
Hoban, Tana *Is It Larger? Is It Smaller?*	E	✓	—	—
Hutchins, Pat *The Very Worst Monster*	E	—	✓	—

	Section	PK–K	1–5	6–12
Karon, Jan *Miss Fannie's Hat*	E	—	✓	—
Lionni, Leo *Swimmy*	E	✓	✓	—
McNaughton, Colin *Suddenly!*	E	—	✓	—
Pilkey, Dav *Dog Breath: The Horrible Trouble with Hally Tosis*	E	—	✓	—
Rathmann, Peggy *Good Night, Gorilla*	E	✓	—	—
Shulevitz, Uri *Snow*	E	—	✓	—
Small, David *George Washington's Cows*	E	—	✓	✓
Tafuri, Nancy *Snowy Flowy Blowy: A Twelve Months Rhyme*	E	✓	—	—
Wells, Rosemary *Noisy Nora*	E	✓	—	—
Wood, Audrey *The Napping House*	E	✓	—	—

GRAMMAR AND SYNTAX

Two- and Three-Word Utterances

	Section	PK–K	1–5	6–12
Alborough, Jez				
It's the Bear!	E	✓	—	—
Where's My Teddy?	E	✓	—	—
Baker, Keith				
Little Green	E	✓	—	—
Bang, Molly				
Ten, Nine, Eight	E	✓	—	—
Barracca, Debra, and Sal Barracca				
The Adventures of Taxi Dog	E	✓	—	—
Barton, Byron				
Airport	E	✓	—	—
Dinosaurs, Dinosaurs	E	✓	—	—
Brown, Margaret Wise				
Goodnight Moon	E	✓	—	—
Carle, Eric				
The Very Busy Spider	E	✓	—	—
The Very Hungry Caterpillar	E	✓	—	—
Carlstrom, Nancy White				
Jesse Bear, What Will You Wear?	E	✓	—	—
Crews, Donald				
Freight Train	E	✓	—	—
Sail Away	E	✓	—	—
School Bus	E	✓	—	—
Truck	E	✓	—	—
Cronin, Doreen				
Click, Clack, Moo: Cows That Type	E	✓	—	—
Degen, Bruce				
Jamberry	E	✓	—	—
Dodds, Dayle Ann				
Sing, Sophie!	E	✓	—	—
Finn, Isabel, and Jack Tickle				
The Very Lazy Ladybug	E	✓	—	—
Fleming, Candace				
Gabriella's Song	E	✓	—	—
Fleming, Denise				
Mama Cat Has Three Kittens	E	✓	—	—
Where Once There Was a Wood	E	✓	—	—
Heller, Ruth				
Many Luscious Lollipops: A Book About Adjectives	E	✓	—	—
Hutchins, Pat				
Rosie's Walk	E	✓	—	—
The Very Worst Monster	E	✓	—	—
Langstaff, John				
Oh, A-Hunting We Will Go	E	✓	—	—
Martin, Bill Jr.				
Brown Bear, Brown Bear, What Do You See?	E	✓	—	—
Polar Bear, Polar Bear, What Do You Hear?	E	✓	—	—
Peek, Merle				
Mary Wore Her Red Dress and Henry Wore His Green Sneakers	E	✓	—	—
Rathmann, Peggy				
Good Night, Gorilla	E	✓	—	—
Riley, Linnea				
Mouse Mess	E	✓	—	—
Rockwell, Anne				
At the Beach	E	✓	—	—
Scheer, Julian, and Marvin Bileck				
Rain Makes Applesauce	E	✓	—	—
Sendak, Maurice				
Alligators All Around: An Alphabet	E	✓	—	—
Shaw, Charles G.				
It Looked Like Spilt Milk	E	✓	—	—
Shaw, Nancy				
Sheep on a Ship	E	✓	—	—
Sloat, Teri				
The Thing That Bothered Farmer Brown	E	✓	—	—

SKILLS

	Section	PK–K	1–5	6–12
Tafuri, Nancy				
Snowy Flowy Blowy: A Twelve Months Rhyme	E	✓	—	—
Waddell, Martin				
Farmer Duck	E	✓	—	—
Williams, Sue				
Went Walking	E	✓	—	—

Noun–Verb Agreement

	Section	PK–K	1–5	6–12
Alborough, Jez				
It's the Bear!	E	✓	—	—
Where's My Teddy?	E	✓	—	—
Baker, Keith				
Little Green	E	✓	—	—
Barracca, Debra, and Sal Barracca				
The Adventures of Taxi Dog	E	✓	—	—
Barton, Byron				
Airport	E	✓	—	—
Brett, Jan				
Annie and the Wild Animals	E	✓	—	—
Brown, Margaret Wise				
Goodnight Moon	E	✓	—	—
Crews, Donald				
School Bus	E	✓	—	—
Truck	E	✓	—	—
Dodds, Dayle Ann				
Sing, Sophie!	E	✓	—	—
Fleming, Denise				
Mama Cat Has Three Kittens	E	✓	—	—
Where Once There Was a Wood	E	✓	—	—
Keats, Ezra Jack				
The Snowy Day	E	✓	—	—
Krauss, Ruth				
A Hole Is to Dig: A First Book of First Definitions	E	✓	—	—

	Section	PK–K	1–5	6–12
Numeroff, Laura				
Chimps Don't Wear Glasses	E	✓	—	—
Rathmann, Peggy				
Good Night, Gorilla	E	✓	—	—
Riley, Linnea				
Mouse Mess	E	✓	—	—
Rockwell, Anne				
At the Beach	E	✓	—	—
Sendak, Maurice				
Alligators All Around: An Alphabet	E	✓	—	—
Shaw, Nancy				
Sheep on a Ship	E	✓	—	—
Sloat, Teri				
The Thing That Bothered Farmer Brown	E	✓	—	—
Tafuri, Nancy				
Snowy Flowy Blowy: A Twelve Months Rhyme	E	✓	—	—
Wells, Rosemary				
Noisy Nora	E	✓	—	—
Waddell, Martin				
Farmer Duck	E	✓	—	—

Singular and Plural Nouns

	Section	PK–K	1–5	6–12
Bang, Molly				
Ten, Nine, Eight	E	✓	—	—
Carle, Eric				
The Very Hungry Caterpillar	E	✓	—	—
Crews, Donald				
School Bus	E	✓	—	—
Hoban, Tana				
Is It Larger? Is It Smaller?	E	✓	—	—
Keats, Ezra Jack				
Over in the Meadow	E	✓	—	—
Shaw, Nancy				
Sheep on a Ship	E	✓	✓	—

SKILLS

Possessive Nouns

Section	PK-K	1-5	6-12
Brown, Marc *Arthur's Nose* E	✓	✓	—
Burningham, John *Mr. Gumpy's Outing* E	✓	✓	—
Carle, Eric *The Mixed-Up Chameleon* E	✓	✓	—
Day, Alexandra *Good Dog, Carl* E	—	✓	—
Henkes, Kevin *Lilly's Purple Plastic Purse* E	✓	✓	—
Hill, Eric *Spot's Birthday Party* E	✓	—	—
Keats, Ezra Jack *Peter's Chair* E	✓	✓	—
McNaughton, Colin *Suddenly!* E	—	✓	—
Marshall, James *George and Martha: Back in Town* E	—	✓	—
Peek, Merle *Mary Wore Her Red Dress and Henry Wore His Green Sneakers* E	✓	—	—

Personal Pronouns

Section	PK-K	1-5	6-12
Ahlberg, Janet, and Allan Ahlberg *Each Peach Pear Plum* E	✓	—	—
Alborough, Jez *It's the Bear!* E	✓	—	—
Brown, Marc *Arthur's Nose* E	✓	✓	—
Brett, Jan *Berlioz the Bear* E	✓	✓	—
Burningham, John *Aldo* E	✓	—	—

Section	PK-K	1-5	6-12
Carlstrom, Nancy White *Jesse Bear, What Will You Wear?* E	✓	—	—
Cazet, Denys *A Fish in His Pocket* E	—	✓	—
de Paola, Tomie *Pancakes for Breakfast* E	✓	✓	—
Fleming, Denise *Mama Cat Has Three Kittens* E	✓	—	—
Freeman, Don *Corduroy* E	✓	✓	—
Heller, Ruth *Mine, All Mine: A Book About Pronouns* E	—	✓	—
Hutchins, Pat *The Wind Blew* E	—	✓	—
Keats, Ezra Jack *Peter's Chair* E	✓	✓	—
Keller, Holly *Geraldine's Blanket* E	✓	—	—
Lear, Edward (Illustrated by Jan Brett) *The Owl and the Pussycat* E	✓	✓	—
McPhail, David *Emma's Pet* E	✓	—	—
Marshall, James *George and Martha: Back in Town* E	—	✓	—
Mayer, Mercer *Hiccup* E	—	✓	—
Palatini, Margie *Piggie Pie* E	✓	✓	—
Peek, Merle *Mary Wore Her Red Dress and Henry Wore His Green Sneakers* E	✓	—	—
Pilkey, Dav *The Hallo-wiener* E	✓	✓	—
Rathmann, Peggy *Good Night, Gorilla* E	✓	—	—
Officer Buckle and Gloria E	✓	✓	—

SKILLS

647

	Section	PK–K	1–5	6–12
Rylant, Cynthia *The Relatives Came*	E	—	√	—
Shulevitz, Uri *Snow*	E	—	√	—
Soto, Gary *Too Many Tamales*	E	—	√	—

Possessive Pronouns

	Section	PK–K	1–5	6–12
Alborough, Jez *It's the Bear!*	E	√	—	—
Where's My Teddy?	E	√	—	—
Barton, Byron *Hester*	E	√	—	—
Brett, Jan *Berlioz the Bear*	E	√	√	—
Brown, Marc *Arthur's Nose*	E	√	√	—
Burningham, John *Aldo*	E	√	—	—
Carlstrom, Nancy White *Jesse Bear, What Will You Wear?*	E	√	—	—
Cazet, Denys *A Fish in His Pocket*	E	—	√	—
de Paola, Tomie *Pancakes for Breakfast*	E	√	√	—
Fleming, Denise *Mama Cat Has Three Kittens*	E	√	—	—
Fox, Mem *Tough Boris*	E	—	√	—
Freeman, Don *Corduroy*	E	√	√	—
Heller, Ruth *Mine, All Mine: A Book About Pronouns*	E	—	√	—
Henkes, Kevin *Lilly's Purple Plastic Purse*	E	√	√	—
Hutchins, Pat *The Wind Blew*	E	—	√	—

	Section	PK–K	1–5	6–12
Keats, Ezra Jack *Peter's Chair*	E	√	√	—
Keller, Holly *Geraldine's Blanket*	E	√	—	—
Lear, Edward (Illustrated by Jan Brett) *The Owl and the Pussycat*	E	√	√	—
McPhail, David *Emma's Pet*	E	√	—	—
Mahy, Margaret *The Seven Chinese Brothers*	E	—	√	—
Marshall, James *George and Martha: Back in Town*	E	—	√	—
Palatini, Margie *Piggie Pie*	E	√	√	—
Peek, Merle *Mary Wore Her Red Dress and Henry Wore His Green Sneakers*	E	√	—	—
Pilkey, Dav *The Hallo-wiener*	E	√	√	—
Rathmann, Peggy *Officer Buckle and Gloria*	E	√	√	—
Rylant, Cynthia *The Relatives Came*	E	—	√	—
Shultevitz, Uri *Snow*	E	—	√	—
Soto, Gary *Too Many Tamales*	E	—	√	—
Teague, Mark *Pigsty*	E	—	√	—

Reflexive Pronouns

	Section	PK–K	1–5	6–12
Brown, Marc *Arthur's Nose*	E	√	√	—
Carlstrom, Nancy White *Jesse Bear, What Will You Wear?*	E	√	—	—

SKILLS

	Section	PK-K	1-5	6-12
Fox, Mem				
Tough Boris	E	—	✓	—
Wilfrid Gordon McDonald Partridge	E	—	✓	—
Freeman, Don				
Corduroy	E	✓	✓	—
Gray, Nigel				
A Country Far Away	E	—	✓	—
Gulbis, Stephen				
I Know an Old Lady Who Swallowed a Fly	E	✓	—	—
Heller, Ruth				
Kites Sail High: A Book About Verbs	E	—	✓	—
Hutchins, Pat				
Rosie's Walk	E	✓	—	—
The Very Worst Monster	E	✓	✓	—
Karon, Jan				
Miss Fannie's Hat	E	—	✓	—
Keats, Ezra Jack				
Over in the Meadow	E	✓	—	—
Peter's Chair	E	✓	✓	—
The Snowy Day	E	✓	—	—
Keller, Holly				
Geraldine's Blanket	E	✓	—	—
Krauss, Ruth				
The Carrot Seed	E	✓	—	—
Lear, Edward (Illustrated by Jan Brett)				
The Owl and the Pussycat	E	✓	✓	—
McDermott, Gerald				
Anansi the Spider: A Tale from the Ashanti	E	—	✓	—
McNaughton, Colin				
Suddenly!	E	—	✓	—
McPhail, David				
Emma's Pet	E	✓	—	—
Mahy, Margaret				
The Seven Chinese Brothers	E	—	✓	—
Marshall, James				
George and Martha: Back in Town	E	—	✓	—
Mayer, Mercer				
Frog on His Own	E	—	✓	—
There's an Alligator Under My Bed	E	✓	✓	—
Meddaugh, Susan				
Martha Speaks				
Miranda, Anne				
To Market, To Market	E	✓	—	—
Numeroff, Laura				
Chimps Don't Wear Glasses	E	✓	✓	—
If You Give a Mouse a Cookie	E	✓	✓	—
Palatini, Margie				
Piggie Pie	E	✓	—	—
Peek, Merle				
Mary Wore Her Red Dress and Henry Wore His Green Sneakers	E	✓	—	—
Pilkey, Dav				
The Hallo-wiener	E	—	✓	—
Prelutsky, Jack				
The Baby Uggs Are Hatching!	P	—	✓	—
Rathmann, Peggy				
Officer Buckle and Gloria	E	✓	✓	—
Riley, Linnea				
Mouse Mess	E	✓	—	—
Rylant, Cynthia				
Night in the Country	E	✓	✓	—
Scheer, Julian, and Marvin Bileck				
Rain Makes Applesauce	E	✓	✓	—
Sendak, Maurice				
Alligators All Around: An Alphabet	E	✓	—	—
Chicken Soup with Rice	E	—	✓	—
Shaw, Nancy				
Sheep on a Ship	E	✓	—	—
Shulevitz, Uri				
Snow	E	—	✓	—
Sierra, Judy				
Counting Crocodiles	E	✓	✓	—

SKILLS

	Section	PK–K	1–5	6–12
Rockwell, Anne *At the Beach*	E	✓	—	—
Rohmann, Eric *Time Flies*	E	—	✓	—
Rylant, Cynthia *The Relatives Came*	E	—	✓	—
Sendak, Maurice *Alligators All Around: An Alphabet*	E	✓	—	—
Chicken Soup with Rice	E	✓	✓	—
Shaw, Nancy *Sheep on a Ship*	E	✓	✓	—
Sierra, Judy *Counting Crocodiles*	E	✓	✓	—
Soto, Gary *Too Many Tamales*	E	—	✓	—
Spier, Peter *Dreams*	E	—	✓	—
London Bridge Is Falling Down	E	—	✓	—
Oh, Were They Ever Happy	E	—	✓	—
Teague, Mark *Pigsty*	E	—	✓	—
Van Allsburg, Chris *The Mysteries of Harris Burdick*	E	—	✓	✓
Viorst, Judith *Alexander and the Terrible, Horrible, No Good, Very Bad Day*	E	—	✓	—
Waddell, Martin *Farmer Duck*	E	✓	✓	—
Weitzman, Jacquiline Preiss *You Can't Take a Balloon Into the Metropolitan Museum*	E	—	✓	—
Wells, Rosemary *Noisy Nora*	E	✓	—	—
Wiesner, David *Sector 7*	E	—	✓	—
The Three Pigs	E	—	✓	✓
Tuesday	E	—	✓	✓

	Section	PK–K	1–5	6–12
Wood, Audrey *The Napping House*	E	✓	—	—
Silly Sally	E	✓	—	—

Past Tense

	Section	PK–K	1–5	6–12
Bang, Molly *The Paper Crane*	F	—	✓	—
Barracca, Debra, and Sal Barracca *The Adventures of Taxi Dog*	E	✓	✓	—
Bennett, Jill *Teeny Tiny*	E	—	✓	—
Berger, Barbara *Grandfather Twilight*	E	✓	—	—
Brett, Jan *Annie and the Wild Animals*	E	✓	—	—
Brown, Margaret Wise *Big Red Barn*	E	✓	—	—
Browne, Anthony *Gorilla*	E	—	✓	—
Bunting, Eve *In the Haunted House*	E	—	✓	—
Burningham, John *Aldo*	E	✓	—	—
Burton, Virginia Lee *Mike Mulligan and His Steam Shovel*	E	✓	—	—
Cazet, Denys *A Fish in His Pocket*	E	—	✓	—
Charlip, Remy *Fortunately*	E	✓	✓	—
Crews, Donald *Freight Train*	E	✓	—	—
Day, Alexandra *Good Dog, Carl*	E	—	✓	—
de Paola, Tomie *The Knight and the Dragon*	E	—	✓	—
Pancakes for Breakfast	E	—	✓	—

	Section	PK–K	1–5	6–12
Demi				
One Grain of Rice: A Mathematical Folktale	F	—	✓	—
Dunrea, Oliver				
Bear Noel	E	—	✓	—
Enderle, Judith, and Stephanie G. Tessler				
Six Creepy Sheep	E	—	✓	—
Feiffer, Jules				
Meanwhile	E	—	✓	✓
Finn, Isabel, and Jack Tickle				
The Very Lazy Ladybug	E	✓	—	—
Fleming, Candace				
Gabriella's Song	E	✓	✓	—
Fleming, Denise				
Where Once There Was a Wood	E	—	✓	—
Fox, Mem				
Tough Boris	E	—	✓	—
Wilfrid Gordon McDonald Partridge	E	—	✓	—
Freeman, Don				
Corduroy	E	✓	✓	—
Gackenbach, Dick				
Harry and the Terrible Whatzit	E	—	✓	—
Gulbis, Stephen				
I Know an Old Lady Who Swallowed a Fly	E	✓	—	—
Hearne, Betsy Gould				
Seven Brave Women	J	—	✓	✓
Heller, Ruth				
Kites Sail High: A Book About Verbs	E	—	✓	—
Henkes, Kevin				
Lilly's Purple Plastic Purse	E	✓	✓	—
Hutchins, Pat				
Good-Night, Owl!	E	✓	✓	—
Rosie's Walk	E	✓	—	—
The Wind Blew	E	—	✓	—
Karon, Jan				
Miss Fannie's Hat	E	—	✓	—

	Section	PK–K	1–5	6–12
Keats, Ezra Jack				
Over in the Meadow	E	✓	—	—
Peter's Chair	E	✓	✓	—
The Snowy Day	E	✓	✓	—
Krauss, Ruth				
The Carrot Seed	E	✓	—	—
Lawrence, Jacob				
Harriet and the Promised Land	F	—	✓	✓
Lear, Edward (Illustrated by Jan Brett)				
The Owl and the Pussycat	E	✓	✓	—
Lobel, Arnold				
Ming Lo Moves the Mountain	E	—	✓	—
McDermott, Gerald				
Anansi the Spider: A Tale from the Ashanti	F	—	✓	—
McNaughton, Colin				
Here Come the Aliens!	E	—	✓	—
Suddenly!	E	—	✓	—
Mahy, Margaret				
The Seven Chinese Brothers	F	—	✓	—
Marshall, James				
George and Martha: Back in Town	E	—	✓	—
Mayer, Mercer				
There's an Alligator Under My Bed	E	✓	✓	—
Frog on His Own	E	—	✓	—
Meddaugh, Susan				
Martha Speaks	E	—	✓	—
Miranda, Anne				
To Market, To Market	E	✓	—	—
Numeroff, Laura				
If You Give a Mouse a Cookie	E	✓	—	—
Palatini, Margie				
Piggie Pie	E	—	✓	—
Peek, Merle				
Mary Wore Her Red Dress and Henry Wore His Green Sneakers	E	✓	—	—

SKILLS

	Section	PK–K	1–5	6–12
Pilkey, Dav				
The Hallo-wiener	E	✓	✓	—
Pinkwater, Daniel Manus				
The Big Orange Splot	E	—	✓	—
Rathmann, Peggy				
Officer Buckle and Gloria	E	✓	✓	—
Rohmann, Eric				
Time Flies	E	—	✓	—
Rylant, Cynthia				
Night in the Country	E	✓	✓	—
The Relatives Came	E	—	✓	—
When I Was Young in the Mountains	E	—	✓	—
Sendak, Maurice				
Where the Wild Things Are	E	—	✓	—
Shaw, Charles G.				
It Looked Like Spilt Milk	E	✓	—	—
Shaw, Nancy				
Sheep on a Ship	E	✓	✓	—
Sierra, Judy				
Counting Crocodiles	E	✓	✓	—
Sloat, Teri				
The Thing That Bothered Farmer Brown	E	✓	✓	—
Small, David				
George Washington's Cows	E	—	✓	✓
Imogene's Antlers	E	—	✓	—
Soto, Gary				
Chato's Kitchen	E	—	✓	—
Too Many Tamales	E	—	✓	—
Spier, Peter				
Dreams	E	—	✓	—
Oh, Were They Ever Happy	E	—	✓	—
Teague, Mark				
Pigsty	E	—	✓	—
Trapani, Iza				
The Itsy Bitsy Spider	E	✓	✓	—

	Section	PK–K	1–5	6–12
Van Allsburg, Chris				
The Mysteries of Harris Burdick	E	—	✓	✓
Viorst, Judith				
The Tenth Good Thing About Barney	E	✓	✓	—
Waddell, Martin				
Farmer Duck	E	✓	✓	—
Wiesner, David				
Sector 7	E	—	✓	—
The Three Pigs	E	—	✓	✓
Tuesday	E	—	✓	—
Williams, Sue				
I Went Walking	E	✓	—	—
Wood, Audrey				
Silly Sally	E	✓	—	—

Future Tense

	Section	PK–K	1–5	6–12
Bang, Molly				
The Paper Crane	F	—	✓	—
Burningham, John				
Hey! Get Off Our Train	E	✓	✓	—
Carlstrom, Nancy White				
Jesse Bear, What Will You Wear?	E	✓	—	—
Cherry, Lynne				
The Great Kapok Tree: A Tale of the Amazon River Forest	J	—	—	✓
Langstaff, John				
Oh, A-Hunting We Will Go	E	✓	—	—
McNaughton, Colin				
Suddenly!	E	—	✓	—
Numeroff, Laura				
If You Give a Mouse a Cookie	E	✓	✓	—
Rathmann, Peggy				
Officer Buckle and Gloria	E	—	✓	—

SKILLS

653

Section	PK-K	1-5	6-12
Small, David *Imogene's Antlers* E	—	✓	—
Soto, Gary *Too Many Tamales* E	—	✓	—
Van Allsburg, Chris *The Mysteries of* *Harris Burdick* E	—	✓	—
Zolotow, Charlotte *Someday* E	—	✓	—

Negative Structures

Section	PK-K	1-5	6-12
Burningham, John *Mr. Gumpy's Outing* E	✓	✓	—
Carle, Eric *The Very Busy Spider* E	✓	—	—
Finn, Isabel, and Jack Tickle *The Very Lazy Ladybug* E	✓	—	—
Guarino, Deborah *Is Your Mama a Llama?* E	✓	✓	—
Numeroff, Laura *Chimps Don't Wear* *Glasses* E	✓	✓	—
Rathmann, Peggy *Officer Buckle and* *Gloria* E	✓	✓	—
Shaw, Charles G. *It Looked Like* *Spilt Milk* E	✓	—	—
Shulevitz, Uri *Snow* E	—	✓	—
Small, David *Imogene's Antlers* E	—	✓	—

Question Structures

Section	PK-K	1-5	6-12
Allen, Pamela *Who Sank the Boat?* E	✓	✓	—
Bennett, Jill *Teeny Tiny* E	—	✓	—

Section	PK-K	1-5	6-12
Burningham, John *Mr. Gumpy's Outing* E	✓	✓	—
Would You Rather? E	—	✓	—
Carle, Eric *The Very Busy Spider* E	✓	—	—
Carlstrom, Nancy White *Jesse Bear, What Will* *You Wear?* E	✓	—	—
de Regniers, Beatrice Schenk *May I Bring a Friend?* E	✓	—	—
Dunrea, Olivier *Bear Noel* E	✓	✓	—
Guarino, Deborah *Is Your Mama a Llama?* E	✓	✓	—
Martin, Bill Jr. *Brown Bear, Brown Bear,* *What Do You See?* E	✓	—	—
Polar Bear, Polar Bear, *What Do You Hear?* E	✓	—	—
Numeroff, Laura *Chimps Don't Wear* *Glasses* E	✓	✓	—
Rathmann, Peggy *Officer Buckle and* *Gloria* E	✓	✓	—
Small, David *Imogene's Antlers* E	✓	—	—
Williams, Sue *I Went Walking* E	✓	—	—

Advanced Syntactic Structures

Section	PK-K	1-5	6-12
Anno, Mitsumasa *Anno's Journey* E	—	—	✓
Anno's Medieval World E	—	—	✓
Burleigh, Robert *Home Run* J	—	✓	✓
Burningham, John *Would You Rather . . .* E	—	✓	—
Cendrars, Blaise *Shadow* P	—	—	✓

SKILLS

	Section	PK–K	1–5	6–12
Small, David				
George Washington's Cows	E	—	√	√
Soto, Gary				
Too Many Tamales	E	—	√	—

	Section	PK–K	1–5	6–12
Stanley, Diane				
The Gentleman and the Kitchen Maid	J	—	—	√
Van Allsburg, Chris				
The Mysteries of Harris Burdick	E	—	√	√

LANGUAGE LITERACY

Relating Personal Experiences

Section	PK-K	1-5	6-12
Barracca, Debra, and Sal Barracca			
The Adventures of Taxi Dog	E	✓	✓	—
Barton, Byron			
Airport	E	✓	—	—
Brett, Jan			
Annie and the Wild Animals	E	✓	—	—
Brown, Margaret Wise			
The Important Book	E	✓	✓	—
Burningham, John			
Aldo	E	✓	—	—
Buscaglia, Leo F.			
The Fall of Freddie the Leaf	E	—	✓	—
Cazet, Denys			
A Fish in His Pocket	E	—	✓	—
Charlip, Remy			
Fortunately	E	✓	✓	—
Crews, Donald			
School Bus	E	✓	—	—
Cronin, Doreen			
Click, Clack, Moo: Cows That Type	E	✓	✓	—
Cuyler, Margery			
That's Good! That's Bad!	E	✓	✓	—
Brett, Jan			
Annie and the Wild Animals	E	✓	—	—
de Paola, Tomie			
Pancakes for Breakfast	E	✓	✓	—
Demi			
The Empty Pot	E	✓	—	—
Dorros, Arthur			
Abuela	E	—	✓	—
Ehlert, Lois			
Planting a Rainbow	E	✓	—	—
Feiffer, Jules			
Meanwhile	E	—	✓	✓

Section	PK-K	1-5	6-12
Fleming, Denise			
Mama Cat Has Three Kittens	E	✓	—	—
Fox, Mem			
Wilfrid Gordon McDonald Partridge	E	—	✓	✓
Freeman, Don			
Corduroy	E	✓	✓	—
Hoban, Tana			
I Read Signs	E	—	✓	—
Shadows and Reflections	E	✓	—	—
Hughs, Shirley			
Alfie Gets in First	E	✓	—	—
Hutchins, Pat			
Don't Forget the Bacon	E	✓	—	—
Keats, Ezra Jack			
Peter's Chair	E	✓	✓	—
The Snowy Day	E	✓	✓	—
Keller, Holly			
Geraldine's Blanket	E	✓	—	—
Krauss, Ruth			
The Carrot Seed	E	✓	—	—
Hines, Anna Grossnickle			
Daddy Makes the Best Spaghetti	E	✓	—	—
McPhail, David			
Emma's Pet	E	✓	—	—
Mayer, Mercer			
Hiccup	E	—	✓	—
Peek, Merle			
Mary Wore Her Red Dress and Henry Wore His Green Sneakers	E	✓	—	—
Rockwell, Anne			
At the Beach	E	✓	—	—
Rylant, Cynthia			
The Relatives Came	E	—	✓	—
When I Was Young in the Mountains	E	—	✓	—
Sakurai, Gail			
Stephen Hawking: Understanding the Universe	N	—	—	✓

	Section	PK–K	1–5	6–12
Say, Allen				
Grandfather's Journey	E	—	√	√
Silverman, Erica				
Don't Fidget a Feather!	E	√	—	—
Sloat, Teri				
The Thing That Bothered Farmer Brown	E	√	√	—
Soto, Gary				
Too Many Tamales	E	—	√	—
Spier, Peter				
Oh, Were They Ever Happy	E	—	√	—
Tafuri, Nancy				
Snowy Flowy Blowy: A Twelve Months Rhyme	E	√	—	—
Teague, Mark				
Pigsty	E	—	√	—
Viorst, Judith				
The Tenth Good Thing About Barney	E	√	√	—
Wells, Rosemary				
Noisy Nora	E	√	—	—
Zion, Gene				
Harry the Dirty Dog	E	—	√	—

Predicting

	Section	PK–K	1–5	6–12
Allen, Pamela				
Who Sank the Boat?	E	√	√	—
Asbjornsen, Peter				
The Three Billy Goats Gruff	E	√	√	—
Bang, Molly				
The Paper Crane	F	—	√	—
Brett, Jan				
Annie and the Wild Animals	E	√	—	—
The Mitten: A Ukrainian Folktale	F	√	√	—
Bunting, Eve				
The Man Who Could Call Down Owls	E	—	√	√

	Section	PK–K	1–5	6–12
Burningham, John				
Hey! Get Off Our Train	E	√	√	—
Mr. Gumpy's Outing	E	√	√	—
Charlip, Remy				
Fortunately	E	√	√	—
Cuyler, Margery				
That's Good! That's Bad!	E	√	√	—
de Regniers, Beatrice Schenk				
May I Bring a Friend?	E	√	—	—
Feiffer, Jules				
Meanwhile	E	—	√	√
Finn, Isabel, and Jack Tickle				
The Very Lazy Ladybug	E	√	—	—
Fleming, Denise				
Mama Cat Has Three Kittens	E	√	—	—
Fox, Mem				
Hattie and the Fox	E	√	—	—
Howe, James				
I Wish I Were a Butterfly	E	√	√	—
Hughs, Shirley				
Alfie Gets in First	E	√	—	—
Leaf, Margaret				
The Eyes of the Dragon	E	—	√	—
Lobel, Arnold				
Ming Lo Moves the Mountain	E	—	√	—
McNaughton, Colin				
Suddenly!	E	—	√	—
Mahy, Margaret				
The Seven Chinese Brothers	F	—	√	—
Mayer, Mercer				
Ah-Choo	E	—	√	—
Frog on His Own	E	—	√	—
Hiccup	E	—	√	—
There's an Alligator Under My Bed	E	√	√	—
Numeroff, Laura				
If You Give a Mouse a Cookie	E	√	√	—

Section	PK–K	1–5	6–12
Ehlert, Lois			
Cucú: Un cuento folklórico mexicano/Cuckoo: A Mexican Folktale E	✓	—	—
Growing Vegetable Soup E	✓	—	—
Planting a Rainbow E	✓	—	—
Emberley, Barbara			
Drummer Hoff E	✓	—	—
Finn, Isabel, and Jack Tickle			
The Very Lazy Ladybug E	✓	—	—
Gulbis, Stephen			
I Know an Old Lady Who Swallowed a Fly E	✓	—	—
Hines, Anna Grossnickle			
Daddy Makes the Best Spaghetti E	✓	—	—
Hogrogian, Nonny			
One Fine Day E	✓	—	—
Hutchins, Pat			
Don't Forget the Bacon E	✓	—	—
Rosie's Walk E	✓	—	—
Keats, Ezra Jack			
The Snowy Day E	✓	✓	—
Krauss, Ruth			
The Carrot Seed E	✓	—	—
Lobel, Arnold			
Ming Lo Moves the Mountain F	—	✓	—
McDermott, Gerald			
Arrow to the Sun F	—	✓	✓
Mayer, Mercer			
Ah-Choo E	—	✓	—
Frog on His Own E	—	✓	—
There's an Alligator Under My Bed E	✓	✓	—
Meddaugh, Susan			
Martha Speaks E	—	✓	—
Miranda, Anne			
To Market, To Market E	✓	—	—
McNaughton, Colin			
Suddenly! E	—	✓	—

Section	PK–K	1–5	6–12
Numeroff, Laura			
If You Give a Mouse a Cookie E	✓	✓	—
Palatini, Margie			
Piggie Pie E	✓	✓	—
Rathmann, Peggy			
Good Night, Gorilla E	✓	—	—
Officer Buckle and Gloria E	✓	✓	—
Riley, Linnea			
Mouse Mess E	✓	✓	—
Rockwell, Anne			
At the Beach E	✓	—	—
Rohmann, Eric			
Time Flies E	—	✓	—
Rylant, Cynthia			
The Relatives Came E	—	✓	—
Scheer, Julian, and Marvin Bileck			
Rain Makes Applesauce E	✓	✓	—
Sendak, Maurice			
Where the Wild Things Are E	—	✓	—
Sierra, Judy			
Counting Crocodiles E	✓	—	—
Silverman, Erica			
Big Pumpkin E	✓	—	—
Sloat, Teri			
The Thing That Bothered Farmer Brown E	✓	✓	—
Slobodkina, Esphyr			
Caps for Sale: A Tale of a Peddler, Some Monkeys and Their Monkey Business E	✓	✓	—
Soto, Gary			
Too Many Tamales E	—	✓	—
Tafuri, Nancy			
Snowy Flowy Blowy: A Twelve Months Rhyme E	✓	—	—
Teague, Mark			
Pigsty E	—	✓	—
Turkle, Brinton			
Deep in the Forest E	—	✓	—

	Section	PK-K	1-5	6-12
Viorst, Judith				
Alexander and the Terrible, Horrible, No Good, Very Bad Day	E	—	✓	—
Weitzman, Jacquiline Preiss				
You Can't Take a Balloon Into the Metropolitan Museum	E	—	✓	—
Wiesner, David				
Sector 7	E	—	✓	—
Wood, Audrey				
King Bidgood's in the Bathtub	E	✓	✓	—
The Napping House	E	✓	—	—
Yorinks, Arthur				
Hey, Al	E	—	✓	—

Cause-and-Effect Relationships

	Section	PK-K	1-5	6-12
Allard, Harry, and James Marshall				
Miss Nelson Is Missing!	E	—	✓	—
Allen, Pamela				
Who Sank the Boat?	E	✓	✓	—
Anno, Mitsumasa				
Anno's Medieval World	E	—	—	✓
Baker, Keith				
Who Is the Beast?	E	✓	✓	—
Brett, Jan				
Berlioz the Bear	E	✓	✓	—
Browne, Anthony				
Piggybook	E	—	✓	—
Bunting, Eve				
The Man Who Could Call Down Owls	E	—	✓	✓
Carle, Eric				
The Mixed-Up Chameleon	E	✓	✓	—
The Very Busy Spider	E	✓	—	—
The Very Hungry Caterpillar	E	✓	—	—
Cazet, Denys				
A Fish in His Pocket	E	—	✓	—

	Section	PK-K	1-5	6-12
Cherry, Lynne				
The Great Kapok Tree: A Tale of the Amazon River Forest	J	—	—	✓
The River Ran Wild: An Environmental History	N	—	—	✓
Corey, Shana				
You Forgot Your Skirt, Amelia Bloomer	E	—	✓	—
Cuyler, Margery				
That's Good! That's Bad!	E	✓	✓	—
Ehlert, Lois				
Cucú: Un cuento folklórico mexicano/Cuckoo: A Mexican Folktale	E	✓	—	—
Enderle, Judith R., and Stephanie G. Tessler				
Six Creepy Sheep	E	—	✓	—
Finn, Isabel, and Jack Tickle				
The Very Lazy Ladybug	E	✓	—	—
Fleming, Denise				
Where Once There Was a Wood	E	—	✓	—
Gulbis, Stephen				
I Know an Old Lady Who Swallowed a Fly	E	✓	—	—
Henkes, Kevin				
Lilly's Purple Plastic Purse	E	✓	✓	—
Hogrogian, Nonny				
One Fine Day	E	✓	—	—
Howe, James				
I Wish I Were a Butterfly	E	✓	✓	—
Hutchins, Pat				
Rosie's Walk	E	✓	—	—
Keats, Ezra Jack				
Peter's Chair	E	—	✓	—
Kraus, Robert				
Leo the Late Bloomer	E	—	✓	—
Leaf, Margaret				
The Eyes of the Dragon	E	—	✓	—
Lionni, Leo				
Frederick	E	✓	—	—

SKILLS

	Section	PK-K	1-5	6-12
McDermott, Gerald *Arrow to the Sun*	F	—	✓	✓
McNaughton, Colin *Suddenly!*	E	—	✓	—
Mahy, Margaret *The Seven Chinese Brothers*	F	—	✓	—
Mayer, Mercer *Ah-Choo*	E	—	✓	—
Frog on His Own	E	—	✓	—
There's an Alligator Under My Bed	E	✓	✓	—
Meddaugh, Susan *Martha Speaks*	E	—	✓	—
Pinkwater, Daniel Manus *The Big Orange Splot*	E	—	✓	—
Rathmann, Peggy *Officer Buckle and Gloria*	E	✓	✓	—
Ringgold, Faith *Aunt Harriet's Underground Railroad in the Sky*	E	—	✓	—
If a Bus Could Talk: The Story of Rosa Parks	N	—	✓	—
Say, Allen *Grandfather's Journey*	E	—	✓	✓
Sloat, Teri *The Thing That Bothered Farmer Brown*	E	✓	✓	—
Trapani, Iza *The Itsy Bitsy Spider*	E	✓	✓	—
Van Allsburg, Chris *The Mysteries of Harris Burdick*	E	—	✓	✓
The Wretched Stone	E	—	✓	✓
Weitzman, Jacquiline Preiss *You Can't Take a Balloon Into the Metropolitan Museum*	E	—	✓	—
Wood, Audrey *The Napping House*	E	✓	—	—

Storytelling

	Section	PK-K	1-5	6-12
Anno, Mitsumasa *Anno's Journey*	E	—	—	✓
Asbjornsen, Peter *The Three Billy Goats Gruff*	E	✓	✓	—
Bang, Molly *The Paper Crane*	F	—	✓	—
Brown, Marc	E	✓	—	—
Arthur's Nose	E	✓	—	—
Buckley, Richard *The Foolish Tortoise*	E	✓	—	—
Burningham, John *Come Away from the Water, Shirley*	E	—	✓	—
Day, Alexandra *Good Dog, Carl*	E	—	✓	—
de Paola, Tomie *Charlie Needs a Cloak*	E	—	✓	—
The Knight and the Dragon	E	—	✓	—
The Legend of Bluebonnet	F	—	✓	—
Pancakes for Breakfast	E	✓	✓	—
Demi *One Grain of Rice: A Mathematical Folktale*	F	—	✓	—
Fisher, Leonard Everett *The Great Wall of China*	E	—	—	✓
Fox, Mem *Wilfrid Gordon McDonald Partridge*	E	—	✓	✓
Freeman, Don *Corduroy*	E	✓	✓	—
Glass, Andrew *Mountain Men: True Grit and Tall Tales*	J	—	—	✓
Goble, Paul *Iktomi and the Boulder*	F	—	✓	✓
Hearne, Betsy Gould *Seven Brave Women*	J	—	✓	✓
Hughes, Shirley *Alfie Gets in First*	E	—	—	—

	Section	PK–K	1–5	6–12
Hutchins, Pat				
Good-Night, Owl!	E	✓	✓	—
Lionni, Leo				
Swimmy	E	✓	✓	—
McDermott, Gerald				
Anansi the Spider: A Tale from the Ashanti	F	—	✓	—
Sun Flight	F	—	✓	—
Mahy, Margaret				
The Seven Chinese Brothers	F	—	✓	—
Marshall, James				
George and Martha: Back in Town	E	—	✓	—
Mayer, Mercer				
Ah-Choo	E	—	✓	—
Frog on His Own	E	—	✓	—
Hiccup	E		✓	—
There's an Alligator Under My Bed	E	—	✓	—
Numeroff, Laura				
If You Give a Mouse a Cookie	E	✓	✓	—
Oughton, Jerrie				
How the Stars Fell Into the Sky: A Navajo Legend	F	—	—	✓
Palatini, Margie				
Piggie Pie	E	—	✓	—
Pinkwater, Daniel Manus				
The Big Orange Splot	E	—	✓	—
Rohmann, Eric				
Time Flies	E	—	✓	—
Scieszka, Jon				
The Stinky Cheese Man and Other Fairly Stupid Tales	E	—	—	✓
The True Story of the Three Little Pigs	E	—	✓	—
Sendak, Maurice				
Where the Wild Things Are	E	—	✓	—
Service, Robert W.				
The Cremation of Sam McGee	P	—	—	✓

	Section	PK–K	1–5	6–12
Sierra, Judy				
Counting Crocodiles	E	—	✓	—
Silverman, Erica				
Don't Fidget a Feather!	E	✓	—	—
Sís, Peter				
Starry Messenger	N	—	—	✓
Small, David				
Imogene's Antlers	E	—	✓	—
Soto, Gary				
Too Many Tamales	E	—	✓	—
Spier, Peter				
Oh, Were They Ever Happy	E	—	✓	—
Stewart, Sarah				
The Gardener	E	—	✓	—
Turkle, Brinton				
Deep in the Forest	E	—	✓	—
Van Allsburg, Chris				
The Mysteries of Harris Burdick	E	—	✓	✓
The Wreck of the Zephyr	E	—	✓	—
The Wretched Stone	E	—	✓	✓
Viorst, Judith				
Alexander and the Terrible, Horrible, No Good, Very Bad Day	E	—	✓	—
The Tenth Good Thing About Barney	E	✓	✓	—
Waddell, Martin				
Farmer Duck	E	✓	✓	—
Weitzman, Jacquiline Preiss				
You Can't Take a Balloon Into the Metropolitan Museum	E	—	✓	—
Wells, Rosemary				
Noisy Nora	E	✓	—	—
Wiesner, David				
Sector 7	E	—	✓	—
Tuesday	E	—	✓	✓
Wood, Audrey				
King Bidgood's in the Bathtub	E	—	✓	—
Zion, Gene				
Harry the Dirty Dog	E	—	✓	—

SKILLS

Problem Solving

	Section	PK-K	1-5	6-12
Baker, Keith *Who Is the Beast?*	E	√	√	—
Brett, Jan *Berlioz the Bear*	E	√	√	—
Brown, Marc *Arthur's Nose*	E	—	√	—
Browne, Anthony *Piggybook*	E	—	√	—
Canfield, Jack; Hansen, Mark Victor; and Kirberger, Kimberly (Eds.) *Chicken Soup for the Teenage Soul III: More Stories of Life, Love and Learning*	YA	—	—	√
Cazet, Denys *A Fish in His Pocket*	E	—	√	—
Cherry, Lynne *The Great Kapok Tree: A Tale of the Amazon River Forest*	J	—	—	√
The River Ran Wild: An Environmental History	N	—	—	√
Corey, Shana *You Forgot Your Skirt, Amelia Bloomer*	E	—	√	—
Cronin, Doreen *Click, Clack, Moo: Cows That Type*	E	√	√	—
de Paola, Tomie *Pancakes for Breakfast*	E	√	√	—
The Legend of Bluebonnet	F	—	√	—
Demi *One Grain of Rice: A Mathematical Folktale*	E	—	√	—
Fisher, Leonard Everett *The Great Wall of China*	E	—	—	√
Fleming, Denise *Where Once There Was a Wood*	E	—	√	—
Fox, Mem *Wilfrid Gordon McDonald Partridge*	E	—	√	√

	Section	PK-K	1-5	6-12
Gackenbach, Dick *Harry and the Terrible Whatzit*	E	—	√	—
Henkes, Kevin *Lilly's Purple Plastic Purse*	E	√	√	—
Hogrogian, Nonny *One Fine Day*	E	√	—	—
Hort, Lenny *The Boy Who Held Back the Sea*	E	—	√	—
Howe, James *I Wish I Were a Butterfly*	E	√	√	—
Hughs, Shirley *Alfie Gets in First*	E	√	—	—
Karon, Jan *Miss Fannie's Hat*	E	—	√	—
Kasza, Keiko *The Rat and the Tiger*	E	√	√	—
Leaf, Margaret *The Eyes of the Dragon*	E	—	√	—
Lionni, Leo *Swimmy*	E	√	√	—
Lobel, Arnold *Ming Lo Moves the Mountain*	E	—	√	—
McDermott, Gerald *Arrow to the Sun*	F	—	√	√
Sun Flight	F	—	√	—
Mahy, Margaret *The Seven Chinese Brothers*	F	—	√	—
Mayer, Mercer *Liza Lou and the Yeller Belly Swamp*	E	—	√	—
There's an Alligator Under My Bed	E	√	—	—
Meddaugh, Susan *Martha Speaks*	E	—	√	—
Palatini, Margie *Piggie Pie*	E	—	√	—

SKILLS

	Section	PK–K	1–5	6–12
Pinkwater, Daniel Manus				
The Big Orange Splot	E	—	✓	—
Say, Allen				
Grandfather's Journey	E	—	—	✓
Service, Robert W.				
The Cremation of Sam McGee	P	—	—	✓
Shaw, Nancy				
Sheep on a Ship	E	—	✓	—
Sís, Peter				
Starry Messenger	N	—	—	✓
Spier, Peter				
London Bridge Is Falling Down	E	—	✓	—
Stanley, Diane				
The Gentleman and the Kitchen Maid	J	—	—	✓
Stewart, Sarah				
The Gardener	E	—	✓	—
Van Allsburg, Chris				
The Wreck of the Zephyr	E	—	✓	—
The Wretched Stone	E	—	✓	✓
Viorst, Judith				
Alexander and the Terrible, Horrible, No Good, Very Bad Day	E	—	✓	—
Waber, Bernard				
Lovable Lyle	E	—	✓	—
Waddell, Martin				
Farmer Duck	E	✓	✓	—
Wiesner, David				
Tuesday	E	—	✓	✓
Wood, Audrey				
King Bidgood's in the Bathtub	E	✓	✓	—

Verbal Expression

	Section	PK–K	1–5	6–12
Berger, Barbara				
Grandfather Twilight	E	✓	—	—

	Section	PK–K	1–5	6–12
Brett, Jan				
Annie and the Wild Animals	E	✓	—	—
Berlioz the Bear	E	✓	✓	—
The Mitten: A Ukrainian Folktale	F	✓	✓	—
Brown, Margaret Wise				
Big Red Barn	E	✓	—	—
The Important Book	E	✓	✓	—
Bunting, Eve				
Scary, Scary Halloween	E	✓	✓	—
Burningham, John				
Would You Rather . . .	E	—	✓	—
Carle, Eric				
The Mixed-Up Chameleon	E	✓	✓	—
Charlip, Remy				
Fortunately	E	✓	✓	—
Crews, Donald				
Truck	E	✓	—	—
Cronin, Doreen				
Click, Clack, Moo: Cows That Type	E	✓	✓	—
Cuyler, Margery				
That's Good! That's Bad!	E	✓	✓	—
Day, Alexandra				
Good Dog, Carl	E	—	✓	—
de Paola, Tomie				
Pancakes for Breakfast	E	—	✓	—
Feiffer, Jules				
Meanwhile	E	—	✓	✓
Feelings, Muriel				
Jambo Means Hello: Swahili Alphabet Book	E	—	✓	—
Fox, Mem				
Tough Boris	E	—	✓	—
Wilfrid Gordon McDonald Partridge	E	—	✓	—
Goble, Paul				
Iktomi and the Boulder	E	—	✓	✓
Gray, Nigel				
A Country Far Away	N	—	✓	—

	Section	PK–K	1–5	6–12
Hoban, Tana				
Shadows and Reflections	E	✓	—	—
Hughs, Shirley				
Alfie Gets in First	E	✓	—	—
Krauss, Ruth				
A Hole Is To Dig: A First Book of First Definitions	E	✓	—	—
McDermott, Gerald				
Anansi the Spider: A Tale from the Ashanti	F	—	✓	—
Martin, Bill Jr., and John Archambault				
Barn Dance!	E	✓	✓	—
Paulsen, Gary, and Ruth Paulsen				
Dogteam	E	—	✓	✓
Peek, Merle				
Mary Wore Her Red Dress and Henry Wore His Green Sneakers	E	✓	—	—
Rylant, Cynthia				
Night in the Country	E	✓	✓	—
Shaw, Charles G.				
It Looked Like Spilt Milk	E	✓	—	—
Siebert, Diane				
Train Song	E	—	✓	—
Spier, Peter				
Dreams	E	—	✓	—
London Bridge Is Falling Down	F	—	✓	—
Waddell, Martin				
Farmer Duck	E	—	✓	—
Weitzman, Jacquiline Preiss				
You Can't Take a Balloon Into the Metropolitan Museum	E	—	✓	—
Wiesner, David				
Tuesday	E	—	✓	✓
Williams, Sue				
I Went Walking	E	✓	—	—

Compare and Contrast

	Section	PK–K	1–5	6–12
Anno, Mitsumasa				
Anno's Journey	E	—	—	✓
Anno's Medieval World	E	—	—	✓
Baker, Keith				
Who Is the Beast?	E	✓	✓	—
Burningham, John				
Would You Rather . . .	E	—	✓	—
Carle, Eric				
The Grouchy Ladybug	E	✓	—	—
The Mixed-Up Chameleon	E	✓	✓	—
The Very Busy Spider	E	✓	—	—
Cendrars, Blaise				
Shadow	P	—	—	✓
Cherry, Lynne				
The River Ran Wild: An Environmental History	N	—	—	✓
Corey, Shana				
You Forgot Your Skirt, Amelia Bloomer	E	—	✓	—
Cowcher, Helen				
Antarctica	N	—	✓	—
Crews, Donald				
Freight Train	E	✓	—	—
de Paola, Tomie				
The Legend of Bluebonnet	F	—	✓	—
Feelings, Muriel				
Jambo Means Hello: Swahili Alphabet Book	E	—	✓	—
Fleming, Candace				
Gabriella's Song	E	—	✓	—
Gray, Nigel				
A Country Far Away	N	—	✓	—
Hearne, Betsy Gould				
Seven Brave Women	J	—	—	✓
Hoban, Tana				
Shadows and Reflections	E	✓	—	—
Kosek, Jane Kelly				
Learning About Courage from the Life of Christopher Reeve	J	—	—	✓

Drawing Inferences

Section	PK–K	1–5	6–12
Jacobsen, Kathy (music and words by Woody Guthrie) *This Land Is Your Land* F	—	—	√
Henkes, Kevin *Lilly's Purple Plastic Purse* E	√	√	—
Hort, Lenny *The Boy Who Held Back the Sea* E	—	√	—
Howe, James *I Wish I Were a Butterfly* E	√	√	—
Hutchins, Pat *Good-Night, Owl!* E	√	√	—
Rosie's Walk E	√	—	—
Kasza, Keiko *The Rat and the Tiger* E	√	√	—
Keats, Ezra Jack *Peter's Chair* E	√	√	—
Krauss, Robert *Leo the Late Bloomer* E	—	√	—
Lawrence, Jacob *Harriet and the Promised Land* F	—	√	√
Lincoln, Abraham (Illustrated by Michael McCurdy) *The Gettysburg Address* N	—	—	√
Lobel, Arnold *Ming Lo Moves the Mountain* E	—	√	—
Macaulay, David *Rome Antics* J	—	—	√
McDermott, Gerald *Anansi the Spider: A Tale from the Ashanti* E	—	√	—
McNaughton, Colin *Suddenly!* E	—	√	—
Marshall, James *George and Martha: Back in Town* E	—	√	—
Mayer, Mercer *Hiccup* E	—	√	—
Liza Lou and the Yeller Belly Swamp E	—	√	—

Section	PK–K	1–5	6–12
Muir, John (Retold by Donnell Rubay) *Stickeen: John Muir and the Brave Little Dog* N	—	—	√
Oughton, Jerrie *How the Stars Fell Into the Sky: A Navajo Legend* F	—	—	√
Pinkwater, Daniel Manus *The Big Orange Splot* E	—	√	—
Ringgold, Faith *Aunt Harriet's Underground Railroad in the Sky* E	—	√	—
Rohmann, Eric *Time Flies* E	—	√	—
Ryan, Pam Muñoz *Amelia and Eleanor Go for a Ride* N	—	—	√
Sakurai, Gail *Stephen Hawking: Understanding the Universe* N	—	—	√
Say, Allen *Grandfather's Journey* E	—	√	√
Scieszka, Jon *The True Story of the Three Little Pigs* E	—	√	√
Service, Robert W. *The Cremation of Sam McGee* P	—	—	√
Siebert, Diane *Train Song* E	—	√	—
Sierra, Judy *Counting Crocodiles* E	—	√	—
Silverman, Erica *Big Pumpkin* E	√	—	—
Sís, Peter *Starry Messenger* N	—	—	√
Sloat, Teri *The Thing That Bothered Farmer Brown* E	√	√	—
Soto, Gary *Chato's Kitchen* E	—	√	—
Stanley, Diane *The Gentleman and the Kitchen Maid* J	—	—	√

SKILLS

	Section	PK–K	1–5	6–12
Stewart, Sarah				
The Gardener	E	—	✓	—
Thayer, Ernest Lawrence				
(Illustrated by Christopher Bing)				
Casey at the Bat: A Ballad of the Republic Sung in the Year 1888	F	—	—	✓
Turner, Ann				
Dakota Dugout	J	—	—	✓
Van Allsburg, Chris				
The Wreck of the Zephyr	E	—	✓	—
The Wretched Stone	E	—	✓	✓
Viorst, Judith				
Alexander and the Terrible, Horrible, No Good, Very Bad Day	E	—	✓	—
The Tenth Good Thing About Barney	E	✓	✓	—
Waddell, Martin				
Farmer Duck	E	✓	✓	—
Wells, Rosemary				
Noisy Nora	E	✓	—	—
Wiesner, David				
Tuesday	E	—	✓	✓
Williams, Vera B.				
A Chair for My Mother	E	—	✓	—
Yorinks, Arthur				
Hey, Al	E	—	✓	—

Point of View

	Section	PK–K	1–5	6–12
Barracca, Debra, and Sal Barracca				
The Adventures of Taxi Dog	E	—	✓	—
Bunting, Eve				
Scary, Scary Halloween	E	—	✓	—
Day, Alexandra				
Good Dog, Carl	E	—	✓	—
Garland, Sherry				
Voices of the Alamo	J	—	—	✓
Goble, Paul				
Iktomi and the Boulder	F	—	✓	✓

	Section	PK–K	1–5	6–12
Hearne, Betsy Gould				
Seven Brave Women	J	—	✓	✓
Muir, John				
(Retold by Donnell Rubay)				
Stickeen: John Muir and the Brave Little Dog	N	—	—	✓
Say, Allen				
Grandfather's Journey	E	—	✓	✓
Scieszka, Jon				
The Stinky Cheese Man and Other Fairly Stupid Tales	E	—	—	✓
The True Story of the Three Little Pigs	E	—	✓	✓
Van Allsburg, Chris				
The Wretched Stone	E	—	✓	✓
Wiesner, David				
The Three Pigs	E	—	✓	✓

Critical Thinking

	Section	PK–K	1–5	6–12
Brown, Marc				
Arthur's Nose	E	—	✓	—
Browne, Anthony				
Gorilla	E	—	✓	—
Bunting, Eve				
The Man Who Could Call Down Owls	E	—	✓	✓
Hort, Lenny				
The Boy Who Held Back the Sea	E	—	✓	—
Keats, Ezra Jack				
Peter's Chair	E	✓	✓	—
McDermott, Gerald				
Arrow to the Sun	F	—	✓	✓
Sun Flight	F	—	✓	—
Turner, Ann				
Dakota Dugout	J	—	—	✓
Van Allsburg, Chris				
The Wreck of the Zephyr	E	—	✓	—
Wiesner, David				
Sector 7	E	—	✓	—

SKILLS

Answering *Why* Questions

Section	PK-K	1-5	6-12
Lawrence, Jacob *Harriet and the* *Promised Land*	F	—	√	√
Yorinks, Arthur *Hey, Al*	E	—	√	—

Retelling Events

Section	PK-K	1-5	6-12
Burleigh, Robert *Home Run*	J	—	√	√
Hearne, Betsy Gould *Seven Brave Women*	J	—	√	√
Kosek, Jane Kelly *Learning About Courage* *from the Life of* *Christopher Reeve*	N	—	—	√
Soto, Gary *Chato's Kitchen*	E	—	√	—
Stewart, Sarah *The Gardener*	E	—	√	—
Strazzabosco, Jeanne *Learning About* *Determination from the* *Life of Gloria Estefan*	N	—	—	√
Learning About *Forgiveness from the* *Life of Nelson Mandela*	N	—	—	√
Wiesner, David *The Three Pigs*	E	—	√	√

Explaining Processes in Detail

Section	PK-K	1-5	6-12
Canfield, Jack; Hansen, Mark Victor; and Kirberger, Kimberly (Eds.) *Chicken Soup for the* *Teenage Soul Journal*	YA	—	—	√
de Paola, Tomi *Pancakes for Breakfast*	E	—	√	—

Section	PK-K	1-5	6-12
Muir, John (Retold by Donnell Rubay) *Stickeen: John Muir* *and the Brave Little Dog*	N	—	—	√
Sís, Peter *Starry Messenger*	N	—	—	√
Wiesner, David *Sector 7*	E	—	√	—

Discussion

Section	PK-K	1-5	6-12
Allard, Harry, and James Marshall *Miss Nelson Is Missing!*	E	—	√	—
Baker, Keith *Who Is the Beast?*	E	√	√	—
Bang, Molly *The Paper Crane*	F	—	√	—
Barracca, Debra, and Sal Barracca *The Adventures of* *Taxi Dog*	E	—	√	—
Brett, Jan *The Mitten: A Ukrainian* *Folktale*	E	√	√	—
Browne, Anthony *Piggybook*	E	—	√	—
Bunting, Eve *The Man Who Could* *Call Down Owls*	E	—	√	√
Scary, Scary Halloween	E	√	—	—
Burleigh, Robert *Home Run*	J	—	√	√
Burningham, John *Aldo*	E	√	—	—
Buckley, Richard *The Foolish Tortoise*	E	√	—	—
Buscaglia, Leo F. *The Fall of Freddie* *the Leaf*	E	√	√	—

SKILLS

PRAGMATIC LANGUAGE

	Section	PK–K	1–5	6–12
Buehner, Caralyn *It's a Spoon, Not a Shovel*	E	√	√	—
Canfield, Jack; Hansen, Mark Victor; and Kirberger, Kimberly (Eds.) *Chicken Soup for the Teenage Soul Journal*	YA	—	—	√
Carle, Eric *The Grouchy Ladybug*	E	√	—	—
Cherry, Lynne *The River Ran Wild: An Environmental History*	N	—	—	√
de Regniers, Beatrice Schenk *May I Bring a Friend?*	E	√	—	—
Ehlert, Lois *Cucú: Un cuento folklórico mexicano/Cuckoo: A Mexican Folktale*	E	√	—	—

	Section	PK–K	1–5	6–12
Fleischman, Paul *Big Talk: Poems for Four Voices*	P	—	—	√
Hutchins, Pat *The Very Worst Monster*	E	√	—	—
Kasza, Keiko *The Rat and the Tiger*	E	√	√	—
Meddaugh, Susan *Martha Speaks*	E	—	√	—
Ryan, Pam Muñoz *Amelia and Eleanor Go for a Ride*	N	—	—	√
Simon, Charnan *Bill Gates: Helping People Use Computers*	N	—	—	√
Stanley, Diane *The Gentleman and the Kitchen Maid*	J	—	—	√
Wiesner, David *Sector 7*	E	—	√	—

PHONOLOGICAL AWARENESS

	Section	PK–K	1–5	6–12
Alborough, Jez				
It's the Bear!	E	√	—	—
Where's My Teddy?	E	√	—	—
Bang, Molly				
Ten, Nine, Eight	E	√	—	—
Barracca, Debra, and Sal Barracca				
The Adventures of Taxi Dog	E	√	√	—
Base, Graeme				
Animalia	E	√	√	—
Bennett, Jill				
Noisy Poems	P	√	√	—
Brown, Marc				
Pickle Things	P	—	√	—
Buehner, Caralyn				
It's a Spoon, Not a Shovel	E	√	√	—
Bunting, Eve				
In the Haunted House	E	√	√	—
Burton, Virginia Lee				
Mike Mulligan and His Steam Shovel	E	√	—	—
Charlip, Remy				
Fortunately	E	√	√	—
Cleary, Brian P.				
Hairy, Scary, Ordinary: What Is an Adjective?	E	—	√	—
Cronin, Doreen				
Click, Clack, Moo: Cows That Type	E	√	—	—
Dodds, Dayle Ann				
Sing, Sophie!	E	√	√	—
Fleming, Candace				
Gabriella's Song	E	√	√	—

	Section	PK–K	1–5	6–12
Fleming, Denise				
Where Once There Was a Wood	E	√	√	—
Florian, Douglas				
Mammalabilia	P	—	√	—
Gulbis, Stephen				
I Know an Old Lady Who Swallowed a Fly	E	√	—	—
Hawkins, Colin, and Jacqui Hawkins				
Old MacDonald Had a Farm	E	√	—	—
Henkes, Kevin				
Lilly's Purple Plastic Purse	E	√	√	—
Langstaff, John				
Oh, A-Hunting We Will Go	E	√	—	—
Lear, Edward (Illustrated by Jan Brett)				
The Owl and the Pussycat	E	√	√	—
Lioni, Leo				
Frederick	E	√	√	—
Martin, Bill Jr., and John Archambault				
Barn Dance!	E	√	√	—
Chicka Chicka Boom Boom	E	√	—	—
Massie, Diane Redfield				
The Baby Beebee Bird	E	√	—	—
Miranda, Anne				
To Market, To Market	E	√	—	—
Moss, Lloyd				
Zin! Zin! Zin! A Violin	E	—	√	—
Numeroff, Laura				
Chimps Don't Wear Glasses	E	√	√	—

SKILLS

	Section	PK–K	1–5	6–12
Palatini, Margie				
Piggie Pie	E	✓	✓	—
Prelutsky, Jack				
For Laughing Outloud: Poems To Tickle Your Funnybone	P	✓	✓	—
The Snopp on the Sidewalk and Other Poems	P	✓	—	—
Raschka, Chris				
Waffle	E	—	✓	—
Riley, Linnea				
Mouse Mess	E	✓	✓	—
Rylant, Cynthia				
Night in the Country	E	✓	✓	—
Scheer, Julian, and Marvin Bileck				
Rain Makes Applesauce	E	✓	✓	—

	Section	PK–K	1–5	6–12
Sendak, Maurice				
Chicken Soup with Rice	E	✓	✓	—
Shaw, Nancy				
Sheep on a Ship	E	✓	✓	—
Sierra, Judy				
Counting Crocodiles	E	✓	✓	—
Sloat, Teri				
The Thing That Bothered Farmer Brown	E	✓	✓	—
Slobodkina, Esphyr				
Caps for Sale: A Tale of a Peddler, Some Monkeys and Their Monkey Business	E	✓	✓	—

ARTICULATION

General Articulation

	Section	PK-K	1-5	6-12
Anno, Mitsumasa *Anno's Journey*	E	—	—	√
Base, Graeme *Animalia*	E	√	√	—
Bennett, Jill *Noisy Poems*	P	√	√	—
Canfield, Jack; Hansen, Mark Victor; and Kirberger, Kimberly (Eds.) *Chicken Soup for the Teenage Soul Journal*	YA	—	—	√
Feiffer, Jules *Meanwhile*	E	—	√	√
Fleischman, Paul *Big Talk: Poems for Four Voices*	P	—	—	√
Florian, Douglas *Mammalabilia*	P	—	√	—
Wiesner, David *Sector 7*	E	—	√	—
The Three Pigs	E	—	√	—

Oral Motor Exercises

	Section	PK-K	1-5	6-12
Crews, Donald *Sail Away*	E	√	—	—
Massie, Diane Redfield *The Baby Beebee Bird*	E	√	—	—

B

	Section	PK-K	1-5	6-12
Massie, Diane Redfield *The Baby Beebee Bird*	E	√	—	—
Prelutsky, Jack *For Laughing Outloud: Poems To Tickle Your Funnybone*	P	√	—	—
Ride a Purple Pelican	P	√	—	—

	Section	PK-K	1-5	6-12
Riley, Linnea *Mouse Mess*	E	√	—	—

P

	Section	PK-K	1-5	6-12
Miranda, Anne *To Market, To Market*	E	√	—	—
Prelutsky, Jack *For Laughing Outloud: Poems To Tickle Your Funnybone*	P	√	—	—
Ride a Purple Pelican	P	√	—	—
Riley, Linnea *Mouse Mess*	E	√	—	—

M

	Section	PK-K	1-5	6-12
Guarino, Deborah *Is Your Mama a Llama?*	E	√	—	—
Numeroff, Laura *Chimps Don't Wear Glasses*	E	√	—	—
Prelutsky, Jack *For Laughing Outloud: Poems To Tickle Your Funnybone*	P	√	—	—
Riley, Linnea *Mouse Mess*	E	√	—	—

N

	Section	PK-K	1-5	6-12
Prelutsky, Jack *For Laughing Outloud: Poems To Tickle Your Funnybone*	P	√	—	—

H

	Section	PK-K	1-5	6-12
Barton, Byron *Hester*	E	—	√	—

SKILLS

Articulation

	Section	PK–K	1–5	6–12
Burningham, John *Hey! Get Off Our Train*	E	—	✓	—
Fox, Mem *Hattie and the Fox*	E	✓	—	—
Mayer, Mercer *Hiccup*	E	—	✓	—
Prelutsky, Jack *For Laughing Out Loud:* *Poems To Tickle Your* *Funnybone*	N	—	✓	—
Waddell, Martin *Farmer Duck*	E	✓	✓	—
Zion, Gene *Harry the Dirty Dog*	E	—	✓	—

K

	Section	PK–K	1–5	6–12
Adams, Pam *This Is the House That* *Jack Built*	E	✓	—	—
Brett, Jan *Annie and the Wild* *Animals*	E	✓	—	—
Brown, Ruth *A Dark, Dark Tale*	E	✓	—	—
Carle, Eric *The Very Hungry* *Caterpillar*	E	✓	—	—
Carlstrom, Nancy White *Jesse Bear, What Will* *You Wear?*	E	✓	—	—
Cronin, Doreen *Click, Clack, Moo:* *Cows That Type*	E	✓	—	—
de Paola, Tomie *Pancakes for Breakfast*	E	✓	—	—
de Regniers, Beatrice **Schenk** *May I Bring a Friend?*	E	✓	—	—
Ehlert, Lois *Cucú: Un cuento folklórico* *mexicano/Cuckoo:* *A Mexican Folktale*	E	✓	—	—

	Section	PK–K	1–5	6–12
Fox, Mem *Hattie and the Fox*	E	✓	—	—
Freeman, Don *Corduroy*	E	✓	—	—
Hutchins, Pat *Don't Forget the Bacon*	E	✓	—	—
Rosie's Walk	E	✓	—	—
Krauss, Ruth *The Carrot Seed*	E	✓	—	—
Martin, Bill Jr., **and John Archambault** *Barn Dance!*	E	✓	—	—
Chicka Chicka *Boom Boom*	E	✓	—	—
Miranda, Anne *To Market, To Market*	E	✓	—	—
Numeroff, Laura *Chimps Don't Wear* *Glasses*	E	✓	—	—
Prelutsky, Jack *For Laughing Outloud:* *Poems To Tickle Your* *Funnybone*	P	✓	—	—
Ride a Purple *Pelican*	P	✓	—	—
Riley, Linnea *Mouse Mess*	E	✓	—	—
Silverman, Erica *Don't Fidget* *a Feather!*	E	✓	—	—
Slobodkina, Esphyr *Caps for Sale: A Tale of a* *Peddler, Some Monkeys* *and Their Monkey* *Business*	E	✓	—	—
Waddell, Martin *Farmer Duck*	E	✓	—	—
Williams, Sue *I Went Walking*	E	✓	—	—
Wood, Audry *King Bidgood's in the* *Bathtub*	E	✓	—	—

G

Section	PK-K	1-5	6-12
Asbjornsen, Peter			
The Three Billy Goats Gruff　E	✓	✓	—
Berger, Barbara			
Grandfather Twilight　E	✓	—	—
Brown, Margaret Wise			
Goodnight Moon　E	✓	—	—
Burningham, John			
Hey! Get Off Our Train　E	✓	—	—
Mr. Gumpy's Outing　E	✓	—	—
Carlstrom, Nancy White			
Jesse Bear, What Will You Wear?　E	✓	—	—
Fox, Mem			
Hattie and the Fox　E	✓	—	—
Hutchins, Pat			
Don't Forget the Bacon　E	✓	—	—
Miranda, Anne			
To Market, To Market　E	✓	—	—
Prelutsky, Jack			
For Laughing Outloud: Poems To Tickle Your Funnybone　P	✓	—	—
Ride a Purple Pelican　P	✓	—	—
The Snopp on the Sidewalk and Other Poems　P	✓	—	—
Rathmann, Peggy			
Good Night, Gorilla　E	✓	—	—
Silverman, Erica			
Don't Fidget a Feather!　E	✓	—	—
Williams, Sue			
I Went Walking　E	✓	—	—
Wood, Audrey			
King Bidgood's in the Bathtub　E	✓	—	—

F

Section	PK-K	1-5	6-12
Brett, Jan			
Annie and the Wild Animals　E	✓	—	—

Section	PK-K	1-5	6-12
Carle, Eric			
The Grouchy Ladybug　E	✓	—	—
Charlip, Remy			
Fortunately　E	✓	—	—
Hawkins, Colin, and Jacqui Hawkins			
Old MacDonald Had a Farm　E	✓	—	—
Hogrogian, Nonny			
One Fine Day　E	✓	—	—
Hutchins, Pat			
Don't Forget the Bacon　E	✓	—	—
Prelutsky, Jack			
For Laughing Outloud: Poems To Tickle Your Funnybone　P	✓	—	—
The Snopp on the Sidewalk and Other Poems　P	✓	—	—
Raschka, Chris			
Waffle　E	—	✓	—
Riley, Linnea			
Mouse Mess　E	✓	—	—
Silverman, Erica			
Don't Fidget a Feather!　E	✓	—	—
Waddell, Martin			
Farmer Duck　E	✓	—	—

V

Section	PK-K	1-5	6-12
Carle, Eric			
The Very Busy Spider　E	✓	—	—
The Very Hungry Caterpillar　E	✓	—	—
Finn, Isabel, and Jack Tickle			
The Very Lazy Ladybug　E	✓	—	—
Hutchins, Pat			
The Very Worst Monster　E	✓	—	—
Prelutsky, Jack			
For Laughing Outloud: Poems To Tickle Your Funnybone　P	✓	—	—

SKILLS

L

	Section	PK–K	1–5	6–12
Brett, Jan *The Mitten: A Ukrainian Folktale*	F	—	✓	—
Brown, Marc *Pickle Things*	P	—	✓	—
Finn, Isabel, and Jack Tickle *The Very Lazy Ladybug*	E	✓	—	—
Guarino, Deborah *Is Your Mama a Llama?*	E	✓	✓	—
Henkes, Kevin *Lilly's Purple Plastic Purse*	E	—	✓	—
Hutchins, Pat *Good-Night Owl!*	E	—	✓	—
Krauss, Robert *Leo the Late Bloomer*	E	—	✓	—
Lobel, Arnold *Whiskers and Rhymes*	P	—	✓	—
Mayer, Mercer *Liza Lou and the Yeller Belly Swamp*	E	—	✓	—
There's an Alligator Under My Bed	E	—	✓	—
McNaughton, Colin *Here Come the Aliens!*	E	—	✓	—
Paulsen, Gary, and Ruth Paulsen *Dogteam*	E	—	✓	—
Prelutsky, Jack *For Laughing Out Loud: Poems To Tickle Your Funnybone*	P	—	✓	—
The Snopp on the Sidewalk and Other Poems	P	—	✓	—
Raschka, Chris *Waffle*	E	—	✓	—
Spier, Peter *London Bridge Is Falling Down*	E	—	✓	—
Waber, Bernard *Lovable Lyle*	E	—	✓	—

	Section	PK–K	1–5	6–12
Weitzman, Jacquiline Preiss *You Can't Take a Balloon Into the Metropolitan Museum*	E	—	✓	—

–er

	Section	PK–K	1–5	6–12
Barton, Byron *Hester*	E	—	✓	—
Brett, Jan *Berlioz the Bear*	E	—	✓	—
Goble, Paul *Iktomi and the Boulder*	E	—	✓	—

R

	Section	PK–K	1–5	6–12
Barton, Byron *Hester*	E	—	✓	—
Brown, Marc *Arthur's Nose*	E	—	✓	—
Pickle Things	N	—	✓	—
Burningham, John *Mr. Gumpy's Outing*	E	—	✓	—
Would You Rather . . .	E	—	✓	—
Gantos, Jack *Rotten Ralph*	E	—	✓	—
Goble, Paul *Iktomi and the Boulder*	F	—	✓	—
Henkes, Kevin *Lilly's Purple Plastic Purse*	E	—	✓	—
Lobel, Arnold *Whiskers and Rhymes*	P	—	✓	—
McDermott, Gerald *Anansi the Spider: A Tale from the Ashanti*	F	—	✓	—
Arrow to the Sun	F	—	✓	—
Marshall, James *George and Martha: Back in Town*	E	—	✓	—

	Section	PK-K	1-5	6-12
Mayer, Mercer				
There's an Alligator Under My Bed	E	—	√	—
Sun Flight	F	—	√	√
Paulsen, Gary, and Ruth Paulsen				
Dogteam	E	—	√	√
Prelutsky, Jack				
For Laughing Out Loud: Poems To Tickle Your Funnybone	P	—	√	—
Scheer, Julian				
Rain Makes Applesauce	E	—	√	—
Sendak, Maurice				
Chicken Soup with Rice	E	—	√	—
Where the Wild Things Are	E	—	√	—
Soto, Gary				
Chato's Kitchen	E	—	√	—
Viorst, Judith				
Alexander and the Terrible, Horrible, No Good, Very Bad Day	E	—	√	—
Zion, Gene				
Harry the Dirty Dog	E	—	√	—

S

	Section	PK-K	1-5	6-12
Allard, Harry, and James Marshall				
Miss Nelson Is Missing!	E	—	√	—
Brett, Jan				
The Mitten: A Ukrainian Folktale	F	—	√	—
Brown, Marc				
Arthur's Nose	E	—	√	—
Pickle Things	P	—	√	—
Bunting, Eve				
Scary, Scary Halloween	E	—	√	—
Burningham, John				
Mr. Gumpy's Outing	E	—	√	—
Would You Rather . . .	E	—	√	—

	Section	PK-K	1-5	6-12
Dodds, Dayle Ann				
Sing, Sophie!	E	—	√	—
Enderle, Judith R., and Stephanie G. Tessler				
Six Creepy Sheep	E	—	√	—
Heller, Ruth				
Many Luscious Lollipops: A Book About Adjectives	E	—	√	—
Hutchins, Pat				
Good-Night Owl!	E	—	√	—
Keats, Ezra Jack				
The Snowy Day	E	—	√	—
Kraus, Robert				
Leo the Late Bloomer	E	—	√	—
Lobel, Arnold				
Whiskers and Rhymes	P	—	√	—
McDermott, Gerald				
Anansi the Spider: A Tale from the Ashanti	F	—	√	—
Sun Flight	F	—	√	√
McNaughton, Colin				
Here Come the Aliens!	E	—	√	—
Mayer, Mercer				
Liza Lou and the Yeller Belly Swamp	E	—	√	—
Paulsen, Gary, and Ruth Paulsen				
Dogteam	E	—	√	√
Prelutsky, Jack				
The Baby Uggs Are Hatching!	P	—	√	—
For Laughing Out Loud: Poems To Tickle Your Funnybone	P	—	√	—
The Snopp on the Sidewalk and Other Poems	P	—	√	—
Scheer, Julian				
Rain Makes Applesauce	E	—	√	—
Sendak, Maurice				
Chicken Soup with Rice	E	—	√	—
Where the Wild Things Are	E	—	√	—

	Section	PK-K	1-5	6-12
Shaw, Nancy *Sheep on a Ship*	E	—	√	—
Shulevitz, Uri *Snow*	E	—	√	—
Soto, Gary *Chato's Kitchen*	E	—	√	—
Viorst, Judith *Alexander and the Terrible, Horrible, No Good, Very Bad Day*	E	—	√	—
Zolotow, Charlotte *Someday*	E	—	√	—

	Section	PK-K	1-5	6-12
Sendak, Maurice *Where the Wild Things Are*	E	—	√	—
Soto, Gary *Chato's Kitchen*	E	—	√	—
Viorst, Judith *Alexander and the Terrible, Horrible, No Good, Very Bad Day*	E	—	√	—
My Mama Says . . .	E	—	√	—
Zolotow, Charlotte *Someday*	E	—	√	—

Z

	Section	PK-K	1-5	6-12
Brett, Jan *Berlioz the Bear*	E	—	√	—
The Mitten: A Ukrainian Folktale	F	—	√	—
Bunting, Eve *Scary, Scary Halloween*	E	—	√	—
Burningham, John *Mr. Gumpy's Outing*	E	—	√	—
Would You Rather . . .	E	—	√	—
Dodds, Dayle Ann *Sing, Sophie!*	E	—	√	—
Heller, Ruth *Many Luscious Lollipops: A Book About Adjectives*	E	—	√	—
Lobel, Arnold *Whiskers and Rhymes*	P	—	√	—
McDermott, Gerald *Anansi the Spider: A Tale from the Ashanti*	F	—	√	√
Mayer, Mercer *Liza Lou and the Yeller Belly Swamp*	E	—	√	—
Prelutsky, Jack *For Laughing Out Loud: Poems To Tickle Your Funnybone*	P	—	√	—
The Snopp on the Sidewalk and Other Poems	P	—	√	—

Sh

	Section	PK-K	1-5	6-12
Burningham, John *Come Away from the Water, Shirley*	E	—	√	—
Cazet, Denys *A Fish in His Pocket*	E	—	√	—
Cendrars, Blaise *Shadow*	P	—	—	√
de Paola, Tomie *Charlie Needs a New Cloak*	E	—	√	—
Enderle, Judith R., and Stephanie G. Tessler *Six Creepy Sheep*	E	—	√	—
Kraus, Robert *Leo the Late Bloomer*	E	—	√	—
Lobel, Arnold *Whiskers and Rhymes*	P	—	√	—
McDermott, Gerald *Anansi the Spider: A Tale from the Ashanti*	F	—	√	—
Martin, Bill Jr., and John Archambault *Barn Dance!*	E	—	√	—
Prelutsky, Jack *The Baby Uggs Are Hatching!*	P	—	√	—
For Laughing Out Loud: Poems To Tickle Your Funnybone	P	—	√	—

	Section	PK-K	1-5	6-12
Shaw, Nancy				
Sheep on a Ship	E	—	✓	—

Ch

	Section	PK-K	1-5	6-12
Charlip, Remy				
Fortunately	E	—	✓	—
de Paola, Tomie				
Charlie Needs a New Cloak	E	—	✓	—
Lobel, Arnold				
Whiskers and Rhymes	P	—	✓	—
Martin, Bill Jr., and John Archambault				
Barn Dance!	E	—	✓	—
Mayer, Mercer				
Ah-Choo	E	—	✓	—
Prelutsky, Jack				
The Baby Uggs Are Hatching!	P	—	✓	—
For Laughing Out Loud: Poems To Tickle Your Funnybone	P	—	✓	—
Sendak, Maurice				
Chicken Soup with Rice	E	—	✓	—
Soto, Gary				
Chato's Kitchen	E	—	✓	—
Viorst, Judith				
My Mama Says . . .	E	—	✓	—

J

	Section	PK-K	1-5	6-12
Lobel, Arnold				
Whiskers and Rhymes	P	—	✓	—
Marshall, James				
George and Martha: Back in Town	E	—	✓	—
Martin, Bill Jr., and John Archambault				
Barn Dance!	E	—	✓	—

	Section	PK-K	1-5	6-12
Spier, Peter				
London Bridge Is Falling Down	E	—	✓	—

Th

	Section	PK-K	1-5	6-12
Brown, Marc				
Arthur's Nose	E	—	✓	—
Burningham, John				
Would You Rather . . .	E	—	✓	—
Crowe, Robert L.				
Tyler Toad and the Thunder	E	—	✓	—
Lobel, Arnold				
Whiskers and Rhymes	P	—	✓	—
McDermott, Gerald				
Arrow to the Sun	F	—	✓	✓
Marshall, James				
George and Martha: Back in Town	E	—	✓	—
Sun Flight	F	—	✓	—
Prelutsky, Jack				
For Laughing Out Loud: Poems To Tickle Your Funnybone	P	—	✓	—
Weitzman, Jacquiline Preiss				
You Can't Take a Balloon Into the Metropolitan Museum	E	—	✓	—
Wood, Audrey				
King Bidgood's in the Bathtub	E	—	✓	—

Carryover for Any Target Sound

	Section	PK-K	1-5	6-12
Anno, Mitsumasa				
Anno's Medieval World	E	—	—	✓
Day, Alexandra				
Good Dog, Carl	E	—	✓	—
de Paola, Tomie				
The Knight and the Dragon	E	—	✓	—

	Section	PK–K	1–5	6–12
Fleischman, Paul *Joyful Noise: Poems for Two Voices*	P	—	√	√
Fox, Mem *Tough Boris*	E	—	√	—
Goble, Paul *Iktomi and the Boulder*	F	—	—	√
Gray, Nigel *A Country Far Away*	N	—	√	—
Hort, Lenny *The Boy Who Held Back the Sea*	E	—	√	—
Scieszka, Jon *The Stinky Cheese Man and Other Fairly Stupid Tales*	E	—	—	√

	Section	PK–K	1–5	6–12
The True Story of the Three Little Pigs	E	—	√	√
Spier, Peter *Oh, Were They Ever Happy*	E	—	√	—
Van Allsburg, Chris *The Mysteries of Harris Burdick*	E	—	√	√
Weitzman, Jacquiline Preiss *You Can't Take a Balloon Into the Metropolitan Museum*	E	—	√	—
Williams, Vera B. *A Chair for My Mother*	E	—	√	—

FLUENCY

	Section	PK–K	1–5	6–12
Adams, Pam *This Is the House That Jack Built*	E	√	—	—
Bang, Molly *Ten, Nine, Eight*	E	√	—	—
Barton, Byron *Hester*	E	—	√	—
Base, Graeme *Animalia*	E	√	√	—
Brown, Ruth *A Dark, Dark Tale*	E	√	—	—
Cuyler, Margery *That's Good! That's Bad!*	E	√	√	—
Fleischman, Paul *Joyful Noise: Poems for Two Voices*	P	—	√	√
Fox, Mem *Hattie and the Fox*	E	√	—	—
Gulbis, Stephen *I Know an Old Lady Who Swallowed a Fly*	E	√	—	—
Hawkins, Colin, and Jacqui Hawkins *Old MacDonald Had a Farm*	E	√	—	—
Langstaff, John *Oh, A-Hunting We Will Go*	E	√	—	—
Martin, Bill Jr. *Brown Bear, Brown Bear, What Do You See?*	E	√	—	—
Polar Bear, Polar Bear, What Do You Hear?	E	√	—	—
Mayer, Mercer *Frog on His Own*	E	—	√	—
Prelutsky, Jack *For Laughing Out Loud: Poems To Tickle Your Funnybone*	P	√	√	—
Rathmann, Peggy *Good Night, Gorilla*	E	√	—	—
Sendak, Maurice *Chicken Soup with Rice*	E	√	√	—
Slobodkina, Esphyr *Caps for Sale: A Tale of a Peddler, Some Monkeys and Their Monkey Business*	E	√	√	—
Spier, Peter *Dreams*	E	—	√	—
London Bridge Is Falling Down	E	—	√	—

SKILLS

VOICE

	Section	PK-K	1-5	6-12
Asbjornsen, Peter *The Three Billy Goats Gruff*	E	√	√	—
Bang, Molly *Ten, Nine, Eight*	E	√	—	—
Barton, Byron *Hester*	E	—	√	—
Base, Graeme *Animalia*	E	√	—	√
Burningham, John *Hey! Get Off Our Train*	E	—	√	—
Ehlert, Lois *Cucú: Un cuento folklórico mexicano/Cuckoo: A Mexican Folktale*	E	√	—	—
Fleischman, Paul *Joyful Noise: Poems for Two Voices*	P	—	√	—

	Section	PK-K	1-5	6-12
Fox, Mem *Hattie and the Fox*	E	—	√	—
Gulbis, Stephen *I Know an Old Lady Who Swallowed a Fly*	E	√	—	—
Hawkins, Colin, and Jacqui Hawkins *Old MacDonald Had a Farm*	E	√	—	—
Mayer, Mercer *Hiccup*	E	—	√	—
Rathmann, Peggy *Good Night, Gorilla*	E	√	—	—
Waddell, Martin *Farmer Duck*	E	√	—	—
Zion, Gene *Harry the Dirty Dog*	E	—	√	—

AUTHOR

Adams, Pam
*This Is the House That
Jack Built,* 222

Ahlberg, Janet, and Allan Ahlberg
Each Peach Pear Plum, 79

Alborough, Jez
It's the Bear! 123
Where's My Teddy? 237

Allard, Harry, and James Marshall
Miss Nelson Is Missing! 387

Allen, Pamela
Who Sank the Boat? 244, 483

Anno, Mitsumasa
Anno's Journey, 515
Anno's Medieval World, 516

Asbjornsen, Peter
The Three Billy Goats Gruff,
222, 461

Baker, Keith
Little Green, 137
Who Is the Beast? 243, 482

Bang, Molly
The Paper Crane, 406
Ten, Nine, Eight, 208

Barracca, Debra and Sal
The Adventures of Taxi Dog,
15, 264

Barrett, Judi
A Snake Is Totally Tail, 445
*Things That Are Most
in the World,* 221, 460

Barton, Byron
Airport, 21
Dinosaurs, Dinosaurs, 77
Hester, 345

Base, Graeme
Animalia, 24, 271

Bennett, Jill
Noisy Poems, 157
Teeny Tiny, 453

Berger, Barbara
Grandfather Twilight, 101

Brett, Jan
Annie and the Wild Animals, 28
Berlioz the Bear, 39, 282
*The Mitten: A Ukrainian
Folktale,* 147, 389

Brown, Marc
Arthur's Nose, 29, 275
Pickle Things, 408

Brown, Margaret Wise
Big Red Barn, 41
Goodnight Moon, 99
The Important Book, 117, 354

Brown, Ruth
A Dark, Dark Tale, 76

Browne, Anthony
Gorilla, 333
Piggybook, 417

Buckley, Richard
The Foolish Tortoise, 83

Bunting, Eve
In the Haunted House, 112, 355
*The Man Who Could Call
Down Owls,* 379, 549
Scary, Scary Halloween,
188, 427

Berger, Barbara
Grandfather Twilight, 101

Buehner, Caralyn
It's a Spoon, Not a Shovel,
120, 359

Burleigh, Robert
Home Run, 347, 542

Burningham, John
Aldo, 21
*Come Away from the
Water, Shirley,* 302
Hey! Get Off Our Train, 105, 346
Mr. Gumpy's Outing, 146, 388
Would You Rather . . ., 486

Burton, Virginia Lee
*Mike Mulligan and His
Steam Shovel,* 142

Buscaglia, Leo F.
The Fall of Freddie the Leaf, 312

Canfield, Jack; Hansen, Mark
Victor; and Kirberger, Kimberly
*Chicken Soup for the Teenage
Soul III: More Stories of Life,
Love and Learning,* 525
*Chicken Soup for the Teenage
Soul Journal,* 526

Carle, Eric
The Grouchy Ladybug, 102
The Mixed-Up Chameleon,
147, 389
The Secret Birthday Message,
190
The Very Busy Spider, 227
The Very Hungry Caterpillar,
228

Carlstrom, Nancy White
*Jesse Bear, What Will
You Wear?* 130

Cazet, Denys
A Fish in His Pocket, 313

Cendrars, Blaise
Shadow, 560

Charlip, Remy
Fortunately, 88, 317

Cherry, Lynne
*The Great Kapok Tree: A Tale of
the Amazon River Forest,*
539
*The River Ran Wild: An
Environmental History,* 554

Cleary, Brian P.
*Hairy, Scary, Ordinary:
What Is an Adjective?* 335

Corey, Shana
*You Forgot Your Skirt,
Amelia Bloomer,* 491

AUTHOR

AUTHOR

AUTHOR

AUTHOR

TITLE

TITLE

References

Adams, M. J. (1990). *Beginning to read: Thinking and learning about print.* Cambridge, MA: Massachusetts Institute of Technology Press.

Adams, M. J., Foorman, B. R., Lundberg, I., & Beeler, T. (1998). *Phonemic awareness in young children: A classroom curriculum.* Baltimore: Brookes.

American Speech-Language-Hearing Association. (2001). *Roles and responsibilities of speech-language pathologists with respect to reading and writing in children and adolescents* (guidelines). Rockville, MD: Author.

Applebee, A. N. (1978). *The child's concept of story.* Chicago: University of Chicago Press.

Arnold, D. S., & Whitehurst, G. J. (1994). Accelerating language development through picture book reading: A summary of dialogic reading and its effect. In D. Dickinson (Ed.), *Bridges to literacy: Children, families and schools* (pp. 103–128). Cambridge, MA: Blackwell.

Brown, F. R., III, Aylward, E. H., & Keogh, B. K. (1996). *Diagnosis and management of learning disabilities: An interdisciplinary/lifespan approach* (3rd ed.). San Diego, CA: Singular.

Carlisle, J. F., & Normanbhoy, D. M. (1993). Phonological and morphological awareness in first graders. *Applied Psycholinguistics, 14,* 177–195.

Catts, H. W., Fey, M. E., Zhang, X., & Tomblin, J. B. (2001). Estimating the risk of future reading difficulties in kindergarten children: A research-based model and its clinical implementation. *Language, Speech, and Hearing Services in Schools, 32,* 38–50.

Catts, H. W., & Kamhi, A. G. (1999). Causes of reading disabilities. In H. W. Catts & A. G. Kamhi (Eds.), *Language and reading disabilities.* Boston: Allyn & Bacon.

Chard, D. J., & Dickson, S. V. (1999). Phonological awareness: Instructional and assessment guidelines. *Intervention in School and Clinic, 34*(5), 261–270.

Cullinan, B., & Bagert, B. (1996). *Helping your child learn to read.* Washington, DC: Office of Educational Research and Improvement, U.S. Department of Education.

Ely, R. (2001). Language and literacy in the school years. In J. B. Gleason (Ed.), *The development of language* (5th ed.). Boston: Allyn & Bacon.

Engelmann, S., Bruner, E., Hanner, S., Osborn, J., Osborn, S., & Zoret, L. (1969–1995). *Reading mastery* (Vols. 1–6). Columbus, OH: SRA/McGraw-Hill.

Ferreira, F., & Morrison, F. J. (1994). Children's metalinguistic knowledge of syntactic constituents: Effects of age and schooling. *Developmental Psychology, 30,* 663–678.

Fey, M. E. (2001, April). *The speech-language pathologist as a team member in reading education.* Short course presented at California Speech-Language-Hearing Association State Conference, Monterey, CA.

Fey, M. E., Catts, H. W., & Larrivee, L. (1995). Preparing preschoolers with language impairment for the academic and social challenges of school. In M. E. Fey, J. Windsor, & S. F. Warren (Eds.), *Language intervention: Preschool through the elementary years.* Baltimore: Brookes.

Fey, M. E., Windsor, J., & Warren, S. F. (Eds.). (1995). *Language intervention: Preschool through elementary years.* Baltimore: Brookes.

Gillon, G. T. (2000). The efficacy of phonological awareness intervention for children with spoken language impairment. *Language, Speech, and Hearing Services in Schools, 31,* 126–141.

References

Goldsworthy, C. L. (1998). *Sourcebook of phonological awareness activities: Childrens classic literature.* San Diego, CA: Singular.

Greene, J. F. (1995). *Sounds and letters for readers and spellers: Phonetic awareness drills for teachers and speech-language pathologists.* Longmont, CO: Sopris West.

Hall, S. L., & Moats, L. C. (1999). *Straight talk about reading: How parents can make a difference during the early years.* Chicago: Contemporary Books.

Hoffman, P. R., Norris, J. A., & Monjure, J. (1990). Comparison of process targeting and preschool children. *Language, Speech and Hearing Services in the Schools, 21,* 102–109.

Juel, C. (1988). Learning to read and write: A longitudinal study of 54 children from first through fourth grades. *Journal of Educational Psychology, 80*(4), 437–437.

Kamhi, A. G., & Catts, H. W. (1999). Reading development. In H. W. Catts & A. G. Kamhi (Eds.), *Language and reading disabilities.* Boston: Allyn & Bacon.

Karweit, N. (1994). The effect of story reading on the language development of disadvantaged prekindergarten and kindergarten students. In D. K. Dickinson (Ed.), *Bridges to literacy: Children, families, and schools.* Cambridge, MA: Basil Blackwell.

Knuth, R. A., & Jones, B. F. (1991, September). *What does research say about reading?* Retrieved August 26, 2001, from the North Central Regional Educational Laboratory Web site: www.ncrel.org/sdrs/areas/stw_esys/str_read.htm

Landauer, T. K., & Dumais, S. T. (1997). A solution to Plato's problem: The latent semantic analysis theory of acquisition, induction, and representation of knowledge. *Psychological Review, 104,* 211–240.

Larson, V. L., & McKinley, N. (1995). *Language disorders in older students: Preadolescents and adolescents.* Eau Claire, WI: Thinking Publications.

Lindamood, P., & Lindamood, P. (1998). *The Lindamood phoneme sequencing (LiPS) program for reading, spelling, and speech.* Austin, TX: PRO-ED.

Lundberg, I., Frost, J., & Peterson, O. (1988). Effects of an extensive program for stimulating phonological awareness in preschool children. *Reading Research Quarterly, 23,* 263–284.

McKinley, N. (2000, September). Charting a new course: Identifying and assessing language disorders in adolescents. *CSHA Magazine, 29*(27). Sacramento, CA: California Speech-Language-Hearing Association.

Moats, L. C. (2000). *Speech to print: Language essentials for teachers.* Baltimore: Brookes.

Moats, L. C., & Smith, C. (1992). Derivational morphology: Why it should be included in language assessment and instruction. *Language, Speech, and Hearing Services in Schools, 23,* 312–319.

Neuman, S. B., Copple, C., & Bredekamp, S. (2000). *Learning to read and write: Developmentally appropriate practices in young children.* Washington, DC: National Association for the Education of Young Children.

O'Connor, R. E., Jenkins, J. R., Leicester, N., & Slocum, T. (1993). Teaching phonological awareness to young children with learning disabilities. *Exceptional Children, 59*(6), 532–546.

O'Connor, R. E., Notari-Syverson, A., & Vadasy, P. F. (1998). *Ladders to literacy: A Kindergarten Activity Book.* Baltimore: Brookes.

Otterman, L. M. (1990). The value of teaching prefixes and word-tools. *Journal of Education Research, 48,* 611–616.

Rose, D. S., Parks, M., Androes, K., & McMahon, S. (2000). Imagery-based learning: Improving elementary students' reading comprehension with drama techniques. *Journal of Educational Research, 94*(1), 55–63.

Rosner, J. (1999). *Phonological awareness skills program.* Austin, TX: PRO-ED.

Snider, V. E. (1995). A primer on phonemic awareness: What it is, why it's important, and how to teach it. *School Psychology Review, 24,* 443–455.

Snider, V. E. (1997). The relationship between phonemic awareness and later reading achievement. *Journal of Educational Research, 90,* 203-211.

Snow, C. E. (1994). Enhancing literacy development: Programs and research perspectives. In D. K. Dickinson (Ed.), *Bridges to literacy: Children, families, and schools.* Cambridge, MA: Basil Blackwell.

Snow, C. E., Burns, M. S., & Griffin, P. (Eds.). (1998). *Preventing reading difficulties in young children.* Committee on the Prevention of Reading Difficulties in Young Children. Washington, DC: National Academy Press.

Stanovich, K. E. (1993). Romance and reality. *The Reading Teacher, 47,* 280-291.

Stanovich, K. E., Cunningham, A. E., & Freeman, D. J. (1984). Assessing phonological awareness in kindergarten children: Issues of task comparability. *Journal of Experimental Child Psychology, 38,* 175-190.

Torgesen, J. K., & Bryant, B. R. (1993). *Phonological awareness for training reading.* Austin, TX: PRO-ED.

Torgesen, J. K., Wagner, R. K., Rashotte, C. A., Lindamood, P., Rose, E., Conway, T., & Garvan, C. (1999). Preventing reading failure in young children with phonological processsing disabilities: Group and individual responses to instruction. *Journal of Educational Psychology, 91,* 579-593.

Uhry, J. K. (1999). Phonological awareness and reading: Research, activities and instructional materials. In J. R. Birsh (Ed.), *Multisensory teaching of basic language skills.* Baltimore: Brookes.

Westby, C. E. (1985). Learning to talk—Talking to learn: Oral-literate language differences. In S. Simon (Ed.), *Communication skills and classroom success.* San Diego, CA: College Hill Press.

Westby, C. E. (1990). The role of the speech–language pathologist in whole language. *Language, Speech and Hearing Services in Schools, 21,* 228-237.

Westby, C. E. (1999). Assessing and facilitating text comprehension problems. In H. W. Catts & A. G. Kamhi (Eds.), *Language and reading disabilities* (pp. 154-223). Boston: Allyn & Bacon.

Whitehurst, G. J., Falco, F. L., Lonigan, C. J., Fischel, J. E., DeBaryshe, B. D., Valdez-Menchaca, M. C., & Caulfield, M. (1988). Accelerating language development through picture book reading. *Developmental Psychology, 24*(4), 552-559.

Whitehurst, G. J., Crone, D. A., Zevenbergen, A. A., Schultz, M. D., Velting, O. N., & Fischel, J. E. (1999). Outcomes of an emergent literacy intervention from Head Start through second grade. *Journal of Educational Psychology, 91*(2), 261-272.

About the Author

Jane L. Gebers received her bachelor's degree in speech communication and her master's degree in communicative disorders from California State University, Northridge. She is a member of the California Speech-Language-Hearing Association, where she has served as editor of *CSHA Magazine.* Most of Ms. Gebers's career has been spent in the public school systems in California and Washington as a speech–language pathologist and special day class teacher. She is currently a speech–language pathologist in the Lafayette School District, Lafayette, California. She is also on the ancillary staff of the Department of Education at St. Mary's College, California, where she teaches a class on language development, assessment, and intervention.